Writtle

D1643825

Biology of Growth of Domestic Animals

Biology of Growth of Domestic Animals

Colin G. Scanes

With contributed chapters

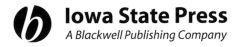

Iowa State Press
A Blackwell Publishing Company

Colin G. Scanes is a professor of Animal Science at Iowa State University. He was educated in the United Kingdom with a B.Sc. from Hull University and Ph.D. from the University of Wales. He was formerly on the faculty at the University of Leeds (UK) and Rutgers—The State University of New Jersey, where he was department chair. He has published extensively in growth biology of domestic animals, with 10 books and over 500 papers. He has also been visiting professor at the Catholic University of Leuven (Belgium) and the Autonomous National University of Mexico (UNAM). He has received numerous awards, including Honorary Professor at the Agricultural University of Ukraine.

©2003 Iowa State Press
A Blackwell Publishing Company
All rights reserved

Iowa State Press
2121 State Avenue, Ames, Iowa 50014

Orders: 1-800-862-6657
Office: 1-515-292-0140
Fax: 1-515-292-3348
Web site: www.iowastatepress.com

Printed on acid-free paper in the United States of America

First edition, 2003

Library of Congress Cataloging-in-Publication Data

Scanes, C.G.
  Biology of growth of domestic animals/Colin G. Scanes.—1st ed.
     p. cm.
Includes bibliographical references (p.).
  ISBN 0-8138-2906-2 (alk. paper)
  1. Domestic animals—Growth. 2. Veterinary physiology. I. Title.
  SF768.S26 2003
  636.089'266—dc21
                    2002155124

The last digit is the print number: 9 8 7 6 5 4 3 2 1

This book is dedicated to people who have made so much difference in my life—teachers, advisors, colleagues, mentors, friends, students, family and—above all—my wife.

Contents

Contributing Authors

Ronald E. Allen
Department of Animal Science
University of Arizona
Tucson, AZ 85721

R. Lee Baldwin
Department of Animal Science
University of California, Davis
Davis, CA 95616

D. H. Beermann
Department of Animal Science
University of Nebraska-Lincoln
Lincoln, NE 68583-0908

Roger E. Calza
School of Molecular BioSciences
Washington State University
Pullman, WA 99164-6310

Archie C. Clutter
Monsanto Company
BB2D
700 Chesterfield Parkway North
Chesterfield, MO 63198

Michael V. Dodson
Department of Animals Sciences
Washington State University
Pullman, WA 99164-6310

Frank R. Dunshea
Natural Resources and Environment
Department of Growth and Development
Victorian Institute of Animal Science
Werribee, Victoria 3030
Australia

Colin Farquharson
Bone Biology Group
Dept of Integrative Biology
Roslin Institute
Roslin EH25 9PS
Scotland, United Kingdom

David J. Flint
Hannah Research Institute
Ayr, KA6 5HL
Scotland, United Kingdom

Darrel E. Goll
Muscle Biology Group
Department of Nutritional Sciences
University of Arizona
Tucson, AZ 85721

Rod A. Hill
Department of Animal and Veterinary Science
University of Idaho
PO Box 442330
Moscow, ID 83844-2330

Elisabeth Huff-Lonergan
Animal Science
Department of Animal Science
Iowa State University
Ames, IA 50011

Steven M. Lonergan
Animal Science
Department of Animal Science
Iowa State University
Ames, IA 50011

Karyn Malinowski
Department of Animal Sciences
Cook College
Rutgers—The State University
New Brunswick, NJ 08903

Dennis Marple
Department of Animal Science
Iowa State University
Ames, IA 50011

Douglas C. McFarland
Department of Animal and Range Sciences
South Dakota State University
Brookings, SD 57007-0392

Jennifer M. Pell
The Babraham Institute
Cambridge
CB2 4AT
United Kingdom

Roberto Sainz
Department of Animal Science
University of California, Davis
Davis, CA 95616

Colin G. Scanes
Department of Animal Science
Iowa State University
Ames, IA 50011

David G. Topel
Department of Animal Science
Iowa State University
Ames, IA 50011

Sandra G. Velleman
Department of Animal Sciences
The Ohio State University
Wooster, OH 44691

Acknowledgments

The invaluable assistance of Ms. Denise Miller in the preparation of some of the chapters is gratefully acknowledged. The encouragement from, and discussions with, colleagues was critically important to the completion of the work.

Preface

Among the fundamental biological processes, growth and reproduction are most important to livestock production. This volume is intended as a textbook for senior undergraduate and graduate classes in animal growth and to be a useful resource for researchers in this field.

This volume covers the fundamental process of growth both from a systems viewpoint (mathematical aspects, modeling, cell and molecular biology, hormones, growth factors, and the extracellular matrix) and at the organ level (muscle, adipose, mammary gland, and bone). The interface of growth with other disciplines—including nutrition, genetics, and environment/management—are considered, as are specific aspects of growth in livestock and companion animal species. Man's relationship with animals is briefly reviewed as an introduction to the importance of domestic animals, which have been critical to human development and provide nutrition, income, transportation, locomotive power, companionship, entertainment, and so forth.

One of the most important hormones related to growth is growth hormone (GH) or somatotropin (ST), but there is often confusion about the name. The term *somatotropin* or *ST* is widely used by animal/dairy scientists and the animal industry. Bovine ST (bST), sold under the name Posilac, is used extensively by dairy farmers to increase milk yield and the efficiency of production. *Growth hormone* or *GH* is the term used by endocrinologists. Opponents of the use of bST (for dairy cattle) use the term bovine *GH*, *BGH* (with the capital *B*), or *BGROWTH HORMONE*. This publication uses the term *growth hormone/somatotropin (GH/ST)*.

Biology of Growth of Domestic Animals

1

Origins of Domestic Animals and Their Importance to Man

Colin G. Scanes

In his classical text, Samuel Brody (1945) stated that "Growth is the basis of and closely related to many productive agricultural processes." This statement included production of eggs, wool, and milk, as well as meat. This book encompasses the biological processes underlying growth in meat-producing animals and companion animals. It also, albeit briefly, considers mammary growth; this being the basis of milk production and neonatal growth/development. The importance of growth of livestock and poultry comes from the high nutritional value of meat together with its popularity in the human diet.

HUMAN POPULATION GROWTH

Thomas Malthus (1798) stated unequivocally "that the power of population is infinitely greater than the power in the earth to produce subsistence for man. Population, when unchecked, increases in a geometrical ratio. Subsistence increases only in an arithmetical ratio." He then brought forward the postulate that it is food restriction that holds the population growth to a low level. World population had been estimated to be growing at a slow rate through history with a doubling time of ~1100 years. In the last 150 years, the rate of increase of the population has accelerated to a doubling rate of ~40 years (Figure 1.1). More recently, the rate of increase is beginning to abate. The "medium" projection for the size of the human population in 2025 is 7.8 billion (United Nations 1999).

The acceleration in the rate of increase in human population in the last two centuries reflects major increases first in the Americas, then in Europe, and subsequently in Asia, Africa, and Latin America. The situation in the United States provides an interesting example of early rapid growth of population. The increase of population in the U.S. is now low and reflects immigration rather than births exceeding deaths. The population growth from that of the thirteen original colonies to the United States of America has been estimated to have been very dramatic (Figure 1.2):

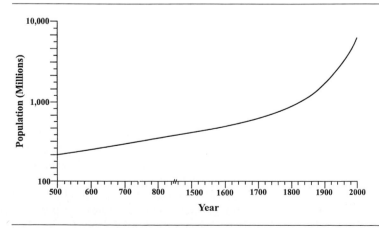

Figure 1.1. Human population growth (using U.N. data).

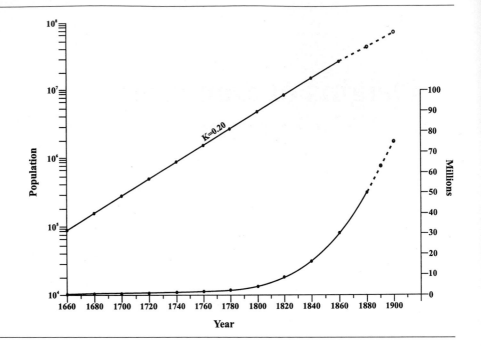

Figure 1.2.
Population growth in U.S.A. (Data adapted from Brody, 1945.)

New England	Doubling time 25 years,
1643– ~1760	Malthzus (1798)
New Jersey,	Doubling time 22 years,
similar period	Malthus (1798)
Thirteen colonies–	Doubling time 24 years,
U.S.A. 1660–1880	Brody (1945)

Malthus (1798), although providing no data, stated that frontier areas had population-doubling times of 15 years, and seaports (well established) had stable populations. Because there was very good information on immigration, the increases in population were largely due to greater births than deaths (Figure 1.3).

The argument put forth by Malthus (1798) was that inadequate food availability (and/or the income to afford to purchase food) acted as a force to countervail the propensity for human population to increase. In reality, the increase in population could be attributed to increased income/wealth, increased food availability, reduced disease, and the potential to increase income/wealth further with children and shifts in ethos.

ORIGIN AND DOMESTICATION OF LIVESTOCK AND POULTRY

Domestication of Sheep and Goats

The probable ancestor of domestic sheep (*Ovis aries*) is the Asian Mouflon (*Ovis orientatis*). Sheep

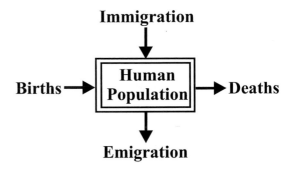

Figure 1.3. Changes in human population.

are thought to have been first domesticated in the fertile crescent (consisting of the land of the present country of Iraq together with contiguous parts of Syria, Iran, and Turkey) about 9000 B.C.E. (11,000 B.P.) (Maijala 1997). Sheep may have been first domesticated as hunting decoys. Another possibility is that young "motherless" lambs were kept as pets by children. Later, the importance of meat, wool, and milk became paramount.

Rearing of sheep during the neolithic period spread from present day Iraq to Europe, Africa, and Asia. Based on archeological evidence (radiocarbon dating of sheep bones at archeological sites), the

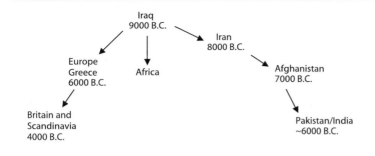

Figure 1.4. The progressive geographical distribution of sheep in antiquity.

progressive geographical distribution of sheep (due to trade, etc.) might be viewed in the manner shown in Figure 1.4 (the names are represented by the present countries).

Similarly, domestic goats (*Capra hircus hirus*) are thought to have been first domesticated about 10,000 years ago in the fertile crescent. Recently, Zeder and Hesse (2000) argued persuasively that goat bones assemblages from ~7900 years B.C.E. (9900 B.P.) were from domesticated goats. These were from the Zagros mountains of western Iran and northeastern Iraq and ^{14}C-dated. The argument for these being domesticated comes from the age/sex ratio (Zeder and Hesse 2000; reviewed Marean 2000)—populations of domesticated goats likely to have young males, not females slaughtered for meat.

Domestication of Cattle

The 800+ breeds for cattle are considered under two species: *Bos indicus* (Indian cattle including Zebu cattle) and *Bos taurus* (European breeds). As there is complete fertility between these, they are perhaps better considered as subspecies, races, or superbreeds. It has long been thought that the ancestors of domestic cattle are the now extinct wild ox or auroch *Bos primigenius*. This species had a wide Old World range. Three separate "races" of the species are known:

- *Bos primigenius namadicus* (Asia)
- *Bos primigenius osisthonomus* (North Africa)
- *Bos primigenius primigenius* (Europe)

Based on information of skeletal remains at archeological sites (including radiocarbon dating), it is believed that European cattle (*Bos taurus*) were domesticated from *B. p. primigenius* in the Near East (in and/or around present day Turkey) (reviewed Loftus et al. 1994). The earliest evidence of cattle is from 5800 B.C.E. (7800 B.P.) in Turkey.

The earliest remains of cattle in the Indian subcontinent, along the Indus, are from 2500 B.C.E. (4500 B.P.). This led to the conclusion, which we now know as false, that *Bos indicus* originated from *Bos taurus*. Based on sequence data from mitachondrial DNA (only inherited from the mother), Loftus and colleagues (1994) concluded that *Bos taurus* and *Bos indicus* are derived from separate populations of the ancestoral wild ox or auroch, these being separated genetically and geographically (Near East and presumably Indian subcontinent).

The cattle of East Africa (Zebu cattle) resemble Indian cattle and have been considered as *Bos indicus*. These are believed to have been introduced by Arab traders 670 A.D. or later. Sequence comparison of mitachondrial DNA clearly demonstrates that these cattle have exclusively *Bos taurus* maternal ancestory (Loftus et al. 1994). However, a relatively small number of *Bos indicus* bulls imported by Arab traders would provide the tropical hardiness of the Zebu cattle. Thus, the offspring would have outcompeted the much earlier introduced "pure" *Bos taurus* (Loftus et al. 1994).

Domestication of Dogs

It has long been surmised that dogs are domesticated gray wolves (*Canis lupus*) (Olsen 1985). The possibility of genetics from other Canids (e.g., the jackal) was, until recently, not precluded. Now it can be! Although there is increasing knowledge of the origins of the domestic dog (*Canis familiaris*), there is not agreement between conclusions from archaeology and those from the application of molecular genetics. Sequence divergence supports the origin of dogs perhaps as early as ~100,000 B.P., but archeological evidence would suggest 14,000 B.P. (Vilà et al. 1997).

There is genetic evidence for dogs having been domesticated multiple times and in multiple locations from gray wolves (Tsuda et al. 1997; Vilà et al.

1997). This is based on parsimony between nucleotide sequences in multiple breeds of dogs from different breeds and geographical locations and multiple wolves. It appears that wolves were domesticated from different populations of gray wolves across Northern Eurasia. On the other hand, very recent mitachondrial DNA evidence suggests a single origin in East Asia between 15,000 (more likely) and 40,000 years ago (Savolainen et al. 2002). Although it is easy to envision spread of dogs throughout Europe, Asia, and Africa, what about Australia and the Americas? There were dogs on both continents prior to European settlement.

The traditional view is that the first people to settle in the Americas came from Asia about 14,000 years ago. They are likely to have brought domesticated dogs with them. However, a divergent view pushes back the first people in the Americas to 20,000 or even 40,000 years ago (for further reading, see review Nemecek 2000). A study on the genetics of a "native" American breed of dogs (the Xoloitzcuitli) does not provide any support for dogs having been domesticated in the Americas (Vila et al. 1999; Leonard et al. 2002). Thus dogs in the Americas came with the first Americans or were the result of some unidentified trade across the Pacific via the Asian-American land bridge in the Bering Sea. Good evidence suggests that domesticated dogs and the Dingo, the feral dog of Australia, arrived via trade with New Guinea and the islands of the Indonesian Archipelago.

Domestication of Horses

Horses (*Equus caballus*) are thought to have been domesticated in the Eurasian grassland steppe about 4000 B.C.E. (6000 B.P.). This is based on the presence of horse bones at archeological sites, for instance, in the land within present-day Ukraine. Domestication may have involved either horses captured from a limited geographical area or multiple capture/domestication events. Based on analysis of mitachondrial DNA, there is strong evidence for multiple matrilines of captured and tamed wild horses (Vilá et al. 2001). The modern horse lineages were estimated to have diverged 0.32–0.63 million years ago (Vilá et al. 2001), well before domestication is conceivable.

The domestication of horses played a critical role in human history because horses were employed for hunting, warfare, and transportation as well as meat and milk. However, prior to the successful use of horses for transportation and warfare, it was essential to use breeding to increase their size. The use of horses in warfare had profound effects in history including:

- The development of chariots/charioteering, superceded (over 2000 years ago) by cavalry
- The invasion/migration of nomadic horse people from the Eurasian steppe (Huns, Turks, Magyars, Mongols, Tatars, and Cossacks)
- The Hispanic conquest of the Empires of Central and South America
- The roles of light and heavy cavalry up until World War I

For further reading, the following excellent books are recommended:

- *A History of Warfare* by John Keegan (1993)
- *Guns, Germs, and Steel* by Jared Diamond (1997)

Domestication of Pigs

The pig (*Sus scrufa domesticus*) was domesticated ~9000 B.P. from the Eurasian wild boar (*Sus scrufa*), of which there are 16 distinct subspecies (reviewed Ruvinsky and Rothschild 1998). Until recent analyses and approaches using molecular genetics, it was not clear whether domestic pigs had one or more genetic origins. Darwin (1871) recognized two species of domestic pigs originating from the wild boar in Europe and Asia. The genetic divergence between European and Asian/Chinese breeds of pigs has been estimated as ~500,000 years ago, well before the consensus time for domestication (Giuffra et al. 2000; Kijas and Andersson 2001; Jiang et al. 2001; Okumura et al. 2001). Moreover, there is much greater genetic similarity between European breeds of pigs and European wild boar (Kiljas and Andersson 2001). There is an analogous situation with the relatedness of Chinese breeds of pigs and the East Asian wild boar (Huang et al. 1999; Jiang et al. 2001; Okumura et al. 2001) with a divergence date of 11,500 B.P. (Jiang et al. 2001). There is also archeological evidence for pigs in the fertile crescent from ~9000 B.P.

Evidence from historical records and supported by molecular genetics indicates that Asian pigs were introgressed into European breeds in the 18th and 19th centuries (Darwin 1868; Giuffa et al. 2000; Okumura et al. 2001).

Domestication of Poultry

Domestic chickens have a monophyletic origin. The ancestral stock for the chicken is the red jungle fowl (*Gallus gallus*), which inhabit the Eastern

Indian subcontinent and the part of Asia that is now Thailand, Malaysia, south China, and Burma. There is strong evidence for monophyletic origin from the red jungle fowl and not other species of jungle fowl (Java or green jungle fowl, Ceylon or Lafayette's jungle fowl, or grey jungle fowl. This is based on morphology, electrophoretic patterns of ovoglobulins (Steven 1991), the presence of an endogenous retrovirus RAV-oDNA in domestic chickens and red jungle fowl but not other species of jungle fowl, and mitachondrial DNA sequences (Fumihito et al. 1994; Akishinonomiya et al. 1996).

The monophyletic origin can be further focused on a subspecies of red jungle fowl (*G.g. gallus*), which presently are found in Thailand, Cambodia, and southern Vietnam. This is based on mitochondrial DNA (Fumihito et al. 1994; Akishinonomiya 1996). It is reasonable to assume that domestication occurred in the geographical range for the ancestoral stock. However, the first archeological evidence for domesticated chickens (or perhaps captive red jungle fowl) is found in sites in northeast China, along the Yellow River (West and Zhou 1989). These sites have been radiocarbon-dated to as early as 5500 B.C.E. (7500 years ago). Domestication probably occurred in northeast China, with captive red jungle fowl from southeast Asia being traded. The possibility of the initial domestication occurring in southeast Asia cannot be precluded. Based on radiocarbon dating of chicken bones at archeological sites, chickens spread from northeast China to Europe (via the silk route or a more northerly route) and elsewhere. The arrival of chickens to Iran, the Near East, and Europe surprisingly preceded their introduction to the Indian subcontinent, as is summarized in the following data of arrival times/first archeological observations from West and Zhou (1989):

Iran	3900–3800 B.C.E.
Ukraine	4000–1000 B.C.E.
Greece	4000–1800 B.C.E.
Turkey	2900–1600 B.C.E.
Syria	2400–1400 B.C.E.
Western Europe	~1500– 500 B.C.E.
U.K.	150– 100 B.C.E.
Japan	200– 100 B.C.E.
Indian Subcontinent	2000–1000 B.C.E.

It has been speculated that chickens were domesticated for food (eggs and meat), religious and ceremonial purposes, and cockfighting (Akishinonomiya et al. 1996). Until the late 1920s, chicken meat was viewed essentially as a by-product of the table egg industry (Cahaner and Siegel 1986). The production of chicken meat transitioned from by-product to dedicated broiler chicken via dual-purpose breeds, with the female reared for egg production and the male for meat. It was not until the advent of broiler chickens that efforts to breed for meat production were undertaken. This was based initially on Barred Plymouth Rock and New Hampshire breeds, but later also using Cornish and Wyandotte germplasm (reviewed Cahaner and Siegel 1986). The resulting synthetic breeds were required to have white plumage for the processor and consumer preference.

Turkeys (*Meleagris gallopavo*) were domesticated more recently in the New World, probably by the pre-Columbian civilizations of present-day Mexico and Central America. The Spanish colonists transported domesticated turkeys to Spain and other Mediterranean countries. The naming of the turkey results from a series of confusions. In Europe, the turkey was confused with the guinea fowl (West African origin). The second mistake was the view that the guinea fowl came from Turkey! This was wrong for two reasons, even if we assume that Turkey/Ottoman empire at that time controlled all of North Africa, the Middle East, and the Balkans in Europe. The original turkeys for the Pilgrim's Thanksgiving celebration were wild turkeys.

Domesticated turkeys were reared on a small scale by farmers and fanciers, particularly in Europe and North America. Interestingly, scientific breeding programs to improve the efficiency of turkey meat production preceded those of the broiler chicken and were initiated in the United Kingdom. Meat breeds were imported to North America in the 1920s (reviewed Cahaner and Siegel 1986). These were crossed with North American turkeys to create the "Broad Breast Bronze" (reviewed Cahaner and Siegel 1986). From the 1950s, breeders succeeded in developing turkeys with white plumage (reviewed Cahaner and Siegel 1986).

CHANGES IN THE ANIMAL INDUSTRY RELATED TO ANIMAL GROWTH

There have been tremendous improvements in animal growth since the publication of the Brody text. In 1945, growth of poultry and livestock raised in conditions as close to the ideal then (in university agricultural research farms) can be summarized by the age to 50% mature weight as the following:

Cattle (Hereford-Shorthorn)	31 months (550 kg)
Pigs (Duroc-Jersey female)	15 months (100 kg)
Sheep (Hampshire or Suffolk)	9 months (~42 kg)
Chicken (Cornish male or female)	3 months (~1.22 kg)

Growth of livestock has been greatly improved by the application of research-based knowledge in genetics, nutrition, disease control, and management, together with the fundamentals of the biology of growth at the molecular, cellular, and physiological/organismic levels. These are addressed in the subsequent chapters in this volume.

REFERENCES

Akishinonomiya, F., Miyake, T., Sumi, S.-I., Takada, M., Shingu, R., Endo, T., Gojobori, T., Kondo, N., and Ohno, S. 1996. Monophyletic origin and unique dispersal patterns of domestic fowls. *Proceedings of the National Academy of Sciences USA* 93:6792–6795.

Brody, S. 1945. *Bioenergetics and Growth*. Baltimore: Waverly Press.

Cahaner, A., and Siegel, P.B. 1986. Evaluation of industry breeding programs for meat-type chickens and turkeys. In *3rd World Congress on Genetics Applied to Livestock*. 337–346.

Darwin, C. 1871. The Descent of Man and Selection in Relation to Sex. London: Murray.

Diamond, J. 1997. *Guns, Germs, and Steel*. New York: W.W. Norton & Company.

Frisby, D.P., Weiss, R.A., Roussel, M., and Stehelin, D. 1979. The distribution of endogenous chicken retrovirus sequences in the DNA of galliform birds does not coincide with avian phylogenetic relationships. *Cell* 17:623–634.

Fumihito, A., Miyake, T., Sumi, S.-I., Takada, M., Ohno, S., and Kondo, N. 1994. One subspecies of the red jungle fowl (*Gallus gallus gallus*) suffice as the matriarchic ancestor of all domestic breeds. *Proceedings of the National Academy of Sciences USA* 91:12505–12509.

Giuffra, E., Kijas, J.M.H., Amarger, V., Carlborg, O., Jeon, J.-T., and Andersson, L. 2000. The origin of the domestic pig: independent domestication and subsequent introgression. *Genetics* 154:1785–1791.

Huang, Y.F., Shi, X.W., and Zhang, Y.P. 1999. Mitochondrial genetic variation in Chinese pigs and wild boars. *Biochemical Genetics* 37:335–343.

Jiang, S.W., Giuffra, E., Andersson, L., and Xiong, Y.Z. 2001. Molecular phylogenetics relationship between six Chinese native pig breeds and three Swedish pig breeds from mitochondrial DNA. *Yi Chuan Xue Bao* 28:1120–1128.

Keegan, J. 1993. *A History of Warfare*. New York: Vintage Books.

Kijas, J.M., and Andersson, L. 2001. A phylogenetic study of the origin of the domestic pig estimated from the near-complete mtDNA genome. *Journal of Molecular Evolution* 52:302–308.

Leonard, J.A., Wayne, R.K., Wheeler, J., Valadez, R., Guillén, S., and Vilá, C. 2002. Ancient DNA evidence for old world origins of new world dogs. Science 298:1613–1616.

Loftus, R.T., MacHugh, D.E., Bradley, D.G., Sharp, P.M., and Cunningham, P. 1994. Evidence for two independent domestications of cattle. *Proceedings of the National Academy of Sciences USA* 91:2757–2761.

Maijala, K. 1997. Genetic aspects of domestication, common breeds and their origin. In *The Genetics of Sheep*. L. Piper and A. Ruvinsky, eds. Oxford, England: CAB International. 13–49.

Malthus, T. 1798. *An Essay on the Principle of Population*. Printed for J. Johnson, in St.Paul's Churchyard, London.

Marean, C.W. 2000. Age, sex and old goats. *Science* 287:2174–2175.

Nemecek, S. 2000. Who were the first Americans? *Scientific American* 280(3):80–87.

Okumura , N., Kurosawa, Y., Kobayashi, E., Watanobe, T., Ishiguro, N., Yasue, H., and Mitsuhashi, T. 2001. Genetic relationship amongst the major non-coding regions of mitochondrial DNAs in wild boars and several breeds of domesticated pigs. Animal Genetics 32:139.

Olsen, S.J. 1985. *Origins of the Domestic Dog*. Tucson: Arizona Press.

Ruvinsky A., and Rothschild, M.F. 1998. Systematics and evolution of the pig. In *The Genetics of the Pig*. A. Ruvinsky and M.F. Rothschild, eds. New York: CAB International.

Savolainen, P., Zhang, Y-p., Luo, J., Lundeberg, J., and Leiter, T. 2002. Genetic evidence for an East Asian origin of domestic dogs. *Science* 298:1611–1613.

Steven, L. 1991. *Genetics and Evolution of the Domestic Fowl*. Cambridge, England: Cambridge University Press.

Tsuda, K., Kikkawa, Y., Yonekawa, H., and Tanabe, Y. 1997. Extensive interbreeding occurred among multiple matriarchal ancestors during the domestication of dogs: evidence from inter- and intraspecies polymorphisms in the D-loop region of mitochondrial DNA between dogs and wolves. *Genes, Genetics and Systematics* 72:229–238.

United Nations. 1999. *World Population Prospects, 1998 Revision*. New York: U.N. Department for Policy Coordination and Sustainable Development.

Vilá, C., Leonard, J.A., Götherström, A., Marklund, S., Sandberg, K., Liden, K., Wayne, R.K., and Ellegren, H. 2001. Widespread origins of domestic horse lineages. *Science* 291:474–477.

Vilá, C., Maldonado, J.E., and Wayne, R.K. 1999. Phylogenetic relationships, evolution, and genetic diversity of the domestic dog. *Journal of Heredity* 90:71–77.

Vilá, C., Savolainen, P., Maldonado, J.E., Amorim, I.R., Rice, J.E., Honeycutt, R.L., Crandall, K.A., Lundberg, J., and Wayne, R.K. 1997. Multiple and ancient origins of the domestic dog. *Science* 276:1687–1689.

West, B., and Zhou, B.-X. 1989. Did chickens go north? New evidence for domestication. *World's Poultry Science Journal* 45:205–218.

Zeder, M.A., and Hesse, B. 2000. The initial domestication of goats (*Capra hircus*) in the Zagros Mountains 10,000 years ago. Science 287:2254–2257.

2
Fundamental Concepts of Growth

Dennis Marple

For centuries, farm animals were selected on the basis of their conformation and size, with some emphasis on their parentage. With the recognition that physical attributes of animals were controlled by both genetic and environmental influences, researchers began to more accurately define factors responsible for differences among animals. The conformation of cattle and swine changed markedly as livestock judges debated the "ideal type" of animals to select and produce. Examples of types of swine and cattle from approximately 1920 and 2001 are demonstrated in Figure 2.1. Swine and cattle in the early 1900s were generally deeper-bodied, fatter, shorter from head to tail, and not as tall as modern swine and cattle.

Those involved in setting standards for the livestock industry through selection of outstanding stock in the show ring were the catalyst for change in the conformation of animals. There were many attempts to alter the proportions of carcasses and thereby increase the amount of meat in the more highly valued cuts. Although differences in conformation may have appeared to exist among animals, Butterfield (1963) and Berg and Butterfield (1976) noted the relatively constant weight relationship among muscles within a carcass. Kempster and coworkers (1982) more specifically reported that the proportion of meat in valued cuts of beef, pork, and lamb carcasses was not influenced by the conformation of animals.

Continental breeds of cattle were introduced to the United States in the 1950s and 1960s, and researchers and livestock producers became more aware of differences in carcass composition between breeds of cattle. Also during the 1960s, the public was advised to reduce their consumption of dietary fats, and the meat industry became aware that excessive fat had little value in meat. Although this was the beginning of a more consumer-oriented livestock industry, the industry continues its efforts to adapt to the needs and expectations of consumers.

The classic experiments of Walton and Hammond (1938) demonstrated the dramatic manner in which genetics and selected offspring can be used to change the size of future generations. The authors made reciprocal crosses of Shire horses and Shetland ponies and their results stimulated decades of research to understand the role of the uterine environment on prenatal growth. The authors noted that birth weight of the foals was influenced more by the body weight of the dam than breed of the sire. As they monitored the growth of the Shire x Shetland offspring, they also noted the interaction of genetic and nutritional factors in the process of animal development (Figure 2.2). Their results demonstrated that the genetic potential for growth would not be realized when nutrition was limited. The impact of nutritional restrictions was most significant when weights and relative growth rates of the crossbred foals were compared. Greater body weight gain was observed in summer months when nutrients were more readily available, compared to more limited growth in winter months. Hammond (1940) also concluded that if the goal is to increase the size of horses, it is important to get good early growth when the foal is young, a goal best achieved by breeding large framed mares and providing adequate nutrition (milk) early in life.

GROWTH AND GROWTH CURVES

For most discussions, growth may be defined as the progressive increase in the size (volume, length, height, or girth) or weight of an animal over time. Hence, growth results from the accretion of nutrients

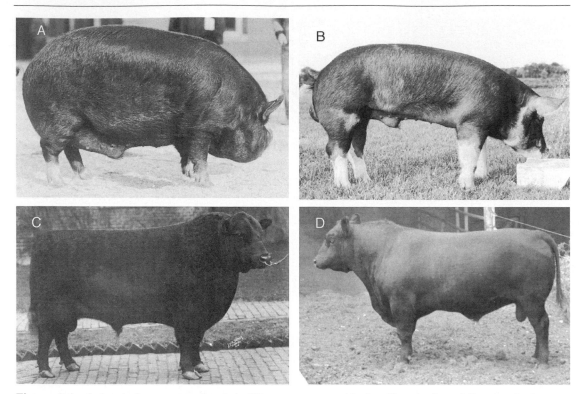

Figure 2.1. Animals from approximately 80 years ago and today. Panels A and C represent examples of deeper-bodied, fatter animals of the past, and panels B and D represent more muscular, leaner animals being selected at this time. (Photos in panels A and C courtesy of the Iowa State University Library/Special Collections Department. Photo in panel B courtesy of M. Peter Hoffman, Ames, Iowa. Photo in panel D courtesy of Gene Rouse and Doyle Wilson, Iowa State University.)

Figure 2.2. Growth of Shetland and Shire cross foals. Shetland X Shetland (solid line), Shire X Shetland (broken line), and Shetland X Shire (dashed line) data represent the patterns of growth of the reciprocal crossbreds compared to the purebred Shetlands. (Data adapted from Walton and Hammond, 1938.)

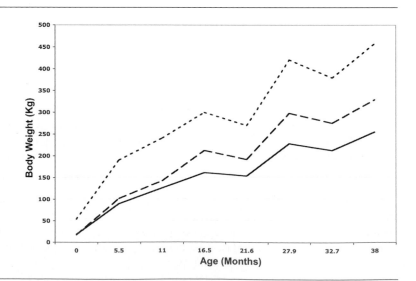

over time. Animal growth is best described by taking measurements of physical characteristics of the animal (weight, height, length, or girth), or attributes of a tissue (backfat thickness or muscle depth), or even a portion of the animal, such as noting changes in the length or girth of a limb as the animal progresses from neonate to maturity.

When body weight is being monitored, the resulting data should not be influenced by possible errors introduced by the ingestion of food or water shortly prior to weighing the animal, because the subsequent increase in weight is not associated with tissues of the body and does not represent a true increase in body weight. Data are easily plotted against the age of the animal or the increments of time over which the data are collected, and the resulting relationship represents a portion of the growth curve for that animal. If body weights are taken at frequent enough times from birth until senescence, the growth curve may achieve a classical sigmoidal shape. However, plotting weight against age until market weight is achieved often results in a graph similar to a linear relationship for cattle and swine (Figure 2.3). Obviously, the time required to reach the point at which growth slows and

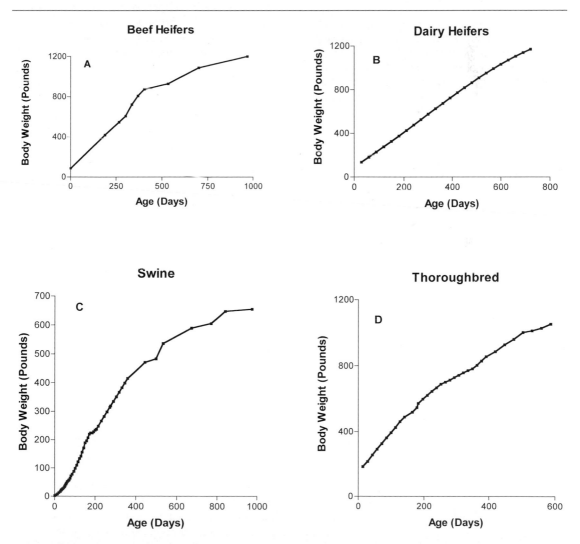

Figure 2.3. Examples of growth curves of livestock. (Data in panels A, B, and C courtesy of Doyle Wilson and Gene Rouse (A), Lee Kilmer (B), and Jack Dekkers (C), Animal Science Department, Iowa State University. Data in panel D adapted from Thompson, 1995.)

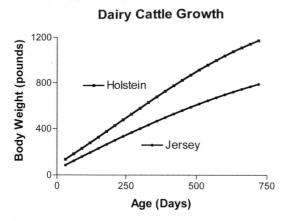

Figure 2.4. Variations in mature size of livestock. Growth curves of Holstein and Jersey dairy heifers demonstrate the more rapid growth and larger mature size of Holstein cattle compared to Jersey cattle. (Data courtesy of Lee Kilmer, Animal Science Department, Iowa State University).

ceases varies across species, and differences in rates of growth may also be found between breeds within species. Some of these differences are easily attributed to differences in ultimate mature size of breeds of animals as well as genetic differences in rates of growth of animals within breeds. (Figure 2.4).

Mature size of normal animals is that stage of the life cycle beyond which the animal essentially ceases to accumulate additional body weight when the animal is allowed to consume food at will. Animals produced for meat typically are slaughtered well before reaching their mature size, and data describing mature size of animals or breeds of animals are typically based on information obtained from breeding stock. Selection for large or mature size is effective and is seen in examples of both miniature cattle and horses that have mature heights approximately 40% or less that of cattle and horses commonly found in livestock production systems. Likewise, cattle may be selected for greater mature size, as demonstrated by the increased size of British breeds of cattle from 1950 to present.

Presentation of growth data vs. time or age is informative, and may be compared to data from other animals in an experiment or production system. Brody (1945) provides an extensive discussion of equations to predict rates of growth and components of growth curves. The equations of Gompertz [Eq.2.1] and Richards [Eq.2.2] have been examined

for their ability to describe animal growth data and are presented as described by

$$W = W_0 exp[\mu_0(1 - e^{-Dt})/D] \qquad \textbf{2.1}$$

$$W = \frac{W_0 W_f}{[W_0^n + (W_f^n - W_0^n)e^{-kt}]^{1/n}} \qquad \textbf{2.2}$$

France and Thornley (1984). In Equations 2.1 and 2.2, W is dry weight, W_0 is the initial dry weight, μ_0 is a proportionality constant at time zero, D is the decay of the specific growth rate, t is time, W_f is the dry weight at the final time, k is a constant > 0, and n is a constant ≥ 0. When $W_0 = 1$, $W_f = 100$, k = .2 and n = 0, the Richards equation yields a growth curve equal to the Gompertz equation.

Lopez and colleagues (2000) derived a generalized Michaelis-Menten equation [Eq. 2.3] to fit a wide range of growth data from 15 animal species and found their model to be superior to the Gompertz equation in many instances and as reliable as the Richards equation in describing postnatal growth data. In their equation, W is weight, W_0 is initial weight, K is a positive constant denoting the time when half-maximal growth is achieved, c is a dimensionless constant >0 (1 in this instance), W_f is the final or maximal weight at infinite time, and t is time or age (days, weeks, months, etc.).

$$W = W_0 K^c + W_f t^c/(K^c + t^c) \qquad \textbf{2.3}$$

Animal weight data are more often expressed in relative terms to describe rates of change, such as average daily gain or weight per day of age. Data in the form of average daily gain or weight per day of age are easily computed and the graphical representation of data is used more to present summary data from groups of animals (Figure 2.5). Examination of relative growth data reveals greater rates of weight gain during the middle and later stages of typical production periods for farm animals, although average daily gain ultimately declines as animals mature. These data may also be compared and analyzed statistically to determine the responses of animals of similar genetic backgrounds to different environmental factors, such as planes of nutrition or management practices. Likewise, similar data are often used to estimate the genetic merit of parents (potential for rapid growth) and/or genetic potential of offspring.

The use of mathematical models to predict postnatal growth has been expanded to optimize man-

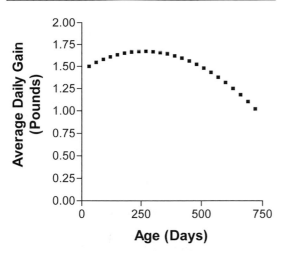

Figure 2.5. Rate of body weight gain changes during growth. Average daily gain (pounds) increases and then decreases during growth of Holstein heifers. (Data courtesy of Lee Kilmer, Animal Science Department, Iowa State University.)

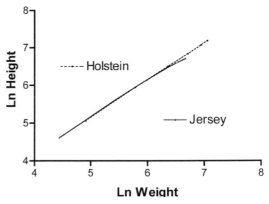

Figure 2.6. Log plot of relative growth. The comparison of data from Holstein and Jersey heifers demonstrates that the increase in height of the Jersey cattle has slowed compared to the continued increase in body weight. Holstein cattle have a larger mature size, and the data demonstrate continued skeletal growth of Holstein cattle as their body weight increases. (Data courtesy of Lee Kilmer, Animal Science Department, Iowa State University.)

agement strategies (de Lange 1992), to predict nutrient needs (Stranks et al. 1988), and to predict daily protein accretion rates in growing swine (Schinckel et al. 1996). Likewise, monitoring growth and production performance by watching for variability in growth patterns has been advocated as a management tool to improve production efficiency of cattle (Menchaca et al. 1996). Similar opportunities exist to improve management strategies by careful monitoring of feed intake as well as milk and egg production of animals.

PATTERNS OF GROWTH

Growth of farm animals generally occurs in a proportional or relative manner rather than at a constant rate for all tissues. If growth was isometric, all tissues would grow in equal dimensions at equal rates, and mature farm animals would look like large versions of newborns. However, growth is allometric or proportional to other tissues and organs of the body. For instance, the head of newborn farm animals is disproportionately large with respect to the remainder of the body, and limbs of newborn animals are relatively thin compared to their mature size. Early efforts to describe allometric growth patterns utilized sketches and photographs to compare changes in shape of portions of the body while holding the size of a limb or part of the body at a constant size.

Huxley (1932) expressed growth of portions of the body on a relative basis using a logarithmic transformation of the data and found the slope of the resulting data described the relative rate of growth of the tissues in question. Huxley's (1932) equation for relative growth

$$y = bx^k \qquad \mathbf{2.4}$$

becomes

$$log\ y = log\ b + k\ log\ x \qquad \mathbf{2.5}$$

for more routine use. In Equation 2.5, y and x are units of weight or size of specific tissues, b is the value of y when x = 0 and k is the rate of growth in x when compared to the growth of y. If k is greater than 1, x is growing more rapidly than y; and if k = 1, the two tissues are growing at the same rate (Figure 2.6). Information obtained using these methods enhanced the understanding of growth, but failed to account for conformational changes due to accumulation of fat.

Hammond (1932) provided the first observation of the orderly progression of growth of tissues defined as 1, nervous tissue; 2, bone; 3, muscle; and 4, fat. These principles of progressive growth of the skeleton followed by growth of muscle and finally,

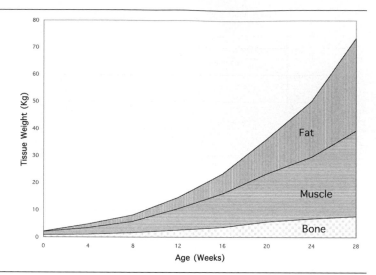

Figure 2.7. Accumulation of bone, muscle, and fat during growth of swine. (Data adapted from McMeekan, 1940.)

accumulation of fat provide the basis for understanding the declining efficiency of growth as animals mature because more energy is required to accumulate fat than to accumulate muscle. In fact, most weight gain by farm animals in the latter days of growth prior to slaughter is due to accumulation of fat (Figure 2.7).

Animals slaughtered at similar points on their relative growth curves tend to have similar body composition, if they have been provided adequate nutrition to allow expression of their genetic potential for growth. For instance, when the mature size of animals is increased, muscle and fat continue to accumulate in a manner proportional to that found in earlier maturing animals, and body composition is similar at similar stages of relative growth. Therefore, the amount of lean in an animal at market weight may be increased by selecting parents who have a much greater mature size and then marketing their offspring at approximately the same weight used prior to the selection process (Figure 2.8). These effects are demonstrated most dramatically in beef cattle since mature sizes of beef cattle increased 30–40% over the past 50 years. The selection for cattle having a larger mature size coupled with genetic selection against excessive external fat has resulted in beef cattle with a greater percentage carcass lean than was present 50 years ago.

Studies of the relative rates of growth of various parts of the body led Huxley (1932) to describe the concept of growth gradients, and he indicated skeletal growth proceeds from the cranium to the posterior and from the distal portion of limbs to the medial

portion of the body. That is, the bones of the cranium undergo less growth during postnatal growth than do bones of the caudal portion of the skeleton. Likewise, the distal portions of the limbs undergo less relative growth during the postnatal period than do the ribs. Allometric studies continue to support the evidence for greater growth of hind limb bones compared to front limb bones in swine (Richmond and Berg 1972; Liu et al. 1999), and similar skeletal growth patterns have also been described for the Thoroughbred horse (Thompson 1995).

THE PROCESS OF GROWTH

Growth is characterized by an increase in the size of individual cells (hypertrophy) as well as an increase in the number of cells in a tissue (hyperplasia). The addition of cells takes place by cell division as well as by the process of differentiation. Although the majority of differentiation takes place during prenatal development, differentiation may be involved in the recruitment of adipocytes in later stages of growth. The biology of differentiation of muscle, bone, and adipose tissue is discussed in more detail in Chapters 8, 9, and 10.

Some tissues, such as skeletal muscle, undergo very little increase in cell number after birth; other tissues, such as adipose tissue, and organs, such as the liver and kidney, are capable of significant increases in cell number during growth. Understanding the factors that regulate growth has long intrigued physiologists. Exercise physiologists have searched for ways to stimulate muscle growth and performance. Likewise, animal scientists have searched for treatments to enhance the growth of

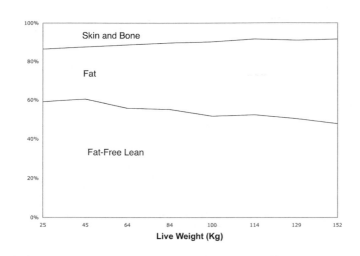

Figure 2.8. Proportions of muscle and fat in carcasses of growing swine. (Data adapted from Wagner et al., 1999.)

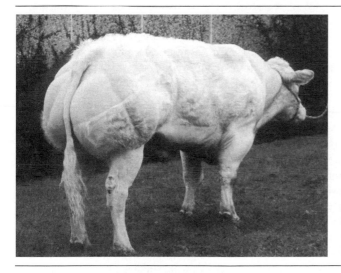

Figure 2.9. Example of muscle hypertrophy. The extensive muscle development and definition between muscles is seen in the photograph of the Belgian Blue bull *Classique de St Lambert*. (Photo courtesy of Linalux, Ciney, Belgium.)

muscle while reducing the accumulation of body fat in meat animals. Although some external treatments, such as dietary supplements and growth-promoting implants, have been effective, the greatest progress in improving meat production has been through genetic selection of animals with less body fat. Selection for muscle size alone has been shown to have its problems as seen in failure of the myostatin gene to adequately restrict muscle growth, which results in the condition commonly referred to as double muscling in cattle. The double-muscled condition is characterized by a dramatic increase in the number of muscle fibers at birth and

is due to specific mutations in the myostatin gene (Grobet et al. 1997; Kambadur et al. 1997; McPherron and Lee 1997; also see Chapter 8). This genetic defect in control of muscle growth results in an increase in the number of muscle fibers present at birth, and the subsequent growth of these cells to their typical mature size during postnatal growth results in a muscle mass greater than that of normal animals (Swatland and Kiefer 1974). The increased conformational thickness due to extensive hyperplasia of muscle fibers is noted in Figure 2.9.

While the double-muscled condition is readily evident at birth and is due to prenatal hyperplasia of

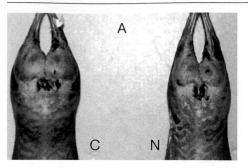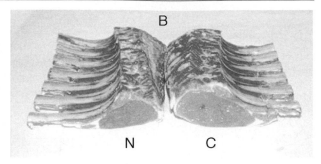

Figure 2.10. Legs and ribs from normal and callipyge lambs. In panel A, a leg from a callipyge lamb (C) is shown on the left and a leg from a normal lamb (N) is on the right. In panel B, the rib on the left is from a normal (N) lamb. The rib on the right has a much greater cross-sectional area and is from a lamb expressing the callipyge (C) gene. (Photo in panel A courtesy of scientists at the U.S. Meat Animal Research Center, Clay Center, Nebraska. Photo in panel B courtesy of Noelle Cockett, Utah State University.)

muscle cells, a condition of sheep known as callipyge (*Gr. calli* for beautiful + *pyge* for buttocks) is characterized by extensive muscular hypertrophy during postnatal growth (Figure 2.10). The condition is not noticeable at birth and does not become evident until approximately 4–6 weeks of age, provided adequate nutrition is available to support accelerated muscle growth (Jackson et al. 1997). The callipyge condition is expressed only in heterozygous lambs that inherit the gene from their sire (Cockett et al. 1996), and the pedigree of all lambs expressing the callipyge condition can be traced to one male in which the genetic mutation occurred. The use of the callipyge gene to enhance muscle content of lamb carcasses has not been widely accepted, because the meat from the loin of lambs expressing the callipyge gene is significantly less tender than that of normal lamb (Ducket et al. 1998).

Changes in body conformation during growth are a combination of the increased muscle mass as well as the accumulation of adipose tissue. The accumulation of fat between muscles is a major factor contributing to an overestimate of muscle present in growing animals (Kauffman et al. 1970). This principle is demonstrated effectively in Figure 2.11 where an extensive amount of fat present between muscles in the hind quarter of cattle adds to the overall thickness in this large muscle region of the body.

Adipose tissue present at birth contains some stored lipid, and the amount of lipid present varies among species (Figure 2.12). With the exception of the human and guinea pig, body fat at birth is gen-

erally low as a percentage of total body weight. Adipose cells, or adipocytes, are found embedded in a matrix of connective tissue and are localized in four major depots in the body in the form of intermuscular fat, subcutaneous fat, perirenal fat, and intramuscular fat. Pigs accumulate subcutaneous body fat by both hyperplasia and hypertrophy of fat cells until approximately 5 months of age with the majority of fat deposition accomplished through hypertrophy of cells thereafter (Anderson and Kauffman 1973). Geneticists have manipulated the amount of subcutaneous fat of pigs effectively because the heritability of subcutaneous fat thickness is approximately 0.5. The swine industry has markedly reduced the amount of fat in pig carcasses because the value of lard declined and because consumers began selecting cuts of pork having little or no external fat. Subcutaneous fat appears in layers in swine and cattle and these layers are most easily observed in swine having excessive fat. With genetic selection against subcutaneous fat, the inner layer of subcutaneous fat has largely disappeared and the middle of the three layers has become markedly less. The outer layer of subcutaneous fat has changed relatively less as a result of selection. Additional information on the biology of adipose tissue and its regulation is explored in greater detail in Chapter 10.

MEASUREMENT OF GROWTH

From the time that Hammond (1932) and McMeekan (1940) noted the orderly progression of growth of tissues (bone, followed by muscle, followed by fat deposition) for sheep and swine,

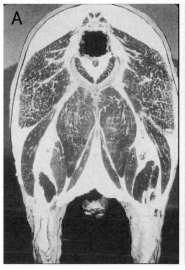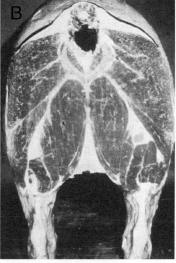

Figure 2.11. Cross-sections through the rounds of beef cattle. Extensive fat is visible in the seams between muscles in panel A compared to panel B. Muscle represents 44% of the cross-section in panel A compared to 60% muscle visible in panel B. (Photos courtesy of the Animal Science Department, Iowa State University.)

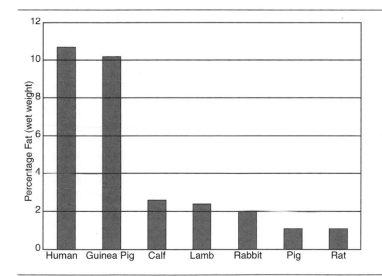

Figure 2.12. Species comparisons of body lipid content at birth. (Data adapted from Widdoson, 1950.)

respectively, animal scientists have wanted to know the relative rates at which muscle and fat were being produced. The serial slaughter technique allowed body composition to be measured by physical dissection of carcasses at specific ages and provided a view of changes taking place in animals under the conditions of specific experiments. The result then had to be extrapolated to related animals if the information was to be valuable in making selection decisions or management recommendations. The value of serial slaughter studies was limited by the obvious loss of the respective animals for further study or breeding.

Carcasses can also yield data such as ribeye area, muscle depth (*Longissimus dorsi*), fat thickness at various locations, lean tissue content, and separable lean, bone, and fat. These results can then be used to predict rates of lean tissue growth or accumulation of body fat. The serial slaughter method certainly had its drawbacks, but when the number of animals slaughtered at each time period of an experiment was great enough, researchers could construct a reasonable picture of changes in lean content of animals in response to specific nutritional or other environmental treatments. The serial slaughter method is extremely expensive in terms of the lost value of meat as well as the extensive labor required to dissect and analyze the many carcasses or portions of carcasses from growth or nutritional experiments. Hence, other methods were sought to estimate the amount of muscle in growing animals.

One of the greatest advances in objective selection of breeding stock was made by Hazel and Kline (1952), who described the direct measurement of subcutaneous fat in live swine using an inexpensive steel ruler. The backfat probe revolutionized selection for meat-type pigs and allowed selection decisions to be based on actual backfat thickness of sires and dams. Estimation of the genetic merit of breeding stock was further enhanced when information describing backfat thickness was added to selection strategies. The concept of the backfat probe was extended to the development of needle probes for measuring backfat thickness in cattle and lambs. However, the amount of backfat on cattle and sheep was markedly less than that on swine, and the thickness of the hide on cattle was more variable than for swine. Hence, the relative error associated with the use of the needle probe was greater than that of the ruler in swine. The cattle industry waited nearly three decades until ultrasound equipment was refined adequately and made suitably portable to provide repeatable and accurate measurements of backfat thickness over the rib of live cattle in field situations.

Because muscle is approximately 80% water, researchers examined many techniques to estimate the amount of total body water and developed predictive equations based on body water content to estimate muscle mass of growing animals. (A more precise value for the water content of muscle is obviously determined during the course of the respective experiment.) Methods to estimate total body water included the use of dye dilution and the dilution of deuterium oxide (heavy water). Other efforts estimated the fractional rates of muscle synthesis and breakdown using biopsy techniques and tissue culture or whole-body infusion of radiolabeled compounds or other compounds that could be monitored during and after the infusion process. The method used most recently with the greatest acceptance to estimate fat thickness and muscle depth and area is real-time ultrasound. Each of the above methods has been useful in constructing growth curves and estimating responses to genetic selection and nutritional treatments. These techniques to measure changes in body and carcass components are discussed in detail in Chapter 3.

Examples of applications of the principles of growth and production outlined above are readily apparent in our livestock industry. Animals have been selected for unique purposes: broiler chickens for meat production and Leghorn chickens for egg production; beef cattle for meat and dairy cattle for milk production; Holstein cattle for volume of milk produced, and Jersey cattle for butterfat content of their milk, small body size, and lower maintenance requirements; and hybrid swine for growth rate and optimal production of pork compared to their predecessors of 25 years ago. Each of these examples has resulted in differences in rates of growth of the animals involved, and research will continue to define mechanisms controlling growth and production of animals to improve the efficiency of producing food from animals.

REFERENCES

Anderson, D.B., and Kauffman, R.G. 1973. Cellular and enzymatic changes in porcine adipose tissue during growth. *Journal of Lipid Research* 14:160.

Berg, R.T., and Butterfield, R.M. 1976. *New Concepts of Cattle Growth*. Sidney: University Press.

Brody, S. 1945. *Bioenergetics and Growth*. New York: Reinhold.

Butterfield, R.M. 1963. Relative growth of the musculature of the ox. In *Carcass Composition and Appraisal of Meat Animals*. D.E. Tribe, ed. East Melborne: CSIRO.

Cockett, N.E., Jackson, S.P., Shay, T.L., Farnir, F., Berghmans, S., Snowder, G.D., Nielsen, D., and Georges, M. 1996. Polar overdominance at the ovine callipyge locus. *Science* 273:236–238.

de Lange, C.F.M. 1992. Practical applications of swine growth simulation models. *Proceedings NPPC Lean Growth Modeling Symposium*. Des Moines: National Pork Producers Council.

Ducket, S.K., Klein, T.A., Dodson, M.V., and Snowder, G.D. 1998. Tenderness of normal and callipyge lamb aged fresh or after freezing. *Meat Science* 49:19–26.

France, J., and Thornley, J.H.M. 1984. *Mathematical Models in Agriculture*. London: Butterworths.

Grobet, L., Royo Martin, L.J., Poncelet, D., Pirottin, D., Brouwers, B., Riquet, J., Schoeberlein, A., Dunner, S., Menissier, F., Massabanda, J., Fries, R., Hanset, R., and Georges, M. 1997. A deletion in the bovine myostatin gene causes the double-muscled phenotype in cattle. *Nature Genetics* 17:71–74.

Hammond, J. 1932. *Growth and Development of Mutton Qualities in Sheep*. London: Oliver and Boyd.

Hammond, J. 1940. *Farm Animals*. London: Edward Arnold & Co.

Hazel, L.N., and Kline, E.A. 1952. Mechanical measurement of fatness and carcass value on live hogs. *Journal of Animal Science* 11:486–494.

Huxley, J.S. 1932. *Problems of Relative Growth*. London: Methuen.Jackson, S.P., Green, R.D., and Miller, M.F.

1997. Phenotypic characterization of rambouillet sheep expressing the callipyge gene: I. Inheritance of the condition and production characteristics. *Journal of Animal Science* 75:14–18.

Kambadur, R., Sharma, M., Smith, TP.L., and Bass, J.J. 1997. Mutations in myostatin (GDF8) in double-muscled Belgian Blue and Piedmontese cattle. *Genome Research* 7:910–915.

Kauffman, R.G., Van Ess, M.D., and Long, R.A. 1970. Bovine topography and its relationship to composition. Proceedings of *23rd Annual Reciprocal Meat Conference*. Gainesville: University of Florida.

Kempster, A.J., Cuthbertson, A., and Harrington, G. 1982. The relationship between conformation and the yield and distribution of lean meat in the carcass of British pigs, cattle and sheep: A review. *Meat Science* 6:37.

Liu, M.F., He, P., Aherne, F.X., and Berg, R.T. 1999. Postnatal limb bone growth in relation to live weight in pigs from birth to 84 days of age. *Journal of Animal Science* 77:1693–1701.

Lopez, S, France, J., Gerrits, W.J.J., Dhanoa, M.S., Humphries, D.J., and Dijkstra, J. 2000. A generalized Michaelis-Menton equation for the analysis of growth. *Journal of Animal Science* 78:1816–1828.

McMeekan, C.P. 1940. Growth and development in the pig, with special reference to carcass quality characteristics. *Journal of Agricultural Science* 30:277–344.

McPherron, A.C., and Lee, S.-J. 1997. Double muscling in cattle due to mutations in the myostatin gene. Proceedings of the *National Academy of Science* 94:12457–12461

Menchaca, M.A., Chase, C.C., Olson, T.A., and Hammond, A.C. 1996. Evaluation of growth curves of Brahman cattle of various frame sizes. *Journal of Animal Science* 74:2140–2151.

Richmond, R.J., and Berg, R.T. 1972. Bone growth and distribution in swine as influenced by live weight, sex, and ration. *Canadian Journal of Animal Science* 52:47–56.

Schinckel, A.P., Preckel, P.V., and Einstein, M.E. 1996. Prediction of daily protein accretion rates of pigs from estimates of fat-free lean gain between 20 and 120 kilograms live weight. *Journal of Animal Science* 74:498–503.

Stranks, M.H., Cooke, B.C., Fairbairn, C.B., Fowler, N.G., Kirby, P.S. McCraken, K.J., Morgan, C.A., Palmer, F.G., and Peers, D.G. 1988. Nutrient allowances for growing pigs. *Research and Development in Agriculture* 5:77.

Swatland, H.J., and Kiefer, N.M. 1974. Fetal development of the double-muscled condition in cattle. *Journal of Animal Science* 38:752–757.

Thompson, K.N. 1995. Skeletal growth rates of weanling and yearling Thoroughbred horses. *Journal of Animal Science* 73:2513–2517.

Wagner, J.R., Schinckel, A.P., Chen, W., Forrest, J.C., and Coe, B.L. 1999. Analysis of body composition changes of swine during growth and development. *Journal of Animal Science* 77:1442–1466.

Walton, A., and Hammond, J. 1938. The maternal effects on growth and conformation in Shire horse-Shetland pony crosses. *Proceedings of the Royal Society of London, Series B, Biological Sciences* 125:311–335.

Widdoson, E.M. 1950. Chemical composition of newly born mammals. *Nature* 166:626–628.

3
Methods to Measure Animal Composition

David G. Topel

One of the oldest and popular research topics for the animal industry is associated with the prediction of carcass characteristics of live animals. Until recent technology was developed, individuals with good evaluation skills could equal—or in some situations, be more accurate than—machines for predicting the dollar value of the carcass. Therefore, visual evaluation of animals was a well-accepted procedure for the purchase of animals, and it is still a method used for the purchase of slaughter animals.

Within the last 10 years, however, the improvements in ultrasound and other methods for estimating body composition described in this chapter have provided the industry with a greater selection of techniques for more accurate predictions. This chapter provides a review of this technology and its application to the animal and meats industry.

REAL-TIME ULTRASOUND
Beef Cattle and Beef Carcasses

Real-time ultrasound has great value for estimating a large number of beef carcass traits in the live animal, including marbling. If ultrasound data are to be considered in genetic evaluation programs, development of an appropriate age adjustment strategy and possible differences in variance components that are due to sex of the animal need to be considered (Hassen et al. 1999).

Feedlot producers can use this technology to sort cattle into uniform groups to produce carcasses with a consistent weight, quality, and composition. Prediction equations could be developed to predict lean weight and composition of carcasses at slaughter based on live real-time ultrasound data obtained early in the feeding period. The data can also be used to predict the number of days needed to reach

a desired weight and compositional end point under a given management system (Hassen et al. 1999).

Marbling Prediction

Ultrasound software systems to predict marbling in beef cattle were compared (Herring et al. 1998). Results from this study indicate that the Iowa State University System (CVIS) and the Kansas State University system (CPEC1-4) were the most precise for predicting intramuscular fat.

Brethour (2000) used the receiver operating characteristic analysis to evaluate the accuracy in predicting future quality grade from ultrasound marbling estimates on beef calves. The use of ultrasound technology on young cattle to predict future quality grades is feasible, but the relative accuracy of 76–78% obtained in this study may not be high enough to impact substantial monetary benefits. More recent research at Iowa State University compared two main types of real-time ultrasound (RTU) machines to capture images for predicting the percentage of intramuscular fat (PIMF) in live cattle. In the comparison of ultrasound equipment, the choice between Aloka 500V and the Classic Scanner 200 does not make a significant difference in the accuracy of predicting the percentage of intramuscular fat when based on algorithms developed by Iowa State University.

Swine and Pork Carcasses

The real-time ultrasound technology has very good potential for on-line estimates of pork carcass composition. Danish researchers developed an on-line pork carcass grading system using the autoform ultrasound concept. The system consists of 16 ultrasound transducers positioned in a frame. The carcass is measured fully automatically at 3,200 positions to a depth of approximately 12 cm with a depth resolution of .19 mm. The ultrasound data form a three-dimensional ultrasound image, which is processed for noise reduction, orientation detection, and extraction of 127 features describing the pork carcass composition. The images are used in a multivariate regression model that is used for on-line predictions of the carcass composition. On-line tests reflect that at line speeds up to 1,150 carcasses per hour, this procedure provides outstanding accuracy (Brøndum et al. 1998).

As the ultrasound technology improves, on-line techniques for development of prediction equations provide the opportunity for estimation of fresh pork carcass yield for a variety of retail and wholesale procurement end points. This process can also be used to provide economic incentive so that the pork industry can use these techniques to better reflect the true value back to the pork producer. The research for these ultrasound techniques were reported by the Texas A&M group (Berg et al. 1999).

Real-time ultrasonic measurements of backfat and loin muscle area in swine using multiple statistical analysis can be used with much success in genetic improvement programs for carcass traits in pigs. Real-time ultrasound seems to be favored over single transducer instruments, because fat and muscle can be visualized in a two-dimensional image rather than at a single point (Moeller and Christian 1998). These technologies are used extensively for pig genetic improvement programs around the world and currently are the preferred method for carcass measurements on live animals for the pork industry.

NUCLEAR MAGNETIC RESONANCE SPECTROSCOPY (NMR)

With nuclear magnetic resonance technology, about 98% of the variability in total body fat content can be explained (Mitchell et al. 1991). The ultrasound technology, however, is almost as good as NMR technology and it is much cheaper and much easier to use. It is also more animal friendly on a partical farm operation (Villé et al. 1997).

DUAL-ENERGY X-RAY ABSORPTIOMETRY

Dual-energy x-ray absorptiometry is based on greater attenuation of the x-rays by lean (water and protein) than by fat. Furthermore, the x-ray is great-ly attenuated by bone or ash, and for that reason, the Angle-Ray is used only for ground meat with little or no bone present. However, dual-energy x-ray absorptiometry (DXA) scans the sample at two x-ray energy levels (i.e., 38 and 70 ke V), which provides a two-dimensional image and measurement of bone minerals, fat, and lean content and total tissue mass.

Difficulties in obtaining a reliable measurement of the fat content of small pigs using DXA were reported (Mitchell et al. 1998). This study indicated, however, that the correlations between DXA and chemical measurements are high enough to suggest that, with proper calibration based on chemical analysis, the DXA measurement could provide a valid measure of body fat in small pigs.

Another study by Mitchell and colleagues (1998) indicated that dual-energy x-ray absorptiometry can be used for determination of the fat, lean, and bone mineral content of pork half-carcasses. The procedure is too slow for compatibility with on-line processing, but has value for research purposes when compared to dissection and chemical analysis.

MAGNETIC RESONANCE IMAGING (MRI)

Magnetic resonance imaging (MRI) is widely recognized as one of the most powerful diagnostic tools of modern medicine. The MRI image is based on the magnetic resonant properties of protons associated with water and lipid molecules of tissues and results in a range of signal intensities capable of distinguishing numerous tissues and organs, including fat and muscle. Magnetic resonance imaging offers a number of possibilities for noninvasive in vivo body composition analysis of the pig, ranging from volumetric measurement of specific organs to prediction of total body fat and lean content (Mitchell et al. 2001). The problem with this technology is that it is too expensive for use in the livestock industry and it is not a practical method for production systems. Using this technology for research has real potential if it is not cost prohibitive.

UREA DILUTION MEASUREMENT OF BODY COMPOSITION IN STEERS

The urea dilution (UD) procedure and ultrasonic measurements of backfat hold much promise for being practical and easily implemented for research as well as on-farm applications. The determination of carcass trait estimates in live animals is of economical importance to the farmers because of the emphasis to predict the value of lean carcasses at slaughter. Also sometimes, reduced financial support available to researchers may prevent them from slaughtering the animal for carcass composition determination. These methods can be helpful in predicting composition without slaughtering the animal. The urea dilution procedure (Preston and Kock 1973; Hammond et al. 1990) holds promise for practical use on farms as well as for research (Wells and Preston 1998).

Visual Assessments of Feeder Lambs and Slaughter Cows

Tatum and colleagues (1998) reported an effective visual grading system for feeder lambs using standardized descriptions for feeder lamb value. Their results indicate that visual assessments of muscle thickness are indicative of eventual differences in carcass lean-meat yield and therefore may be used for describing value differences among feeder lambs.

O'Mara and colleagues (1998) indicated that visual cutability end points for slaughter cows can be accurately predicted using practical live animal and carcass predictors. Therefore, the potential to redefine yield grade standards for slaughter cows and their carcasses is feasible and could provide a more meaningful reporting system for the slaughter cow industry. Apple and colleagues (1999) reported similar results for edible by-products from body composition scores on cull beef cows.

COMPUTER MODEL TO PREDICT COMPOSITION OF EMPTY BODY WEIGHT

Mathematical models have been developed to predict body composition in growing and mature animals (Notter 1977; Oltjen et al. 1986; Keele et al. 1992). Arnold and Bennett, 1991, reported that many models were more accurate in predicting empty body weight than body composition. Williams and colleagues (1992) showed that the model accurately predicted absolute treatment means for fatness and some of the nutritional effects on fatness, not associated with changes in empty body weight. In 1997, Williams and Jenkins developed a model that was based on a different mathematical formulation from that used by Keele and colleagues (1992), to predict composition of empty body weight changes in mature cattle. Williams and Jenkins (1998) proposed that as cattle grow from

birth to maturity, the mathematical formulation to predict composition of gain changes at some point in the life cycle from that used by Keele and colleagues (1992) and that used by Williams and Jenkins (1997). Therefore, Williams and Jenkins (1998) reported on results that integrated the models resulting in an increase in accuracy of predicting composition of gain in compensatory growth experiments.

BIOELECTRICAL IMPEDANCE

Research using bioelectrical impedance has shown promising results with rats (Hall et al. 1989), lamb carcasses (Cosgrove et al. 1988; Berg and Marchello 1994), and live swine and pork carcasses (Swantek et al. 1992). Velazco and colleagues (1999) indicated that bioelectrical impedance analysis (BIA) has potential for use in estimating carcass fat-free mass in Holstein steers, but is not as accurate for results from smaller animals such as rats and lambs. Swantek and colleagues (1999) reported that bioelectrical impedance methodology may be used to accurately assess compositional changes of finishing pigs weighing 50–130 kg. This technique has value for research and genetic selection of breeding animals.

The four-terminal BIA is based on a constant alternating current of 800μA at 50kHz into the body via the sending terminals and is received by the detecting terminals. Impedance is a measurement of voltage reduction as an electrical current passes through an object. This decrease depends on the object's geometric configuration and volume and the strength and frequency of the signal. Assuming a relatively constant geometry for all pigs and using a constant electrical signal, impedance (resistance and reactance) differences should be dependent on the body composition (fat and fat-free mass). The conductivity of an animal is affected by body composition; thus a fat animal has a higher impedance value than a lean animal (Lukaski et al. 1985).

COMPUTER IMAGE ANALYSIS

The most important step in image analysis is to obtain a correct threshold value that divides lean and marbling. Kuchida and colleagues (1997a,b) developed a software for image analyses using the contour comparison method. This software draws contours of marbling particles for a specified area on the computer screen that displays the original color image of the ribeye area. The ratio of fat area to area of the ribeye muscle obtained from the program could be used as a linear covariate to predict crude fat percentage in the ribeye muscle with high precision ($r^2 = .91$) and accuracy. Kuchida and colleagues (2000) improved on the methodology of marbling predicting by computer image analysis.

Dual-Component Computer Vision System (CVS)

In the Dual-Component CVS, one video camera obtains an image of the outside surface and contour of unribbed beef sides as they pass by on the rail before or after chilling. After the carcass has been chilled and ribbed, a second video camera records an image of the exposed 12th/13th rib interface. Computer analyses of the two video camera images are used in calculations of the total carcass dimensions, carcass shape, carcass fat distribution, 12th–13th rib fat thickness, and ribeye area. From these calculations, predictions are made of the whole-sale subprimal yield. The Dual Component Computer Vision System was developed as an alternative to subjective yield grading by the USDA graders. The CVS-predicted wholesale cut yields are more accurate than current online subjective yield grading by USDA graders (Cannell et al. 2002).

LINEAR CARCASS MEASUREMENTS

An inexpensive ruler to measure fat thickness, length, or width of the longissimus dorsi muscle is a historical method to estimate body composition or value of the carcass. The now classical work in this area was reported by Palsson (1939) on lamb carcasses, Hirzel (1939) for beef carcasses, and McMeekan (1941) for pork carcasses. From these early studies have come more than 250 papers relating linear measurements to carcass characteristics. The most popular linear measurements, backfat, and depth of the longissimus muscle are considered good, but not excellent predictors of body composition. Their big advantage is ease of measurement and low costs.

BACKFAT PROBE FOR LIVE ANIMALS

The backfat probe was developed by Hazel and Kline (1952). Until the current ultrasound technology was developed, the simple probe had been the most common and practical measurement for backfat or subcutaneous fat prediction in pigs and cattle.

To measure the actual fat depth, a small incision is made in the skin with a scalpel and a narrow metal ruler is forced through the fat layers, or a ruler containing a needle point is forced directly through the skin and fat layers. Some people use a local anesthesia in the area where the probe is inserted. When the fat depth is known, it can be used in a previously developed regression equation with other variables, such as live weight and muscling measurements, to estimate composition. Fat depth alone usually accounts for most of the variation in composition, but live weight and degree of muscling improves the accuracy for composition estimates (Fahey et al. 1977).

LIVE WEIGHT AND GROWTH CURVES

The development of growth curves from the animal's live weight provides a practical and simple method for estimating body and production traits of animals if the genetic history for body composition is known (Brody 1945; Kaps et al. 2000). As animals grow, their carcass composition changes and the proportion of fat increases at the expense of muscle and bone (Rouse et al. 1970). When comparing animals of similar type grown in the same environment, live weight normally shows a high positive correlation with the percentage of fat in the carcass. Moreover, because of the close relationship between muscle and bone, live weight also shows a high negative correlation with the proportion of muscle in the carcass (Busch et al. 1969).

Live weight of cattle, swine, and sheep is still the major—and in many markets, the only—factor used in deciding when animals are sold for slaughter. Therefore, livestock breeders and farmers must select for cattle, swine, and sheep that have the genetic traits for low fat and high muscle percentage at live weights, which will provide conveniently sized cuts of meat for the consumer and meet the standards established by the packing industry to operate economically.

FAT-O-MEAT'ER OR REFLECTANCE PROBE

The Fat-O-Meat'er is a handheld optical probe used to measure fat and muscle thickness in predefined locations on the pork carcass. The Fat-O-Meat'er is a reflectance probe, and the concept was developed by researchers at the Danish Meat Research Institute (Barton 1983). The Fat-O-Meat'er measures the difference in light reflectance of fat and lean tissue. The probe records light reflectance every 0.5 mm as it passes through backfat and muscle. The probe is usually placed between the third and fourth last ribs. The Fat-O-Meat'er was the first semiobjective pork carcass grading system, and it has the capacity of 1,200 carcasses per hour.

WHOLE-BODY ^{40}K COUNTING

Extensive research on this technique was reported in the 1960s, and it is summarized in a National Academy of Science publication (Breidenstein et al. 1968). Estimating the body composition of living animals by whole-body ^{40}K counting is feasible because of the direct relation of potassium to lean body mass and its indirect relation to fat. Potassium is the only single element found in body tissue in significant amounts that has any predictive value of body composition. The ^{40}K method has proven useful in research projects where the research center has a ^{40}K Whole Body Counter. These are expensive units, and the technology is not often used because other methods are just as good and less expensive.

BODY DENSITY

Body density measurements for estimating body composition of animals is one of the older methods, and it is not very practical when compared to more modern methods. The major problem in determining density is the measurement of volume. Although this would appear to be a simple procedure, it is not, especially in live animals. Empty-body specific gravity in beef was correlated (P<0.05) with the percentage of carcass fat (Kraybill et al. 1951), and Garrett (1968) reported that variation in predicting pork carcass composition is similar to cattle and sheep when density measurements are used. The accuracy of specific gravity for estimating body composition traits varies from average to good. At the 1986 meeting of the American Society of Animal Science Miller and colleagues (1986) reported an average relationship for specific gravity in predicting carcass fat.

Density techniques are slow and have no commercial value, but the techniques may still have some limited use in certain research fields.

TISSUE SAWDUST TECHNIQUE

Vance and colleagues (1970) reported a correlation (P<0.01) between the chemical components of beef carcass sides and the meat sawdust from sawing through the frozen round, loin, rib, and chuck at 2.54 cm intervals. Williams and colleagues (1974) reported more extensive comparisons of the tissue sawdust technique using bull carcasses and carcasses from Holstein calves. The reliability of the sawdust procedure was the greatest from frozen carcasses sawed every 2.54 cm. Chemical composition of the meat sawdust can provide a good estimate of the chemical composition of beef carcasses when the sawdust samples are collected by cutting every 2.54 cm from the frozen carcass. This method has value only as a research tool.

TOTAL BODY ELECTRICAL CONDUCTIVITY (TOBEC)

The accuracy of electromagnetic scanning to estimate body composition of pork carcasses has been studied extensively at Purdue University. The Purdue researchers used an Ag Med, Inc. HA-2 scanner at 64 equidistant intervals, providing an asymmetric bell-shaped curve. The curve peaks when maximum lean mass is in the electromagnetic field. The height and area of the curve segments are analyzed to determine relationships to various carcass components and composition. The Purdue results suggest that electromagnetic scanning accurately estimates total carcass lean as well as yield and composition of carcass primal cuts. Therefore, this technology has potential to predict carcass value (Kuei et al. 1989).

CONCLUSIONS

Significant advances in technology have occurred in the last 10 years for predicting carcass composition in cattle, pigs, and sheep. This technology has been adapted for establishing carcass value by many packing plants for payment to farmers based on percentage of muscle. The technology has also been adapted to predict carcass traits in live animals for genetic selection programs. This has resulted in much improvement in carcass value in the last 5–6 years.

REFERENCES

Apple, J.K., Davis, J.C., and Stephenson, J. 1999. Influence of body composition score on by-product yield and value from cull beef cows. *Journal of Animal Science* 77:2670–2679.

Arnold, R.N., and Bennett, G.L. 1991. Evaluation of four simulation models of cattle growth and body composition: II. Simulation and comparison with experimental growth data. *Agricultural Systems* 36:17–41.

Barton, P. 1983. Quality traits of pork carcasses. In *Annual Report of the Danish Meat Research Institute*. Copenhagen: Danish Meat Research Institute.

Berg, E.P., Grams, D.W., Miller, R.K., Wise, J.W., Forrest, J.C., and Savell, J.W. 1999. Using current on-line carcass evaluation parameters to estimate boneless and bone-in pork carcass yield as influenced by trim level. *Journal of Animal Science* 77:1977–1984.

Berg, E.P., and Marchello, M.J. 1994. Bioelectrical impedance analysis for the prediction of fat-free mass in lamb and lamb carcasses. *Journal of Animal Science* 72:322–329.

Breidenstein, B.C., Lohman, T.G., and Norton, H.W. 1968. Comparison of potassium-40 method with other methods of determining carcass lean muscle mass in steers.In *Body Composition in Animals and Man*. Washington, D.C.: National Academy of Sciences.

Brethour, J.R. 2000. Using receiver operating characteristic analysis to evaluate the accuracy in predicting future quality grade from ultrasound marbling estimates on beef calves. *Journal of Animal Science* 78:2263–2268.

Brody, S. 1945. *Bioenergetics and Growth*. New York: Reinhold Publishing.

Brøndum, J., Egebo, M., Agerskov, C., and Busk, H. 1998. On-line pork carcass grading with the Autoform ultrasound system. *Journal of Animal Science* 76:1859–1868.

Busch, D.A., Dinkel, C.A., and Minyard, J.A. 1969. Body measurements, subjective scores and estimates of certain carcass traits as predictors of edible portion in beef cattle. *Journal of Animal Science* 29:557–566.

Cannell, R.C., Belk, K.E., Tatum, J.D., Wise, W.J., Chapman, P.L., Scanga, J.A., and Smith, G.C. 2002. Online evaluation of a commercial video image analysis system (Computer Vision System) to predict beef carcass red meat yield and for augmenting the assignment of USDA yield grades. *Journal of Animal Science* 80:1195–1201.

Cosgrove, J.R., King, J.W.B., and Brodie, D.A. 1988. A note on the use of impedance measurements of the predictions of carcass composition in lambs. *Animal Production* 47:311–319.

Fahey, T.J., Schaefer, D.M., Kauffman, R.G., Epley, R.J., Gould, P.F., Romans, J.R., Smith, G.C., and Topel, D.G. 1977. A comparison of practical methods to estimate pork carcass composition. *Journal of Animal Science* 44:8–17.

Garrett, W.N. 1968. Expenses in the use of body density as an estimator of body composition of animals.In Body *Composition in Animals and Man*. Washington D.C.: National Academy of Sciences.

Hall, C.B., Lukaski, H.C., and Marchello, M.J. 1989. Determination of rat body composition using bioelectrical impedance analysis. *Nutrition Reports International* 39:627–633.

Hammond, A.C., Waldo, D.R., and Rumsey, T.S. 1990. Prediction of body composition in Holstein steers using urea space. *Journal of Dairy Science* 73:3141–3145.

Hassen, A., Wilson, D.E., Amin, V.R., Rouse, G.H., and Hays, C.L. 2001. Predicting percentage of intramuscular fat using two types of real-time ultrasound equipment. *Journal of Animal Science* 79:11–18.

Hassen, A., Wilson, D.E., and Rouse, G.H. 1999a. Evaluation of carcass, live, and real-time ultrasound measures in feedlot cattle: I. Assessment of sex and beef effects. *Journal of Animal Science* 77:273–282.

Hassen, A., Wilson, D.E., and Rouse, G.H. 1999b.

Evaluation of carcass, live and real-time ultrasound measures in feedlot cattle: II. Effects of different age and points on the accuracy of predicting the percentage of retail product, retail product weight, and hot carcass weight. *Journal of Animal Science* 77:283–290.

Hazel, L.N., and Kline, E.A. 1952. Mechanical measurement of fatness and carcasses value of live hogs. *Journal of Animal Science* 11:313–319.

Herring, W.O., Kriese, L.A., Bertrand, J.K., and Crouch, J. 1998. Comparison of four real-time ultrasound systems that predict intramuscular fat in beef cattle. *Journal of Animal Science* 76:364–370.

Hirzel, R. 1939. Factors affecting quality in mutton and beef with special reference to the proportions of muscle, fat and bone. *Onderstepoort Journal of Veterinary Science* 12:379–408.

Kaps, M., Harring, W.O., and Lamberson, W.R. 2000. Genetic and environmental parameters for traits derived from the Brody growth curve and their relationships with weaning weight in Angus cattle. *Journal of Animal Science* 78:1436–1442.

Keele, J.W., Williams, C.B., and Bennett, G.L. 1992. A computer model to predict the effects of level nutrition on composition of empty body gain in beef cattle. I. Theory and development. *Journal of Animal Science* 70:841–857.

Kraybill, H.F., Bitter, H.L., and Hankins, O.G. 1951. Body composition of cattle. II. Determination of fat and water content from measurement of body specific gravity. *Journal of Applied Physiology* 4:575–582.

Kuchida, K., Kono, S., Konishi, K., VanVleck, L.D., Suzuki, M., and Miyoshi, S. 2000. Prediction of crude fat content of longissimus muscle of beef using the ratio of fat area calculated from computer image analysis: Comparison of regression equations for prediction using different input devices at different stations. *Journal of Animal Science* 78:799–803.

Kuchida, K., Kurihara, A., Suzuki, M., and Miyoshi, S. 1997a. Computer image analysis method for evaluation of marbling of ribeye area. *Animal Science and Technology (Japan)* 68:878–882.

Kuchida, K., Kurihara, A., Suzuki, M., and Miyoshi, S. 1997b. Development of accurate method for measuring fat percentage on ribeye area by computer image analysis. *Animal Science and Technology (Japan)* 68:853–859.

Kuei, C.H., Forrest, J.C., Orcutt, M.W., Judge, M.D., and Schinckel, P.A. 1989. Evaluation of electromagnetic scanning in predicting pork carcass composition and primal cut yield. In *Proceedings of the Reciprocal Meat Conference, Guelph*, Canada 42:198.

Kuei, C.H., Forrest, J.C., Schinckel, A.P., and Judge, M.D. 1991. Total body electrical conductivity in lieu of dissection for pork carcass composition research. *Journal of Animal Science* 69 (Suppl. 1): 339.

Lukaski, H.C., Bolonchuk, W.W., Hall, C.B., and Siders, W.A. 1985. Validation of tetrapolar bioelectrical impedance method to assess human body composition. *Journal of Applied Physiology* 60:1327–1332.

McMeekan, C.P. 1941. Growth and development in the pig with special references to carcass quality characteristics. *Journal of Agricultural Science* 31:1–27.

Miller, M.F., Cross, H.R., Smith, G.C., Baker, J.F., Byers, F.M., and Recio, H.A. 1986. Evaluation of live and carcass techniques for predicting beef carcass composition. *Journal of Animal Science* 63 (Suppl. 1): 234.

Mitchell, A.D., Scholz, A.M., and Conway, J.M. 1998. Body composition analysis of small pigs by dual-energy x-ray absorptiometry. *Journal of Animal Science* 76:2392–2398.

Mitchell, A.D., Scholz, A.M., Pursel, V.G., and Evock-Clover, C.M. 1998. Composition analysis of pork carcasses by dual-energy x-ray absorptiometry. *Journal of Animal Science* 76:2104–2114.

Mitchell, A.D., Scholz, A.M., Wang, P.C., and Song, H. 2001. Body composition analysis of the pig by magnetic resonance imaging. *Journal of Animal Science* 79:1800–1813.

Mitchell, A.D., Wang, P.C., Elsasser, T.H., and Schmidt, W.F. 1991. Application of NMR spectroscopy and imaging for body composition analysis and related to sequential measurement of energy deposition. *12th Energy Symposium of Farm Animals*. Kartausen-Ittinger, September: 4–7.

Moeller, S.J., and Christian, L.L. 1998. Evaluation of the accuracy of real-time ultrasonic measurements of backfat and loin muscle area in swine using multiple statistical analysis procedures. *Journal of Animal Science* 76:2503–2514.

Notter, D.R. 1977. Simulated efficiency of beef production for a cow-calf–feedlot management system. *Ph.D. Dissertation*. University of Nebraska, Lincoln.

Oltjen, J.W., Bywater, A.C., Baldwin, R.L., and Garrett, W.N. 1986. Development of a dynamic model of beef carcass growth and composition. *Journal of Animal Science* 62:86–97.

O'Mara, F.M., Williams, S.E., Tatum, J.D., Hilton, G.G., Pringle, T.D., Wise, J.W., and Williams, F.L. 1998. Prediction of slaughter cow composition using live animal and carcass traits. *Journal of Animal Science* 1594–1603.

Palsson, H. 1939. Meat quality in sheep with special reference to Scottish breeds and crosses. *Journal of Agricultural Science* 29:544–549.

Preston, R.L., and Kock, S.W. 1973. In vivo prediction of body composition in cattle from urea space measurements. *Proceedings of the Society of Experimental Biology Medicine* 143:1057–1061.

Rouse, G.H., Topel, D.G., Vetter, R.L., Rust, R.E., and Wickersham, T.W. 1970. Carcass composition of lambs at different stages of development. *Journal of Animal Science* 31:846–855.

Swantek, P.M., Crenshaw, J.D., Marchello, M.J., and Lukaski, H.C. 1992. Bioelectrical impedance: A nondestructive method to determine fat-free mass of live market swine and pork carcasses. *Journal of Animal Science* 70:169–177.

Swantek, P.M., Marchello, M.J., Tilton, J.E., and Crenshaw, J.D. 1999. Prediction of fat-free mass of pigs from 50 to 130 kilograms live weight. *Journal of Animal Science* 77:893–897.

Tatum, J.D., Sember, J.A., Gillmore, B.R., LeValley, S.B., and Williams, F.L. 1998. Relationship of visual assessments of feeder lamb muscularity to differences in carcass yield traits. *Journal of Animal Science* 76:774–780.

Vance, R.D., Ockerman, H.W., Cahill, V.R., and Plimpton, R.F. 1970. Carcass composition as related to meat sawdust and analysis. *Journal of Animal Science* 31:192.

Velazco, J., Morrill, J.L., and Grunewald, K.K. 1999. Utilization of bioelectrical impedance to predict carcass composition of Holstein steers at 3, 6, 9 and 12 months of age. *Journal of Animal Science* 77:131–136.

Villé, H., Rombouts, G., VanHecke, P., Perremans, S., Maes, G. Spencemaille, G., and Geers, R. 1997. An evaluation of ultrasound and nuclear magnetic resonance spectroscopy to measure in vivo intramuscular fat content of longissimus muscle of pigs. *Journal of Animal Science* 75:2942–2949.

Wells, R.S., and Preston, R.L. 1998. Effect of repeated urea dilution measurement on feedlot performance and consistency of estimated body composition in steers of different breed types. *Journal of Animal Science* 76:2799–2804.

Williams, C.B., and Jenkins, T.G. 1997. Predicting empty body composition and composition of empty body weight changes in mature cattle. *Agricultural Systems* 53:1–25.

Williams, C.B., and Jenkins, T.G. 1998. A computer model to predict composition of empty body weight changes in cattle at all stages of maturity. *Journal of Animal Science* 76:980–987.

Williams, C.B., Keele, J.W., and Bennett, G.L. 1992. A computer model to predict the effects of level of nutrition on composition of empty body weight gain in beef cattle: II. Evaluation of model. *Journal of Animal Science* 70:858–866.

Williams, D.B., Topel, D.G., and Vetter, R.L. 1974. Evaluation of a tissue-sawdust technique for predicting beef carcass composition. *Journal of Animal Science* 39:949–854.

4

Approaches to Assess Animal Growth Potential

Roger E. Calza and Michael V. Dodson

Animal growth is a complex, integrated process involving numerous levels of regulation. Historically, animal scientists have selected domestic animals based on reproductive performance, ability to withstand extremes in heat or cold, or amount of muscling, to name only a few criteria. Therefore, the animals that are seen in pastures, feedlots, dairies, or even in the backyard have experienced hundreds of years of selective fine-tuning for specific characteristics desirable by owners. Does this mean that domestic animals have experienced maximum gains in the expression of desired traits? Likely not—especially since, during the past few decades, modern technology has made rapid advances in developing techniques that can be used to make animal growth performance even more efficient. The focus of this chapter is to summarize some of these methods in order to aid students of animal growth when they read the scientific literature or delve into later chapters of this book. For this purpose we have identified and detailed some of the most common to least common methods presently being used for facilitating animal growth research.

PERFUSED ORGAN/TISSUE SYSTEMS

In numerous studies related to animal growth there is a need to identify the flow, absorption, interaction, conversion, and metabolic rates of biological compounds within an isolated organ or tissue. To that end, methods have been devised to isolate living organs and tissues (Freshney 1986). Isolation might refer to either the complete physical isolation of an organ or the compartmentalization of the organ/tissue away from the rest of the body. When isolated, the organ or tissue is subjected to perfusion, which is the process of introducing a stream of

test materials to the organ or tissue via an entrance route and recovering the test materials via a different exit route. Usually these routes are major arteries and veins of the organ or tissue of interest. Although perfused organ/tissue systems are complex to use and interpret, they have been invaluable to the animal growth field.

EXPLANT (TISSUE) CULTURE

The process of removing a piece of living tissue from an animal and placing it into an incubation medium within a test tube or plastic culture dish is termed explant or tissue culture (Freshney 1986; Resau et al. 1991). Although not as complex a system as perfusion, this method requires skill in order to ensure that the tissue explants are uniform (Bach et al. 1996). The culture of tissue in this manner implies a short-term in vitro process that mimics the in vivo environment as much as possible, as long as the tissue is physiologically active. Tissue culture methods have been devised for evaluating numerous physiological events, such as adipogenesis, amino acid uptake, and the production of secretory agents from the tissue (Trowell 1959; Rodbell 1964; Vernon 1979).

CELL CULTURE

Unlike tissue culture, cell culture refers to isolating populations of living cells from an animal and growing them in a plastic dish (Figure 4.1; Freshney 1994). Cell culture is a method that receives mixed reviews in terms of application to studying whole animal growth, because the physiology of the animal may have more of an effect on the activity of cells immediately isolated (Allen et al. 1997) than on cells allowed to grow for lengthy periods of time. Another problem associated with the use of cell culture for

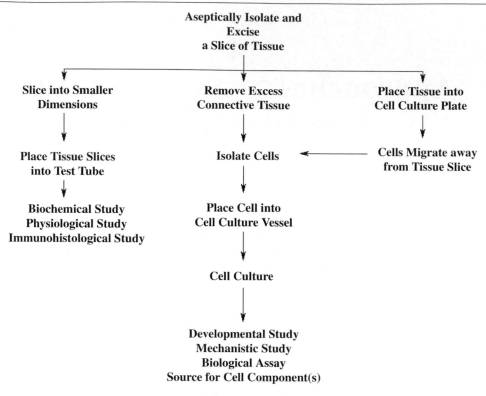

Figure 4.1. Relative differences in initial events and applicability between tissue culture and cell culture.

extrapolation of data to whole animals is the fact that the environment to which the cells are exposed in vitro does not mimic the complex environment to which similar cells are exposed in vivo (Reeds 1991). In addition, cells from different types of animals appear to perform divergently in cell culture, some types of cells require specialized media requirements in order to grow in vitro, and contamination of cultures by bacteria is a constant possibility (Figure 4.2). These challenges suggest that cell culture data need to be scrutinized carefully before being applied to an in vivo model.

In spite of the above limitations, cell culture methods are used extensively for other types of studies. Cell culture technology is quite well received when it is used for defining specific aspects of cell development (Dodson and Schaeffer 2000). For example, cell culture systems have provided a plethora of important basic data on specific mechanisms involved in cellular proliferation and differentiation. Further, it has been primarily through the use of cell culture systems that animal biologists

have defined numerous intrinsic and extrinsic factors involved in making cells alter their physiological status, as well as the specific binding dynamics of important growth factors to cells.

In Vivo Versus In Vitro Environment

Can an animal biologist formulate an in vitro environment that is similar to that in which the cells would be exposed in vivo? Consider the tremendous number of soluble factors impinging upon a normal cell at any given time in vivo, as well as the highly organized manner in which these cells are physically aligned and tied to one another by elements of the basement membrane and extra cellular matrix. It would be impossible to replicate this environment in a cell culture system, let alone replicate the changing environment to which a proliferating or differentiating cell is exposed in vivo. However, to a limited degree this is what has been tried, and in some instances, tried successfully (Dodson et al. 1996; Zimmerman et al. 2000). Over the course of the past twenty years, numerous defined cell culture

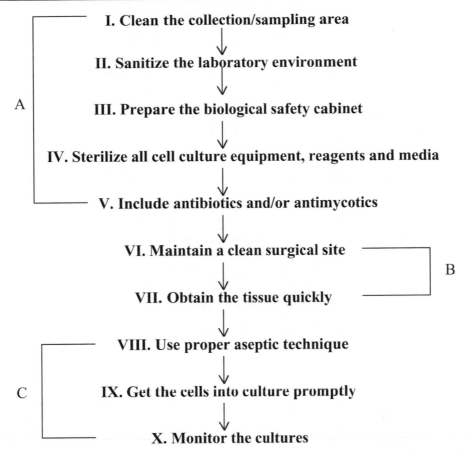

Figure 4.2. Ten commandments for preventing contamination of primary cell cultures. A. Steps involved prior to surgery/tissue collection. B. Steps involved in collection of tissue from the animal and transportation to the laboratory. C. Steps involved in obtaining the cells from the tissue and placing them into culture. (Reprinted with permission from *Methods in Cell Science* 22:33–41, 2000.)

systems have been reported for a number of different cell types (Dodson et al. 1996; Burton et al. 2000; Zimmerman et al. 2000). Common elements of all of these defined systems include the following:

- Some form of substratum coating of the plastic dish in order to mimic basement membrane adhesion
- A defined treatment medium with known vitamins, minerals, and growth factors to keep the cells in a desired physiological state (proliferative or differentiative for example Figure 4.3)
- Cells of known origin that may or may not be homogeneous in their developmental stage (Adams 1980; Dodson et al. 1990, 1996; Burton et al. 2000)

Types of In Vitro Studies

There are at least four types of studies in which cell culture systems have proven to be a powerful tool: developmental studies, mechanistic studies, assays, and the use of cells as a source for other cellular components. A good example of the use of cell cultures for a developmental study is deciphering the regulation of myogenesis in muscle cell development. Myogenesis may be defined as the proliferation, differentiation, fusion, and maturation of muscle cells to form a contractile, competent myofiber. Using muscle cell cultures, one can study any or all compartment(s) in the myogenesis scheme. An example of a mechanistic study is the use of muscle cell cultures to define the specific mechanisms involved when a

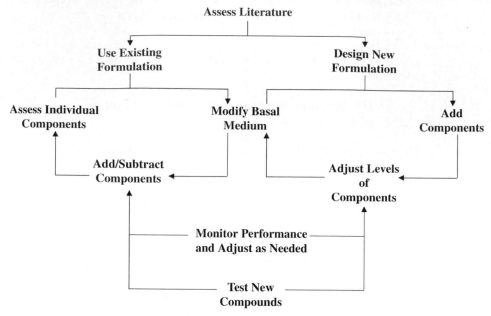

Figure 4.3. Flow chart illustrating pathways for devising a new defined medium or adapting an existing medium to suit one's intended culture system. (Reprinted with permission from *Methods in Cell Science* 22:43–49, 2000.)

growth factor binds to a cellular receptor, and then when the growth factor:receptor complex signals the cells to change physiological compartments. Cell cultures may also be used for assay systems. It is common for muscle cell cultures to be used to assess the relative potency of serum derived from a treated animal when compared to serum from an untreated animal. An example of this would be the investigation of how a specific feeding regimen, genetic pattern, and/or steroid treatment alters the blood composition (Dodson et al. 1996). Cell cultures are also commonly used as a source for cellular components. For example, specific cell types may display high levels of hormone receptors. In order to determine the physical binding of the hormone to the receptor, the cells might be grown to high numbers and then processed to isolate the receptors for subsequent binding studies (Dodson et al. 1987; Mathison et al. 1989). As an example of the isolation of another component, muscle cells are commonly stripped of their myofibrils in order to subsequently isolate myofibrillar proteins for use in biochemical or other types of studies.

Common Cell Culture Systems

Major tissues of interest in studying meat animal growth are muscle, bone, and fat. Cell culture systems have been developed for all these cell types, as well as for numerous other cells from other tissues (Adams 1980; Freshney 1986; Vierck et al. 1996; Komaki et al. 1996; Neville et al. 1998; Gannon and Bader 1998; Pauly et al. 1998; Kubo et al. 2000; Rosen and Spiegelman 2000). Most cell cultures start out with cells derived directly from the tissue. These cultures usually possess a mixture of cell types and are called primary cell cultures (Dodson 2000; McFarland 2000). Each time that cells are removed from the dish and replated, the resultant culture is termed secondary, tertiary, etc. (Freshney 1994). Primary cell cultures have proven to be somewhat successful for increasing knowledge about how specific tissues of animals grow. However, in some instances, it is important to use homogeneous cultures of cells (McFarland 2000). In this case, cells of one type are isolated from other cells of the culture, allowed to proliferate, and then are used in either treatment or propagation cultures.

Cells that are derived from one maternal cell are called clones (McFarland 2000). Clones displaying differences in physiological activity are termed cell strains (Vierck et al. 1995). Clones and strains of cells are useful in a number of studies investigating developmental processes.

Recently, there has been a move to utilize co-cultures of two divergent cell types in order to define mechanisms of intercellular communication (Dodson et al. 1997; Hossner et al. 1997). This in vitro system might be used as a model for muscle and fat communication, as in the case of marbling production (Dodson et al. 1997).

Assessment of Cell Culture Physiology

Because of the importance of muscle in animal growth regimens, the following discussion focuses on current systems that utilize muscle cell cultures. Proliferating muscle cells in culture may be enumerated by methods as simple as manually counting the cells in a hemocytometer or using dyes to determine the amount of DNA in a cell culture, or as complex as labeling cells with an isotope and counting incorporated isotopes as a measure of cell number (Adams 1980; Freshney 1994; Stewart et al. 2000; Table 4.1). Recently, a method was devised to determine cell number while the cells resided in the plate (Byrne et al. 1998). This procedure involved exposing the cultured cells to a dye and using a micro-plate reader to quantify the amount of stain assimilated by the cells. This method has proven successful for counting proliferating myogenic cells (Byrne et al. 1998), but differentiated cell cultures have been more difficult to evaluate (Stewart et al. 2000). Time-consuming counting techniques have been utilized to determine the differentiation state of a muscle cell culture. However, digital cameras married to an inverted microscope and coupled with appropriate software packages are now being employed to allow more automated counting of differentiated cultures.

Other methods are available for determining differentiation in cell culture (Stewart et al. 2000). Examples of these include immunocytochemistry and enzyme-linked immunoculture assay (ELICA) (Stewart et al. 2000, 2001). Immunocytochemistry involves exposing cells to an antibody against a specific protein, and then subsequently reacting the antibody:protein complex with a secondary antibody tagged with a fluorescent dye. Quantitation of the level of protein expression is done either through microscopy or by image analysis. ELICA entails reacting cells with antibodies directed against specific proteins, solubilizing the protein:antibody complex, and performing the colorization and analysis steps in a different vessel or micro-plate (Figure 4.4; Stewart et al. 2000, 2001). Another method, fluorescence activated cell sorting (FACS), is available to quantitate cell compartmentalization within the cell cycle and may differentiate cells from one another (Byrne 2000). With the addition of a sorter unit, a FACS machine may physically sort cells into homologous populations for subsequent use in cell culture or in a number of biochemical/molecular applications (Blanton et al. 2000).

BIOCHEMICAL METHODS

Physiological samples derived from animals, tissue cultures, or cell cultures may be analyzed by a number of biochemical methods (Adams 1980; Mir et al. 2000). In some cases the sample may need to be processed prior to analysis. This processing might involve the removal of connective tissue from lean meat samples prior to harvesting the cells for cell culture, allowing whole blood to clot and centrifuging it before use, or any other means in order to get the sample primed for analysis. Although a number of biochemical methods may be used to analyze physiological samples, the following represent some of the most commonly used in the field of animal growth.

Radioimmunoassays (RIA) and Radioreceptor Assays (RRA)

Rosalyn S. Yalow was awarded the 1977 Nobel Prize in physiology or medicine for devising a radioimmunoassay (RIA) for peptide hormones (Yalow 1977). Widely used by animal scientists from the 1960s to the present, RIA helped shape our current understanding of hormone patterns in both animals and plants (Goldsmith 1975; Burrin et al. 1987; Hedden 1993; Krum 1994). A typical RIA utilizes the direct competition between a radiolabeled antigen, an unlabeled antigen in the test sample and a specific antibody. Binding of the radiolabeled antigen to the antibody is in direct competition with the unlabeled antigen. Consequently, the amount of bound radiolabeled antigen is inversely proportional to the amount of unlabeled antigen. For example, if a large amount of radiolabeled antigen binds to the antibody, the implication is that there is only a small amount of unlabeled antigen in the test sample. By quantifying the amount of radiolabel present in the assay tubes, one may determine the specific amount of unknown in the test sample to a sensitivity of (in some cases) 10^{-15} moles of protein (Krumm 1994). In addition to protein hormones, radioimmunoassays have been developed for steroid hormones, dipeptides such as thyroid hormone, and numerous other growth factors and growth factor binding proteins (Yalow 1977; Goldsmith 1975; Burrin et al. 1987; Hedden 1993; Krum 1994).

Table 4.1. Summary of techniques used for analysis of cells

Category	Name of Technique (Application)	Equipment Required	Functional Limits	Advantages/Drawbacks
Manual Assays	Hemocytometer (cell suspensions)	Microscope, Hemocytometer	$<10^4$, $>10^7$ cells/ml	Inexpensive/Labor intensive Cells must be in suspension
	Phase Contrast Microscopy (living adherent cells)	Phase Contrast Microscope	>200 cells/HPF	Visualize living cell structure/ Labor intensive, inaccurate
	Cell Staining (fixed adherent cells)	Light Microscope	>200 cells/HPF	Enhanced visualization/ Labor intensive
	Ab/Enzyme/Precipitating Substrate (fixed adherent cells)	Light Microscope	>200 cells/HPF	Visualization of Marker/ Labor intensive
	Immunofluorescent Assay (IFA) (fixed adherent cells)	Fluorescent/Confocal Microscope	>300 cells/HPF (3-D = increased #)	Colocalization, high detail, 3-D/ Expensive instrument
Automated Assays	Stained Optical Density (fixed adherent cells)	Densitometric 96 Well Plate Reader	$<10^3$, $>10^4$ cells/well	Rapid, simple/Lower accuracy, reliability
	New Methylene Blue (fixed adherent cells)	Spectrophotometric 96 Well Plate Reader	$<10^3$, $>10^4$ cells/well	Rapid, reliable/Only for cell proliferation
	Creatine Kinase (fixed adherent cells)	Spectrophotometric 96 Well Plate Reader	$<10^3$, $>10^4$ cells/well	Rapid, reliable/Only for myogenic cell differentiation
	DNA Quantification (fixed adherent cells)	Fluorometric 96 Well Plate Reader	$<10^3$, $>10^4$ cells/well	Rapid, reliable/Only for DNA, dividing cells alter results
	Electronic Cell Counting (living cells in suspension)	Electronic Cell Counter (Coulter counter)	$<10^3$, $>10^7$ total cells	Rapid, reliable, counting and sizing/Cells must be in suspension
	Flow Cytometry (living cells in suspension)	Flow Cytometer (FACS)	$<10^3$, $>10^7$ total cells	Rapid, reliable, counting, precision separation of marked cells/expensive instrument
	Magnetic Cell Sorting (living cells in suspension)	Electromagnetic Cell Sorting Chamber	$<10^2$, $>10^8$ total cells	Reliable counting and separation of marked cells/ Cells must be in suspension

Method	Equipment	Sensitivity	Advantages/Disadvantages
Image Analysis (fixed adherent cells)	CCD Camera or Scanner	$<1, >50$ cells/mm^2	Improved image quality, analysis capabilities/Expensive equipment
Chemiluminescence (fixed adherent cells)	+/- SDS-PAGE/Western Blot Apparatus	$\sim 1, >10^4$ cells/well	High sensitivity/Complex procedure
Radioisotope Labeling (fixed adherent cells)	Radioactivity Shields, Dedicated Hood, Geiger Counter	$<10^3, >10^4$ cells/well	High sensitivity/Dangerous reagents
Precursor Incorporation (living/fixed adherent cells)	Radioactivity Shields, Dedicated, Hood, Geiger Counter	$<10^3, >10^4$ cells/well	High sensitivity/Dangerous reagents
In Situ Hybridization/Ligand Binding (fixed adherent cells)	Radioactivity Shields, Dedicated Hood, Geiger Counter mRNA	$<10^2, >10^4$ cells/well	High sensitivity, ability to detect specific markers/Dangerous reagents
Enzyme-Linked Immuno-Culture Assay (fixed adherent cells)	Spectrophotometric 96 Well Plate Reader	$<10^2, >10^4$ cells/well	High sensitivity, rapidity, reliability, cells intact/New technique

Reprinted with permission from *Methods in Cell Science* 22:67–78, 2000.

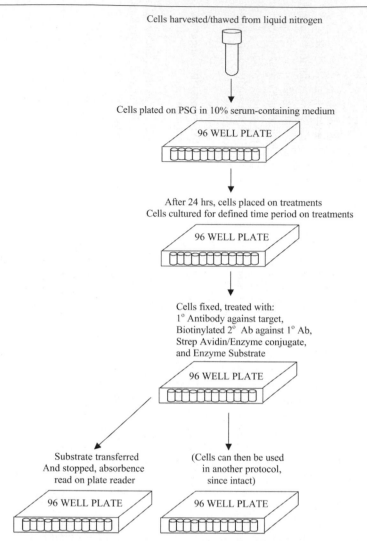

Cells harvested/thawed from liquid nitrogen

Cells plated on PSG in 10% serum-containing medium

96 WELL PLATE

After 24 hrs, cells placed on treatments
Cells cultured for defined time period on treatments

96 WELL PLATE

Cells fixed, treated with:
1° Antibody against target,
Biotinylated 2° Ab against 1° Ab,
Strep Avidin/Enzyme conjugate,
and Enzyme Substrate

96 WELL PLATE

Substrate transferred
And stopped, absorbence
read on plate reader

(Cells can then be used
in another protocol,
since intact)

96 WELL PLATE   96 WELL PLATE

Figure 4.4. Flow diagram of the ELICA protocol. A. Cells are harvested for primary cultures, or thawed from liquid nitrogen for clonal or cell line cultures, plated into a 96-well cell culture plate coated with a PSG substratum, and supplied with a 10% serum-containing medium for the first 24 hours. B. Cultures are then placed on treatments, and grown for the length of time that has been set in the experimental design. C. Cultures are next fixed in methanol and treated with the primary antibody to the marker of interest, the biotinylated secondary antibody specific for the species or subtype of the primary antibody, and the avidin conjugated enzyme. Blocking agents are used to prevent nonspecific binding, and extensive washing steps remove any unbound reagents. The enzyme substrate is then incubated in the wells, which contain the labeled cells. D. Next, the enzyme substrate is transferred to a second 96-well plate, which contains the pre-measured stop solution to stop the reaction. The absorbence of the stopped substrate in this plate is read using the spectrophotometric plate reader set at the correct wavelength for the reaction. The original cell culture plate still contains the adherent cells, which can be further analyzed using other protocols, including morphological and marker localization, since the cellular structure remains intact. (Reprinted with permission from *Methods in Cell Science* 22:67–78, 2000.)

RRA are similar to RIA, except that either cells or a known amount of receptors are used instead of blood or other test samples. A radiolabeled hormone (or growth factor) of interest and a known amount of highly purified hormone standard are added to the cell culture plate or tube containing the isolated receptor fraction (Dodson et al. 1987). Following a specified incubation time, the hormone:receptor complexes are chemically bonded through the use of a crosslinking agent, which prevents the release of the bound molecules. The amount of radionuclide activity in the binding assay can then be determined by counting the pelleted fraction in a gamma, or scintillation, counter. Like RIA, the amount of radiolabel bound to the cells/receptors is inversely proportional to the amount of binding sites. From RRA experiments, the total receptor numbers and the affinity of receptor association/disassociation can be calculated through the use of Scatchard analysis (Dodson et al. 1987).

Polyacrylamide Gel Electrophoresis (PAGE)

PAGE is another biochemical method that is commonly used for analyzing biological samples, especially in protein quantification and purification (see sidebar, page 36). PAGE refers to the placement of purified or partially purified protein solutions onto a bed of acrylamide resin; subjecting the protein to an electrical field, which allows the protein to migrate through the resin; staining the resin; and analyzing the pattern of protein migration. Although commonly used as a step in protein purification, this method is also definitive in the molecular weight determination of proteins. A slightly different form of PAGE called SDS-PAGE utilizes the principle of adding negatively charged moieties to proteins that have been reduced to their basic units and has been used extensively in animal growth research. After proteins are resolved by PAGE or SDS-PAGE, they may be isolated from the gels for biochemical analyses or further characterized by methods such as Western immunoblotting, Western ligand blotting, or dot immunoblotting (Krabbenhoft et al. 1997; Vierck et al. 2001).

Blotting Methods

Western immunoblot methods share several steps in common with other types of blotting techniques (Krabbenhoft et al. 1997). Proteins are separated through the use of PAGE or SDS-PAGE gel systems and then are physically transferred to a blotting membrane, such as a cellulose membrane. After the protein is transferred, the membrane is first exposed to primary antibodies against the protein of interest, then to secondary antibodies directed against the first antibody, and (finally) a colorizing substrate, which enables visualization of the protein bands (Krabbenhoft et al. 1997). System factors like the gel matrix, blotting membrane type, and color developer characteristics may be manipulated in order to obtain the desired sensitivity and resolution (Krabbenhoft et al. 1997).

Western ligand blots are slightly different from Western immunoblots. In Western ligand blotting, a radioactive ligand is employed to identify specific interactions between, for example, hormones and receptors or binding proteins. In this procedure, a radiolabeled hormone might be incubated with a cellular preparation or a purified preparation of cell-derived receptors. Following incubation, the radiolabeled hormone is physically bound to the hormone receptor through the use of numerous commercially available crosslinking agents. The hormone:receptor complex is separated from other components by PAGE or SDS-PAGE, and then the dried gel is exposed to x-ray film. After an incubation period, the x-ray film is developed, and an autoradiogram is produced, with which one may analyze band presence or intensity. Through the use of potential inhibitors of hormone binding, one can perform the initial binding steps and determine if specific factors aid, or inhibit, binding of the radiolabeled hormone to its cellular receptor.

Dot blotting refers to the placement of a small amount of protein directly on to a Western blot membrane, usually with the aid of a vacuum suction device like a blotting manifold hooked to an aspirator. Because the protein is already incorporated on the blotting membrane, there is no need to run a PAGE or SDS-PAGE gel first. Consequently, the blotting membrane can be exposed immediately to the primary antibody, secondary antibody, and colorizing substrate regimen (Krabbenhoft et al. 1997). After they have been optimized, all three blotting methods are easily performed and quite repeatable.

GENOMICS, PROTEOMICS, AND BIOINFORMATICS

The scientific research areas of genomics, proteomics, and bioinformatics promise to revolutionize our understanding of—and our ability to manipulate–biological entities. These are very active research

POLYACRYLAMIDE GEL ELECTROPHORESIS (PAGE)

PAGE has proved to be a powerful method used as a component during a protein purification regimen or when characterizing purified proteins. The procedure involves placing a protein into an electric field. Due to the charged nature of the protein, it will migrate toward the electrode of the opposite sign at a rate determined by interactions of the protein with the surrounding gel matrix (Garfin 1990). Therefore, proteins separate from one another due to sizes, shapes, and net charges of each protein (Hames and Rickwood 1981; Garfin 1990). In order to obtain optimum resolution of protein bands, especially when attempting to separate numerous proteins from within one cocktail\sample, it is important to load the PAGE gel with the correct amount of protein. As such, it is important to perform some sort of a protein assay prior to conduct of PAGE (Figure A). Setup of PAGE equipment is relatively simple (Figure B), as is preparing the gel (Figure C). When actually running the gel, a critical eye should be focused on the rate of migra-

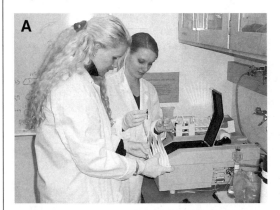

tion of proteins through the gel matrix (Figure D). Proteins migrating too fast or slow will result in distortion of the final banding pattern (Hames and Rickwood 1981; Andrews 1987; Garfin 1990).

When protein migration has reached the limits of the gel, the gel is stained through a variety of dyes including silver stain as one option (Patel et al. 1988), destained, dried, and evaluated. Protein migration relative to one another, as well as to standard preparations, may then be quantitated (Figure E). Prior to staining, the gel may be used for Western blotting.

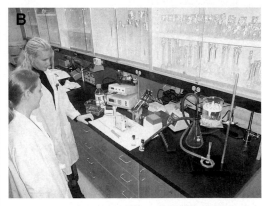

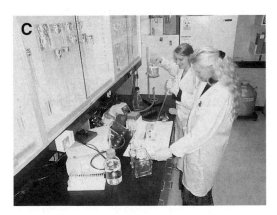

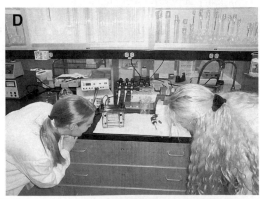

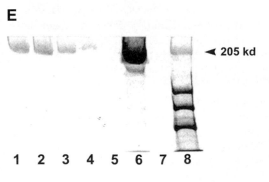

◀ 205 kd

1   2   3   4   5   6   7   8

areas, as illustrated by the fact that there are dozens of research journals where scientists might publish such information. These three research areas are closely related, differing only in the degree or level of scrutiny. For this chapter, however, we discuss each topic as a distinct line of study.

Genomics

Genomics is the field of study devoted to identifying genes and determining gene sequences. This area also includes the elucidation of gene functon (Kannan et al. 2001), the relationship of genes to disease, and an understanding of gene regulation. Genomics attempts to accomplish several goals including

1. Creation of genetic and physical maps of the chromosomes of an organism (Bihoreau et al. 2001; Soejima et al. 2001) or animal
2. Identification of sets of genes and their precise mapping to areas of chromosomes
3. Identification of genes in DNA sequences
4. Determination of the entire DNA base sequence that comprises the organism's genome
5. Analysis of genetic variation between animal species
6. Comparison of sequence information with other organisms or animals
7. Development of appropriate laboratory and computing technologies to facilitate analysis and understanding of gene function and structure
8. Dissemination of such information among scientists, clinicians, and the public
9. Discussion of the legal, ethical, and social issues that such information creates

To fully appreciate the difficulties and the creative aspects of working with genes (Boyer 1971; Wainwright 1993) it is necessary to define a number of basic terms and protocols (Calza et al. 1987; Eschenlauer et al. 1998; McEwan et al. 2000a, 2000b). Genetic engineering is the use of chemical and physical "tricks of the trade" to manipulate segments of nucleic acids (usually DNA) in an effort to improve or understand gene function. In the manipulation of genes, there are several useful or essential tools. By far the most important components relate to the ability to precisely cut the DNA, stick it back together onto a movable object, and make it express the genes it possesses (Dahm et al. 2001; Ishisaki et al. 2001).

Packaging DNA Clones into Vectors

Vehicles (or vectors) are molecular shuttles or buses that provide a way to duplicate the DNA, allow passage to cloning hosts, and afford gene regulation (turned on or off) on demand (Perbal 1988). This procedure, or slight alteration thereof (e.g., cosmids), provides a very powerful cloning vector based on the genome of a bacterial virus called lambda bacteriophage (gt 11 phage). The gt 11 system of cloning genes is very useful because the bacteriophage possesses a high efficiency of bacterial infection and because the assembly of virulent particles can occur in the test tube. Insertion of the cloned DNA fragment into the phage causes inactivation of a gene that otherwise colors the plaque blue. Therefore, the white or clear plaques contain potentially useful gene fragments. The gt 11 cloning vehicle, as well as most others, contains a multicloning site (MCS), which is the site or position within cloning vectors where the foreign DNA can be inserted. The MCS region contains numerous (up to 30) different restriction endonuclease sites (Figure 4.5). The phage vehicle also contains an origin of replication area to cause the replication of the DNA fragments.

To specifically utilize the gt 11 system, scientists place the gene of interest into naked virus DNA, allow the formation of the virus (wrapping in protein) and add it to the cloning host (cell). The virus acts like a molecular syringe or needle and pushes its DNA into the cell. Cellular protein synthesizing components use the virus DNA to make more viruses. When the host is to be screened for the clones of interest, the cells are lysed and gene detection methods are applied. Ordinarily the virus would kill the cell, but gt 11 is rendered harmless. The vector simply serves as a molecular syringe to get foreign DNA into a cell (Elis 1987).

Genomic Library

A genomic library is a collection of clones typically made from a set of randomly generated and overlapping DNA fragments that represent the entire genome of the organism (Blattner and Shao 1997; Fraser and Venter 1998; Adams and Venter 2000; *Arabidopsis* Genome Initiative 2000; Mouchel et al. 2001; Mullikin and Bentley 2000; Wines et al. 2001) or animal. Alternatively, a gene library is a collection of genes cloned in a certain vehicle or host. Similar to books on a shelf, the gene library contains numerous volumes possessing different information. A gene or

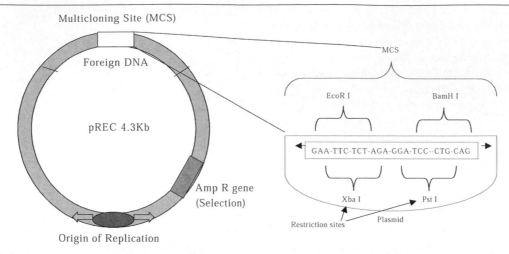

Figure 4.5. Plasmid cloning vector. Shown here is a small (4.3 Kb) plasmid cloning vector containing the origin of replication, selectable antibiotic gene, and multicloning site. Also depicted are sequences of the MCS that list the restriction endonuclease cleavage locations.

clone bank is a physical storage location where embryos, stem cells, genes, or DNA fragments are kept for reference, research, or therapeutic use (see sidebar, page 39).

Sequencing DNA

Sequencing DNA is the determination of the order and identity of the base pairs in DNA. Regardless of the procedure used, numerous sequencing reactions, each starting from a different reference point on the DNA, must be performed to gain reliable sequence information. This overlap of necessity forces the scientist to carry out dozens of reactions to determine the sequence of each DNA fragment (Sanger and Coulson 1975; Howe and Ward 1989). It is necessary to sequence more than a thousand bases to gain reliable sequence information about 100 or 200 bases. Fully equipped laboratories can sequence several thousand bases per week. Several biotechnology companies also provide a sequencing service and at present charge about US$1-2 per base. Such automated systems are said to handle several thousand bases per hour or day. Most systems rely on the use of high performance liquid chromatography (HPLC) to determine the molecular weights of the DNA fragments. Such analyses can be accomplished in a continuous manner.

After a gene library of interest has been prepared, the work of analysis and sequencing can begin.

Many advanced chemical and enzyme-based methods exist to unambiguously order the bases within the gene sequence. The most common and useful method resembles the Sanger dideoxy method. The Sanger method utilizes interruption DNA synthesis to sequence DNA (Figure 4.6). The procedure involves the use of primer/template DNA, polymerase, and a small percentage of dideoxy nucleotide bases to cause the partial synthesis of the region of DNA to be sequenced. The dideoxy analogs of bases are not normal, in that they do not allow the phosphodiester backbone bonds of DNA to be formed. These partial sequences represent the interruption attempts caused by the dideoxy base placed here and there (but opposite the complementary base) within the DNA. PAGE is used to determine the molecular weight of the partial fragments, and the size is correlated with the reaction mixture. If a mixture (one different mixture for each of the bases) has the ddT (dideoxy thymine), the synthesis can occur normally only up to and including that base. The gel tells where interruptions occur and pinpoints where an A is in the sequence. One simply reads up the ladder of the gel. This process is repeated, and a single gel (and lane of gel) can provide the location of hundreds of adenines, cytosines, guanines, or thymines. To successfully utilize this method, one must couple a determination of a single-strand length of DNA with the interrupted

---

WHAT IT MIGHT INVOLVE TO CONSTRUCT AN ANIMAL GENOME IN A CONSTRUCT LIBRARY

Estimates of the number of clones necessary to contain all the genetic information of an organism or animal can be calculated using a simple formula. Let's say that one wants to place all the sequence information from an animal containing approximately 3 million kilobases of DNA into a vehicle that can receive 40 kilobases (such as the gt 11 phage). In order to do so, one would first begin by performing the following calculation:

Divide 1 minus the logarithm of the desired likeliness (for example, 99%) by 1 minus the logarithm of insert size divided by total genome size.

The scientist, then, must obtain (and sequence) more than 300,000 genes to represent the entire animal genome in this library (Fossey et al. 2001). That is many fewer than the total size of the human genome in kilobases; but it nevertheless remains a formidable job, will take up to 20 years if more than a dozen laboratories cooperate, and will likely cost several billion dollars to perform.

---

synthesis of the DNA helix. From a single sequencing gel, thousands of bases can be ordered on a sequence of DNA.

Most scientists now rely on the use of automated sequencing protocols. By analyzing a nested array of fragments each containing a different fluorescent label on the 3' terminating base, it is possible to perform laser-based scanning as the fragment passes through a detector. The color order of the migrating bands is simultaneously translated into sequence data by a computer (Doolittle 1991; Forcellino and Derreumaux 2001).

Polymerase Chain Reaction (PCR)

PCR synthesis shares certain methodological aspects of other cloning methods, such as synthesis of DNA and the use of polymerases, but accomplishes very different results (Mullis and Faloona 1987; Innis et al. 1990; Burden and Whitney 1995). The starting template material in the PCR reaction is a primed (partially double-stranded) fragment of DNA. The result of the PCR reaction is millions of complementary, double-stranded, partial-length DNA fragments (Figure 4.7).

To drive the PCR reaction, it is necessary to use a heat stable enzyme in a cyclic incubation of high and low temperatures. *Thermus aquaticus* is the species of bacteria from which the Taq I enzyme is usually isolated. The Taq I enzyme allows the denaturation step to be done repeatedly without

inactivation of the enzyme. The repeated primer renaturation to the template DNA (at low temperature), the procession DNA synthesis done by the Taq I enzyme (at moderate temperature), and the denaturation of the double-stranded DNA (at high temperature) cause the amplification. A thermocycler is the incubator used for the reaction. This device is little more than a heater or incubator that can be programmed to change the temperature and time of incubation. The low, moderate, and high temperature settings are repeated dozens of times before the reaction of amplification is considered complete. Some thermocyclers will simultaneously mix or shake the samples.

cDNA Synthesis

The making of complementary DNA involves the synthesis of DNA by a precise pairing of bases with a messenger RNA (Figure 4.8). This procedure is perhaps the most powerful cloning approach used by scientists today. Cells transmit (or pass on) the information for the making of proteins from their DNA through an intermediate called RNA. The type of RNA called messenger RNA (or mRNA) actually contains the precise instruction for the cell to make enzymes or proteins. The cell must first manipulate the mRNA before sending it to the protein synthesis factory (e.g., ribosomes), but nevertheless, within mRNA are the ordering directions for amino acid placement into the polypeptide.

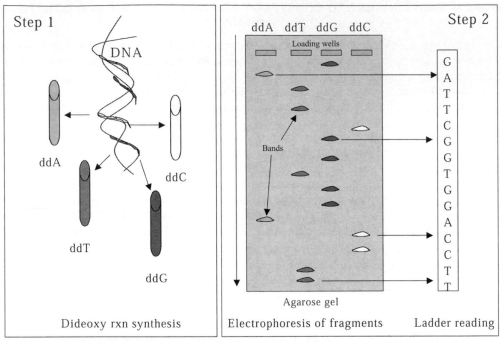

Figure 4.6. DNA sequencing method. The panel to the left shows the four reaction tubes containing sequences of interest and dideoxy nucleotide bases. The panel to the right shows the banding results after DNA sequencing gel separations. The "ladder" of sequence is read from the bottom of the gel, and each band differs by one base in length.

Unfortunately, mRNA is unstable in the hands of most scientists, and so conversion to a more stable cDNA allows cloning of most genes. The conversion process makes use of nearly a dozen cloning enzymes, such as ligase, reverse transcriptase, and ribonuclease. Ligase, for example, is the enzyme used to join cut ends of DNA. This enzyme is the molecular glue that forms the contiguous backbone of the DNA fragments. The overall process copies the ordering of the mRNA and builds a very similar molecule, but using DNA bases. These bases utilize the sugar deoxyribose instead of ribose (it has one more oxygen), and there are several slight chemical changes within the nitrogenous component in the building block. The cDNA, like all DNA molecules, is double-stranded (double tape) making it distinct from the ordinarily single-stranded structure of RNA. This cDNA structure, therefore, contains all the protein-making information that the mRNA possessed, but because it is now a type or form of DNA, it is stable and very useful for cloning.

Differential Hybridization (DH)

Hybridization yields a comparison of base sequences by measuring the success of pairing between nucleic acid polymers. This is a very useful tool to sort for the presence of a particular sequence of DNA or RNA (Ausubel et al. 1992). The procedure involves attempting to bind complementary nucleic acids and takes advantage of the natural tendency of complementary DNA strands to associate together. The cell requires different species of mRNA at different times of metabolism. Using the correct probes, one can gain a measure of which mRNA is present by their ability to stick to the probe (which is generally fixed onto a filter). The procedure is broadly called autoradiography, if scientists utilize radioactive probes to locate (and bind to) the nucleic acid fragments (Figure 4.9). For instance, one would expect the mRNA for the enzyme cellulase to be present in a cell only when cellulose is being utilized as a carbon source. One

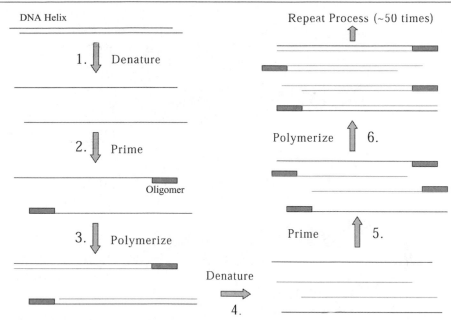

Figure 4.7. Polymerase chain reaction. Steps 1 through 3 represent a single cycle of replication of the target DNA. Each successful replication (doubling of DNA) must involve association of the primer with the DNA, polymerization of the complementary sequence by Taq I, and the denaturation of the completed double-stranded DNA in preparation for the next round of priming, etc.

may test for its presence and approximate concentrations by probing with the gene for cellulase. This procedure therefore determines relatedness of two populations of nucleic acids. Two preparations of cDNA libraries made to such mRNA may be used to distinguish concentration differences. A dot blot is a convenient protocol for determining relatedness of two sequences of nucleic acids. Application of DNA or RNA onto a filter or other solid matrix is done in such a way as to allow hundreds of different samples to be selected or compared. A dot blot is simply a DNA or RNA hybridization reaction.

DNA Microarray

A DNA microarray is a tool that combines the microprocessing of computer chip (microchip) manufacturing with the chemical methods of DNA sequencing and complementary base pairing of helixes (Taniguchi et al. 2001). The microarray is little more than a tiny piece of plastic support matrix that can bind thousands of different sequences of DNA within precise and distinct locations (Figure 4.10). The preparation of the microarray involves the placement on, or printing of, regions of the support matrix with tiny droplets containing different fragments of DNA. Each exact spot on the array can then represent a distinct allele or gene and provide information as to its activity (or expression) within a cell. To use the array, the scientist labels the DNA sample of interest with fluorescent chemicals, heats it to separate (denature) the two strands of DNA, bathes the chip in this material to allow complementary binding, gently rinses the chip, and finally views the chip using a fluorescence-detecting microscope. A computer compares the areas of high fluorescence with the known positions and identities of the DNA array checkerboard. This checkerboard pattern of microscopic blocks of DNA might, in fact, represent all the genes expressed in a particular cell or throughout an organism. In theory, it will soon be possible to place a person's entire gene complement onto a piece of plastic less than one inch square, providing a precise and unambiguous description of each human (or animal) on the planet (sidebar, page 44).

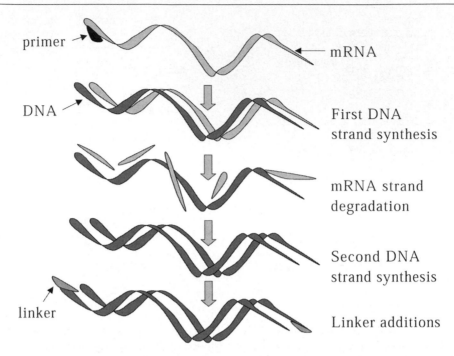

Figure 4.8. Complementary DNA synthesis. Shown are the events leading to the conversion of a single-stranded molecule of RNA into a double-stranded DNA molecule. At the top of this figure is the starting mRNA. The enzymatic reactions include "reverse transcriptase" synthesis of a single strand of DNA complementary to the mRNA, degradation of the original mRNA, second DNA strand synthesis by a polymerase, and finally addition of cloning linkers using ligase.

Blots

Northern blots involve the attachment of RNA molecules onto a solid support, such as a nitrocellulose filter, and subsequently hybridizing the filter with radioactive DNA or other RNA. This is a very useful procedure for the determination of messenger RNA (mRNA) copy number or abundance. Scientists can use this procedure to determine if a gene is transcriptionally active. Southern blotting is a filter-binding method used to screen or select for gene clones (Southern 1975). The method is named after the scientist who first used the method to secure fragments of DNA onto an insoluble matrix, while nevertheless allowing the hybridization reaction to occur. This method allows for the detection of a gene sequence even if it is only one sequence in a billion. It is also possible to locate a bacterial colony containing the gene of interest by probing with a few radioactive base pairs of a related, but not identical, gene from other organisms.

Gene Therapy

Gene therapy attempts to replace a defective or faulty gene with a normal one. Efforts are underway to determine the entire DNA sequence of several higher animals.

Such information combined with methods for isolating individual genes likely will allow clinicians, in the near future, to correct genetic defects in humans, animals, and plants (Collins 1992; Koller and Smithies 1992; Harris and Lemoine 1996). The human genome project (HGP) hopes to sequence the entire DNA complement and provide information about how gene therapy methods may benefit humans (Palladino 2002). The same type of concerted effort is also being exerted toward important domestic animals.

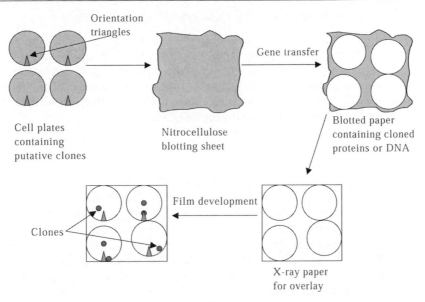

Figure 4.9. Autoradiography. Shown is the blotting and detection of gene sequences using a radioactive (or fluorescent) and complementary probe. The final development of the "signal" is typically done on standard x-ray photographic emulsion film. The original blot (or touch) may be of colonies on a growth plate, tissue culture piles, spots of various sequences of nucleic acids, etc.

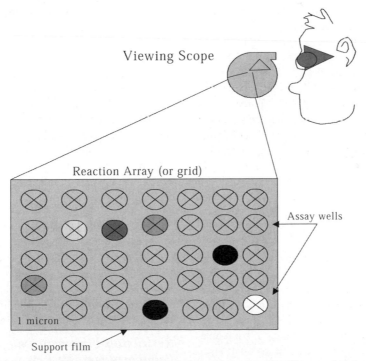

Figure 4.10. Microarray. The drawing shows observation of a tiny film containing a large number of organized spots where different nucleic acid sequences have been immobilized. The signal of detection is typically a hybridization probe, but antibodies may also be used.

REPETITIVE SEQUENCES—IMPORTANT OR JUNK?

Human DNA contains a large number of repetitive sequences, but it was not until scientists possessed the genetic map that they fully realized that the placement of the so-called junk DNA was apparently nonrandom and at an even predictable location throughout the chromosomes. Before the crude genetic map was reported, most researchers talked of discovering 100,000 genes on human chromosomes. It now seems clear that the number of functional genes in humans is less than one-half of that, and maybe only one-third.

In order to efficiently conduct gene therapy, at the very least it is necessary to clone the normal gene, develop vectors to introduce it into the afflicted patient, and cause the normal and timely functioning of the replacement gene. The smallpox virus, adenovirusm and HIV are examples of DNA cloning vectors that are potentially useful for gene replacements. Scientists believe that it may be possible to "add" the resistance to devastating animal diseases—such as hoof-and-mouth, scours, trypanosomiasis, and rabies—and to parasites, such as tapeworms and liver flukes.

Gene therapy is particularly difficult, because it is often necessary to place the normal gene within a precise control region near a specific gene on the proper chromosome within all the cells of the affected individual. It is sobering to be reminded that the adult human contains trillions of cells. The use of reporter genes has greatly assisted in the development of this methodology.

Many scientists are hopeful that stem cells will provide a means of replacing genes in humans. The strategy involves placing the normal gene into the appropriate stem cells of the affected individual, forcing (or allowing) those cells to mature or differentiate and carry with them the replacement gene. "Therapy" genes must be expressed within the appropriate tissues, at the proper stage of animal development, and be synthesized in the correct amounts to correct the genetic defect. The first successful experiment of gene replacement was performed in the early 1980s (Palmiter and Brinster 1985). In these experiments, rat growth hormone was expressed in mice, and the mouse growth could be controlled using dietary components. In these experiments, a small amount of zinc in the diet allowed the inserted gene control region (from metallothionein) to greatly increase the production of growth hormone. Since then, similar experiments have been attempted in several domestic animals. For example, rapidly growing fish have been produced by using the same technology (Devlin et al.

1994). Equipped with up-regulated Sockeye salmon growth hormone genes, Coho salmon can grow 11 times as rapidly as wild-type Coho.

Large animal breeding studies to measure production traits is a very time-consuming activity. A single pedigree analysis typically takes several years to complete, and a limited number of offspring are produced. To develop useful models to study genetic interactions, scientists have devised the strategy of targeted mutagenesis and gene replacement in mice (Figure 4.11).

Mus musculus (the common house mouse) lends itself to breeding studies because its fecundity is high and analogous genetic abnormalities can be induced. If a gene known to be a problem in animals is available in the mouse, it is possible to replace the normal mouse gene with a mutated gene. The gene switching process involves several steps of manipulation. The scientist must first clone the mouse gene thought to be responsible for the phenotype. A cloning vector containing a gene knockout function and selectable marker (usually conferring antibiotic resistance) must then be constructed. Collection of stem cells contained within mouse blastocysts and growth of these undifferentiated cells in cell culture is carried out. Transfection/transformation of those stem cells containing the cloned mutant gene is next accomplished, followed by placement of the recombined gene sequence into a recipient blastocyst. Surrogate mothers via mouse embryo transplantation must then be used, and finally, genetic crossing is performed to select for mutant mouse strains. The method essentially replaces the wild-type gene with the laboratory-constructed mutant gene. Animals containing the mutant gene should exhibit the characteristic phenotype of affected individuals.

Restriction Fragment Length Polymorphism (RFLP)

This procedure results in the comparison of DNA sequences (fragments) from one member of a species to the next. To measure fragment length dif-

Cloning and Stem Cell Culture   **Embryo Implantation and Breeding**

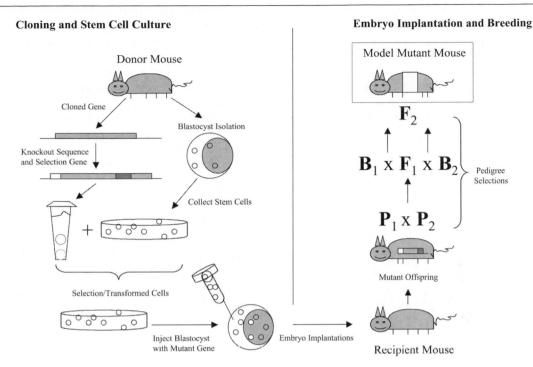

Figure 4.11. Mouse model for disease. Shown is a diagram representing the recovery of a gene of interest from one mouse, its cloning and inactivation, its placement into stem cells isolated from blastocysts, and the gene's eventual placement into a population of mice. Classical methods of crossing are used to select the mutated gene. The process therefore replaces the wild-type gene with a mutant gene. Mice containing such mutant genes are expected to be physiologically similar to higher animals.

ferences, a scientist isolates the organism's DNA, cuts it with nucleases (restriction enzymes), separates the fragments using polyacrylamide gel electrophoresis, and finally hybridizes the fragments to a gene probe.

Restriction endonucleases are the DNA cutting enzymes (or molecular knives). These enzymes are used because they are able to recognize a few orderly bases in the DNA sequence and break the sequence precisely at those points. Sticky ends are the terminal regions of a cloning vehicle or DNA fragment resulting from nuclease cutting. Sticky ends allow fragment base pairing and ligation. If the correct area of DNA sequence is chosen to compare, it will be possible to distinguish, by differences, one person or one animal from billions of others. This procedure is commonly used in forensic medicine to determine parental ownership or location at a crime scene. A few skin cells or cells from the base of a single hair follicle will provide enough DNA to compare individuals. The process of RFLP mapping

generally involves the use of DNA amplification using PCR methods (Feinberg and Vogelstein 1983). The random primer method of amplifying regions of DNA is also dependent on PCR methods. The primers used are, however, produced in the laboratory to resemble sequences likely used throughout the genome.

RAPD is the abbreviation for random amplified polymorphic DNA. This closely related procedure allows genome comparisons using only the most basic of cloning methods and primer synthesis. This method is also frequently used in laboratories doing forensic analysis, and the gel banding patterns of the amplified DNA provide the basis for comparison.

Clonal Screening

Screening is the scrutiny process for a gene library as one looks for a gene of interest. Screening for gene isolation typically amounts to playing the game of looking for the needle in the haystack. Most of the thousands of genes in a cell are present in only one or two copies each. To find the particular gene of interest, the scientist might probe the library with radioactive DNA or RNA from a matching gene. It may be helpful to probe using related sequences, or, if the gene is active, to use an activity assay. If the gene is synthesized but not active, the scientists might use antibodies against the protein of interest. It is possible to tag the antibody and follow antibody binding to the protein that serves as the antigen. It also may be helpful to isolate the mRNA and sort the mRNA population using differential hybridization, size fractionation, or immuno-purification exclusion before making the library. This can greatly enrich the sequences of interest and increase the probability of obtaining the needed clone.

Screening for, or determination of, gene location on chromosomes is done using painting and walking procedures. Chromosomal painting is a procedure that colors each chromosome or chromosome region with a different fluorescent probe. The DNA sequence probes used are selected because they hybridize to distinct regions of the chromosome arms. Chromosome walking is possible if adequate painting methods are available. This procedure involves the positioning of genes relative to others on a chromosome. Both procedures are dependent and based on reference DNA sequences on the chromosomes.

Site-Specific Mutagenesis

Mutagenesis is an intentional laboratory method used to cause precise changes in the DNA of cloned fragments or genes. The procedure is based on the use of the M13 bacterial phage cloning system that involves a virus capable of existing in both single- and double-stranded forms. Scientists ligate the gene of interest into the single M13 virus, place artificially synthesized and mutated single-stranded sequences into the plasmid, force *E. coli* to replicate the plasmid containing the mutated sequence, select for the replicative form of plasmid and test the mutated form for function. The mutated sequences provided are usually less than 30 bases in length and typically contain 1–3 altered bases. This many altered bases will not inhibit the necessary and temporary hydrogen bonding to form the double helix used by the cloning host to replicate a perfectly complementary copy of the mutated DNA.

Protein engineering refers to the manipulation of gene sequences to change the activity of enzymes encoded by these genes (Bastolla et al. 2001). When a gene of interest is cloned, it is possible to mutate the DNA sequence and test the effects of that mutation on enzyme activity. Considerable success has been achieved in modifying proteases. Many such proteases have been made more active, heat stable, and less site-specific by changing just one or two bases in the sequence. By performing such experiments, scientists gain valuable information about the positional importance of certain amino acids. Such information will be invaluable in the development of useful and unique biotechnological products.

High Performance Liquid Chromatography (HPLC)

Of the numerous methods devised to separate macromolecules, high performance liquid chromatography is best suited to high output (speed) DNA sequencing. The instrumentation includes multiple piston pumps, an in-line column containing a separation matrix (e.g., aliphatics attached to silica), a detection monitor (usually a light detection photomultiplier), and a computer to precisely control liquid flow rates (Figure 4.12).

Samples are injected into the elution liquid or buffers just before the column, and separated molecules (e.g.,, DNA fragments possessing different fluorescently labeled bases) are monitored using the detector as they elute from the column (Ausubel et al. 1992). Rapid and precise separation of DNA fragments can be achieved; because HPLC minimizes diffusion of macromolecules, only tiny amounts of sample (e.g., less than one millionth of a liter) are required for analysis, and separation matrices are available or can be synthesized that will specifically bind or separate the molecules.

Maxicell Procedure

In an effort to produce or synthesize adequate amounts of a cloned protein for in vitro study, scientists have devised ways of forcing the cloning host (e.g., *E. coli*) to specifically synthesize large amounts of the protein encoded by cloned genes. The method is dependent on the destruction of the host chromosome (the large circular DNA), the multiplication of the cloning plasmid containing the cloned gene of interest, specific selection for only those cloning hosts containing the gene of interest, and the stimulation of protein synthesis by the cell but using only the cloned DNA sequence for transcription (Figure 4.13).

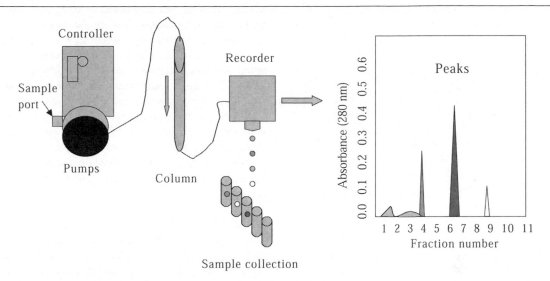

Figure 4.12. High performance liquid chromatography. Shown are the major components of the apparatus used for this type of chromatography. Sample collections can be accomplished simultaneously.

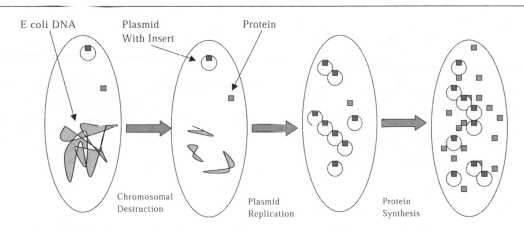

Figure 4.13. Maxicell production of proteins. Shown are the steps involved with the in vivo production of cloned genes in *E. coli*. Chromosomal destruction is mediated by enzymes in the cell after ultraviolet irradiation caused damage in the chromosome. Only cells containing cloning vectors endure the antibiotic selection, and protein synthesis is promoted using transcription promoters.

Researchers devised this procedure to utilize the protein-synthesizing apparatus of the cloning host and limit and direct such synthesis to those proteins encoded on the vector (e.g., genes of interest; Sancar et al. 1979). Application of this procedure has made it possible to overproduce otherwise very low copy numbered proteins. This procedure has evolved into related (and now routine) protocols used in industry, medicine, and research.

Submarine Gel Electrophoresis

The separation of nucleic acids using electrophoresis is similar to that of proteins. Submarine electrophoresis is a procedure for the separation of DNA fragments and differs from PAGE mainly in that the gel is submerged or floating under a buffer. The simple apparatus involves a device for holding the gel (usually made of agarose or polyacrylamide) and samples in a well at the end of the gel, connectors to the high-voltage power source, and the running buffer (e.g., salts) that is flooded over the gel. The migration (separation) of fragments is based on molecular weight (or fragment size). The smaller the DNA pieces, the farther they will migrate into the gel. For maximum fragment separation, this system is set up to avoid overheating of the gel by the large amount of current that must be applied within the buffer. Using special sequencing gels, it is possible to separate up to several hundred fragments of DNA that differ in only one base in length.

Proteomics

Proteomics is the field of study dedicated to determining what certain proteins do and how they provide normal cellular function (Zhou and Shan 2001) or metabolism. Efforts are directed to study the full set of proteins encoded by a genome:

1. Elucidation of information describing protein function
2. Determination of protein domain structure (Szuztakowski and Weng 2000)
3. Mapping subcellular location of proteins
4. Identification of posttranslational modifications and effects on protein function
5. Determination of sequence variants and sequence alignments
6. Determination of sequence similarities to other proteins and homology modeling

This research field must therefore identify every protein in the cell, determine the sequence of each protein and enter that information into a databank, and analyze globally the proteins in cells at different stages of development and growth. Scientists generally rely on two-dimensional (2-D) gel electrophoresis to map the protein varieties, use other procedures to isolate each protein in a pure form, and perform mass spectrometry on such isolates to analyze the sequence.

Ordinarily, amino acid sequence data are inferred from the nucleic acid sequence information and are based on codon usage. Sequence alignment of polypeptides and nucleic acids is a key end point during the initial analysis within the study of proteomics (Taylor 1989). By comparing the sequences of unknown proteins to well-defined sequences, scientists immediately gain hints to 3-D conformation, function, cellular importance, and molecular systematics, (or evolutionary relatedness—Miyoshi et al. 2001). The presence of a zinc-binding motif, for instance, might imply that the protein serves as a DNA binding protein, hormone receptor, or transcriptional control factor. Such nucleic acid and protein interactions are apparently common in nature (Figure 4.14).

Methods to determine the importance of peptide modifications—such as glycosylation, phosphorylation, and acetylation—and their locations with respect to active sites are advanced and beyond the scope of this chapter. Our understanding of protein "action" or movement (such as allosteric changes—Luque and Freire 2000) will be increased greatly as scientists develop more powerful algorithms (mathematical and procedural instructions) along with more flexible computer graphing software (Sauder et al. 2000; Figure 4.15). Progress will also benefit from improved instrumentation, such as synchrotron and position sensitive x-ray defraction spectroscopy, megahertz NMR spectroscopy, and mass spectroscopy such as matrix-assisted lazar desorption ionization (MALD/I).

By combining these procedures, several basic protein characteristics including structure, protein folding (Ferrara et al. 2000), active site allosteric movements, functional relationships of nonadjacent sequences, catalysis reactions, and likely actions as regulation controllers become possible. Even the simple fact of a protein's molecular weight, if precisely determined, can provide evidence for its ability to function within an enzymatic process such as DNA synthesis where nearly two dozen different proteins are typically involved. Scientists often rationalize the interaction of a protein with a sequence of nucleic acid if it will simply fit. Scattering (electron) data can yield important hints to conformational folding and provide the "fit" data necessary. It has been shown that many stem cell growth factors work as a consort of proteins and are often dependent on cell-to-cell contacts. If details of protein-to-protein interactions were completely tabulated, inferences to cell differentiation might be apparent.

One of the earliest examples of protein engineering nicely proves the usefulness of understanding amino acid sequence and protein folding structure.

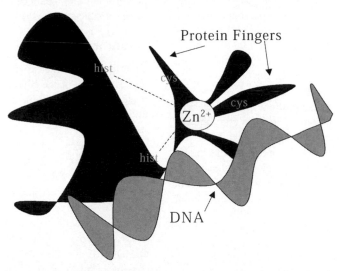

Figure 4.14. Zinc finger motifs. Shown is a positional representation of a zinc ion, DNA helix, and a polypeptide sequence. This structure is present at, or near, the active sites of many proteins and may allow close, important, and specific interactions between nucleic acids and proteins.

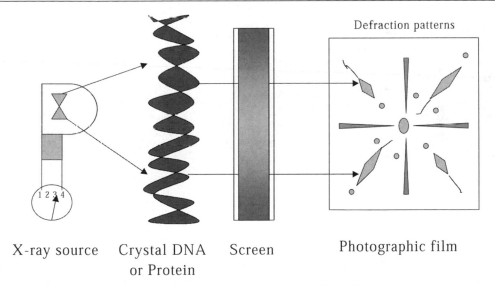

Figure 4.15. X-ray crystallography. Shown is a representation of the components necessary to carry out diffraction pattern analysis of a macromolecule. This procedure is typically useful to determine the shape of DNA and possibly the structure of proteins that interact with DNA.

Scientists using what is now considered rather primitive cloning techniques were nevertheless able to change the protein sequence in the laboratory and dramatically change the activity of a protein that degrades (breaks) other proteins. These proteases are very useful enzymes and have been shown to work as detergents for cleaning clothes, as a natural method of tenderizing meat, and as effective digestive aids in both animals and humans. They have also been shown to protect animals against pathogen invasion, reduce the formation of blood clots in people suffering heart attacks, reduce the swelling of damaged or bruised tissues, and function as therapeutic agents in the treatment of leukemia.

Subtilism BPN' is a protease that has been the subject of considerable protein engineering. This enzyme is originally from *Bacillus*, a common soil bacteria, and has been cloned and shown to be very useful as a cloning model. By precisely altering the DNA sequence of this gene, scientists have been able to determine the importance of certain amino acids within the active site. When a single amino acid near the active (catalytic) site within the entire sequence of more than 220 amino acids of the BPN' protease was replaced, the activity was shown to increase by 100-fold. After other substitutions, activity decreased greatly to the point where the enzyme classification was appropriately changed. Some amino acid changes may even change the enzyme sequence specificity and create a completely different activity. Such information has allowed scientists to assign the importance of certain electron configurations to enzyme function in other nonrelated proteins.

Many proteins are apparently involved with the process of cell differentiation, and so it is essential to elucidate their mode of action. Of the known cellular protein components that stimulate cellular development and physiology, several have been studied in some detail including hormones, interleukins (Kauppi et al. 2001) and lymphokines (types of cytokines produced by localized cells; Miyajima et al. 1993), and tissue or event-specific growth factors. Many of these proteins range in molecular weight between 8KD and 80KD and function as monomers (single polypeptides). By determining their sequence and 3-D structure, it will be possible to determine their mode of action. With a detailing of mode of action, scientists will possess the information to tailor new and improved stem cell signals. In humans, the genes that encode these proteins have been found on all but six chromosomes. However, it is expected that after a more detailed study, scientists will find such genes on all the chromosomes of humans. These protein components have been shown to cause tissue proliferation, cell renewal and growth, cell commitment to tissue-specific differentiation, cell maturation, and rapid cell death. The replacement of certain cell lineages by stem cell maturation is therefore closely related to the presence of such growth components and their changes in concentrations and cell-to-cell contacts.

Bioinformatics

Bioinformatics is the expert annotation, interpretation, and evaluation of the genome and in particular of the proteome. The proteome is a comprehensive set or collection of expressed proteins within the cell at a particular time. That annotation includes adding pertinent information such as genes coded for, amino acid sequences, or other commentary to the database entry of raw sequence DNA bases. The field must provide a framework to process and store enormous amounts of sequence information generated by sequencing and microarray machines and provide adequate modeling of protein structure-function relationships of genes. Because of the complexity of the more pertinent genomes, informatics is, therefore, the science of managing and analyzing biological data using advanced computing techniques and software. Many software packages are created each year in an effort to keep up with the avalanche of biological data being generated daily. To succeed, this interdisciplinary pursuit must include the practical tools of mathematics and computer science. This will be especially important during the detailed analyses of genomic research data (Yuwaraj et al. 2001).

Bioinformatics is the centerpiece in the field of functional genomics. Functional genomics attempts to elucidate the functions of all genes in the entire genome, including the study of gene expression and control. Unlike most historic approaches to studying gene activities based on phenotypic observation of gene activity, scientists within this area must work "backward" in that they are provided the gene sequence but have little or no information about the gene action and must infer the function. Laboratory experiments and sophisticated computer analysis must therefore fuse biology, mathematics, and computer science to

1. Discover sequences responsible for genes within the genome.
2. Align these sequences to putative genes in well-studied databases and make matches.
3. Predict the structure and activity of the gene products encoded by these sequences.
4. Outline the likely interactions between genes, and gene products between cells.
5. Relate such interactions to organismal function.
6. Postulate relatedness of one sequence to others to create a phylogenetic basis.

Within the relatively new research area of molecular systematics, scientists have gained revolutionary evolution data relating the newt to cattle and to man. It fact, there lies an underlying relatedness of most complex mammals never before suspected, based only on physical appearance or even simply on analysis of DNA sequences from the housekeeping genes. The RAPD procedure rapidly provides DNA sequence relatedness data by applying PCR techniques, but this abundance of information was of little use until informatics analysis proved its utility in speciation. The analysis can even apply codon usage to generate definitive individual locations within an evolutionary tree (see sidebar below).

APPLICATION OF METHODS TOWARD STEM CELLS AND GENE REGULATION

By combining the experimental protocols, described in this chapter, it will be possible to detail the molecular events leading to cell differentiation of stem cells (Clark and Frisen 2001). We have outlined one feasible analysis that demonstrates the utility of the approach. Stem cells may be isolated from animal muscle and prepared in vitro, and over a time course exposed to cell growth promotants (Buckingham 2001; Simian et al. 2001). At different stages of cell differentiation, mRNA is isolated from these cell populations, and cDNA is synthesized and finally sequenced. DNA sequence data is recorded, and typical proteomics and bioinformatics annotations are performed (Pletcher et al. 2001). When sufficient information of this kind is accumulated, it will be useful in the rational development of animal breeding and nutritional programs that optimize performance (Dworkin and Losick 2001).

Generalized microinjection techniques (a very small needle is used to deliver tiny quantities of liquid) with cell tissues provide very low levels of gene recombination into the genome. This greatly limits the number of experiments that scientists can perform with cell lines. The transfer of pluripotent embryonic stem cells containing an altered gene via microinjection into blastocysts produces a transgenic animal possessing cells descended from the stem cell lineage (Brinster 1993; Deutsch et al. 2001; Watt 2001). The heterozygous animal can then be interbred to produce offspring homozygous for the altered gene. Using these procedures, relatively high levels of success in chimera production allow scientists to study important but rare events.

Even though only a crude human DNA sequence map is currently available, scientists have gained key insights into gene control. The human genome project is the multinational research effort to determine the sequence of the entire DNA complement of the human chromosomes. Similar efforts are underway for all important meat animal species. Regardless of animal type, however, researchers have suspected that most genes are controlled from locations adjacent to the gene of interest. Low-resolution maps provide proof that gene regulatory elements (called enhancers) are usually spread across vast regions of DNA sequences and often are located on different chromosomes. Such information will greatly assist efforts to create transgenic animals producing useful proteins and provide key insights into gene activities during the enormously complex events of stem cell differentiation.

In the near future, as the entire human DNA genome sequence is determined, increased insights into a number of important cellular processes will become apparent. Certain stem cells destined to become key players in the immune response are able to precisely reorganize their DNA as they commit to producing and secreting antibodies. Often during the treatment of cancer, patients must endure a compromised immune system. If physicians fully understood the process of β-cell antibody gene regulation, it might be possible to provide patients with certain factors to promote antibody productions by these cells (Huff and Saunders 1993). It may be necessary to genetically engineer stem cells to induce their differentiation toward specific lineages.

Alternatively, the successful cells may need to be "trained" by surrounding and neighboring cells to act and function appropriately.

STEM RESEARCH YET TO BE DONE

The procedures listed above will speed the acquisition of several fundamental questions about stem cells. A partial list of the items yet to be answered include the following:

- To quantify the tissue populations of adult stem cells
- To determine locations and abundance of stems cells within body tissues
- To measure the plasticity of adult stem cells
- To determine if adult stem cells can provide an experimental alternative to embryonic-derived stem cells

In addition, it will be important to decide if all stem cells possess the ability to self renew and determine their capacity to develop into different types of differentiated cells. Also, this research will determine if lineage stem cells are really limited to muscle, nerve, blood, epidermis, intestine, bone-marrow, liver, and pancreatic tissues, or whether stem cells might generate cell types other than those types with which they reside. In other words, might stem cells readily dedifferentiate and redifferentiate as the need arises? If so, what precisely are the cellular factors that decide a differential pathway for stem cells (Wang et al. 2001a, 2001b). Finally, it will be important to determine the specific therapeutic capabilities of stem cells.

APPLICATIONS IN THE FUTURE

What might we do with stem cells if we possessed a full understanding of their function? A few examples might include the therapeutic repair of nerve, muscle, or bone tissue, including clinical stem cell transplantation to combat degenerative diseases. In addition, it might be possible to devise precise methods of management (hormonal control) of diseases such as diabetes (Kim and Hebrok 2001; Rogner et al. 2001; Fossey et al. 2001), or to inhibit neoplastic transformation and discover how mutations in such genes like sonic hedgehog, patched, meis, and smad, might promote cancer growth (Weinberg 1991). It seems feasible to produce rare or novel products by cell translation of proteins requiring posttranslation modifications such as glycosylation, phosphorylation, and acetylation. We may be in a position to outline evolutionary systematics and species ancestral organizations, or to perform rational protein engineering and modeling (for analysis). From a physiological perspective, we will likely be capable of precisely defining cell maturation and differentiation control events, to formulate animal disease control measures (via gene therapy) and repair viral damage to cells. Alternatively, we will be able to alter reproduction management, spermatogenesis, or embryo development. In clinical settings we might conduct carryout eye lens repair and burned tissue reconstructions, promote plans of nutritional well-being of individuals through cell health, or determine intercellular signaling pathways that govern embryonic development.

Cellular development and physiological regulation are very complex processes. For instance, in the maturation of pancreatic cells, the binding of the hormone insulin to its cell-surface receptor, possessing tyrosine kinase activity stimulates autophosphorylation of amino acids and cytosolic proteins (Miyajima et al. 1992, Bowen et al. 2000, de Longh et al. 2001). This cascade of events is required for proper development of the pancreatic cells. These cellular\cytosolic events first occur during gestation and persist into neonatal periods, but are essential for proper β-cell growth.

Several cellular products related to stem cell development and growth have been cloned and produced in large amounts for use in research and medicine. For instance, tissue plasminogen activator (TPA) dissolves blood clots, human growth hormone (hGH) is used to treat dwarfism, transforming growth factor-beta (TGF-β) stimulates new blood vessel and epidermal cell growth, and platelet-derived growth factor (PDGF) is used to lessen ulceration in people with diabetes. Many growth factors are usually a protein (maybe acting like a hormone) that mediates much of what the cell must do to grow. A hormone is a compound that triggers a response in cells located some distance from where it was synthesized. Farmers are using BST (bovine somatotropin) to promote rapid or efficient muscle (meat) development in pigs and greater feed conversion in milk-producing cattle. These production changes increase animal performance efficiency and, in turn, the profit margin. By administering tiny amounts of such hormones (one-millionth of one-millionth of a pound) one can cause the animal to produce one-third more muscle, and therefore less fat, or 10–20% more milk from the same amount of food consumed. Because the consumer wishes to eat less fat and pay less for milk, it makes good business sense. We suggest that the future looks very bright indeed.

SUMMARY

Stem cell research relates to several important areas of human endeavors, including animal production. Use of pluripotent stem cells grown in culture will accelerate advances in drug development and toxicity testing, provide useful tissues for therapy and replacements, and lead to key discoveries in studies of gene control and regulation (Figure A).

The recent increase in research efforts and publications within molecular biology suggests that our level of understanding of biological systems is maturing at an exponential rate. However, problems within the agricultural, medical, and environmental areas will require much more detailed information for defining and resolving the problems than are presently available. It is hoped that, armed with such information, innovative biotechnological products and services will soon be available to increase food production, treat animal and human diseases, and attend to environmental pollution concerns. More than 100 million humans in the U.S. alone are

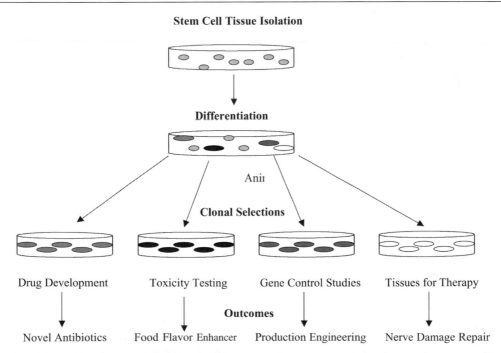

Figure A. The potential usefulness of stem cell products. Several potential biotechnological products are listed that would find application in agriculture and medicine.

affected by serious health problems, such as cancer, cardiovascular disease, autoimmune disease, diabetes (Rogner et al. 2001), osteoporosis, Alzheimer's, spinal cord injuries, and various birth defects. In many nations, food production lags behind population growth. Animals with characteristics that resist disease or enhance performance will provide a more abundant and plentiful food supply. The use of animal models such as diabetic dogs, obese mice, and double muscling and superovulation in sheep should provide important clues to genetic regulation of stem cells. In turn, these discoveries will be the keys to gene replacement therapies, and ultimately, to greatly enhanced animal production. Evidence exists to suggest that stem cell research and the application of such pluripotent cells might greatly lessen the suffering caused by disease or may even provide a cure to a disease. To carry out stem cell analysis, it will be necessary to determine the importance of cell regulatory signals during differentiation (Figure B). It is suggested that it will also be important to utilize molecular biology to timely and fully accomplish that goal.

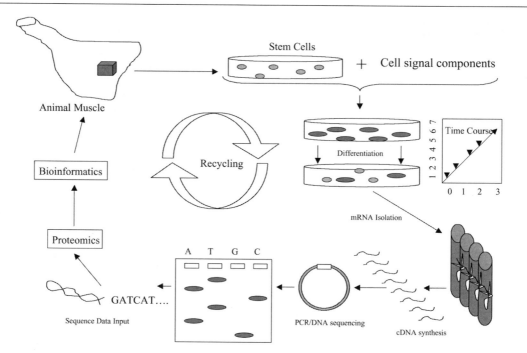

Figure B. Stem cell analysis. Shown is the relationship of stem cell products to the fields of molecular biology. The experimental analysis is explained within the text of this chapter. It is possible that such experimentation will lead to useful products or therapies to increase animal well-being.

GLOSSARY

Clone (or copy) is an artificial and perhaps self-replicating fragment of DNA able to be passed from one place or organism to another.

Cosmids are powerful cloning vehicles that contain components from bacterial viruses, bacteria, yeast, and plasmids. These vehicles can carry large amounts of foreign DNA.

DNA is the abbreviation for deoxyribonucleic acid. It is a double-stranded structure and serves as the genetic material for most organisms.

Fluorescence is the generation of a long wave-length of light during the movement of electrons from one atomic orbital to another.

Gene is the unit of heredity or a segment of DNA encoding a protein. Often the gene is represented as a contiguous sequence, or segment, of DNA.

Gene splicing is the combination or joining two genes together, usually within a cloning vector.

Gene transfer is the use of physical manipulation to introduce foreign genes into host cells. It is the movement of genetic information from one organism to another.

Genome is the total genetic endowment of an organism; that is, the complete complement of all nitrogenous base sequences.

Housekeeping genes are responsible for activities that are common and particularly important to the cell. Examples include carrying oxygen transport (hemoglobin) or energy formation (kinase).

Knockout gene is a DNA sequence used in cloning to inactivate the function of a gene. Normally it is placed within or near a gene of interest.

Ligation is the process of combining fragments of nucleic acids. Most often scientists use the ligase isolated from T4 phage.

Recombinant DNA is the hybrid DNA produced by joining different pieces of DNA. Sometimes this term is abbreviated as rDNA.

Reporter genes indicate the presence of a trans-genic animal or the chromosomal insertion of a particular gene. Reporter genes (e.g. luciferase) are closely associated with placement of the gene.

Restriction map is a drawing or diagram of a DNA region containing the precise location of the restriction endonucleases incisions.

Reverse transcriptase is properly called RNA directed DNA polymerase and "reads" a template of RNA and synthesizes a complementary strand of DNA. The Taq I enzyme is an example.

Shuttle vector is a cloning vehicle that can move DNA through a variety of different hosts. For example, the BKV cloning plasmid can function within *E.coli*, yeast, or certain plant cells.

Subcloning is the process of taking the original clone and manipulating it further, usually for enhanced expression.

Totipotent cell is a single cell or tissue that is capable of providing all the genetic coding information necessary for the creation of a complete and adult organism.

X-ray crystallography is an imaging procedure for determining molecular structure. This procedure is dependent on pure crystal formations of proteins (or nucleic acids) and diffraction of electrons onto a photographic emulsion.

Zinc finger motifs are locations and structures found within many proteins and contain zinc or similar metals. These deep pocket structures promote catalysis of these enzymes.

REFERENCES

Adams, M.D., and Venter, J.C. 2000. The genome sequence of *Drosophila melanogaster. Science* 287:2185–2215.

Adams, R.L.P. 1980. In Cell Culture for Biochemists. New York: Elsevier/North Holland Biomedical Press.

Allen, R.E., Temm-Grove, C.J., Sheehan, A.M., and Rice, G. 1997. Skeletal muscle satellite cell cultures. *Methods in Cell Biology* 52:155–176.

Andrews A., ed. 1987. In *Electrophoresis: Theory, Techniques and Biochemical and Clinical Applications.* New York: Oxford University Press.

Arabidopsis Genome Initiative. 2000. Analysis of the genome sequence of the flowering plant Arabidopsis thaliana. *Nature* 408:796–815.

Ausubel, F., Brent, R., Kingston, R., Moore, D., Seidman, J., Smith, J., and Struhl, K. 1992. In *Short Protocols In Molecular Biology.* 2d ed. New York: Greene Publishing Associates and John Wiley & Sons.

Bach, P.H., Vickers, A.E.M., Fisher, R., Baumann, A., Brittebo, E., Carlile, D.J., Koster, H.J., Lake, B.G., Salmon, F., Sawyer, T.W., and Skibinski, G. 1996. The use of tissue slices for pharmacotoxicological studies. *Alternatives to Laboratory Animals* 24:893–923.

Bastolla, U., Farwer, J., Knapp, E.W., and Vendruscolo, M. 2001. How to guarantee optimal stability for most representative structures in the protein data bank. *Proteins: Structure, Function, and Genetics* 44:79–96.

Bihoreau, M-T., Sebag-Montefiore, L., Godfrey, R.F., Wallis, R.H., Brown, J.H., Danoy, P.A., Collins, S.C., Rouard, M., Kaisaki, P.J., Lathrop, M., and Gauguier, D. 2001. A high-resolution consensus linkage map of the rat, integrating radiation hybrid and genetic maps. *Genomics* 75:57–58.

Blanton Jr., J.R., Robinson, J.P., Gerrard, D.E., Bidwell, C.A., and Grant, A.L. 2000. Rapid purification of transfected porcine muscle cells. *Methods in Cell Science* 22:217–223.

Blattner, F.R., and Shao, Y. 1997. The complete genome sequence of *Escherichia coli* K-12. *Science* 277:1453–1463.

Bowen, M.A., Aruffo, A.A., and Bajorath, J. 2000. Cell surface receptors and their ligands: In vitro analysis of CD6-CD166 interactions. *Proteins: Structure, Function, and Genetics* 40:420–428.

Boyer, H.W. 1971. DNA restriction and modification mechanisms in bacteria. *Annual Review Microbiology* 25:153–176.

Brinster, R. L. 1993. Stem cells and transgenic mice in the study of development. *International Journal Developmental Biology* 37:89–99.

Buckingham, M. 2001. Skeletal muscle formation in vertebrates. *Current Opinion in Genetics and Development* 11:440–448.

Burden, D., and Whitney, D. 1995. In *Biotechnology, Proteins to Biotechnology*. Boston: Ed. Birkhauser.

Burrin, J.M., Uttenthal, L.O., McGregor, G.P. and Bloom, S.R. 1987. Aspects of measurement and analysis of regulatory peptides. *Experientia* 43:734–741.

Burton, N.M., Byrne, K.M., Vierck, J.L., and Dodson, M.V. 2000. Methods for satellite cell culture under a variety of conditions. *Methods in Cell Science* 22(1):51–61

Byrne, K.M., guest ed. 2000. Applications of flow cytometry across species. *Methods in Cell Science* 22:165–252.

Byrne, K.M., Cheng, X., Vierck, J.L., Greene, E.A., Duckett, S.K., and Dodson, M.V. 1998. Use of a 96-well plate reader to evaluate proliferation of equine satellite cells in vitro. *Methods in Cell Science* 19(4):311–316.

Calza, R., Huttner, E., Vincentz, M., Rouze, P., Galangau, F., Vaucheret, H., Cherel, I., Meyer, C., Kronenberger, J., and Caboche, M. 1987. Cloning of DNA fragments complementary to tobacco nitrate reductase mRNA and encoding epitopes common to the nitrate reductases from higher plants. *Molecular General Genetics* 209:552–562.

Clark, D., and Frisen, J. 2001. Differentiation potential of adult stem cells. *Current Opinion in Genetics and Development* 11:575–580.

Collins, F. 1992. Cystic fibrosis: Molecular biology and therapeutic implications. *Science*. 256:774–779.

Dahm, K., Nielsen, P.J., and Muller, A.M. 2001. Transcripts of *Fliz1*, a nuclear zinc finger protein, are expressed in discrete foci of the murine fetal liver. *Genomics* 73:194–202.

de longh, R.U., Lovicu, F.J., Overbeek, P.A., Schneider, M.D., Joya, J., Hardeman, E.D., and McAvoy, J.W. 2001. Requirement for TGFB receptor signaling during terminal lens fiber differentiation. *Development* 128:3995–4010.

Deutsch, G., Jung, J., Zheng, M., Lora, J., and Zaret, K.S. 2001. A bipotential precursor population for pancreas and liver within the embryonic endoderm. *Development* 128:871–881.

Devlin, R.H., Yesaki, T.Y., Biagi, C.A., Donaldson, E.M., Swanson, P., and Chan, W.K. 1994. Extraordinary salmon growth. *Nature* 371:209–210.

Dodson, M.V., guest ed. 2000. Basic cell culture methods. *Methods in Cell Science* 22(1):25–81.

Dodson, M.V., Hossner, K.L., Vierck, J.L., Mathison, B.A., and Krabbenhoft, L.A. 1996. Correlation of serum IGF-I and GH to satellite cell responsiveness in targhee rams. *Animal Science* 62(1):89–96.

Dodson, M.V., Mathison, B.A., and Hossner, K.L. 1987. Interaction of ovine somatomedin-C/IGF-I and IGF-I with specific IGF-I receptors on cultured muscle-derived fibroblasts. *ACTA Endocrinologica*. 116:186–192.

Dodson, M.V., Mathison, B.A., and Mathison, B.D. 1990. Effects of medium and substratum on ovine satellite cell attachment, proliferation and differentiation in vitro. *Cell Differentiation and Development* 29(1):59–66.

Dodson, M.V., McFarland, D.C., Grant, A.L., Doumit, M.E., and Velleman, S.J. 1996. Extrinsic regulation of domestic animal-derived satellite cells. *Domestic Animal Endocrinology* 13(2):107–126.

Dodson, M.V., and Schaeffer, W.I. 2000. Generation of viable cell-culture data. *Methods in Cell Science* 22(1):27–28.

Dodson, M.V., Vierck, J.L., Hossner, K.L., Byrne, K., and McNamara, J.P. 1997. The development and utility of a defined muscle and fat co-culture system. *Tissue & Cell* 29:517–524.

Doolittle, R. F. 1991. Computer analysis of protein and nucleic acid sequences, *In Methods of Enzymology*. vol. 183. San Diego: Academic Press.

Dworkin, J., and Losick, R. 2001. Linking nutritional status to gene activation and development. *Genes and Development* 15:1051–1054.

Elis, R.J. 1987. Proteins as molecular chaperones. *Nature* 328:378–379.

Eschenlauer, S.C.P., McEwan, N.R., Calza, R.E., Wallace, R.J., and Newbold, C.J. 1998. Phylogenetic position and codon usage of two centrin genes from the rumen ciliate protozoan *Entodinium caudatum*. *Federation of European Microbiological Societies Letters* 166:147–154.

Feinberg, A.P., and Vogelstein, B. 1983. A technique for radiolabeling DNA restriction endonuclease fragments to high specific activity. *Analytical Biochemistry* 132:6–13.

Ferrara, P., Apostolakis, J., and Caflisch, A. 2000. Computer simulations of protein folding by targeted molecular dynamics. *Proteins: Structure, Function, and Genetics* 39:252–260.

Forcellino, F., and Derreumaux, P. 2001. Computer simulations aimed at structure prediction of supersecondary motifs in proteins. *Proteins: Structure, Function, and Genetics* 45:159–166.

Fossey, S.C., Mychaleckyj, J.C., Pendleton, J.K., Snyder, J.R., Bensen, J.T., Hirakawa, S., Rich, S.S., Freedman, B.I., and Bowden, D.W. 2001. A high-resolution 6.0-megabase transcript map of the type 2 diabetes susceptibility region on human chromosome 20. *Genomics* 76:45–57.

Fraser, C.M., and Venter, J.C. 1998. Complete genome sequence of Treponema pallidum, the syphilis spirochete. *Science* 281:375–388.

Freshney, R.I. 1986. *Animal Cell Culture: A Practical Approach*. Washington D.C.: IRL Press.

Freshney, R.I. 1994. *Culture of Animal Cells: A Manual of Basic Technique*. 3d ed. New York: Wiley-Liss.

Gannon, M., and Bader, D. 1998. Avian cardiac progenitors: Methods for isolation, culture and analysis of differentiation. *Methods in Cell Biology* 52:117–132.

Garfin, D.E. 1990. One-dimensional gel electrophoresis. *Methods in Enzymology* 182:425–441.

Goldsmith, S.J. 1975. Radioimmunoassay: Review of basic principles. *Seminar Nuclear Medicine* 5:125–152.

Hames, B.D., and Rickwood, D., eds. 1981. In *Gel Electrophoresis of Proteins: A Practical Approach*. Washington, D.C.: IRL Press.

Harris, J.D., and Lemoine, N.R. 1996. Strategies for targeted gene therapy. *Trends in Genetics* 12:400–405.

Hedden, P. 1993. Modern methods for the quantitative analysis of plant hormones. *Annual Reviews* (plant physiology and plant molecular biology) 44:107–129.

Hossner, K.L., Yemm, R., Vierck, J., and Dodson, M.V. 1997. Insulin-like growth factor (IGF)-I and -II and

IGFBP secretion by ovine satellite cell strains grown alone or in co-culture with 3T3-L1 preadipocytes. In *Vitro Cellular & Developmental Biology* 33:791–795.

Howe, C.J., and Ward, E.S. 1989. *In Nucleic Acids Sequencing: A practical approach.* Oxford, U.K.: IRL Press.

Huff, V., and Saunders, G. 1993. Wilm's tumor genes. *Biochemistry Biophysics Acta* 1155:295–306.

Innis, M.A., Gelfand, D.H., Sninsky, J.J., and White, T.L. 1990. In *PCR Protocols: A Guide to Methods and Applications.* San Diego: Academic Press.

Ishisaki, Z., Takaishi, M., Furuta, I., and Huh, N. 2001. Calmin, a protein with calponin homology and transmembrane domains expressed in maturing spermatogenic cells. *Genomics* 74:172–179.

Kannan, N., Selvaraj, S., Gromiha, M.M., and Vishveshwara, S. 2001. Clusters of a/b barrel proteins. Implications for protein structure, function, and folding. *Proteins: Structure, Function, and Genetics* 43:103–112.

Kauppi, P., Lindblad-Toh, K., Sevon, P., Toivonen, H.T.T., Rioux, J.D., Villapakkam, A., Laitinen, L.A., Hudson, T.J., Kere, J., and Laitinen, T. 2001. A second-generation association study of the 5q31 cytokine gene cluster and the interleukin-4 receptor in asthma. *Genomics* 77:35–36.

Kim, S.K., and Hebrok, M. 2001. Intercellular signals regulating pancreas development and function. *Genes and Development* 15:111–127.

Koller, B.H., and Smithies, O. 1992. Altering genes in animals by gene targeting. *Annual Review Immunology* 10:705–730.

Komaki, M., Katagiri, T., and Suda, T. 1996. Bone morphogenetic protein-2 does not alter the differentiation pathway of committed progenitors of osteoblasts and chondrocytes. *Cell Tissue Research* 28:9–17.

Krabbenhoft, E.A., Shultz, K., Brannon-O'Reilly, B.A., Chen, Y., Stewart, N.T., and Dodson, M.V. 1997. A simplified method of analysis of cell conditioned medium for IGF activity. *Methods in Cell Science* 19:129–135.

Krumm, R. 1994. Radioimmunoassay: A proven performer in the lab. *The Scientist* 8:17.

Kubo, Y., Kaidzu, S., Nakajima, I., Takenouchi, K., and Nakamura, F. 2000. Organization of extracellular matrix components during differentiation of adipocytes in long-term culture. *In Vitro Cellular and Developmental Biology* 36:38–44.

Luque, I., and Freire, E. 2000. Structural stability of binding sites: Consequences for binding affinity and allosteric effects. *Proteins: Structure, Function, and Genetics* 4:63–71.

Mathison, B.D., Mathison, B.A., McNamara, J.P., and Dodson, M.V. 1989. IGF receptor analyses of satellite cell-derived myotubes from two lines of Targhee rams selected for growth rate. *Domestic Animal Endocrinology* 6(3):191–201.

McEwan, N.R., Eschenlauer, S., Calza, R., Wallace, and J., Newbold, J. 2000a. The 3 prime end untranslated region of messages in the rumen protozoan *Entodinium caudatum. Protist* 151:139–146.

McEwan, N.R., Gatherer, D., Eschenlauer, S.C.P., McIntosh, F.M., Calza, R.E., Wallace, R.J., and Newbold,

C.J. 2000b. An unusual codon usage pattern in the ciliate family *Ophryoscolecidae* and its implications for determining the source of cloned DNA. *Anaerobe* 6:21–28.

McFarland, D.C. 2000. Preparation of pure cell cultures by cloning. *Methods in Cell Science* 22:63–66.

Mir, P.S., Vierck, J.L., Mir, Z., and Dodson, M.V. 2000. Quantification of lipid in cultured 3T3-L1 adipocytes. *Animal Science* 71:521–526.

Miyajima, A., Kitamura, T., Harada, N., Yokota, T., and Arai, K. 1992. Cytokine receptors and signal transduction. *Annual Review Immunology* 10:295–331.

Miyajima, K., Ochijo, H., and Heldin, C-H. 1993. Enhanced bFGF expression in response to transforming growth factor-b stimulation of AkR-23 cells. *Growth Factors* 8:11–22.

Miyoshi, K., Cui, Y., Riedlinger, G., Robinson, P., Lehoczky, J., Zon, L., Oka, T., Dewar, K., and Hennighausen, L. 2001. Structure of the mouse stat 3/5 locus: Evolution from *Drosophila* to zebrafish to mouse. *Genomics* 71:150–155.

Mouchel, N., Tebbutt, S.J., Broackes-Carter, F.C., Sahota, V., Summerfield, T., Gregory, D.J., andHarris, A. 2001. The sheep genome contributes to localization of control elements in a human gene with complex regulatory mechanisms. *Genomics* 76:9–12.

Mullikin, J.C., and Bentley, D.R. 2000. An SNP map of human chromosome 22. *Nature* 407:516–520.

Mullis, K.B., and Faloona, F.A. 1987. Specific synthesis of DNA in vitro via a polymerase-catalyzed chain reaction. *Methods Enzymology* 155:335–350.

Neville, C., Rosenthal, N., McGrew, M., Bogdanova, N., and Hauschka, S. 1998. Skeletal muscle cultures. *Methods in Cell Biology* 52:85–116.

Palladino, M.A. 2002. *Understanding the Human Genome Project.* San Francisco: Benjamin Cummings Publishing.

Palmiter, R.D., and Brinster, R.L. 1985. Transgenic mice. *Cell* 41:343–345.

Patel, K., Easty, D.J., and Dunn, M.J. 1988. Detection of proteins in polyacrylamide gels using an ultrasensitive silver staining technique. In *Methods in Molecular Biology #3: New Protein Techniques.* J.M. Walker, ed. Clifton, N.J.: Humana Press.

Pauly, R.P., Bilato, C., Chenge, L., Monticone, R., and Crow, M.T. 1998. Vascular smooth muscle cell cultures. *Methods in Cell Biology* 52:133–154.

Perbal, B. 1988. In *A Practical Guide to Molecular Cloning.* 2d ed. New York: John Wiley & Sons.

Pletcher, M.T., Wiltshire, T., Cabin, D.E., Villanueva, M., and Reeves, R.H. 2001. Use of comparative physical and sequence mapping to annotate mouse chromosome 16 and human chromosome 21. *Genomics* 74:45–54.

Reeds, P.J. 1991. Future trends in growth biology research. *Journal of Animal Science* 69 (suppl 3):1–23.

Resau, J.H., Sakamoto, K., Cottrell, J.R., Hudson, E.A., and Meltzer, S.J. 1991. Explant organ culture: a review. *Cytotechnology* 7(3):137–149.

Rodbell, M. 1964. Metabolism of isolated fat cells. *Journal of Biological Chemistry* 239:375–380.

Rogner, U.C., Boitard, C., Morin, J., Melanitou, E., and Avner, P. 2001. Three loci on mouse chromosome 6 influence onset and final incidence of type 1 diabetes in NOD.C3H congenic strains. *Genomics* 74:163–171.

Rosen, E.D., and Spiegelman, B.M. 2000. Molecular regulation of adipogenesis. *Annual Review Cell Developmental Biology* 16:145–171.

Sancar, A., Hack, A., and Rupp, W. 1979. A method for the production of cloned gene products. *Journal of Bacteriology*, 137:692–699.

Sanger, F., and Coulson, A.R. 1975. A rapid method for determining sequences in DNA by primed synthesis with DNA polymerase. *Journal Molecular Biology* 94:441–448.

Sauder, J.M., Arthur, J.W., and Dunbrack, R.L., Jr., 2000. Large-scale comparison of protein sequence alignment algorithms with structure alignments. *Proteins: Structure, Function, and Genetics* 40:6–22.

Simian, M., Hirai, Y., Navre, M., Werb, A., Lochter, A., and Bissell, M. 2001. The interplay of matrix metalloproteinases, morphogens and growth factors is necessary for branching of mammary epithelial cells. *Development* 128:3117–3131.

Soejima, H., Kawamoto, S., Akai, J., Miyoshi, O., Arai, Y., Morohka, T., Matsuo, S., Niikawa, N., Kimura, A., Okubo, K., and Mukai, T. 2001. Isolation of novel heart-specific genes using the bodymap database. *Genomics* 74:115–120.

Southern, E.M. 1975. Detection of specific sequences among DNA fragments separated by gel electrophoresis. *Journal Molecular Biology* 98:503–517.

Stewart, N.T., Byrne, K.M., Ragle, C., Vierck, J., and Dodson, M.V. 2001. Patterns of expression of muscle-specific markers of differentiation in satellite cell cultures: Determination by enzyme-linked immunoculture assay (ELICA) and confocal immunofluorescent microscopy (CIFA). *Cell Biology International* 25(9):873–884.

Stewart, N.Y., Byrne, K.M., Vierck, J.L., Hosick, H., and Dodson, M.V. 2000. Traditional and emerging methods for analyzing cell activity in cell cultures. *Methods in Cell Science* 22(1):67–78.

Szuztakowski, J.D., and Weng, Z. 2000. Protein structure alignment using a genetic algorithm. *Proteins: Structure, Function, and Genetics* 38:428–440.

Taniguchi, M., Miura, K., Iwao, H., and Yamanaka, S. 2001. Quantitative assessment of DNA microarrays-comparison with northern blot analyses. *Genomics* 71:34–39.

Taylor, W.R. 1989. A flexible method to align large numbers of biological sequences. *Journal Molecular Evolution* 28:161–169.

Trowell, O.A. 1959. The culture of mature organs in synthetic medium. *Experimental Cell Research* 16:118–147.

Vernon, R.G. 1979. Metabolism of adipose tissue in tissue culture. *International Journal of Biochemistry* 10:57–60.

Vierck, J., Byrne, K.M., and Dodson, M.V., with technical assistance from L. Krabbenhoft and Y. Chen. 2001. Assessing dot and western blots through the use of image analysis and pixel quantification of electronic images. *Methods in Cell Science* 23(4):313–318.

Vierck, J., McNamara, J.P., and Dodson, M.V., with technical assistance from B.D. Mathison. 1996. Proliferation and differentiation of progeny of ovine unilocular fat cells (adipofibroblasts). In *Vitro Cellular and Developmental Biology* 32(10):564–572.

Vierck, J., McNamara, J., Hossner, K., and Dodson, M.V. 1995. Characterization of ovine skeletal muscle satellite cell strains in a defined culture medium formulated to enhance differentiation: fusion and the IGF-I system. *Basic and Applied Myology* 5(1):12–21.

Wainwright, B.J. 1993. The isolation of disease genes by positional cloning. *Medical Journal Australia* 159:170–174.

Wang, A., Johnson, D.G., and MacLeod, M. 2001b. Molecular cloning and characterization of a novel mouse epidermal differentiation gene and its promoter. *Genomics* 73:284–290.

Wang, Q., Green, R.P., Zhao, G., and Ornitz, D.M. 2001a. Differential regulation of endochondral bone growth and joint development by FGFR1 and FGFR3 tyrosine kinase domains. *Development* 128:3867–3876.

Watt, F.M. 2001. Stem cell fate and patterning in mammalian epidermis. *Current Opinion in Genetics and Development* 11:410–417.

Weinberg, R.A. 1991. Tumor suppressor genes. *Science* 254:1138–1145.

Wines, M.E., Lee, L., Katari, M.S., Zhang, L., DeRossi, C., Shi, Y., Perkins, S., Feldman, M., McCombie, W.R., and Holdener, B.C. 2001. Identification of mesoderm development (mesd) candidate genes by comparative mapping and genome sequence analysis. *Genomics* 72:88–98.

Yalow, R.S. 1977. Radioimmunoassay: A probe for fine structure of biologic systems. Nobel Lecture, 8 December 1977. From *Nobel Lectures* 1971–1980.

Yuwaraj, S., Ding, J.W., Liu, M., Marsden, P.A., and Levy, G.A. 2001. Genomic characterization, localization, and functional expression of FGL2, the human gene encoding fibroleukin: A novel human procoagulant. *Genomics* 71:330–338.

Zhou, H-X., and Shan, Y. 2001. Prediction of protein interaction sites from sequence profile and residue neighbor list. *Proteins: Structure, Function, and Genetics* 44:336–343.

Zimmerman, A.M., Vierck, J.L., O'Reilly, B.A., and Dodson, M.V. 2000. Formulation of a defined medium to maintain cell health and viability. *Methods in Cell Science* 22(1):43–49.

5
Hormones and Growth

Colin G. Scanes

Growth in livestock is under the control of multiple hormones. This chapter considers the following hormones: growth hormone (GH), insulin-like growth factors, corticosteroids, thyroid hormones, sex steroids, insulin, and other hormones (leptin, prolactin, and erythropoietin).

GROWTH HORMONE/ SOMATOTROPIN (GH)

A major pituitary hormone influencing growth is growth hormone (GH). The effects of GH on growth (bone, cartilage, and muscle) are mediated by insulin-like growth factor-I (IGF-I). IGF-I is produced predominantly by the liver but also locally. The hypothalamo-pituitary GH-IGF-I-growth axis is summarized in Figure 5.1.

The somatotropes of the anterior pituitary gland synthesize and release GH. The hypothalamus (within the central nervous system, CNS) controls the release and synthesis of GH by peptides (neurosecretory peptides or releasing hormones/factors). These are released from neurosecretory nerve terminals in the median eminence of the hypothalamus. The peptides are transported to the anterior pituitary gland through the hypophyseal portal blood vessels.

Hypothalamic Control of GH Secretion

The release of GH from the somatotropes is under the control of hypothalamic releasing hormones. This is summarized in Table 5.1. Immunocytochemistry has allowed the localization of GHRH and SRIF neurons in the hypothalamus of cattle and pigs (Leshin et al. 1994). See Figure 5.2 for the hypothalamic distribution of releasing factors that affect GH. Until recently, it appeared that two hypothalamic peptides were the releasing hormones for GH. These are growth hormone releasing hormone (GHRH), which stimulates GH release, and somato-statin (SRIF), which inhibits the release of GH. Recently, the natural ligand for the GH secretagogue receptor (GHS-R) was identified as ghrelin (Kojima et al. 1999). This appears to be another hypothalamic releasing hormone for GH. Moreover, other factors influence GH release (see Table 5.2). For instance, thyrotropin releasing hormone (TRH) stimulates GH release in some species, at least under some physiological circumstances.

There is a balance between stimulatory and inhibitory hypothalamic inputs to GH release. Evidence for this between stimulatory and inhibitory control in livestock comes from hypophysial stalk sectioning in pigs. This results in reduced GH in the pituitary and increased responsiveness to GHRH (Anderson et al. 1991). The reduced pituitary GH probably reflects lack of stimulation of GH synthesis by GHRH. The increased responsiveness to GHRH reflects removal of the inhibitory effects of endogenous SRIF.

Episodic GH Secretion

Episodic release of GH has been observed in all species examined (reviewed, e.g., Shaffer Tannenbaum and Epelbaum 1999). Pulse intervals are between one to four hours with the following frequencies reported: ~0.2 pulses/hr in cattle (Ohlson et al. 1981), 0.66 pulses/hr in cattle (Wheaton et al. 1986), 0.4–0.9 pulses/hr in chickens (e.g. Johnson, 1988) 0.4–0.5 pulses/hr in pigs (Dubreuil et al. 1988), 0.3–0.4 pulses/hr in sheep (Dodson et al. 1983; Klindt et al. 1985) and 0.3–0.7 pulses/hr in turkeys (Bacon et al. 1989). Pulsatile GH release varies with species, age, genetics, and sex. The available evidence in rodent models suggests that GHRH and/or other GH secretagogues is primarily responsible for the peaks with SRIF responsible for the troughs (reviewed, e.g., Shaffer Tannenbaum and Epelbaum

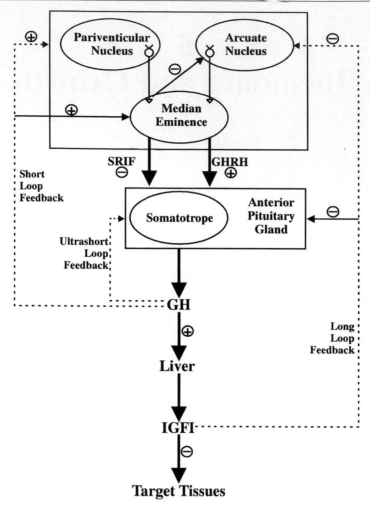

Figure 5.1. Schematic diagram of the hypothalamic-pituitary growth hormone/somatotropin (GH)-insulin-like growth factor-I (IGF-I) axis.

1999). The applicability of this to sheep is supported by increased "basal" or trough concentrations of GH receiving anti-SRIF (Varner et al. 1980). The relationship between GH pulses and hypothalamo-hypophyseal portal blood concentrations of GHRH and SRIF have been examined in conscious pigs. Secretory pulses of GH were associated with increasing GHRH and/or decreasing SRIF (Drisko et al. 1998).

Growth Hormone Releasing Hormone (GHRH)

Growth hormone releasing hormone (GHRH) is a polypeptide with 40–44 amino-acid residues with an N terminal amide (Figure 5.3). The major func-

tion of GHRH is to stimulate the release of GH from the somatotrope. Based on studies in primates and rodents, GHRH is expressed in the hypothalamus together with other tissues, including the gastrointestinal tract, gonads, immune tissues, and the placenta (reviewed Frohman and Kineman 1999). The function of GHRH outside the hypothalamic-pituitary axis is not fully understood. In domestic animals, GHRH is expressed in the placenta of sheep (Lacroix et al. 1996).

The *GHRH* gene consists of five exons (reviewed Frohman and Kineman 1999). This gene is a member of the glucagon/VIP gene family. GHRH is translated as preproGHRH (107/108 amino-acid residues). The C terminal signal peptide (30 amino-

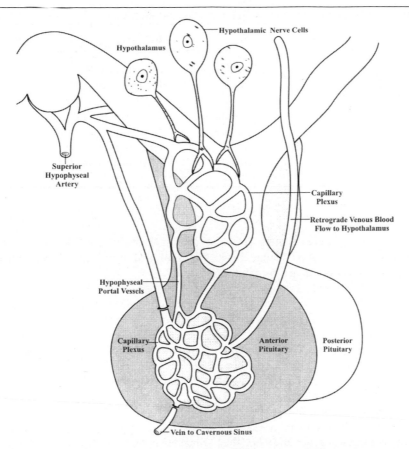

Figure 5.2. Schematic diagram of hypothalamic-pituitary axis showing neuroendocrine cells in the hypothalamus terminating on the hypophyseal portal blood vessels in the median eminence and hence transporting releasing hormones to the anterior pituitary gland.

Table 5.1. Hypothalamic peptides that influence the release of GH

Peptide Name	Structure	Stimulates⇑/ Inhibits⇓	Receptor	Species
Growth hormone releasing hormone (GHRH)	Polypeptide with 40–44 amino-acid residues [GHRH (1–44) amide]	⇑	GHRH receptor (GHRH-R)	All (but GHRH not isolated in birds yet)
Somatostatin (SRIF)	Polypeptide with 14 amino-acid residues (SRIF-14); SRIF-28 also exists	⇓	SRIF receptor (SRIF-R)	All
Ghrelin	Acylated peptide	⇑	GH secretagogue receptor (GHS-R)	All mammals examined
Thyrotropin releasing hormone (TRH)	Modified tripepeptide	⇑	TRH receptor (TRH-R)	Some

Table 5.2. Factors influencing release of GH in cattle and sheep

Factor	Species	GH	Level	Reference
GHRH	Sheep	⇑⇑⇑	Pituitary	Silverman et al., 1989
GHRH	Cattle	⇑⇑⇑	Pituitary	Plouzek et al., 1988
TRH	Sheep	⇒	-	Wrutniak et al., 1987
TRH	Cattle	⇑	Pituitary	Convey et al., 1973; Johke, 1978
SRIF	Sheep	⇓	Pituitary	Silverman et al., 1989
$PGF_{2\alpha}$	Cattle	⇑		Haynes et al., 1978
IGF-I	Sheep	⇓	Pituitary	Silverman et al., 1989
DES	Cattle	⇑		Martin et al., 1979

acid residues) is cleaved to yield pro-GHRH. The N terminal peptide (32 amino-acid residues) is cleaved, followed by amidation of the N-terminal amino-acid residue (reviewed Frohman and Kineman 1999).

The GHRH-receptor has been characterized by sequencing cDNA from the pig (Hsiung et al. 1993) together with human and rodent. The *GHRH-receptor* gene is a member of the calcitonin/parathyroid hormone/VIP/secretin receptor gene subfamily. As with the other members of the subfamily, the GHRH-R consists of an extracellular domain, seven transmembrane domains, and an intracellular G_s-binding domain (reviewed Frohman and Kineman 1999). The mechanism (signal transduction) for GHRH based on Frohman and Kineman (1999) involves the following steps:

1. GHRH binding to the GHRH-R, leading to the activation of the G_s-protein
2. The G_s-protein activating adenylate cyclase (isoform II and/or IV) and, hence, causing the synthesis of cyclic AMP (3',5'adenosine monophosphate) (cAMP)
3. cAMP activating protein kinase A
4. The catalytic subunit of protein kinase A phosphorylating the transcription factor, cAMP-response element binding protein (CREB) in the nucleus
5. CREB binding to cAMP-response elements (CRE) within the promoter regions of GH, GHRH-R, and Pit-1 genes to activate transcription

GHRH binding increases intracellular Ca^{++} concentrations (and thereby stimulating GH release) both by stimulating influx of Ca^{++} (via L- and T-type voltage sensitive Ca^{++} channels into the somatotrope and by phospholipase C hydrolysis of phosphatidyl inositol and hence mobilizing intracellular Ca^{++} stores.

The release of GHRH from the hypothalamic nerve terminals is under nervous control. The details of this are not well understood. The available evidence supports SRIF inhibiting GHRH release (reviewed, e.g., Shaffer Tannenbaum and Epelbaum 1999), but ghrelin/GH secretagogues stimulate GHRH release (see below).

Somatostatin (SRIF)

Somatostatin (SRIF) is a cyclic 14 or 28 amino-acid residue containing peptide (Figure 5.4). The structure of SRIF-14 is identical (see Figure 5.4) in all mammals and birds together with other vertebrates examined (reviewed Shaffer Tannenbaum and Epelbaum 1999). The gene encoding SRIF has been located to chromosome 1q23-q25 in cattle (Thue and Schutz 1995). The coding region of the gene has two exons. Upstream from the coding region are a variant TATA box, a CRE, and binding sites/promoters for both transcription factors and enhancers (reviewed Shaffer Tannenbaum and Epelbaum 1999). As is the case with GHRH, SRIF is translated as a preproform, which undergoes proteolyic cleavage to ultimately yield SRIF-14 or –28 (reviewed Shaffer Tannenbaum and Epelbaum 1999):

Pre-Pro-SRIF⇒Pro-SRIF (+ signal peptide) ⇒SRIF-28 (minor→SRIF-14) (pathway 1)

Or

Pre-Pro-SRIF⇒Pro-SRIF (+ signal peptide) ⇒ SRIF-14 (pathway 2)

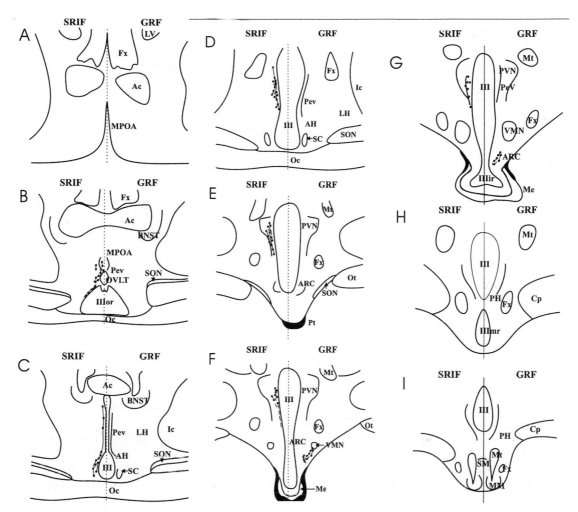

Figure 5.3. Hypothalamic distribution of releasing factors that affect GH release. Immunocytochemical localization of somatostatin (SRIF) and GHRH (GRF, growth hormone releasing factor) neurons in bovine hypothalamus (adapted from Leshin et al., 1994).

SRIF immunostaining depicted in the left section half and GHRH immunostaining depicted in the right section half. Letters (A–I) indicate representative sections anterior to posterior, with numbers indicating approximate distance (mm) from the first section (A). Circles indicate perikarya; fine lines indicate fibers. Ac = Anterior commissure; AH = anterior hypothalamus, ARC = arcuate nucleus; BNST = bed nucleus of stria terminalis; Cp = cerebral peduncle; Fx = fornix; Ic = internal capsule; LH = lateral hypothalamus; LS = lateral septum; LV = lateral ventricle; Me = median eminence; MM = medial mammillary nucleus; MPOA = medial preoptic area; MS = medial septum; Mt = mammilothalamic tract; Oc = optic chiasm; Ot = optic tract; OVLT = organum vasculism of the lamina terminalis; PH = posterior hypothalamus; Pt = pars tuberalis; PEV = periventricular nucleus; PVN = paraventricular nucleus; SC = suprachiasmatic nucleus; SM = supramammillary nucleus; SON = supraoptic nucleus; VMN = ventromedial nucleus; III = third ventricle; IIIir = infundibular recess of the third ventricle; IIImr = mammillary recess of the third ventricle; IIIor = optic recess of the third ventricle (redrawn from Frohman and Kineman, 1999).

Pathway 1 is found in the gastrointestinal tract because most of SRIF activity there is SRIF-28. Pathway 2 predominates in nervous tissue because 70% of SRIF is SRIF-14 (Benoit et al. 1987). Not only do multiple tissues synthesize SRIF, but there also are many effects of SRIF throughout the

Preprosomatostatin 1

```
        1          10        20        30        40        50
Human   ML SCRLQCALAAL.SIVLALGCVTGAPS DP RLRQFLQKSLAAAAGKQELAKY
Bovine  ML SCRLQCALAAL.SIVLALGGVTGAPS DP RLRQFLQKSLAAAAGKQELAKY
Rat     ML SCRLQCALAAL.CIVLALGGVTGAPS DP RLRQFLQKSLAAATGKQELAKY
Chicken ML SCRLQCALALL.SLA LAVGTVSA APS DP RLRQFLQKSLAAAAGKQELAKY

            60        70        80        90        100       110
Human   F LAELL.SEPN QTEN DALEP EDLSQAAEQDEM RLE LQRSANSNPA MAPRERKAGCKNFFWKTFTSC
Bovine  F LAELL.SEPN QTE I DALEP EDLSQAAEQDEM RLE LQRSANSNPA MAPRERKAGCKNFFWKTFTSC
Rat     F LAELL.SEPN QTEN DALEP EDLPQAAEQDEM RLE LQRSANSNPA MAPRERKAGCKNFFWKTFTSC
Chicken F LAELL.SEP S QTEN EALES EDLSRGAEQDE V RLE LERSANSNPA L APRERKAGCKNFFWKTFTSC
```

Figure 5.4. Structure of SRIF precursor.

animal. Somatostatin is produced by multiple cell-types (reviewed Tannenbaum and Epelbaum 1999), including hypothalamic cell bodies whose neurosecretory terminals release SRIF into the hypophyseal portal blood (and thus inhibiting release of GH and thyrotropin from the pituitary); cell bodies distributed widely in the brain (with effects on feeding, arousal, and sleep); D cells in the gastrointestinal tract (inhibiting release of gastric secretions) and pancreas (inhibiting release of insulin, glucagon, etc.); C-cells of thyroid (inhibiting release of thyroid hormones) and cells in the reproductive system (including gonads and placenta), kidneys, and adrenal medulla.

One of the major functions of SRIF is to inhibit the release but not synthesis of GH acting at the level of the pituitary gland (reviewed Shaffer Tannenbaum and Epelbaum 1999). In addition, SRIF acts at the level of the hypothalamus to inhibit release of GHRH.

The SRIF receptor (sst) is encoded by five different but intronless genes (*sst*1-5) (reviewed, e.g., Tannenbaum and Epelbaum 1999). Based on studies in the human, the dominant sst in the anterior pituitary gland is sst-5, and then sst-2. In the rat anterior pituitary gland, the major SRIF receptor type is sst-2 (Reed et al. 1999). The sst are members of the G-protein coupled superfamily of receptors in an extracellular domain, seven transmembrane domains, and an intracellular G-binding domain. Signal transduction for SRIF consists of binding to SRIF receptors (sst) and subsequently G-protein coupled reduction in L- and T-type voltage sensitive Ca^{++} influx/channels and increased K^+ channels

(reviewed, e.g., Shaffer Tannenbaum and Epelbaum 1999).

The release and synthesis of SRIF in the hypothalamus is under control by neurotransmitters and hormones. Neurotransmitters can either stimulate or inhibit SRIF release and synthesis. For instance, GABA inhibits SRIF release and synthesis, dopamine, neuropeptide Y, and noradrenergic agents stimulate SRIF release (reviewed, e.g., Shaffer Tannenbaum and Epelbaum 1999). SRIF appears to play a critical role in the feedback control of GH release, because both GH (short-loop feedback) and IGF-I/IGF-II (long-loop feedback) stimulate SRIF synthesis and release (reviewed Shaffer Tannenbaum and Epelbaum 1999).

GH Secretagogue (GHS)/Ghrelin

A series of synthetic peptides and non-peptide analogues have been found to stimulate the release of GH (reviewed Bowers 1999). The receptor (GHS-R) for the synthetic GH secretagogues (GHS) was characterized (Howard et al. 1996) before the identification of the natural endogenous ligand. Recently, this ligand for the GHS-R was characterized as an acylated peptide with 28 amino-acid residues, ghrelin (Kojima et al. 1999). The name *ghrelin* comes from the Proto-Indo-European word for "grow" (Kojima et al. 1999).

Ghrelin was first identified in the stomach where it affects gastric acid secretion and gut motility (Masuda et al. 2000). It has also been found in the small intestine and in the central nervous system, including the hypothalamus (Kojima et al. 1999; Lee et al. 2002). In addition to effects on GH release (direct effects on somatotropes and indirect via GHRH), ghrelin influences feed intake (Asakawa et al. 2001; Nakazato et al. 2001).

Ghrelin acts by binding to the GHS receptor (GHS-R). The GHS-R is a 7-transmembrane domain G-protein coupled receptor (Howard et al. 1996). The signal transduction mechanism involves

1. Binding to receptor
2. Activation of phospholipase C (via G-protein)
3. Hydrolysis of membrane phospholipid to generate inositol phosphate and diacyl glycerol
4. Increases in intracellular Ca++ (reviewed Bowers 1999)

There is evidence in domestic animals, as well as rodents, that ghrelin stimulates GH release both directly acting at the level of the anterior pituitary gland and by enhancing GHRH release. Administration of a presumed ghrelin agonist, the hexapeptide GH releasing peptide, to sheep enhanced both release of GH and portal blood concentrations of GHRH/release of GHRH (Guillaume et al. 1994). Moreover, another GHS, the non-peptidal secretagogue L-692,585, was observed to be much less effective in eliciting GH release in pigs where the hypophyseal stalk had been surgically cut/sectioned (hence drastically reducing GHRH and SRIF bathing the pituitary (Hickey et al. 1996).

Other GH Secretagogues (e.g., TRH)

The modified tripeptide, TRH, stimulates the release of thyrotropin (see section below). In addition, TRH stimulates the release of GH. However, this effect is seen only in some species and under some, but not all, physiological conditions. For instance, TRH stimulates GH release in cattle (Convey et al. 1973; Johke 1978) and young chickens (Harvey et al. 1978a), but has little effect in sheep (Wrutniak et al. 1987).

Neurotransmitters/Neuropeptides

Neurotransmitters/neuropeptides also influence GH secretion acting at the level of the hypothalamus. For instance, there is evidence for endogenous opioids influencing GH secretion based on effects of morphine administration; morphine increases GH secretion in pigs (Barb et al. 1992a), but decreases release of GH in chickens (Harvey and Scanes 1987). Studies in the chicken show respectively marked decreases and increases in circulating concentrations of GH with pharmacological agents that inhibit the synthesis or release or receptor binding

of norepinephrine (Buonomo et al. 1984) or serotonin (Rabii et al. 1981). This is consistent with noradrenergic and serotonergic innervation of the putative GHRH and/or SRIF neurons.

Nutrients and GH Secretion

There are profound effects of nutritional status, nutrients, and metabolites on GH secretion in domestic animals. There are, however, marked differences in both the magnitude and even direction of the responses between different domestic animals. This is summarized in, respectively, Table 5.3 for cattle and sheep, Table 5.4 for pigs, and Table 5.5 for chickens. Nutritional status influences GH secretion via the hypothalamus.

Peripheral Hormones and GH Secretion (Feedback Control)

Peripheral hormones affect the rate of release of GH. This can be negative feedback control, as is the case with IGF-I. A direct effect of IGF-I on the pituitary gland is supported by inhibition of GH release by IGF-I in vitro in fetal and neonatal sheep (Blanchard et al. 1988) and in chickens (Perez et al. 1987), and in vivo studies in chickens (Buonomo et al. 1987). An inhibitory effect at the level of the hypothalamus is also likely (discussed in the section "Somatostatin (SRIF)," above).

In contrast to the situation in rodents, thyroid hormones inhibit GH secretion in poultry due to reduced responsiveness to secretagogues (e.g., Scanes and Harvey 1989) and decreased GH synthesis/expression (Radecki et al. 1994). Similarly, GH expression by bovine somatotropes is reduced by either triiodothyronine (T_3) or the glucocorticoid, dexamethasone (Silverman et al. 1988).

Somatotropes

Growth hormone is synthesized and released from the somatotropes in the anterior pituitary gland. Other tissues also synthesize GH including mammary gland (progesterone-treated dog) and eye (chick embryo).

Somatotropes undergo differentiation and proliferation. The genesis of the somatotropes (GH producing cells) involves the following:

- Formation of Rathke's pouch, an invagination of the oral ectoderm, which makes contact with the overlying neural epithelium (reviewed Dasen et al. 1999; Scully and Rosenfeld 2002). These cells will form adenohypophysial cells, which will ultimately go on to form the anterior pituitary gland (pars

Table 5.3. Nutritional factors influencing release of GH in ruminants

Factor	Species	GH	Level	Reference
Fasting	Cattle	⇓	Hypothalamic	Rule et al., 1985
Feeding	Sheep	⇓	Hypothalamic	Bassett, 1974
Feeding	Cattle	⇓	Hypothalamic	Vasilatos and Wangsness, 1980
Fat (infusion)	Sheep	⇓	Hypothalamic	Estienne et al., 1990
Agents that depress FFA	Sheep	⇑	Hypothalamic	Hertelendy and Kipnis, 1973
Butyrate (infusion)	Sheep	⇓	Hypothalamic	Hertelendy et al., 1969
Glucose infusion	Cattle	⇑?	Hypothalamic	Sartin et al., 1985a
Propionate (infusion)	Cattle	⇑	Hypothalamic	Sartin et al., 1985b
Low protein diets	Cattle	⇑	Hypothalamic	Martin et al., 1979
Arginine (infusion)	Sheep	⇑⇑⇑	Hypothalamic	Hertelendy et al., 1969
Arginine (infusion)	Cattle	⇑	Hypothalamic	McAtee and Trenkle, 1971

Table 5.4. Factors influencing release of GH in pigs

Factor	GH	Level	Reference
Fasting	⇑	Hypothalamic?	Machlin et al., 1968; Buonomo et al., 1988
Insulin	⇑[1]	Hypothalamic?	Machlin et al., 1968; Bonneau, 1993
Arginine	⇑	Hypothalamic	Atinmo et al., 1978; Wangsness et al., 1977; Anderson et al., 1991
Glucose	⇑[2]	Hypothalamic?	Machlin et al., 1968; Wangsness et al., 1977
Free fatty acids	⇑[3]⇓	Hypothalamic?	Barb et al., 1991
Streptozotocin induced diabetes GH	⇑[4]	Hypothalamic?	Barb et al., 1992b

[1]In Yorkshires, but not Meishans (Bonneau 1993).
[2]Delayed increase observed lean or commercial lines, but no effect in obese line of pigs.
[3]Sensitivity to GHRH reduced, but basal pulse amplitude increased.
[4]Increased pulse frequency and amplitude.

Table 5.5. Factors influencing release of GH in chickens

Factor	GH	Level	Reference
Fasting	⇑	Hypothalamic?	Harvey et al., 1978b
Chronic nutritional (e.g., calorie and/or protein) deprivation	⇑	Hypothalamic?	Engster et al., 1979; Scanes et al., 1981
Insulin	⇓	Hypothalamic?	Harvey et al., 1978b
Glucose	⇑	Hypothalamic?	Harvey et al., 1978b
Epinephrine	⇓	Hypothalamic?	Harvey and Scanes, 1978

distalis) and intermediate lobe (pars intermedia). Cell-cell contact between the oral ectoderm and the ventral diencephalon neural epithelium is required for differentiation. Pituitary development involves signaling by growth factors [bone morphogenic factors (BMF), fibroblast growth factor 10 (FGF10), and *Wnt* gene family products [from the developing brain (ventral diencephalon) and Sonic hedgehog (Shh) from the oral ectoderm] (reviewed Scully and Rosenfeld 2002).

- Growth factors are intimately involved in the organogenesis of the pituitary gland. BMP4 is required for the initial phase of organ commitment, with BMP2 and FGF8 gradients affecting development of cell phenotype (reviewed Dasen et al. 1999; Scully and Rosenfeld 2002).
- Pit-1 is the critical pituitary-specific POU-1 domain DNA binding factor that induces differentiation of somatotrophs, lactotrophs, and thyrotrophs and is essential for the expression of GH, prolactin, and the β-subunit of TSH.
- Pit-1 expression is initially activated by PROP-1 (Prophet of Pit-1) (Sornson et al. 1996).
- Proliferation of somatotrophs is stimulated by GHRH (Billestrup et al. 1986).
- Proliferation/differentiation of somatotrophs can also be stimulated by glucocorticoids based on studies with chicken embryos (e.g., Porter and Dean 2001; Porter et al. 2001).

There is information on Pit-1 in domestic animals. DNA sequences for Pit-1 for cattle and pigs have been reported (reviewed Tuggle and Trenkle 1996). Alternative splicing can give different forms of Pit-1. There is also genomic variation in Pit-1 with Pit-1 alleles associated with growth and fatness in pigs (Yu et al. 1999). Several distinct Pit-1 sequences are found in the anterior pituitary of the chicken and turkey (Wong et al. 1992; Kurima et al. 1998; Tanaka et al. 1999; Van As et al. 2000). Expression of Pit-1 is first detected on day 5 of incubation in the chicken (Van As et al. 2000) prior to the first reported observation of the development/differentiation of lactotrophs (Jozsa et al. 1979). During development and at other physiological phases, there are cells that synthesize both GH and prolactin. These are the somatomammotropes.

GH Gene

There is a single gene for GH, both in rodents (reviewed Cooke and Liebhaber 1999) and in all domestic animals examined. In contrast, in the human, there are five GH genes; one expressed in the pituitary

gland and four in the placenta (reviewed Cooke and Liebhaber 1999). Knowledge of the GH gene stems largely from studies in the human and rat. The coding region consists of five exons. In addition, upstream there is a CRE and binding site(s) for the trans-acting factor, Pit-1 (reviewed Cooke and Liebhaber 1999). In view of the presence of CRE upstream from the coding region of the GH gene and the cAMP signal transduction mechanism of GHRH, it is not surprising that GHRH increases GH expression by somatotropes (cattle: Silverman et al. 1988; chickens: Vasilatos-Younken et al. 1992; Radecki et al. 1994).

Predominantly, pituitary expression of GH yields a single mRNA. In the human pituitary gland, there is alternatively spliced GH mRNA, which on translation produces 20K Da GH (reviewed Cooke and Liebhaber 1999). There is also evidence for alternative splicing of GH with different translational products in the bovine pituitary gland (Hampson et al. 1987) and the chick eye (Takeuchi et al. 2001).

Genetics and GH

A polymorphism exists in exon V of the bovine GH gene (Lucy et al. 1991, 1993). This results in the expression of the GH with either leucine or valine at position 127. In New Zealand sheep, variation on the number of GH genes have been reported. Some sheep are homozygous, having a single GH gene at the GH allele (oGH-N). Some are homozygous for two GH genes separated by 3.5 Kb at the GH allele (oGH-Z); Other are heterozygous (Valinsky et al. 1990; Gootwine et al. 1993; Fleming et al. 1997). Lean sheep with the oGH-N allele have higher pituitary contents than those with oGH-Z alletes, but no difference in body weight is apparent (Fleming et al. 1997). A positive correlation has been reported for the GH secretory response to GHRH and postweaning growth (Auchtung et al. 2001a, 2001b).

GH Structure

The crystal structure of porcine GH has been established by X-ray crystallography (Abdel-Meguid et al. 1987); there are four helical domains arranged in an anti-parallel manner. Moreover, GH has two distinct binding sites (Cunningham et al. 1991). Site-specific mutations in binding 2 have enabled the design and construction of specific antagonists to bovine and other GH (e.g., Chen et al. 1990).

GH Isoforms (Post-Translational Variants)

There is substantial evidence that GH can undergo post-translational modification. This includes glycosylation (e.g., chicken: Berghman et al. 1987), phosphorylation (sheep: Liberti et al. 1985; chicken: Aramburo et al. 1992), dimerization/oligomerization (e.g., chicken: Houston and Goddard 1988; Aramburo et al. 2000), and proteolytic cleavage (e.g., chicken Arámburo et al. 2001). The physiological significance of post-translational modification is not well understood. It is possible that modification may represent degradation pathway(s). Alternatively, post-translational variants may be secreted and may have biological activities distinct from that of unmodified GH. There is evidence that a cleaved product of chicken GH is angiogenic (Arámburo et al. 2001).

GH Receptors

The GH receptor is a member of the class I of the cytokine receptor superfamily (see Figure 5.5) (reviewed, e.g., Finidori and Kelly 1995; Waters 1999). Cytokine receptors do not contain a tyrosine kinase but are closely associated with a member of the Janus Kinase (JAK) family, which in turn activates specific transcription factors, signal transducers, and activators of transcription (STATs).

Transcription of GHR Gene

There are two GHR mRNAs. These result from alternative splicing and initiation of transcription from promoters 1 and 2. These transcribe, respectively, GHR 1A and GHR 1B (cattle: Heap et al. 1996; pigs: Liu et al. 1999, 2000). Expression of mRNA for GHR 1A is restricted to the liver and is developmentally controlled, not occurring until postweaning. In contrast, mRNA for GHR 1B is found in multiple tissues and in early and later stages of postnatal development (Liu et al. 2000).

Regulation of GHR

GHR expression is autoregulated. The total number of GHR (both occupied and unoccupied) in the liver is affected by GH status. In some species, GHR is up-regulated by GH (GHR number, sheep: Sauerwein et al. 1991); GHR number and mRNA, pigs: Chung and Etherton 1980; Brameld et al. 1996). In other species, GHR is down-regulated by GH (GHR number, chicken: Vanderpooten et al. 1991). Other factors/hormones also influence GHR/expression. Fetal mammals are poorly respon-

---

Classes of Cytokine Receptors

Class I includes:
   Receptors for IL-1, IL-3, IL-4, IL-5, IL-6, IL-7, IL-9, IL-11, IL-12, IL-13, IL-15,
granulocyte colony-stimulating factor (G-CSF), granulocyte/macrophage-stimulating factor (GM-CSF),
LIF, CNTF, EPO, GH and PRL

Class II
   Receptors for IL-10, IFNα/β, IFNγ

Ligand binding leads to receptor homo- or heterodimerization
Homodimers
   Receptors for: GH, PRL, EPO, G-CSF

Heterodimers
   Other members of the heterodimeric receptor cytokine complex, involving gp 130 module in the case of the receptors for IL-6, LIF, CNTF, and IL-11 and the gp 190 molecules for LIF and CNTF.

Receptor associated with member of JAK family of tyrosine kinases
JAK1	LIF, CNTF, IL-2, IL-4, IL-7, IL-9
	IFNα/β, IFNγ
JAK2	IFNγ, EPO, GH, PRL, IL-3, IL-5, IL-6, LIF, CNTF
JAK3	IL-2, IL-4, IL-7, IL-9
Tyk2	IFNα/β, IL-6, LIF, CNTF, IL-12

Figure 5.5. The cytokine receptor gene family (based on Finidori and Kelly, 1995)

sive to GII due to the low numbers of GHR. In sheep, GHR numbers markedly increase at birth (Breier et al. 1994). This is due to parturition-related factors, possibly the hypothalamic-pituitary adrenal axis.

Growth Hormone Receptor Mutations

Mutations in the GHR gene exist in domestic animals as in Laron dwarfism in humans. Both the sex-linked dwarf chicken and a line of miniature *Bos indicus* cattle have such mutations. Growth rate is reduced in the sex-linked dwarf chicken (e.g., Scanes et al. 1983). This is not due to an absence of GH; sex-linked dwarf chickens have elevated circulating concentrations of GH (Scanes et al. 1983) (see Table 5.6) and show little response to exogenous GH (Marsh et al. 1984a). The dwarfism is associated with low circulating concentrations of IGF-I (see Table 5.6) (Huybrechts et al. 1985) and with nonexistent/very low expression of GHR (Leung et al. 1987; Vanderpooten et al. 1991). This is due to a mutation in an intron immediately downstream from a cleavage site leading to inappropriate splicing and destabilization of the full length transcript (Burnside et al. 1991, 1992; Huang et al. 1993). There are also low circulating concentrations of T_3 (hypotriodothyronemia) (Scanes et al. 1983) due to the absence of GH-stimulated hepatic monodiiodination of T_4 (Berghman et al. 1989). Administration of T_3 or thyroxine (T_4) or IGF-I can partially restore growth rate in sex-linked chickens (Marsh et al. 1984b; Tixier-Boichard et al. 1992).

A line of miniature Brahman cattle exhibits similar characteristics with reduced growth, circulating concentrations of IGF-I together with hepatic IGF-I mRNA expression and elevated circulating concentrations of GH (Hammond et al. 1991; Liu et al. 1999) (see Table 5.6). This is due to aberrantly low expression of GHR 1A but not GHR1B in the liver (Liu et al. 1999) (see Table 5.6). It is probable that miniature cattle have a mutation in a critical promoter for GHR 1A.

Signal Transduction Pathways of GH

The mechanism of action of GH is summarized in Figure 5.6. The mechanism involves the following: GH binding to two GHR molecules, GHR dimerization, activation of JAK2, phosphorylation of a Stat (Stat6), and expression of specific genes. The GHR dimerization brings two JAK2 molecules together and allows transphosphorylation.

GH and Growth

In postnatal animals, GH is required for the full expression of growth. Table 5.7 summarizes observed effects of surgical removal of the pituitary (hypophysectomy) on growth in livestock and poultry. The major pituitary hormone required for growth is GH (reviewed, e.g., Scanes 1992).

GH and Growth—Mediation by IGF-I

The concept that a circulating factor mediated the effects of GH on growth of cartilage was initially proposed in 1957 (Salmon and Daughaday 1957). This became known as the "Daughaday hypothesis." The circulating factor was initially called sulfation factor but was later identified as insulin-like growth factor-I (IGF-I) (reviewed Hintz 1999). Although the liver is the major source of IGF-I in the circulation, IGF-I is also produced locally by cells, including muscle and cartilage, where IGF-I can exert both autocrine and paracrine effects. This is the "dual effector" theory (reviewed Ohlsson et al. 1999). The major hormone controlling IGF-I expression is GH. Direct evidence of GH stimulating IGF-I production also carries from in vitro studies with cultured chick hepatocytes (Houston and O'Neill, 1991). Moreover, hypophysectomy reduces circulating concentrations of IGF-I in domestic animals (Table 5.7) as well as rodents (reviewed Hintz, 1999). Administration of GH can restore IGF-I levels. There is considerable evidence that GH increases IGF-I in domestic animals (see the section "GH and IGF-I," below).

GH and Growth in Pigs

The administration of GH increases the growth rate of pigs (see Table 5.8); the percentage increases in average daily gain (ADG) are 14.7% (Machlin 1972), 9.9% (Chung et al. 1985), 11.1% (Etherton et al. 1986), and 16.7% (Campbell et al. 1988). Accompanying the increased ADG are improved feed:gain conversion ratios (see Table 5.9). These improvements to performance range from 3.7–23.7% (Machlin 1972; Chung et al. 1985; Etherton et al. 1986; Campbell et al. 1988). Either pituitary derived porcine GH (pGH) or recombinant pGH are effective in improving ADG and feed:gain efficiency (McLaren et al. 1990). Moreover, there are also improvements in carcass composition including reduced fat and increased protein with GH administration (see Table 5.8 for examples). Adverse effects of pGH treatment were reported in early studies. which used very high doses of pGH

Biology of Growth of Domestic Animals

Table 5.6. Endocrine parameters in GHR-deficient dwarf chickens and cattle

	Control		GHR-Deficient Dwarf (% Control)	Reference
A. Sex-linked dwarf male chickens				
GH ng/ml (throughout growth)	90	*	121 (134%)	Scanes et al., 1983
IGF-I (6 weeeks)	1.34	*	0.50 (37%)	Huybrechts et al., 1985
T_3 (ng/ml) (throughout growth)	1.63	*	0.58 (36%)	Scanes et al., 1983
T_4	18.0	NS	19.7 (109%)	Scanes et al., 1983
18-week-old (~adult) body weight (kg)	1.43	*	0.9 (64%)	Scanes et al., 1983
18-week-old size—shank toe (mm)	87	*	59 (68%)	Scanes et al., 1983
Liver—GH binding	2.94	*	0.40 (14%)	Leung et al., 1987
B. Miniature Brahman cattle				
GH (calf) ng/ml	6.2	*	38 (613%)	Hammond et al., 1991
IGF-I (calf) ng/ml	209	*	35 (17%)	Hammond et al., 1991
T_3 (calf) ng/ml	2.5	*	1.8 (72%)	Hammond et al., 1991
T_4 (calf) ng/ml	89	*	56 (63%)	Hammond et al., 1991
Adult body weight kg	472	*	314 (67%)	Chase et al., 1998
Adult size (hip height) meters	1.41	*	1.16 (82%)	Chase et al., 1998
Hepatic IGF-I mRNA (arbitary units)	0.26	*	0.03 (12%)	Liu et al., 1999
Hepatic GHR mRNA (arbitary units)	4.85	*	0.83 (17%)	Liu et al., 1999
Hepatic GHR 1A (arbitary units)	0.53	*	0.10 (19%)	Liu et al., 1999
Hepatic GHR 1B (arbitary units)	0.91	NS	0.97	

*$p<0.01$.
NS = Nonsignificant.

(Machlin 1972). A comprehensive study compared different doses of pituitary and recombinant pGH. No effects on "soundness" were observed (McLaren et al. 1990).

GH and Adipose Growth

The administration of GH reduces carcass fat and lipid accretion in pigs (e.g., Etherton et al. 1986; Campbell et al. 1988, 1989) (see Tables 5.8 and 5.10). Among the specific effects of GH on porcine adipose tissue are reduced or complete suppressed insulin induced lipogenesis (fatty acid synthesis) (Walton and Etherton 1986; Walton et al. 1986) and down-regulating fatty acid synthase (Donkin et al. 1996). There is no effect of GH in lipolysis in vitro (Walton and Etherton 1986) and on circulating concentrations of free fatty acids (Chung et al. 1985). In vitro studies also indicate that GH can inhibit both proliferation and differentiation of preadipocytes (Gerfault et al. 1999). As might be expected, GH influences adipocyte size. Chronically, GH reduced adipocyte volume: vehicle 4.2, GH injected for 10 weeks 1.9 ($p<0.001$) (Lee et al. 1994).

GH and Protein Metabolism

Both carcass protein and accretion are increased with GH treatment in pigs (Tables 5.8, 5.10, and 5.11). The effect of GH requires adequate nutrition with protein level and limiting amino acids (e.g., lysine) being particularly critical. For instance, GH had no effect on protein accretion with a low protein diet (9 g lysine per day). However, at approximately 22–23 g lysine per day, GH increased protein accretion by 42% (Krick et al. 1993) (also see Table 5.11).

GH and Carbohydrate Metabolism

Chronic administration of GH increases circulating of glucose and insulin (Chung et al. 1985; Gopinath and Etherton 1989a). The insulin response to glucose is greater following GH treatment (Gopinath

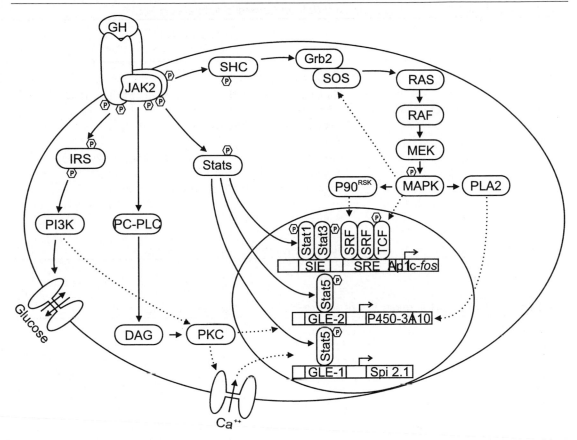

Figure 5.6. Signal transduction pathways of GH (adapted from Arzetsinger and Carter-Su, 1996).

and Etherton 1989b). On the other hand, the glucose response to insulin is reduced (Gopinath and Etherton 1989b).

GH and Appetite

In many—but not all—studies in which GH is administered to pigs, there are reductions in feed intake (e.g., observed reduced in Machlin, 1972 and Campbell et al., 1988, but not by Chung et al., 1985). Changes in carcass composition (Table 5.8) may reflect changes in nutrient availability as the result of feed intake differences and not GH effects on tissues per se.

GH and IGF-I

In pigs, in vivo administration of GH influences the expression of IGF-I and GHR in a manner dependent on both the tissue and the level of protein in the diet. There are increases in the expression of the fol-

lowing: IGF-I in the liver (independent of dietary protein), GHR in the liver (dependent on dietary protein), GHR in skeletal muscle, IGF-I in some but not all muscles, and IGF-I in adipose tissue (Brameld et al. 1996).

GH and Neonatal Growth

Growth of neonatal pigs is refractory to exogenous GH. Administration of GH did not influence growth of piglets (3 days–6 weeks) (Carroll et al. 1999). There were, however, increases in circulating concentrations of IGF-I and hepatic IGF-I mRNA (Carroll et al. 1999).

GH and Growth in Cattle

Exogenous GH can increase growth in cattle, but the effects are somewhat inconsistent. No effect of GH implants on ADG were observed in feedlot steers (Dalke et al. 1992) (see Table 5.12). In contrast, ADG

Table 5.7. Effect of hypophysectomy on growth in domestic animals

Species Growth	Hx (% Control)	Reference
Cattle	32%	Anderson, 1977
Pigs	30%	Ford and Anderson, 1967; Anderson et al., 1976, 1981
Sheep	58%	Young et al., 1989
Chickens	54%	King and Scanes, 1986; Scanes et al., 1986
Limb growth		
Pigs	74%	Ford and Anderson, 1967; Anderson et al., 1981
Sheep	46%	Young et al., 1989
Chickens	41%	King and Scanes, 1986; Scanes et al., 1986
Plasma IGF-I		
Pigs	16%	Ramsey et al., 1989
Sheep	21%	Young et al., 1989
Chickens	38%	Scanes et al., 1986

Table 5.8. Effect of GH administration[1] on growth in pigs and carcass quality

Parameter	Control		GH	Reference
Average daily gain (ADG)-kg	0.75	*	0.86	Machlin, 1972
ADG-kg	0.91	*	1.00	Chung et al., 1985
ADG-kg	0.90	*	1.00	Etherton et al., 1986
ADG-kg	0.90	*	1.05	Campbell et al., 1988
Carcass fat				
Back fat thickness (cm)	3.52	*	3.01	Machlin, 1972
Back fat thickness (cm)	2.7	NS	2.8	Chung et al., 1985
Average back fat thickness	22.7	*	17.3	Campbell et al., 1988
Ham fat content %	21.0	*	13.6	Machlin, 1972
Carcass adipose tissue (kg)	8.4		8.7	Chung et al., 1985
Carcass fat %	29	*	24	Etherton et al., 1986
Carcass fat %	28	*	20	Campbell et al., 1988
Carcass protein				
Loin-eye area (cm^2)	25.8	*	31.0	Machlin, 1972
Loin-eye area (cm^2)	18.6	NS	19.0	Chung et al., 1985
Carcass muscle mass (kg)	21.1	*	22.4	Chung et al., 1985
Carcass protein %	14.7	*	15.9	Etherton et al., 1986
Carcass protein %	14.5	*	16.1	Campbell et al., 1988
Carcass water %	34	*	58	Etherton et al., 1986
Carcass water %	54	*	59	Campbell et al., 1988

*$p<0.05$.
[1]In the studies of Machlin (1972), 0.13 mg pituitary derived porcine GH/kg body weight was injected intramuscularly (i.m.) daily between 46 and 94 kg body weight; in those of Chung et al., 22 µg pituitary derived porcine GH/kg body weight injected i.m. daily from 32 kg to ~60 kg; in those of Etherton et al., 30 µg pituitary derived porcine GH was injected daily i.m. from 50 kg to ~77 kg; and in those of Campbell et al., 22 µg/kg/day were injected i.m. between 25 and 58 kg body weight.
NS = Nonsignificant.

was increased in Hereford steers (10 months old) (GH injections for 112 days): vehicle 1.30 kg/d; bovine GH 1.50 kg/d (p<0.01) (Early et al. 1990a). Carcass weight or protein tended to increase, but fat tended to be decreased (Early et al. 1990b). Bovine GH (daily injections to 9-month-old Friesen steers) enhanced

Table 5.9. Effect of GH on feed:gain in pigs[1]

GH Dose	Control		GH	Δ as %	Reference
130	3.49	*	2.96	Δ15.2%	Machlin, 1972
22	2.7	*	2.6	Δ 3.7%	Chung et al., 1985
30	3.01	*	2.44	Δ18.9%	Etherton et al., 1986
22	2.57	*	1.96	Δ23.7%	Campbell et al., 1988
9 mg/pig/d[2]	3.75		2.70	-	McLaren et al., 1990
9 mg/pig/d[3]	3.75		2.91		McLaren et al., 1990

*Difference p<0.05.
[1]In the studies of Machlin, 0.13 mg pituitary derived porcine GH/kg body weight was injected intramuscularly (i.m.) daily between 46 and 94 kg body weight; in those of Chung et al., 22 μg pituitary derived porcine GH/kg body weight injected i.m. daily from 32 kg to ~60 kg; in those of Etherton et al., 30 μg pituitary derived porcine GH was injected daily i.m. from 50 kg to ~77 kg; and in those of Campbell et al., 22 μg/kg/day were injected i.m. between 25 and 58 kg body weight.
[2]Pituitary derived porcine GH.
[3]Recombinant porcine GH.

Table 5.10. Effect of GH administration[1] on the accretion (net synthesis) of protein and fat in the pig carcass (data from Campbell et al., 1988)

	Control		GH
Protein accretion	110	*	151
Fat accretion	283	*	193

*Difference p<0.05.
[1]Pituitary derived porcine GH was administered at a dose of 22 μg/kg/day i.m. for 3 days between 25 and 55 kg body weight.

Table 5.11. Influence of dietary protein on the ability of porcine GH to affect growth together with protein and lipid accretion in pigs (data from Campbell et al., 1990)

Protein in Diet	Average Daily Gain kg/d[1]		Protein Accretion g/d[1]		Lipid Accretion g/d[2]	
%	Vehicle	GH	Vehicle	GH[1]	Vehicle	GH[2]
8.3	0.60	0.58	72	71	234	186
11.4	0.71	0.75	108	111	208	175
14.5	0.76	0.91	122	152	210	162
17.6	0.87	1.00	144	166	200	133
20.7	0.79	1.01	146	173	192	123
23.8	0.87	1.00	139	174	182	98

[1]Significant effects (p<0.01): GH, protein, and interaction.
[2]Significant effect (p<0.01): GH.

ADG (vehicle 0.95 kg/d; GH 1.00 kg/d) and improved feed:gain efficiency (vehicle 1:7.9; GH 1:7.6) (Enright et al. 1990). Similarly, ADG is increased by ~8.5% in bovine GH treated veal calves (Kirchgessner et al. 1987). GH also repartitions nutrients with reduced fat and increased protein (Table 5.12).

GH and Protein Metabolism

Chronically, GH increases muscle gain (e.g., see Table 5.12). GH stimulates skeletal muscle development and carcass lean with larger muscles: longissimus (Dalke et al. 1992; Vann et al. 1998) and

Table 5.12. Effect of GH implants[1] on growth in feedlot performance in steers (data from Dalke et al., 1992)

	0	40	80	160 bGH mg/week	
Average daily gain (kg/d)	1.70	1.68	1.72	1.79	NS
Feed:gain	6.20	5.91	5.85	5.45	Linear, $p<0.01$
Hot carcass weight (kg)	331	331	336	337	NS
Backfat depth	1.40	1.37	1.38	1.13	Linear, $p<0.05$
Longissimus muscle area (cm²)	80.6	83.5	82.6	83.9	NS
9,10,11 rib protein %	14.0	14.7	14.6	15.3	Linear, $p<0.001$
9,10,11 rib fat %	39.5	37.4	35.8	34.8	Linear, $p<0.001$

[1]377 kg steers received GH via weekly implants for 12 weeks.
NS = Nonsignificant.

Table 5.13. Effect of GH on nitrogen metabolism of beef steers (data from Eisemann et al., 1989)

Parameter	Vehicle		bGH
Nitrogen metabolism			
Intake (g/d)	144		147
Fecal (g/d)	57		56
Urinary (g/d)	59	+	53
Retained (g/d)	29	*	38
Protein metabolism			
Leucine oxidation (μmol/min)	105	*	70
Whole-body protein synthesis (kg/d)	1.27	+	1.41
Whole-body protein degradation (kg/d)	1.11		1.18
Circulating urea (mM)	1.61	*	1.24

+$p<0.1$.
*$p<0.05$.

semitendinous (Vann et al. 2001), the latter with more fast twitch muscle fibers (Vann et al. 2001).

Exogenous GH also has a positive effect on nitrogen/protein metabolism. For instance, GH administration increased nitrogen retention in Holstein steers (Moseley et al. 1982), Hereford heifers (Eisemann et al. 1986a, 1986b), and Hereford x Angus steers (Eisemann et al. 1989) (Table 5.13). In growing Holstein heifers, there are dose-dependent increases in nitrogen retention and decreases in urinary nitrogen (Crooker et al. 1990) (Table 5.14). Circulating concentrations of urea nitrogen are decreased in heifers receiving GH (Crooker et al. 1990).

GH and Adipose Growth

Exogenous GH exerts some nutrient repartitioning effect of reducing adipose tissue in cattle. For instance, subcutaneous fat thickness has been reported to be decreased in finishing steers receiving GH injections (Dalke et al. 1992) (see Table 5.12). GH acts to reduce lipid accretion in adipose tissue (decreasing triglyceride synthesis and/or increasing breakdown of triglyceride).

It is assumed that GH has a similar effect in growing cattle as in adult cows and growing sheep (see the section "GH and Growth in Sheep," below), not directly affecting lipolysis but changing the

Table 5.14. Effect of GH on nitrogen retention and circulating concentrations of IGF-I in cattle (data from Crooker et al., 1990)

Parameter	Vehicle	GH(mg/kg)	
		33	100
Nitrogen retention (%)	26.7[a]	30.4[b]	31.1[b]
Serum IGF-I (ng/ml)	154[a]	217[b]	249[b]

[a,b]Different superscript letters indicate different p<0.05.

response to lipolytic or antilipolytic agents. In the lactating cow, GH increases the lipolytic response to β-adrenergic agonists (Sechen et al. 1990; Houseknecht et al. 1995a, 1995b; Houseknecht and Bauman 1997). In vitro GH does not affect basal lipolysis, but it reduces the inhibitory effects of adenosine (Lanna and Bauman 1999).

GH and Glucose Metabolism

GH exerts a diabetogenic effect, shifting glucose-insulin homeostasis in cattle. GH increases circulating concentrations of glucose (from 99.5 mg/dl to a maximum of 107.4 mg/dl) and tends to increase those of insulin (Crooker et al. 1990).

GH and IGF-I

The effect of GH on growth/protein metabolism is mediated by IGF-I. Administration of GH increases circulating concentrations of IGF-I in growing Holstein steers (Crooker et al. 1990) (Table 5.14).

GH and Growth in Sheep

Growth and performance of lambs is improved by GH administration (see Table 5.15). Treatment with GH increases ADG (Johnsson et al. 1987; Zainur et al. 1989; Beermann et al. 1990; Pell et al. 1990), feed:gain (e.g., Muir et al. 1983; Zainur et al. 1989), dressed carcass weight (Zainur et al. 1989), carcass protein (e.g., Muir et al. 1983), and nitrogen retention, with concomitant reductions in urinary nitrogen and plasma urea nitrogen (Beermann et al. 1991).

GH and Lipid Metabolism in Sheep

Accompanying the effects of GH on the growth/protein metabolism is reduction of carcass adipose tissue (Johnsson et al. 1987; Zainur et al. 1989; Beerman et al. 1990; Pell et al. 1990) (also see Table 5.15). Although GH is not per se lipolytic, it affects the response to lipolytic agents. In vitro GH per se

does not affect lipolysis by sheep adipose tissue (Duquette et al. 1984). In vivo concentrations of glycerol are elevated in the plasma of GH injected sheep [vehicle 205 μM, GH treated 268 μM (p<0.001)] and in an adipose tissue microdialysis perfusate [vehicle 55 μM, GH treated 76 μM (p<0.001) (Doris et al. 1996). Chronic administration of GH enhances the lipolytic response to the β-adrenergic agonist, isoproterenol by increasing β-adrenergic receptors and reducing the antilipolytic effect of adenosine (Doris et al. 1996).

GH and Carbohydrate Metabolism

Chronic administration of GH markedly affects glucose homeostasis (Table 5.15). Beerman and colleagues (1991) reported elevated plasma concentrations of both glucose and insulin in GH treated lambs [glucose: vehicle ~3.5 mmol/liter, GH treated ~4.3 (↑24%) mmol/liter (p<0.01); insulin: vehicle 1.13 mmol/l, GH treated 1.4 mmol/l (p<0.001)]. Thus, GH is diabetogenic, reducing tissue sensitivity to insulin.

GH and IGF-I in Sheep

It is reasonable to assume that GH exerts its effects on growth/protein metabolism via IGF-I. Certainly GH increases circulating concentrations of IGF-I in sheep (Beerman et al. 1990).

GH and Growth in Chickens

Exogenous GH does not stimulate growth in broiler chickens (reviewed Vasilatos-Younken et al. 1999). Studies in which chicken GH is administered between hatch and broiler market weight (~7 weeks), clearly show that GH does not influence growth rate or feed to gain efficiency. This is irrespective of whether the chicken GH was purified from pituitary glands, is recombinant, or is administered daily by a single injection (Burke et al. 1987; Peebles et al. 1988; Cogburn et al. 1989), as a con-

Table 5.15. Effect of GH on growth/performance in lambs (data from Zainur et al. 1989)

Parameter	Vehicle	GH(μg/kg/d) 50	150	250	
Average daily gain (g/d)	180	27 (21%)	238 (32%)	261 (45%)	Linear, $p<0.001$
Feed conversion	5.7	5.0	4.7	4.0	Linear, $p<0.001$
Carcass (kg)	14.4	16.4	16.6	16.8	Linear, $p<0.01$
Loin-eye area square (mm)	1352	1869	1500	1492	NS
Glucose homeostasis					
Plasma insulin (μU/ml)	44	58	92	224	Linear, $p<0.01$

Note: Recombinant bovine GH was injected for 60 days.
NS = Nonsignificant.

tinuous infusion, or in a pulsatile manner (Moellers and Cogburn, 1995). A transitory increase in growth was observed in one study (Leung et al. 1986).

In older chickens, administration of GH appears to have some stimulatory effect on growth rate. Pulsatile administration of GH intravenously (i.v.) between 8 and 11 weeks old increased ADG by 20.7% ($p<0.05$) (Table 5.16) (Vasilatos-Younken et al. 1988). Continuous administration of GH (via osmotic pump implanted subcutaneously) stimulated ADG between 12 and 15 weeks of age (Scanes et al. 1990) [vehicle 32 g/d, GH (50 μg/kg/d)—52.0 g/d ($p<0.05$)]. Growth is, however, not affected by either continuous administration of GH (8–11 weeks) (Vasilatos-Younken et al. 1988) or daily injections of GH between 8 and 12 weeks of age (Scanes et al. 1990).

Administration of chicken GH has no effect on feed:gain ratios in broiler-aged chickens (e.g., Burke et al. 1987). Combining the studies of Larry Cogburn's laboratory, identical feed efficiency is observed with control or GH treated broiler chickens: vehicle 1.65, GH 1.67 (Cogburn et al. 1989; Moellers and Cogburn 1995).

GH and Carcass Protein

Exogenous GH does not increase deposition of protein in muscle in chickens younger than about 11 weeks old. No increases (and in some cases, decreases) in carcass protein percentage and/or breast muscle weight were reported in broiler chickens receiving chicken GH as a daily injection (e.g., Burke et al. 1987; Cogburn et al. 1989) or continuous or pulsatile infusion (Moellers and Cogburn 1995). Similarly in 8–11-week-old chickens, neither continuous nor pulsatile infusion of GH increased

carcass protein or breast muscle weight (Vasilatos-Younken et al. 1988; Rosenbrough et al. 1991). In other studies of older chickens, GH did affect breast muscle weight (Scanes et al. 1990).

GH and Carcass Fat

GH does not reduce adipose tissue in broiler-aged chickens. Indeed in some studies, GH treated chickens had more adipose tissue (e.g., Cogburn et al. 1989). Intravenous infusions of recombinant chicken GH increased carcass fat 12.9% to 14.6% with continuous infusion and to 15.1% with pulsatile infusion (Moellers and Cogburn et al. 1989). In older chickens (8–11 weeks), the effect of GH on adiposity differed markedly with mode of administration. Pulsatile administration of GH reduced abdominal fat weight (Vasilatos-Younken et al. 1988, Rosebrough et al. 1991). There was no effect with either continuous infusion of GH (Vasilatos-Younken et al. 1988; Rosebrough et al. 1991) or daily injections of GH (Scanes et al. 1990). Infusion of GH to 12–15-week-old chickens increased abdominal fat-pad weight (Scanes et al. 1990).

GH and Lipid Metabolism

The effect of GH in adipose weight with pulsatile GH administration is explicable by an 81% decrease in hepatic lipogenesis (Rosebrough et al. 1991). Harvey and colleagues (1978) established that GH could suppress insulin-induced lipogenesis by chicken hepatic tissue in vitro. Although GH exerts a lipolytic effect with adipose tissue from adult chickens (Campbell and Scanes 1985; Campbell et al. 1995) and acutely in vivo (Scanes 1992), chronic administration of GH does not have a consistent effect on circulating concentrations of free fatty acids. For instance, circulating

Table 5.16. Effect of pulsatile administration of chicken GH on 4–7-week-old and 8–11-week-old chickens and turkeys (data from, respectively, Moellers and Cogburn 1995; Vasilatos-Younken et al. 1988; Bacon et al. 1995)

Parameter	4–7 Weeks Old Control		GH	8–11 Weeks Old Chicken Control		GH	Turkey Control		GH
Average daily gain (g)	77		84	34		41	107	NS	106
Feed:gain	1.70	*	1.93	4.3	*	3.2	2.44	NS	2.33
Carcass weight (kg)	-		-	1.90		1.78	3.99	NS	3.77
Carcass fat %	12.9	*	15.1	23.2		15.9	19.0	*	15.7
Carcass protein %	18.5	*	17.9	16.6		16.6	30.6	NS	30.3
Carcass water %	65.6	*	63.8	51.2		59.5	45.9	*	48.2
Breast muscle (g)	-		-	585		530	489	NS	468
Abdorant fat pad (g)	66		63	99		55	27*		8
Plasma FFA (μmoles/ml)	0.66		0.73	0.86		1.10	0.13	*	0.24
Plasma glucose (mg/dl)	266		281	212		229	253	NS	248
Plasma IGF-I (ng/ml)	191		196	51	*	92	8.81	NS	9.72
Plasma T$_4$ (ng/ml)	5.5	*	6.5	6.7	*	3.6	5.2	*	2.3
Plasma T$_3$ (ng/ml)	2.6		2.7	2.2		3.3	2.8	*	3.7
Hepatic GH receptor specific GH binding	8.8	*	4.2	-		-			

*$p<0.05$.
NS = Nonsignificant.

concentrations of free fatty acids are unaffected by GH (e.g., Vasilatos-Younken et al. 1988; Moellers and Cogburn 1995) or elevated by GH (Scanes et al. 1990)

GH and Carbohydrate Metabolism

There does not appear to be a diabetogenic effect of GH in chickens. Plasma concentrations of glucose are not affected acutely by GH (Scanes 1992). Similarly, chronic administration of GH does not influence circulating concentrations of glucose or insulin (Vasilatos-Younken et al. 1983; Cogburn et al. 1989; Moellers and Cogburn 1995).

GH and IGF-I

GH elevates IGF-I in chickens (reviewed McMurtry et al. 1997). Chronic administration of GH increases circulating concentrations of IGF-I even where no stimulation of growth was observed (Vasilatos-Younken et al. 1988; Moellers and Cogburn 1995). Moreover, the secretion of IGF-I from the liver is controlled by both GH and insulin based on in vitro studies (Houston and O'Neill 1991)

GH and Growth in Turkeys

Pulsatile administration of GH to turkeys does not affect growth (Bacon et al. 1995) (see Table 5.16). This is in contrast to the stimulation of growth rate and major increases in muscles and decreases in adipose tissue in turkeys receiving androgen treatment (reviewed Scanes 1999).

GH and Growth in Fish

Discussion of effects of GH on growth in meat animals is not complete without mention of effects of GH in fish. There is increasing interest in fish as a source of animal protein in diet due to health claims and to cost. The ability to raise fish by aquaculture or mariculture has the potential of increasing production efficiency while reducing pressure on fish populations. GH stimulates growth rate (see Table 5.17 for examples) markedly in salmon (e.g., Higgs et al. 1975; Down et al. 1988, 1989; McLean et al. 1990) and trout (e.g., Agellon et al. 1988; Schulte et al. 1989; Garber et al. 1995). Interactions with environment exist with no effect of GH on growth

Table 5.17. Effect of GH on growth in fish

Species	GH Effect as $\Delta\%$ Increase over Controls	Reference
A. *Rainbow trout*		
Trout (initial weight 2g)[1]		
Specific growth rate	132%	Schulte et al., 1989
Average daily gain[2] 0–14 days	44.8%	Garber et al., 1995
0–28 days	30.4%	Garber et al., 1995
B. *Coho salmon*		
Yearling (initial weight ~11g)		
Specific growth rate3	0107%	Higgs et al., 1975

[1]bGH injected alternate weeks.
[2]Single injection of bGH on day 0.
[3]bGH injected three times per week.

observed in trout reared at relatively warm temperatures (Danzmann et al. 1990). The future commercial application of GH in fish may involve either administration of GH in slow release forms or transgenic fish expressing high levels of GH. There is concern on the latter approach that transgenic fish might escape and adversely affect wild populations.

Other Actions

GH and Calcium Metabolism

There are changes in calcium metabolism with GH administration. The effects of GH are probably not secondary to GH induced increases in bone growth. Chronically, GH in growing pigs increases circulating concentrations of 1,25 dehydroxy vitamin D and phosphate, small intestine and kidney weights, and decreases the number of unoccupied 1,25 $(OH)_2$ vitamin D receptors in the kidney (Goff et al. 1990).

GH and Gastrointestinal Functioning

Growth hormone affects intestinal functioning. For instance in the pig, GH reduces pancreatic amylase while not affecting either pancreatic trypsin or chymotrypsin (Hibbard et al. 1992).

GH and Thyroid Hormones

The Leuven (Belgium) group of Decuypere, Kühn, and colleagues has demonstrated profound effects of GH on thyroid hormones. In chick embryos, GH increases circulating concentrations of T_3. This is due to increased conversion of T_4 to T_3 by 5 monodeiodination in the liver (Berghman et al. 1989;

Darras et al. 1990, 1993) and/or decreased inactivation of T_3 by hepatic type III monodeiodinase (Darras et al. 1993).

INSULIN-LIKE GROWTH FACTOR I (IGF-I)

The two insulin-like growth factors (IGFs) were initially purified from conditioned media or serum, with nonsuppressible insulin activity (active in the presence of antisera to insulin) being IGF-I and IGF-II. In subsequent studies, IGF-I was found to be identical to sulfation factor (reviewed Hintz 1999). Multiplication stimulating activity and IGF-II were synonomous (reviewed Lund 1999). In both mammals and birds, there are two IGFs: IGF-I and IGF-II.

IGF-I and IGF-II Genes/Chemistry

The *IGF-I* gene is complex with 6 exons and ~80 kilobases; the *IGF-II* gene contains 9 exons and ~30 kilobases (reviewed Lund 1999). The amino-acid sequences for IGF-I and II have been reported for domestic animals and foul (e.g., cattle: Francis et al. 1988; chickens: Dawe et al. 1988; Kajimoto and Rotwein 1989; Ballard et al. 1990; Upton et al. 1995).

Genetics and IGF-I

In cattle, although circulating concentrations of IGF-I are heritable, there is a negative correlation between these circulating concentrations and growth rate (Davis and Simmen 1997)

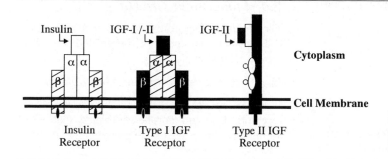

Figure 5.7. IGF and insulin receptors (adapted from Richman, 1999)

IGF-I and IGF-II Expression/ Translation

There is remarkable variation in the size of IGF-I mRNA due to alternative splicing. For instance in the rat liver, there are multiple IGF-I mRNA with sizes between 0.8 and 8 kilobases (reviewed Lund 1999). The IGF-I mRNA can be assigned to class 1 or 2 [based on 5'sequences (including part of the leader squence)] or Ea or Eb type [based on 3'sequences (including part of the E domain sequence)] (reviewed Lund 1999). Similarly, there are multiple forms of IGF-II mRNA.

The translational product (pre-pro-IGF-I) consists of the mature IGF-I with B, C, A, D domains together with an N-terminal leader sequence and a C-terminal E sequence (reviewed Lund 1999). A similar situation exists for IGF-II with pre-pro-IGF-II. The signal peptide is cleaved to yield pro-IGF-II.

IGF-I Expression

A major site of IGF-I production is the liver. In addition, multiple tissues synthesize IGF-I, including the developing muscle (e.g., in pigs, myoblasts—Hembree et al. 1996), cartilage (e.g., Burch et al. 1986), developing eye (Caldes et al. 1991; Zackenfels et al. 1995), etc. The role of GH in the control of IGF-I expression is discussed elsewhere (see above and below). In addition, there are binding sites in the promoter region for other transcription factors.

Structure of IGF-I and IGF-II

IGF-I is a peptide with 70 amino-acid residues in the B, C, A, and D coding regions/domains. It shows marked homology to IGF-II, which is a peptide with 67 amino-acid residues with the same domain structure (B, C, A, and D coding regions). This provides a ready explanation for the ability of IGF-II to evoke identical effects to IGF-I by binding to the IGF-IR, albeit with a lower potency/affinity in mammals. In addition, IGF-I and IGF-II show homology to proinsulin (reviewed Lund 1999). The ability of proinsulin/insulin to bind to the IGF-IR is also not surprising.

IGF-I Receptor (IGF-IR)

There are two insulin-like growth factor receptors in mammals; the IGF-I receptor (IGF-IR) and the IGF-II receptor (IGF-IIR). The IGF-IR is a transmembrane tyrosine kinase. With four subunits (two α and two β subunits) and substantial homology, the IGF-IR shows marked similarity to the insulin receptor (Figure 5.7). In mammals, the mannose-6-phosphate receptor is also the IGF-IIR.

Biology of IGF-I

There is strong evidence of the effectiveness of IGF-I in stimulating growth in rodent modents and either a physiological or transgenic/gene in "knockout" approaches. For instance with the former, IGF-I enhances growth of the GH deficient (and hence IGF-I deficient) Snell's dwarf mouse (e.g., van Buul-Offers et al. 1986) and hypothesized rats (Fiedler et al. 1996). There have been few physiological studies that demonstrate effects of IGF-I and II on growth in domestic animals except in growing chickens. Administration of IGF-I stimulates growth only in sex-linked dwarf chickens, but not in control line chickens (Tixier-Boichard et al. 1992).

In studies using chick embryos, IGF-I and/or IGF-II (presumably locally produced) have been shown to profoundly influence development. There are increases in the following

- Growth (Girbau et al. 1987)
- Fibroblast protein accretion (Cynober et al. 1985; Kallincos et al. 1990)

- Eye and neural development (Caldés et al. 1991; Zackenfels et al. 1995)
- Cell proliferation of preadipocytes (Butterwith and Goddard 1991), chondrocytes (Leach and Rosselet 1992), and heart mesenchymal cells (Balk et al. 1982)

IGF-I and Development

Postnatally, IGF-I is the mediator for GH's effects on growth. Prenatally, autonomous release of IGF-I (either endocrine or paracrine/autocrine) is important for growth. Chick embryo growth can be retarded by ex ovo incubation, and there is a concomitant absence of the mid-embryonic peak in circulating concentrations of IGF-I (Robcis et al. 1991).

IGF-I may be involved in growth of multiple tissues, including muscle cells (myocyte differentiation cell multiplication), cartilage (chondrocyte colony formation, sulfate uptake, alkaline phosphatase activity), bone (osteoblast division and proliferation), and hematopoietic cells (e.g., erythroid differentiation) (reviewed Zapf and Froesch 1999).

IGF-II and Growth

IGF-II is proposed as "the regulator of fetal growth in some species" (Richman 1999). The mitotic effects of IGF-II are mediated via the IGF-I receptor, and other actions of IGF-II are mediated via the type II IGF receptor/mannose-6-phosphate receptor.

IGF-I and IGF-II and Fetal Growth

There is a relationship between circulating concentrations of IGF-I or IGF-II and growth in the fetus. Placental development can be restricted by removal of uterine endometrial caruncles prior to mating. Under these circumstances, fetal growth is greatly impaired and there is a concomitant decline in both IGF-I and IGF-II in the fetal circulation (Owens et al. 1994). Fetal hypoxia for 24 hours similarly reduces the circulating concentrations of IGF-I (McLellan et al. 1992).

IGF-I and Muscle Growth

IGF-I and IGF-II stimulate muscle growth. Examples are considered under GH of effects of GH in domestic animals; these GH effects are mediated by IGF-I. In vitro studies have demonstrated that IGF-I can stimulate proliferation of muscle satellite cells from, for instance, chicken (Wilkie et al. 1995). In view of the proposed relationship between IGF-II and muscle development, the observed high level of IGF-II expression on fetal bovine muscle is expected (Listrat et al. 1994).

IGF-I and Antler Growth

The presence of specific receptors for IGF-I but not GH in antler tips supports a role for IGF-I in antler growth (Elliott et al. 1992).

IGF-I and Carbohydrate Metabolism

In view of the ability of IGF-I to bind to the insulin receptor, it should not be surprising that IGF-I administration induces hypoglycemia in pigs (Walton et al. 1989).

Controls on IGF-I and IGF-II Expression

Development and IGFs

There are profound changes of circulating concentrations of both IGF-I and IGF-II during growth and development. In mammals, circulating concentrations of IGF-II are very high during fetal development (sheep: e.g., Carr et al. 1995). Changes in plasma concentrations of IGF-I and IGF-II have also been determined during development in the chicken; IGF-I is high during mid–posthatch growth (Huybrechts et al. 1985; McGuinness and Cogburn 1990; McMurtry et al. 1994) but there are only relatively minor changes for IGF-II (Scanes et al. 1989, 1997).

Nutrition and IGFs

There are profound effects of inadequate nutrition on IGFs. These effects are frequently independent of pituitary GH secretion. Circulating concentrations of IGF-I and IGF-I mRNA expression are depressed in fasted or chronically nutritionally restricted animals and are increased upon refeeding (e.g., chickens: Lauterio and Scanes 1987; Rosebrough et al. 1989; pigs: Charlton et al. 1993; Dauncey et al. 1993). Similarly, circulating concentrations of IGF-I are reduced, for instance, in protein restricted chickens (Lauterio and Scanes 1987). Lambs on a restricted diet show reduced expression of IGF-I (Rhoads et al. 2000).

Hormones and IGF-I/II Expression

The major hormonal control of IGF-I expression is GH (see above). In addition, epidermal growth factor (EGF) may influence synthesis/release of IGF-I as administration of EGF in mini-pumps to pigs reduced the circulating concentrations of IGF-I (Vinter-Jensen et al. 1996). Expression of the *IGF-II* gene in the liver and skeletal muscle of fetal lambs is reduced by infusion of cortisol (F) (Li et al.

1993). Evidence that this is a physiological effect comes from the increase in IGF-II mRNA following adrenalectomy of the fetus (Li et al. 1993).

Environment and IGF-I

There are temperature/humidity effects on circulating concentrations of IGF-I in cattle (Sarko et al. 1994) and pigs (Dauncey et al. 1993).

Anesthesia and IGF-I

Anesthesia acutely reduces circulating concentrations of IGF-I in young lambs (Lord et al. 1994).

Insulin-Like Growth Factor Binding Proteins

Both IGF-I and IGF-II, in the circulation, are largely bound to IGF-binding proteins (IGFBP)—namely, IGFBP1-6 (see Table 5.18). IGFBP-2 has been isolated and its cDNA sequenced in cattle (Upton et al. 1990). IGFBP-3 has been isolated and characterized in pigs and sheep (Walton and Etherton 1989; Carr et al. 1994). IGFBP-4 has been isolated and its cDNA sequenced in sheep (Carr et al. 1994). IGFBP-3 is normally the most abundant IGFBP. Each IGFBP is the gene product of a specific gene. Protease exists in the plasma that specifically cleaves IGFBPs and particularly IGFBP-3. In the sheep, circulating concentrations of IGFBP-2, 3, and 4 increased during fetal development and fetal weight (Carr et al. 1995).

Role of IGFBPs

IGFBP-1–6 bind both IGF-I and II and, thereby, act to exert the following:

- Inhibits the action of IGFs/sequesters IGFs
- Prolongs the half-life of IGFs in the circulation
- Enhances the effectiveness of IGFs
- May allow different effects of IGFs to be manifest

In addition, the IGFBP may have inherent biological activity. These effects are explicable at least in the cases of IGFBP-1 and IGFBP-2 by their capability of associating with the surface of cells due to the presence of a cell membrane integrin-binding region (reviewed Shen et al. 2001). In addition, IGFBPs bind to the extracellular matrix and thereby bring IGFs in close proximity to specific cells where proliferation/differentiation is required during development. Binding either to the cell or extracellular matrix or IGF may protect the IGFBP from protease degradation.

There are numerous examples of IGFBPs binding either IGF-I or II and inhibiting the action of the IGF by sequestering the IGF. In the area of growth biology, IGF-I stimulation of growth in Snell dwarf mice is reduced in the presence of either IGFBP-3 or IGFBP-1 (van Buul-Offers et al. 1995, 2000). In domestic animals, IGFBP-3 has been shown to inhibit the effects of IGF-I on glucose metabolism by porcine adipose tissue (Walton and Etherton 1989) and on chick embryo fibroblasts (Blat et al. 1989).

There are examples of IGFBPs enhancing the activity of IGFs. The administration of IGFBP-1 with IGF-I enhances IGF-I's effectiveness in increasing growth of the spleen in Snell dwarf mice (van Buul-Offers et al. 2000). In domestic animals,

Table 5.18. The names of the members of the IGFBP superfamily (from Baxter et al., 1998)

Recommended Names	Previous Names
High-affinity IGFBPs	
IGFBP-1	PP12; pregnancy-associated endometrial alpha1-globulin; BP-28
IGFBP-2	
IGFBP-3	BP-53
IGFBP-4	
IGFBP-5	
IGFBP-6	
IGFBP-related proteins	
IGFBP-rP1	mac25, TAF, PSF
IGFBP-rP2	CTGF
IGFBP-rP3 (provisional)	nov
IGFBP-rP4 (provisional)	cyr61

IGFBP-3 enhances IGF-I induced proliferation of either porcine skin fibroblasts (Coleman and Etherton 1994) or bovine mammary epithelial cells (Romagnolo et al. 1994).

Evidence exists that IGFBPs have inherent biological activity. For instance, IGFBP-1 alone or bound to IGF-I evokes a similar increase in kidney growth in Snell dwarf mice (van Buul-Offers et al. 2000). Similarly, IGFBP-5 alone influences bone formation stimulating alkaline phosphatase activity and osteocalcin production by human osteoblasts in vitro and in mice in vivo (Richman et al. 1999).

IGFBP-3

IGFBP-3 is the GH dependent IGFBP (e.g., in pigs: Walton and Etherton 1989). The complex of IGF-I or IGF-II with IGFBP-3 is further bound to an 85-kDA acid-labile protein (ALP).

Acid-Labile Protein (ALP)

The complex of IGF-I or IGF-II with IGFBP-3 is further bound to an 85-kDA acid-labile protein (ALP).

$$IGF\text{-}I/II + IGFBP\text{-}3 + ALP \Rightarrow$$
$$IGF\text{-}I/II{\sim}IGFBP\text{-}3{\sim}ALP$$

The ALS is large glycoprotein (~578 amino acid residues) that stabilizes the circulating IGF-IGFBP-3 complex and hence extends its half-life (reviewed Clemmons 1999). The function of the ALP is not fully understood. Transgenic mice that are overexpressing ALP do not show changes in the circulating concentrations of IGF-I or IGFBP-3, but do exhibit a slight reduction in growth rate (Silha et al. 2001). Hepatic ALS expression is reduced in slow growing sheep fetuses (Rhoads et al. 2000).

Location of IGFBP Synthesis

Multiple tissues produce IGFBPs. For instance, IGFBP-3 is synthesized predominantly in the liver. IGFBP-2 is synthesized by porcine fibroblasts. Both IGFBP-2 and IGFBP-3 are synthesized by porcine myogenic/myoblast cells, with TGFβ-1 stimulating synthesis of IGFBP-3 but not IGFBP-2 (Hembree et al. 1996).

Control of IGFBPs

The synthesis and release of IBFBPs is influenced by factors such as nutrition, physiological conditions, and hormones. The following sections discuss these influences for each IGFBP.

Control of IGFBP-1

NUTRITION AND IGFBP-1. Nutritional state/fasting depresses fetal growth but increases circulating concentrations/expression of IGFBP-1. For instance, fasting pregnant sheep increases circulating concentrations of IGFBP-1 and hepatic expression of IGFBP-1 in the mother and, to a greater extent, in the fetus (Osborn et al. 1992). The change in IGFBP-1 expression is overcome by glucose infusion (Osborn et al. 1992). Similarly, fasting acutely increases circulating concentrations of IGFBP-1 in pigs (McCusker et al. 1985).

HYPOXIA AND IGFBP-1. Reducing fetal oxygen in fetal sheep availability increases both circulating concentrations of and expression in fetal liver of IGFBP-1 (McLellan et al. 1992). The effect of hypoxia on IGFBP-1 may be mediated by release of epinephrine (E) and norepinephrine (NE) (Hooper et al. 1994). In a perhaps analogous manner, halothane anesthesia increases IGFBP-1 in young lambs (Lord et al. 1994).

HORMONES AND IGFBP-1. Hormones influence IGFBP-1 expression. In fetal lambs, IGF-I increases IGFBP-1 and insulin decreases IGFBP-1 (Shen et al. 2001). Similarly, IGF-I stimulates release of IGFBP-1 from bovine fibroblasts (Conover 1990). This effect of IGF-I may provide the explanation for the reduction in circulating concentrations of IGFBP-1 following hypophysectomy in fetal pigs (lack of GH and hence of IGF-I) (Latimer et al. 1993). Thyroxine increases circulating concentrations of IGFBP-1 in hypophysectomized pig fetuses (Latimer et al. 1993). In addition, the catecholamines, E or NE, increase circulating concentration and hepatic expression of IGFBP-1 in fetal sheep (Hooper et al. 1994). Administration of EGF to pigs increases the circulating concentrations of IGFBP-1 (Vinter-Jensen et al. 1996).

Control of IGFBP-2

There appears to be an inverse relationship between the IGFBP-2 and growth rate, but this is not totally consistent.

HORMONES AND IGFBP-2. GH increases growth but decreases circulating concentrations of IGFB-2 in growing pigs (Coleman and Etherton 1991). In contrast, hypoxia (also depressing growth) decreases both the circulating concentrations of IGFBP-2 and fetal liver expression of IGFBP-2 mRNA in sheep (McLellan et al. 1992). Catecholamines do not appear to affect circulating concentrations of IGFBP-2 (Hooper et al. 1994). IGF-I increases IGFBP-2 release from bovine fibroblasts (Conover 1990). The relationship between pituitary hormones and IGFBP-2 expression is not fully established. Circulating concentrations of IGFBP-2 are reduced in decapitated or hypophysectomized pig fetuses but increased in postnatally hypophysectomized pigs (McCusker et al. 1985; Latimer et al. 1993). Thyroxine Administration of T_4 increases circulating concentrations of IGFBP-2 in hypophysectomized pig fetuses (Latimer et al. 1993). Administration of EGF to pigs increases circulating concentrations of IGFBP-2 (Vinter-Jensen et al. 1996).

NUTRITION AND IGFBP-2. Inadequate nutrition can be associated with elevated circulating concentrations of IGFBP-2 (pigs: e.g., Dauncey et al. 1993) and elevated IGFBP-2 expression in sheep (Rhoads et al. 2000). A relationship between IGFBP-2 and growth is indicated by the elevated expression of IGFBP-2 in growth restricted fetal pigs (Kampman et al. 1993).

Control of IGFBP-3

HORMONES AND IGFBP-3. Circulating concentrations/expression of IGFBP-3 are under control by GH, acting directly or indirectly via IGF-I. For instance, circulating concentrations of IGFBP-3 are increased by GH in pigs (Coleman and Etherton 1991) reduced by hypophysectomy (McCusker et al. 1985). IGF-I increases circulating concentrations of IGFBP-3 in fetal sheep (Shen et al. 2001). Similarly IGF-I stimulates release at IGFBP-3 by bovine fibroblasts (Conover et al. 1990) and mammary cells (Romagnolo et al. 1994). Growth factors also influence IGFBP-3 expression. Synthesis of IGFBP-3 by porcine myogenic cells/myoblasts is stimulated by TGFβ-1 (Hembree et al. 1996). Circulating concentrations of IGFBP-3 are reduced by EGF in pigs (Vinter-Jensen et al. 1996).

NUTRITION AND IGFBP-3. Circulating concentrations of IGFBP-3 are depressed in pigs chronically on a low plane of nutrition (Dauncey et al. 1993) or acutely following fasting (McCusker et al. 1985). However, sheep on a nutritionally restricted diet show no change on IGFBP-3 expression (Rhoads et al. 2000).

Gender and IGFBPs

Circulating concentrations of IGFBPs may be influenced by gender. For instance, the circulating concentration of the 44 kDa IGFBP-3, but not other IGFBPs, are lower in gilts than barrows/boars (Clapper et al. 2000).

CORTICOSTEROIDS AND GROWTH

The Hypothalamo-Pituitary-Adrenal-Stress axis

Glucocorticoid hormones—cortisol (F) in domestic mammals; corticosterone (B) in poultry—are released in response to stress and other influences from the adrenal cortex. This is under stimulatory control by the hypothalamo-pituitary-adrenal axis (Figure 5.8) (see the next sections). Corticotropin releasing hormone (CRH) increases ACTH secretion and hence the synthesis of cortisol. The effect of CRH is potentiated by arginine vasopressin. This has been demonstrated, for instance in domestic animals, in calves (Veissier et al. 1999). Based on studies in sheep, acute stress (insulin induced hypoglycemia) increases the release of both CRH and AVP from the median eminence into the hypophyseal portal blood (Engler et al. 1989).

Corticotropin Releasing Hormone (CRH)

CRH is a 41 amino-acid residue containing peptide. CRH acts via binding to the CRH receptor (a G_s coupled receptor with 7 transmembrane spanning domains). There are several types of CRH receptors, including the type 1 or CRH-R1 (found in the pituitary) and type 2 CRH-R2 (found in the CNS). Unlike any other releasing factor, CRH is transported and probably also released with a binding protein, CRH-BP.

Glucocorticoid Synthesis by the Adrenal Cortex

Production of F by adrenocortical cells is under stimulatory control by ACTH. Other factors influence glucocorticoid synthesis. Using bovine adrenocortical cells, in vitro, IGF-I was found to stimulate. TGFβ1 reduced both basal- and ACTH-induced F secretion, cAMP production together with the gene expression for ACTH receptors, steroidogenic enzymes, and a key protein, Steroidogenic Acute Regulatory Protein.

Circulating Binding Proteins for Glucocorticoids

In domestic mammals, F is transported in the circulation largely bound to a high affinity specific binding protein, corticosteroid-binding globulin (CBG)

Stress, etc.
⇓
Hypothalamus
⇓
Corticotropin releasing hormone (CRH)
and other hypothalamic factors, e.g., arginine vasopressin
⇓
Anterior Pituitary gland
⇓
Adrenocorticotropic hormone (ACTH)
⇓
Adrenal cortex
⇓
Glucocorticoid hormones – cortisol (F) in domestic mammals; corticosterone (B) in poultry)
⇓
Metabolic effects, e.g., catabolism

Figure 5.8. The hypothalamo-pituitary-adrenal axis.

(Table 5.19). In addition, plasma albumin represents a low affinity but very high capacity (~0.6 mM) binding site for a glucocorticoid (Gayrard et al. 1996) (Table 5.19). Similarly in birds, B is transported in the blood stream bound to an avian CBG or to albumin (reviewed Carsia and Harvey 2000) (Table 5.19). The consensus is that only a free steroid hormone affects cells, diffusing down a concentration gradient into cells.

Genetics and the Hypothalamo-Pituitary-Adrenal Axis

There are examples of genetics influencing the adrenal axis. For instance, in halothane-sensitive pigs (porcine stress syndrome due to a mutation in skeletal ryanodine receptors), basal circulating concentrations of ACTH and F are high (Marple et al. 1974; Weaver et al. 2000b). Moreover, meat quality relates to muscle glucocorticoid receptor concentrations; paler meat is associated with lower free glucocorticoid receptor numbers (Lundström et al. 1983). Lines of pigs selected for rate of gain and reduced backfat thickness have differences in adrenal cortical hormones (reduced circulating concentrations of F and CBG in the lean line) (Lundström et al. 1983). There are breed effects on circulating CBG concentration and association constant (Aberle et al. 1976).

Glucocorticoids and Growth

Glucocorticoids markedly depress growth. This is seen, for instance, in rodent models (e.g., Tomas et

al. 1984) and livestock, poultry, and horses (see Chapter 21). Accompanying this effect on growth is a reduction in muscle weight that occurs in both young and adult animals. The changes in protein metabolism provide precursors for hepatic gluconeogenesis. Glucocorticoids also increase liver size. Muscle protein accretion is reduced by glucocorticoids (Table 5.20). In vitro muscle protein synthesis is inhibited by glucocorticoids (e.g., with rodents, cells in culture with the synthetic glucocorticoid dexamethasone: Desler et al. 1996; chick muscle: Klasing et al. 1987). Effects on muscle protein degradation are less consistent, with no effect observed with chicken tissue (Klasing et al. 1987).

Glucocorticoids and Growth in Poultry

Glucocorticoids depress growth in chickens. Discussion will be limited to studies that employed B, the endogenous glucocorticoid in birds. The growth depressing effect of exogenous B is observed irrespective of whether the hormone is injected (Bartov et al. 1980; also see Table 5.21), administered orally and mixed in the feed (Gross et al. 1980; Siegel et al. 1989; also see Table 5.22), or infused (Donker and Beuving 1989). The effect is observed in the embryo (reviewed Scanes 2000), immediately following hatching (Table 5.22) and later in growth (Table 5.22). The inhibitory effect of glucocorticoids appears to be physiological because doubling circulating concentrations of B; $\Delta B = \sim 2$ ng/ml for 7 days reduces growth rate by 23%

Table 5.19. Transportation of glucocorticoids in the circulation in domestic animals

Species	Glucocorticoid	CBG		Albumin		Glucocorticoid (nm)	Reference
		K_d (nm)	B_{max} (nm)	K_d (mM)	B_{max} (mM)		
Cattle	Cortisol	13	110	0.9	0.6	21	Gayrard et al., 1996
Chicken	Corticosterone	56–82	14–220	-	-	~5	Reviewed Carsia and Harvey, 2000
Dog	Cortisol	8	82	0.5	0.5	23	Gayrard et al., 1996
Horse	Cortisol	19	220	0.4	0.5	130	Gayrard et al., 1996
Sheep	Cortisol	9	78	0.5	0.6	50	Gayrard et al., 1996

Table 5.20. Effect of glucocorticoids on protein metabolism in rats

Parameter	Name	Dose	Response (as % Vehicle)		Reference
Muscle protein accretion	Triamcinolone acetonide	5 mg/kg/d	<0%	*	Waterlow et al., 1978
Protein fractional synthesis rate in vivo	Triamcinolone acetonide	5 mg/kg/d	84%	*	Waterlow et al., 1978
Protein synthesis in vitro	Triamcinolone acetonide	1 μM	69%	*	McGrath and Goldspink, 1982
	Corticosterone	1 μM	76%		McGrath and Goldspink, 1982
Protein degradation in vivo as indicated by urinary N^τ-methyl histidine	Corticosterone	30mg/kg/d	186%		Tomas et al., 1984
Protein degradation in vitro	Triamcinolone acetonide	1 μM	52%		McGrath and Goldspink, 1982
	Corticosterone	1 μM	63%		McGrath and Goldspink, 1982

*$p < 0.05$.

(Donker and Beuving 1989). Moreover, B in the diet at 20 and 40 mg/kg feed increases circulating concentrations of B by, respectively, ~4 and ~8 ng/ml, while reducing growth and relative muscle weight and increasing adiposity and circulating concentrations of glucose (Davison et al. 1983). Similarly, continuous infusion of ACTH via osmotic minipump reduces growth rate of chickens (Puvadolpirod and Thaxton 2000); ACTH acts presumably to increase B production. In growing chicks, consumption of feed is increased by B. This is associated with elevated retention of energy but decreased retention of nitrogen (Siegel and Van Kampen 1984).

Physiological doses of B reduce muscle growth (Table 5.22). There is a 21% decrease in relative muscle weight and even larger reductions in absolute muscle weight (56% and 64% decrease with, respectively, 20 mg/kg and 30 mg/kg B in the diet) (Siegel et al. 1989). Glucocorticoid's effects on protein metabolism are summarized in Table 5.20. Glucocorticoids increased glucogenesis from precursors such as amino-acids increases in hepatic glucose production in vitro, and are observed in

Table 5.21. Effect of corticosterone injections in heavy (broiler type) chickens (between 26 and 36 days of age)

Parameter	Control		Corticosterone[1]
Average daily gain (g/d)	4.9±0.2	*	3.4±0.2
Abdominal fat pad (% BWt)	2.4±0.2	*	5.2±0.3
Liver weight (% BWt)	25.0±1.3	*	47.5±2.3
Liver lipid (% wet Wt)	3.5±0.1	*	20.7±1.2

* $p<0.05$.
[1]600 µg/day.

Table 5.22. Effect of the glucocorticoid, corticosterone, administration on growth of chickens (data from Siegel et al. 1989)

		Corticosterone[+]	
	Control	20	30
Heavy (meat type) chicken)			
Average daily gain (g/d) (% of control)			
1–8 days	14[a] (100)	12[b] (83)	10[c] (72)
8–15 days	28 (100)	14 (51)	11 (38)
15–22 days	39 (100)	16 (41)	13 (32)
Breast muscle weight (g/kg body wt.)	153[a]	117[c]	95[b]
Liver weight (g/kg body wt.)	28[a]	82[b]	91[b]
Abdominal fat (g/kg body wt.)	9[a]	22[c]	16[b]
Light (Leghorn) type			
Average daily gain (g/d) (% of control)			
1–8 days	5.6[a] (100)	4.7[b] (85)	4.0[c] (72)
8–15 days	8.4 (100)	5.0 (59)	4.3 (51)
15–22 days	10.7 (100)	5.0 (47)	3.7 (35)
Breast muscle weight (g/kg body wt.)	137[a]	108[b]	108[b]
Liver weight (g/kg body wt.)	29[a]	41[b]	53[c]
Abdominal fat (g/kg body wt.)	6[a]	13[b]	14[b]

[+]Administered in the feed at either 20 or 30 mg/kg feed.
[a,b,c]Different superscript letters indicate different $p<0.05$.

chickens implanted with corticosterone (Kafri et al. 1988). In chickens, B increases adipose tissue weights (Table 5.22) and hepatic lipid content (e.g., Bartov et al. 1980). Implants of B in growing chickens increases the activities of lipogenic enzymes and the rate of lipogenesis as measured in vitro (Kafri et al. 1988). Similarly, B increases abdominal fat pad weight and reduces growth rate in lean or fat lines of chickens (Saadoun et al. 1987). Growth is also depressed by glucocorticoid treatment in turkeys (e.g., Huff et al. 1999).

Glucocorticoids and Differentiation

Glucocorticoids influence terminal differentiation of some cells. Effects of glucocorticoids on adipocyte differentiation are considered in Chapter 10. Another example is the effect of glucocorticoids on the production of the lung surfactant. Circulating concentrations of B peak at the time of hatching in chicks (chicken: Kalliecharan and Hall 1974; Scott et al. 1981; turkey: Wentworth and Hussein 1985). One of the functions of this peak in B is to induce the synthesis of surfactant phospholipids in the avian lung that are critical to air breathing (Hylka and Doneen 1983). Similarly, B is the hormone responsible for the large developmental increase in the activity of hepatic detoxifying enzymes (UDP-glucuronyltransferase and aniline hydroxylase) prior to hatching in the chicken (Wishart and Dutton 1974; Leakey and Dutton 1975).

Other Effects in Poultry

Glucocorticoids reduce gut transit time in young chickens (Tur et al. 1989).

Glucocorticoids and Growth in Pigs

Glucocorticoids suppress growth in pigs. The administration of F (hydrocortisone acetate) to piglets has been observed to stunt growth (Chapple et al. 1989a) (Table 5.23). There is also disproportionately high liver growth (Chapple et al. 1989a) (see Table 5.23). Increasing doses of F exert greater effects on body and liver growth (Chapple et al. 1989b). Growth between days 14 and 26 for piglets receiving vehicle were 175 g/d; for 8 mg F-151 g/d (or 86% of control); 16 mg F 156 g/d (or 89% of control); and 24 F-114 g/d (or 65% of control).

Glucocorticoids and Carbohydrate Metabolism

Glucocorticoids also influence the activity of a key enzyme involved in carbohydrate metabolism/glu-coneogenesis, increasing the activity of glutamate-oxaloacetate (Chapple et al. 1989a).

Glucocorticoids and Gastrointestinal Functioning

Glucocorticoids can affect gastrointestinal tract in the pig. The administration of F to piglets has been observed to increase the activity of amylase in the pancreas (Chapple et al. 1989b, 1989c). Neither dexamethasone nor F treatment affected protease activity in the gastric mucosa of piglets (Pelletier et al. 1983).

Neonatal Acute Stress and Growth

Pigs exposed to the stress of handling neonatally exhibit long-term changes, including reduced growth, elevated circulating CBG levels, and, hence, reduced circulating concentrations of free F in the adult and changes in adult behavior (Weaver et al. 2000a). This would suggest that neonatal stress induces a permanent change (shifting a "set-point") in the pig and presumably in the hypothalamic-pituitary-adrenal cortical axis. Arguably in a similar manner, neonatal administration of a single dose of the glucocorticoid, dexamethasone, evokes a long-term change (an increase) in growth rate (Seaman et al. 2001). Again this mitigates for a long-term shift in the setpoint for the adrenal axis mediated by a component of the axis.

Glucocorticoids and Growth in Cattle and Sheep

Growth in ruminants is relatively refractory to the inhibitory effects of elevated concentrations of glu-

Table 5.23. Effect of cortisol[1] on growth in pigs (data from Chapple et al., 1989a)

Parameter	Control	C
Body weight at 56 days	14.7*	11.7
Average daily gain (g/d)		
Lactation period		
14–21	281	214
21–28	274	160
28–35	70	−1
Nursery period		
35–42	199	147
42–49	348	266
49–56	423	289

*p<0.05.
[1]Administered alternate days from day 14 to day 26 with 25 mg. cortisol per kg body weight

cocorticoids. Effects on protein and fat metabolism are, however, still manifest. In early studies in sheep, cortisone acetate either had no effect on growth (e.g., Harter and Vetter, 1967) or enhanced growth (e.g., Spurlock and Clegg 1962). There is no effect on fat free carcass weight, reduced percentage protein, and increased percentage fat in carcass (Spurlock and Clegg 1962). The reduced percentage protein may reflect decreased net protein accretion. Glucocorticoids exert the same effects in ruminants as nonruminants, stimulating use of amino-acids as gluconeogenic precursors at the expense of protein synthesis. High doses of cortisone have been found to increase urinary nitrogen loss (Harter and Vetter 1967). Moreover in the ovine fetus, F infusion induces hepatic gluconeogenic enzymes (Fowden et al. 1993). Dexamethasone, early in gestation, has a delayed effect reducing fetal weight (Moritz et al. 2002).

Administration of the synthetic glucocorticoid, dexamethasone, at low doses has little effect on growth (ADG) (Brethour 1972). There were, however, improvements in marbling score and carcass grade (Brethour 1972). This reflects increased lipid deposition in response to glucocorticoid. Recently, dexamethasone has been found to improve dressing percentage as well as affecting other aspects of meat quality but being without effect on average daily gain in cattle also implanted with estradiol benzoate and progesterone (Corah et al. 1995) (Table 5.24). The administration of either dexamethasone or F reduced the proteolytic activity of abomasal fundic mucosa of calves (Pelletier et al. 1983).

THYROID AND GROWTH

The Hypothalamo-Pituitary-Thyroid Axis

The major thyroid hormone thyroxine (T_4) is secreted under control of the glycoprotein thyrotropin (thyroid stimulating hormone-TSH). This is, in turn, under the control of the hypothalamic releasing factor, thyrotropin releasing hormone (TRH) (see Figure 5.9). TRH is a modified tripeptide, L-pyroglutamyl-L-histidyl-L-proline amide. TRH is produced as a protein/precursor molecule containing 5 copies of the TRH progenitor sequence.

This "classical" hypothalamic-pituitary axis was established by studies predominantly in rodent models. There is abundant evidence that the system is applicable to domestic animals. For instance, TRH stimulates TSH release (e.g., in sheep: Borger and Davis 1974; cattle: Hurley et al. 1981). The role of thyrotropin in enhancing thyroidal secretion of T_4 in domestic animals is supported by the precipitous drop in circulating concentrations of T_4, accompanying a decrease of TSH release (Kahl et al. 1992) and the increase in circulating T_4 concentrations after TRH administration (Hurley et al. 1981). Thyrotropin is secreted in a pulsatile manner in livestock (cattle: Ohlson et al. 1981; sheep: Davis et al. 1978), presumably reflecting the effects of TRH and SRIF. Secretion of TSH has been shown also to be elevated by estrogens (diethylstilbesterol) (sheep: Davis et al. 1978).

Secretion of TSH is under negative feedback control by T_3. As might be expected, circulating concentrations for TSH have been found to be elevated

Table 5.24. Effect of the glucocorticoid, dexamethasone[1], on performance on cattle[2] (data from Corah et al, 1995)

Parameter	Control		Dexamethasone
Average daily gain (kg)	1.25		1.32
Dressing percentage	62.5	*	64.4
Subcutaneous fat thickness (cm)	0.81	*	1.14
Longissumus muscle (as cm[2])	70.0	*	75.9
Marbling score	488		411
Lipid content of Longissumus muscle %	4.6		3.8

*$p<0.05$.
[1]Implanted with 100 mg dexamethasone. This releases ~0.5 mg dexamethasone per day.
[2]430 kg steers also implanted with estadiol benzoate (20mg) progesterone (200 mg); duration of the study: to liveweight 545–567 kg.

Metabolic requirements
⇓
Hypothalamus
⇓
Thyrotropin releasing hormone (TRH) +ve
Somatostatin (SRIF)-ve
⇓
Anterior Pituitary gland
⇓
Thyrotropin (thyroid stimulating hormone) (TSH)
⇓
Thyroid
⇓
Thyroxine (T$_4$)
⇓
Liver
⇓   ⇒   ⇒   ⇒ Reverse T$_3$ (inactive metabolite)
⇓
Triiodothyronine(T$_3$)
⇓
⇓
Metabolic effects/growth

Figure 5.9. The hypothalamo-pituitary-thyroid axis.

by over 100-fold in thyroidectomized lambs (Borger and Davis 1974). Moreover, T$_3$ exerts a negative feedback effect reducing circulating concentrations of TSH (e.g., in cattle: Kahl et al. 1992).

Control of Growth of the Thyroid Gland

The growth of the thyroid involves both cell proliferation and differentiation. There are multiple growth factors/hormones that affect the proliferation of the thyroid follicular cells. These stimulatory and inhibitory factors are listed in summary form in Table 5.25. Excess iodine has a toxic effect on the thyroid gland. High levels of iodine impair thyroidal functioning and cause a "breakdown" of thyroid tissue by the process of apoptosis.

Other Factors Influencing Thyroid Function

Thyroid function can be influenced by multiple factors, including nutrition. Circulating concentrations of T$_4$ have been reported to be depressed with a low plane of nutrition (e.g., Fitzgerald et al. 1982). Similarly circulating concentrations of both T$_3$ and T$_4$ are reduced with feed restriction in cattle (Blum and Kuntz 1981; Blum et al. 1985). In cattle fed the organophosphate ronnel, there is some elevation in the circulating concentrations of T$_4$ but not T$_3$ (Rumsey et al. 1983).

Thyroid Hormone Metabolism and Mechanism of Action

The pro-hormone, T$_4$, is metabolized to its active form, T$_3$, by monodeiodination. Alternatively, T$_4$ can be metabolized to an inactive form, reverse T$_3$.

The mechanism of action of T$_3$ involves binding to a nuclear receptor. It turns out that proto-oncogene *c-erb A* encodes a protein that binds T$_3$ and is the thyroid hormone receptor (TR). Moreover the TR is a member of the nuclear receptor superfamily of transcription factors containing a C terminal ligand binding domain, a DNA binding domain with two zinc fingers and an N terminal transcription activation domain (reviewed Koenig 1999). There are two *TR* genes: TRα and TRβ, with the avian erythroblastus virus, *v-RrbA*, more closely related to TRα (reviewed Koenig 1999). There are also gene products that result from alternative splicing: TRα1, TRαv2 and TRαv3, which do not bind T$_3$ but inhibit T$_3$ action, TRβ1, and TRβ2. TRα, TRβ1, and TRβ2 can dimerize to form homodimers or, with the

Table 5.25. Stimulators and inhibitors of thyroid follicular proliferation in domestic animals

Proliferation (Growth)		Reference
Stimulators		
IGF-I	Pig	Tsushima et al., 1988
TSH	Pig	Cowin et al., 1996
EGF	Pig	Tsushima et al., 1988; Cowin et al., 1996
T_3 *via local production of EGF*	Bovine	Fulvio et al., 2000
Inhibitors		
Iodide	Pig	Cowin and Bidey, 1995
Plasmin	Pig	Cowin and Bidey, 1995
TGFβ1	Pig	Tsushima et al., 1988; Cowin and Bidey, 1995
Iodide Uptake (Functioning)		
Stimulator		
TSH	Pig	Tsushima et al., 1988
IGF-I[a] (potentiating TSH)	Sheep	Becks et al., 1992
Cortisol (potentiating TSH)	Sheep	Becks et al., 1992
Inhibitor		
TGFβ1	Pig	Tsushima et al. 1988

[a]No effect alone, but potentiated TSH effect.

gene products of the *retinoid X receptor* genes (RXRα, RXRβ, RXRγ), to form heterodimers (reviewed Koenig 1999). Both TRα and β are expressed in cartilage (chondrocytes) in the epiphyseal growth plate but TRα is more important.

Catabolism

Although T_3 and T_4 are metabolized predominantly by monodeiodination, there is significant sulfation of both T_3 and T_4 (Wu et al. 1992).

Circulating Binding Proteins for Thyroid Hormones

Thyroid hormones are transported in the blood and cerebral spinal fluid bound to transthyretin, synthesized by the liver and the choroid plexus.

Thyroid Hormones and Growth

Evidence that the thyroid is necessary for growth in domestic animals comes from studies in the chicken, pig, and sheep. In chickens, growth (average daily gain and skeletal growth) is retarded greatly following thyroidectomy (chemical thyroidectomy by goitrogen administration: King and King 1973, 1976; Raheja and Snedecor 1970; radiothyroidecto-

my: Raheja and Snedecor 1970; surgical thyroidectomy: Harvey et al. 1983; Moore et al. 1984). Replacement therapy with T_3 or T_4 restores growth (Raheja and Snedecor 1970; King and King 1973, 1976). The thyroid hormones are important for muscle growth, in particular, fast-phasic muscles but not slow tonic muscles (Moore et al. 1984). Similarly, thyroidectomy of fetal lambs reduces growth as indicated by body weight and length (Hopkins and Thorburn 1972). Similarly, treating the pregnant ewe with the goitrogen methylthiouracil reduced growth of the fetus (Lascelles and Setchell 1959). In growing pigs, growth was markedly depressed by feeding the goitrogen potassium thiocyanate (an inhibitor of thyroid functioning) and elevated by iodide supplementation, as can be seen from the following ADG: goitrogen—176 g/d, control—486 g/d, and iodine supplemented—526 g/d (Cromwell et al. 1975). Similar effects have been observed with another goitrogen, methimazole (Sihombing et al. 1974).

There is not good evidence that increasing circulating thyroid hormone concentration enhances growth in normal euthyroid domestic animals. For instance, administration of T_4 to lambs did not affect growth (Hatch et al. 1972; Rosemberg et al. 1989). Similarly, addition of thyroprotein to the diet increases circulating concentrations of T_4 (and T_3 to a less extent) did not affect growth (ADG) or carcass composition in either lean or obese pigs (Yen and Pond 1985) but depressed growth in sheep (Ely et al. 1976).

Other Effects of Thyroid Hormones

T_4 induces a shift from slow-tonic to fast-twitch myofibers in muscle (Moore et al. 1984; Carpenter et al. 1987). In vitro studies with chick embryo cartilage provide strong support for T_3 directly affecting cartilage growth (Burch and Lebovitz 1982).

Thyroid hormones are necessary for wool growth. Thyroidectomy decreases wool growth and T_4 replacement therapy restores wool growth (Maddocks et al. 1985). Development of wool follicles is retarded in thyroidectomized fetal lambs (Hopkins and Thorburn 1972).

Genetic Differences in Thyroid Function

Marked genetic differences in thyroid function have been reported. For instance, large framed steers have higher circulating concentrations of T_4 than small framed steers, but with no difference in T_3 observed (Verde and Trenkle 1987). Similarly, when comparing Angus and Brangus cattle, the former had somewhat higher growth rates and also greater circulating concentrations of T_3 and T_4 (Beaver et al. 1989). Halothane-sensitive (stress-susceptible) pigs exhibit changes in thyroid function, with reduced circulating concentrations of T_4 and increased metabolic clearance rates for T_3 and T_4 (Marple et al. 1977).

Another example of genetics influencing thyroid functioning is a chicken model for autoimmune thyroiditis. The obese line of chickens is susceptible to thyroiditis and the parent line exhibits low susceptibility; susceptibility is increased as dietary iodine levels are raised (Bagchi et al. 1985).

Environment and Thyroid Hormones

The thyroid hormone T_3, and also T_4 to a less extent, increases the rate of metabolism. For instance, T_3 administration has been reported to elevate oxygen consumption (sheep: Kennedy et al. 1977). This provides a basis for the conventional wisdom that circulating concentrations of T_3 and T_4 will be inversely related to temperature, because they are high in cold environments and low in warm envi-

ronments. Studies in calves are consistent with this. The following are circulating concentrations of T_3 and T_4: cool (10–13°) T_3 1.9±0.2 ng/ml, T_4 87±3.7 ng/ml; moderate (21–23°) T_3 1.4±0.1 ng/ml, T_4 71±5.6 ng/ml and hot (34–35°) T_3 1.1±0.1 ng/ml, T_3 74±2.1 ng/ml (Hurley et al. 1981). The physiological mechanism for this probably reflects shifts in peripheral deiodination, because there were no differences in either basal or TRH stimulated circulating concentrations of TSH (Hurley et al. 1981). In an analogous manner, circulating concentrations of both T_3 and T_4 are depressed in young pigs in a tropical (hot) environment (Christon 1988). However, circulating concentrations of neither T_3 nor T_4 were consistently affected by either high or low environmental temperatures in finishing pigs (Becker et al. 1993).

SEX STEROIDS AND GROWTH

The effects of gonadal hormones on growth are considered elsewhere in this book (see Chapter 17).

Circulating Binding Proteins Gonadal Hormones

Both estrogens (estradiol) and androgens are transported in the plasma bound to specific protein, sex steroid binding globulin (SSBG). This binding is high affinity and regulates the amount of estradiol or testosterone that is available to influence a target tissue. It is present in humans and rabbits, but not rats or mice postnatally. This is a similar protein to testicular androgen binding protein.

Cellular Mechanism of Action of Gonadal Hormones

Estrogens act by binding to estrogen receptors (ER). Estrogen receptors are nuclear transcription factors, members of the nuclear receptor superfamily along with the thyroid hormone receptors and androgen receptors. There are various isoforms of ER: ERα, ERβ, and truncated estrogen receptor product-1 (TERP-1).

INSULIN AND GROWTH

It is difficult to differentiate between the growth promoting, metabolic, and pharmacological effects of insulin. In the case of the latter, insulin at very high concentrations binds to the IGF-I receptor. Effects of insulin on growth have been reported predominantly from clinical studies in the human and use of rodent models. There is relatively little information on the role of insulin in growth in domestic animals, but it is reasonable to assume similarities with the human, rat, and mouse. Insulin stimulation of growth may reflect the following:

- The ability of insulin to substitute for IGF-I, albeit as a poor agonist
- In the absence of insulin, metabolism is disrupted
- Insulin per se stimulates growth (reviewed Martin et al. 1984; Messina 1999)

It is not clear which mechanism is responsible for the ability of insulin to increase growth in hypophysectomized rats (Salter and Best 1953). The inherent insulin effect on growth involves its binding to the insulin receptor, a transmembrane tyrosine kinase, and phosphorylation of the insulin receptor substrate 1 (IRS-1). In the absence of insulin receptors, growth is reduced—e.g., in Leprechanism (extreme insulin resistance) in man and knock out (null) mice (reviewed Messina 1999).

　The preponderance of the evidence favors insulin being required for normal fetal/neonatal growth at least in rodent models. Insulin administration improves growth and particularly growth of the intestine in newborn mice (Menon and Sperling 1996). Conversely in rats, nutritional deprivation of the dam results in intrauterine growth retardation due to probable fetal insulin insufficiency (Gruppuso et al. 1994). This is more definitive evidence for a role for insulin in an ingenious study in which fetal rat paws were transplanted under the kidney capsule of a syngeneic host; paw growth was decreased with insulin deficiency (streptozotocin induced diabetes) and restored by insulin replacement therapy (Cooke and Nicoll 1984). There is evidence for insulin stimulating growth in domestic animals.

Insulin and Growth in Chick Embryos

Administration of insulin to very early chick embryos (2 days of development) enhances growth (de Pablo et al. 1985) and overcomes the growth retarding effect of phorbol ester (Girbau et al. 1989). Similarly, insulin in vitro stimulates both proliferation and protein synthesis by chick embryo cells (Pérez-Villamil et al. 1994). There is evidence that endogenous insulin is exerting growth promoting via insulin receptors because the administration of antisera against either insulin or insulin receptors reduces growth/weight of early chick embryos (de Pablo et al. 1985; Girbau et al. 1988). Insulin expression is observed prior to pancreatic β cell differentiation (see the previous section).

Insulin and Growth in Fetal Pigs and Sheep

The reduction in growth following pancreatectomy in fetal lambs supports a requirement for insulin in fetal growth (Gluckman et al. 1987). In fetal domestic animals, administration of additional insulin fails to affect growth. For instance, Spencer and colleagues (1983) reported insulin infusion had no effect on the lengths (indicating skeletal growth) or weight of pig fetuses (weights: control 823±34 g; insulin-treated 855±42 g). Similarly in fetal lambs infused with insulin, there was no effect on growth (length) or body weight (Milley 1986).

Insulin and IGFs and IGFBPs

Insulin may influence by influencing the expression of IGFs and IGFBPs. There is good evidence that insulin increases the production of IGF-I. For instance, streptozotocin induction of diabetes in growing pigs shows decreased growth and circulating concentrations of IGF-I/hepatic IGF-I mRNA (Leaman et al. 1990). Moreover, elevated circulating concentrations of IGF-I are observed of fetal pigs with insulin infusion (Spencer et al. 1983) (IGF-I as a % of control: control 100±10; insulin 175±15). Insulin stimulates IGF-I production by chick hepatocytes, particularly in the presence of GH (Houston and O'Neill 1991). Insulin also affects expression of at least one IGFBP, IGFBP-1, inhibiting IGFBP-1 expression (Ooi et al. 1992; Shen et al., 2001).

Insulin and Cell Proliferation/Differentiation

Insulin is involved in cell proliferation/differentiation (also see Chapters 8–10). Insulin stimulates proliferation of hepatocytes acting via the insulin receptor (Krett et al. 1987; Gruppuso 1989; Gruppuso et al. 1994). Insulin can exert a synergistic effect, with specific growth factors increasing the number of cells moving from Go/G to S phase in the cell cycle (Shipley and Ham 1983a, 1983b). The evidence is equivocal as to whether insulin affects liver growth in vivo. Hypoinsulinemia (maternal fasting) in the rat fetus decreases liver weight and DNA (Gruppuso et al. 1994). In contrast, there is no effect of hyperinsulinemia in liver weight or DNA in fetal lambs (Milley 1986).

Insulin and Protein Metabolism Postnatally

It is now clear that insulin has a profound stimulatory effect on growth in the neonatal animal. Studies in neonatal pigs have demonstrated that net protein synthesis (protein accretion/deposition) is very high following birth. Insulin plays an important role in this postnatal protein synthesis (Davis et al. 2001). One technique that has been employed in a series of elegant studies is the insulin infusion euglycemic and amino acid clamp. This entails insulin infusion while maintaining circulating concentrations of both glucose and branched chain amino-acids constant (e.g., Wray-Cahen et al. 1997, 1998; Davis et al. 2001). Insulin infusion enhanced the fractional rate of protein synthesis, particularly in skeletal muscles of 7-day-old piglets. The effect was much reduced by 1 month of age (Davis et al. 2001). The increase in muscle protein synthesis was observed in both myofibrillar and sarcoplasmic proteins (Davis et al. 2001).

Insulin Expression

Postnatally, insulin gene expression is restricted to the β cells of the pancreas. However during embryonic/fetal development, extra-pancreatic insulin expression is observed in the chick embryo before β cell differentiation (Serrano et al. 1989; Pérez-Villamil et al. 1994).

Control of Insulin Release

In monogastic animals, the secretion of insulin is stimulated by increases in the circulating concentration of glucose. In ruminants, the predominant control is exerted by volatile fatty acids. There are also hormones from the small intestine (released in response to glucose or fat in the digesta) that stimulate insulin release. These gut hormones are glucose-dependent insulinotropic polypeptide (GIP) (from the K cells) and glucagon-like pepide-1 (GLP-1) (from the L cells). Other hormones influence insulin secretion. Leptin decreases insulin release, and prolactin stimulates insulin secretion in vitro—an effect that is reversed by glucocorticoids.

Effects of Hormones on β Cell Growth

During growth, the mass of β cells increases, as does the capacity to produce insulin. Islet β cells undergo both hyperplasia and hypertrophy. In the case of the former, the rate of cell division exceeds the rate of cell death during growth. In the adult, the two rates are approximately equal except when there is a chronic demand for more insulin (prolonged hyperglycemia after injury to the panceas/ loss of β cells).

OTHER HORMONES

Leptin

Leptin is the product of the *ob* gene discovered by Zhang and colleagues (1994). Leptin is not present in the obese (ob) mouse, and this deficiency is responsible for the increased fat mass. The leptin receptor is absent/nonexpressed in the db/db mouse.

Chemistry

Leptin is a 167 amino-acid residue containing protein.

Site of Production

The major site of leptin production is the adipose tissue (white adipose tissue). There are other sites for leptin production, including the stomach and specific neurons in the hypothalamus (Hoggard et al. 1997).

Control of Leptin Release

The leptin release (and also the circulating concentrations) is related to the following: Leptin release is proportional to the mass of adipose tissue (the fatter the animal, the higher the circulating concentrations of leptin). Leptin release is decreased with fasting in both thin and obese animals. The secretion of leptin is under the control of energy balance. Other hormones influence the release of leptin. Cholecystokinin (CCK) (released from I cells of the duodenum in response to digesta) stimulates the release and synthesis of leptin by adipose tissue. In addition, the cytokine interleukin-1β stimulates leptin release from adipose tissue, with this effect mediated via receptors of the class I of the cytokine receptor family.

Role

Leptin is involved predominantly with energy homeostasis, but it has other effects also, including effects on reproduction. Leptin functions as a hormonal messenger from adipocytes signaling the brain (the hypothalamus) on status of adipose tissue (volume/mass⇑) and thereby reducing food consumption (⇓) (Figure 5.10).

Administration of leptin close to the hypothalamus (by intracerebroventricular injection) reduces food intake in pigs (Barb et al. 1998) (Figure 5.11).

Leptin and Anterior Pituitary Functioning

There is also a role for leptin affecting anterior pituitary functioning and affecting the secretion of hor-

Blood
Glucose ⇒ Adipose cells ⇒ Leptin ⇒ Brain Barrier
⇓
⇓
Hypothalamic Leptin Receptors
⇓
⇓
Appetite/Feeding ⇓
Via NeuropeptideY⇓

Figure 5.10. Schematic diagram of the physiology of leptin.

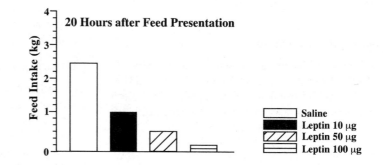

Figure 5.11. Effect of leptin administration on feed intake in pigs (adapted from Barb et al., 1998)

mones related to both growth and reproduction. Intracerebroventricular injection of leptin is followed by a marked increase in circulating concentrations of GH in pigs (Barb et al. 1998). Much of this effect is presumed to be at the hypothalamic level. However, leptin can directly increase GH release based on studies of pig anterior pituitary cells in vitro (Barb et al. 1998). In fasted sheep, plasma concentrations of luteinizing hormone (LH) are depressed, due to a much fewer number of pulses of LH release. Leptin administration overcomes the effect of fasting. It is presumed that leptin is a major signal that informs the hypothalamus on the energy state of the animal and thereby affects appetite and the neuroendocrine control of reproduction.

Other Direct Actions of Leptin

Leptin can influence adipose tissue metabolism, increasing lipolysis in mono-gastric animals—e,g., pigs (Ramsay 2001), but not with ruminants. Neither lipolysis nor lipogenesis by sheep adipose tissue in vitro are affected by leptin (Newby et al.

2001). Leptin also affects adrenal cortical functioning. Prolonged exposure of either human or rat adrenal cortical cells in vitro is accompanied by reduced secretion of glucocorticoid (human: cortisol; rat: corticosterone) (Pralong et al. 1998). Leptin stimulates lung growth (increasing cell proliferation) during development based on studies with human and rodent cells (Tsuchiya et al. 1999) and angiogenesis (Sierra-Honigmann et al. 1998).

Indirect Actions of Leptin

Leptin indirectly affects bone mass (via the hypothalamus), based on studies with ob/ob (leptin deficient), db/db (leptin receptor deficient), and control mice (Ducy et al. 2000).

Leptin and Embryonic/Fetal Growth

Leptin has recently been observed to stimulate the development of early stage embryos (Kawamura et al. 2002). However, leptin reduces fetal growth rate, as demonstrated by the increased birth weight of db/db mouse in which the leptin receptor is absent/nonexpressed and reduced birth weight after leptin administration to control but not in db/db mice (Yamashita et al. 2001).

Leptin Receptors

The leptin receptor (Ob-R) is a member of the superfamily of cytokine receptors—class I (forming homodimers with itself after ligand binding). It is the product of the *db* gene. There are at least five splicing variants, with the long form, Ob-Rl, being the predominant signaling form (Mercer et al. 1996). This long form is expressed in multiple tissues in the pig, including the hypothalamus, other brain regions, pituitary gland, adrenal, lung, liver, muscle, adipose tissue, bone marrow, and ovary (Lin et al. 2000).

Prolactin and Growth

Until recently, there was no definitive evidence that the hormone, prolactin, was required for growth, and there is still a lack of information in livestock. However, studies have been conducted in mice without the prolactin receptor (prolactin receptor knock-out mice). Growth (body weight gain postnatally) is reduced 70 and 40% in female and male prolactin receptor knock-out mice. Moreover, adipose tissue is markedly decreased, again to a greater extent in females than males (49% in females and 34% in males) (Freemark et al. 2001). In contrast, neither bovine nor porcine prolactin stimulates growth (weight gain) in rats (McLaughlin et al. 1997). These studies had the distinct advantage of employing preparations of recombinant prolactin, which unlike prolactin purified from pituitary tissue will not have any cross contamination with GH. These preparations of biosynthetic prolactin did not affect growth of pigs but did reduce voluntary feed intake (McLaughlin et al. 1997).

Erythropoietin

Erythropoietin (EPO) plays a critical role in controlling the number of red blood cells and hence oxygen delivery to tissues, growing or otherwise. Until recently, studies on EPO have focused on rodent models, rabbits, and the human clinical situation; EPO production and hence the production of red blood cells reducing with kidney disease (for recent review, see Fisher 1997). Porcine EPO and the EPO receptor cDNA have recently been cloned and characterized (David et al. 2001; Pearson et al. 2000).

The physiology of EPO is summarized in Figure 5.12.

Chemistry

Circulating EPO is a glycoprotein with 166 amino-acid residues and a molecular weight of ~30 K Da (reviewed Jelkman 1992). The difference between this and the molecular weight of the peptide (18 K Da) is due to the heavy glycosylation; there are three N-linked and one O-linked oligosaccharides (Sasak et al. 1987). The glycosylation greatly reduces the rate of clearance of EPO from the circulation and prolongs its biological effectiveness (Tsuda et al. 1990).

Site of Production

Postnatally, erythropoietin is produced predominantly by the kidney, specifically the interstitial cells of the peritubular capillary bed (Koury et al. 1989). The liver synthesizes some EPO. Table 5.26 summarizes the relative levels of EPO RNA in tissues. The liver is frequently considered as the major site of EPO production in the fetus. There are, however, species differences, with a major source of EPO in the sheep fetus being the mesonephric kidney (the metanephric kidney developing later in development) (Wintour et al. 1996).

Low oxygen tension $\Rightarrow$ kidney $\Rightarrow$ erythropoietin⇑

$\Downarrow$

erythroid precursor cells
in bone marrow or liver (fetus)

$\Downarrow$

red blood cell formation

Figure 5.12. Schematic diagram of the physiology of erythropoietin.

Table 5.26. Quantitation of EPO mRNA in kidneys, liver, and testes from five-week-old piglets (adapted from David et al., 2001)

	EPO-mRNA/RNA$_{total}$ (amol/μg)	EPO-mRNA/Organ (fmol)
Kidneys	7.2[a] (2.7–12.7)	184[a] (171–192)
Liver	0.05[a] (0.04–0.08)	16.3[a] (12.7–18.7)
Testes	0.13[a] (0.08, 0.17)	0.74[a] (0.47, 1.01)

[a]The means are based on figures calculated individually for each animal.

Control of Erythropoeitin Synthesis and Release

EPO is synthesized and released in response to low oxygen tension in the blood. This low circulating oxygen tension may be the result of anemia (following, for instance, blood loss or dietary iron deficiency) or decreased ambient oxygen tension due to increased altitude or the increased utilization of oxygen (reviewed, e.g., Fisher 1997).

Role of Erythropoietin

EPO increases the production of new red blood cells (erythrocytes) by action on the committed erythrogenic cells (reviewed, e.g., Fisher 1997).

Erythropoietin Receptor

The EPO receptor is a member of the cytokine receptor superfamily—class I (forming homodimers with itself after ligand binding). The amino-acid residues sequence of the pig EPO receptor is ~85% identical to that of the human EPO receptor and ~80% identical to the rat and mouse EPO receptors (Pearson et al. 2000). The EPO receptor has a molecular weight of 66–78 K Da (Bazan 1989; reviewed Fisher 1997) and is found in the cell membrane. The EPO receptor is expressed in erythrogenic tissues, including committed erythrogenic cells in the bone marrow and the fetal liver (reviewed Fisher 1997). Hepatic expression of the EPO receptor in the fetal pig increases markedly between 24 and 30 days of gestation (Pearson et al. 2000).

Erythropoietin Mechanism of Action

The mechanism of action of EPO involves the following:

1. EPO binding to two EPO receptors
2. Receptor dimerization
3. Activation of the Janus tyrosine kinase 2
   (JAK2)-signal transducer
4. Activation of transcription factor (STAT) 5
   (STAT is a substrate of JAK)
5. Activation of *ras*-mitogen activated protein kinase (MAPK) pathways (Ihle and Kerr 1995).

REFERENCES

Abdel-Meguid, S.S., Shieh, S.-H., Smith, W.W., Dayringer, H.E., Vialand, B.N., and Bentle, L.A. 1987. Three dimensional structure of a genetically engineered variant of porcine growth hormone. *Proceedings of the National Academy of Sciences of the USA* 84:6434–6437.

Aberle, E.D., Riggs, B.L., Alliston, C.W., and Wilson, S.P. 1976. Effects of thermal stress, breed and stress susceptibility on corticosteroid binding globulin in swine. *Journal of Animal Science* 43:816–820.

Agellon, L.B., Emery, C.J., Jones, J.M., Davies, S.L., Dingle, A.D., and Chen, T.T. 1988. Promotion of rapid growth of rainbow trout (Salmo gairdneri) by a recombinant fish growth hormone. *Canadian Journal of Fisheries and Aquatic Sciences* 45:146–151.

Anderson, L.L. 1977. Development in calves and heifers after hypophyseal stalk transection or hypophysectomy. *American Journal of Physiology* 232:E497–E503.

Anderson, L.L., Bohnker, C.R., Parker, R.O., and Kertiles, L.P. 1981. Metabolic actions of growth hormone in pigs. *Journal of Animal Science* 53:363–370.

Anderson, L.L., Feder, J., and Bohnker, C.R. 1976. Effect of growth hormone on growth in immature hypophysectomized pigs. *Journal of Endocrinology* 68:345–346.

Anderson, L.L., Ford, J.J., Klindt, J., Molina, J.R., Vale, W.W., and Rivier, J. 1991. Growth hormone and prolactin secretion in hypophysial stalk-transected pigs as affected by growth hormone and prolactin-releasing and inhibiting factors. *Proceedings of the Society of Experimental Biology and Medicine* 196:194–202.

Arámburo, C., Carranza, M, Reyes, M., Luna, M., Coria, H., Berúmen, L., and Scanes,C.G. 2001. Characterization of a bioactive 15 kda fragment produced by proteolytic cleavage of chicken growth hormone. *Endocrine* 15:231–240.

Arámburo, C., Luna, M., Carranza, M., Reyes, M., Martinez-Coria, H., and Scanes, C.G. 2000. Growth Hormone Size Variants: Changes in the Pituitary During

Development of the Chicken. *Proceedings of the Society for Experimental Biology and Medicine* 223:67–74.

Arámburo, C., Montiel, J.L., Proudman, J.A., Berghman, L.R., and Scanes, C.G. 1992. Phosphorylation of prolactin and growth hormone. *Journal of Molecular Endocrinology* 8:181–191.

Argetsinger, L.S., and Carter-Su, C. 1996. Mechanism of signaling by growth hormone receptor. *Physiological Reviews* 76:1089–1107.

Asakawa, A., Inui, A., Kaga, T., Yuzuriha, H., Nagata, T., Ueno, N., Makino, S., Fujimiya, M., Niijima, A., Fujino, M.A., and Kasuga, M. 2001. Ghrelin is an appetite-stimulatory signal from stomach with structural resemblance to motilin. *Gastroenterology* 120:337–345.

Atinmo, T., Baldijao, C., Houpt, K.A., Pond, W.G., and Barnes, R.H. 1978. Plasma levels of growth hormone and insulin in protein malnourished vs normal growing pigs in response to arginine or glucose infusion. *Journal of Animal Science* 46:409–416.

Auchtung, T.L., Barao, S.M., and Dahl, G.E. 2001b. Relation of growth hormone response to growth hormone-releasing hormone before weaning and postweaning growth performance in beef calves. *Journal of Animal Science* 79:2217–2223.

Auchtung, T.L., Connor, E.E., Barao, S.M., Douglass, L.W., and Dahl, G.E. 2001a. Use of growth hormone response to growth hormone-releasing hormone to determine growth potential in beef heifers. *Journal of Animal Science* 79:1566–1572.

Bacon, W.L., Long, D.W., and Vasilatos-Younken, R. 1995. Responses to exogenous pulsatile turkey growth hormone by growing 8-week-old female turkeys. *Comparative Biochemistry and Physiology* 111B:471–482.

Bacon, W.L., Vasilatos-Younken, R., Nestor, K.E., Andersen, B.J., and Long, D.W. 1989. Pulsatile patterns of plasma growth hormone in turkeys: effects of growth rate, age, and sex. *General and Comparative Endocrinology* 75:417–426.

Bagchi, N., Brown, T.R., Urdanivia, E., and Sundick, R.S. 1985. Induction of autoimmune thyroiditis in chickens by dietary iodine. *Science* 230–327.

Balk, S.D., Shiu, R.P.C., La Fleur, M.M., and Young, L.L. 1982. Epidermal growth factor and insulin cause normal chicken heart mesenchymal cells to proliferate like the Rous sarcoma virus-infected counterparts. *Proceedings of the National Academy of Sciences* 79:1154–1157.

Ballard, F., Johnson, R., Owens, P., Upton, F., McMurtry, J., and Wallace, J. 1990. Chicken insulin-like growth factor-I: amino acid sequence, radioimmunoassay, and plasma levels between strains during growth. *General and Comparative Endocrinology* 79: 459–468.

Barb, C.R., Cox, N.M., Carlton, C.A., Chang, W.J., and Randle, R.F. 1992b. Growth hormone secretion, serum, and cerebral spinal fluid insulin and insulin-like growth factor-I concentrations in pigs with streptozotocin-induced diabetes mellitus. *Proceedings of the Society of Experimental Biology and Medicine* 201:223–228.

Barb, C.R., Kraeling R.R., Barrett J.B., Rampacek G.B., Campbell R.M., and Mowles T.F. 1991). Serum glucose and free fatty acids modulate growth hormone and luteinizing hormone secretion in the pig. *Proceedings of the Society of Experimental Biology and Medicine* 198:636–642.

Barb, C.R., Kraeling, R.R., and Rampacek. G.B. 1992a. Opioid modulation of FSH, growth hormone and prolactin secretion in the prepuberal gilt. *Journal of Endocrinology* 133:13–19.

Barb, C.R., Yan, X., Azain, M.J., Kraeling, R.R., Rampacek, G.B., and Ramsay, T.G. 1998. Recombinant porcine leptin reduces feed intake and stimulates growth hormone secretion in swine. *Domestic Animal Endocrinology* 15:77–86.

Bartov, I., Jensen, L.S., and Veltmann, J.R. 1980. Effect of corticosterone and prolactin on fattening in broiler chicks. *Poultry Science* 59:1328–1334.

Bassett, J.M. 1974. Early changes in plasma insulin and growth hormone levels after feeding in lambs and adult sheep. *Australian Journal of Biological Science* 27:157–166.

Baxter, R.C., Binoux, M.A., Clemmons, D.R., Conover,C.A., Drop, S.L.S., Holly, J.M.P., Mohan, S., Oh, Y., and Rosenfeld, R.G. 1998. Recommendations for nomenclature of the insulin-like growth factor binding protein superfamily. *Endocrinology* 139:4036.

Bazan, J.F. 1989. A novel family of growth factor receptors: a common binding domain in the growth hormone, prolactin, erythropoietin and IL-6 receptors, and the p74 IL-2 receptor β-chain. *Biochemical and Biophysical Research Communication* 164:788–795.

Beaver, E.E., Williams, J.E., Miller, S.J., Hancock, D.L., Hannah, S.M., and O'Connor, D.L. 1989. Influence of breed and diet on growth, nutrient digestibility, body composition and plasma hormones of Brangus and Angus steers. *Journal of Animal Science* 67:2415–2425.

Becker, B.A., Knight, C.D., Veenhuizen, J.J., Jesse, G.W., Hedrick, H.B., and Baile, C.A. 1993. Performance, carcass composition, and blood hormones and metabolites of finishing pigs treated with porcine somatotropin in hot and cold environments. *Journal of Animal Science* 71:2375–2387.

Becks, G.P., Buckingham, K.D., Wang, J.-F., Phillips, I.D., and Hill, D.J. 1992. Regulation of thyroid hormone synthesis in cultured ovine thyroid follicles. *Endocrinology* 130:2789–2794.

Beermann, D.H., Hogue, D.E., Fishell, V.K., Aronica, S., Dickson, H.W., and Schricker, B.R. 1990. Exogenous human growth hormone releasing factor and ovine somatotropin improve growth performance and composition of gain in lambs. *Journal of Animal Science* 68:4122–4133.

Beermann, D.H., Robinson, T.F., Byrem, T.M., Hogue, D.E., Bell, A.W., and McLaughlin, C.L. 1991. Abomasal casein infusion and exogenous somatotropin enhance nitrogen utilization by growing lambs. *Journal of Nutrition* 121:2020–2028.

Benoit, R., Ling, N., and Esch, F. 1987. A new prosomatostatin-derived peptide reveals a pattern for prohormone cleavage at monobasic sites. *Science* 238:1126–1129.

Berghman, L., Darras, V.M., Huybrechts, L.M., Decuypere, E., Kuhn, E.R., and Vandesande, F. 1989. Evidence for chicken GH as the only hypophyseal factor responsible for the stimulation of hepatic 5′-monodeiodination activity in the chick embryo. *Reproduction, Nutrition et Development* 29:197–202.

Berghman, L.R., Lens, P., Decuypere, E., Kuhn, E.R., and Vandesande, F. 1987. Glycosylated chicken growth hormone. *General and Comparative Endocrinology* 68:408–414.

Billestrup, N., Swanson, L.W., and Vale, W. 1986. Growth hormone-releasing factor stimulates proliferation of somatotroph in vitro. *Proceedings of the National Academy of Sciences* 83:6854–6857.

Blanchard, M.M., Goodyer, C.G., Charrier, J., and Barenton, B. 1988. In vitro regulation of growth hormone (GH) release from ovine pituitary cells during fetal and neonatal development: effects of GH-releasing factor, somatostatin, and insulin-like growth factor I. *Endocrinology* 122:2114–20.

Blat, C., Delbe, J., Villaudy, J., Chatelain, P.G., Golde, A., and Harel, L. 1989. Inhibitory diffusible factor-45 bifunctional activity as a cell growth inhibitor and as an insulin-like growth factor I-binding protein. *Journal of Biological Chemistry* 264:12449–12454.

Blum, J.W., and Kuntz, P. 1981. Effects of fasting on thyroid hormone levels and kinetics of reverse triiodothyronine in cattle. *Acta Endocrinologica* 98:234–239.

Blum, J.W., Schnyder, W., Kunz, P.L., Blom, A.K., Bickel, H., and Schurch, A. 1985. Reduced and compensatory growth: endocrine and metabolic changes during food restriction and refeeding in steers. *Journal of Nutrition* 115:417–424.

Bonneau, M. 1993. Growth hormone response to GRF and insulin-induced hypoglycemia in Yorkshire and Meishan pigs. *American Journal of Physiology* 264:E54–E59.

Borger, M.L., and Davis, S.L. 1974. Development of a specific ovine thyrotropin (TSH) radioimmunoassay from non-specific antisera. *Journal of Animal Science* 39:768–774.

Bowers, C.Y. 1999. Growth hormone-releasing peptides. In *Handbook of Physiology.* J.L. Kostyo, ed. New York and Oxford: Oxford University Press.

Brameld, J.M., Atkinson, J.L., Saunders, J.C., Pell, J.M., Buttery, P.J., and Gilmour, R.S. 1996. Effects of growth hormone administration and dietary protein intake on insulin-like growth factor I and growth hormone receptor mRNA expression in porcine liver, skeletal muscle, and adipose tissue. *Journal of Animal Science* 74:1832–1841.

Breier, B.H., Ambler, G.R., Sauerwein, H., Surus, A., and Gluckman, P.D. 1994. The induction of hepatic somatotrophic receptors after birth in sheep is dependent on parturition-associated mechanisms. *Journal of Endocrinology* 141:101–108.

Brethour, J.R. 1972. Effects of acute injections of dexamethasone on selective deposition of bovine intramuscular fat. *Journal of Animal Science* 35:351–356.

Buonomo, F.C., Grohs, D.L., Baile, C.A., and Campion, D.R. 1988. Determination of circulating levels of insulin-like growth factor II (IGF-II) in swine. *Domestic Animal Endocrinology* 5:323–329.

Buonomo, F.C., Lauterio, T.J., Baile, C.A., and Daughaday, W.H. 1987. Effects of insulin-like growth factor I (IGF-I)

on growth hormone-releasing hormone (GRF) and thyrotropin-releasing hormone (TRH) stimulation of growth hormone (GH) secretion in the domestic fowl (Gallus domesticus). *General and Comparative Endocrinology* 66:274–279.

Buonomo, F.C., Zimmerman, N.G., Lauterio, T.J., and Scanes, C.G. 1984. Catecholamines involvement in the control of growth hormone secretion in the domestic fowl. *General and Comparative Endocrinology* 54:360–371.

Burch, W.M., and Lebovitz, H.E. 1982. Triiodothyronine stimulation of in vitro growth and maturation of embryonic chick cartilage. *Endocrinology* 111:462–468.

Burch, W.M., Weir, S., and Van Wyk, J.J. 1986. Embryonic chick cartilage produces its own somatomedin-like peptide to stimulate cartilage growth in vitro. *Endocrinology* 119:1370–1376.

Burke, W.H., Moore, J.A., Ogez, J.G., and Builder, S.E. 1987. The properties of recombinant chicken growth hormone and its effects on growth, body composition, feed efficiency, and other factors in broiler chickens. *Endocrinology* 120:651–658.

Burnside, J., Liou, S.S., and Cogburn, L.A. 1991. Molecular cloning of the chicken growth hormone receptor complementary deoxyribonucleic acid: mutation of the gene in sex-linked dwarf chickens. *Endocrinology* 128:3183–3192.

Burnside, J., Liou, S.S., Zhong, C., and Cogburn, L.A. 1992. Abnormal growth hormone receptor gene expression in the sex-linked Dwarf chicken. *General and Comparative Endocrinology* 88:20–28.

Butterwith, S.C., and Goddard, C. 1991. Regulation of DNA synthesis in chicken adipocyte precursor cells by insulin-like growth factors, platelet-derived growth factor and transforming growth factor-β. *Journal of Endocrinology* 131:203–209.

Caldés, J., Alemany, J., Robcis, H.L., and DePablo, F. 1991. Expression of insulin-like growth factor I in developing lens is compartmentalized. *Journal of Biological Chemistry* 266:20786–20790.

Campbell, R.G., Johnson, R.J., King, R.H., Taverner, M.R., and Meisinger, D.J. 1990. Interaction of dietary protein content and exogenous porcine growth hormone administration on protein and lipid accretion rates in growing pigs. *Journal of Animal Science* 68:3217–3225.

Campbell, R.G., Steele, N.C., Caperna, T.J., McMurtry, J.P., Solomon, M.B., and Mitchell, A.D. 1988. Interrelationships between energy intake and endogenous porcine growth hormone administration on the performance, body composition and protein and energy metabolism of growing pigs weighing 25 to 55 kilograms live weight. *Journal of Animal Science* 66:1643–1655.

Campbell, R.G., Steele, N.C., Caperna, T.J., McMurtry, J.P., Solomon, M.B., and Mitchell, A.D. 1989. Effects of exogenous porcine growth hormone administration between 30 and 60 kilograms on the subsequent and overall performance of pigs grown to 90 kilograms. *Journal of Animal Science* 67:1265–1271.

Campbell, R.M., Chen, W.Y., Wiehl, P., Kelder, B., Kopchick, J.J., and Scanes, C.G. 1995. A growth hormone (GH) analog that antagonizes the lipolytic effect but retains full insulin-like (antilipolytic) activity of GH. *Proceedings of Society for Experimental Biology and Medicine* 203:311–316.

Campbell, R.M., and Scanes, C.G. 1985. Lipolytic activity of purified pituitary and bacterially derived growth hormone on chicken adipose tissue in vitro. *Proceedings of Society for Experimental Biology and Medicine* 184:456–460.

Carpenter, C.E., Greaser, M.L., and Cassens, R.G. 1987. Accumulation of newly synthesized myosin heavy chain during thyroxine-induced myofiber type transition. *Journal of Animal Science* 64:1574–1587.

Carr, J.M., Grant, P.A., Francis, G.L., Owens, J.A., Wallace, J.C., and Walton, P.E. 1994. Isolation and characterization of ovine IGFBP-4:protein purification and cDNA sequence. *Journal of Molecular Endocrinology* 13:219–236.

Carr, J.M., Owens, J.A., Grant, P.A., Walton, P.E., Owens, P. C., and Wallace, J.C. 1995. Circulating insulin-like growth factors (IGF's), IGF binding proteins (IGFBP's) and tissue mRNA levels of IGFBP-2 and IGFBP-4 in the ovine fetus. *Journal of Endocrinology* 145:545–557.

Carroll, J.A., Buonomo, F.C., Becker, B.A., and Matteri, R.L. 1999. Interactions between environmental temperature and porcine growth hormone (pGH) treatment in neonatal pigs. *Domestic Animal Endocrinology* 16:103–113.

Carsia, R.V., and Harvey, S. 2000. Adrenals. In Sturkie's *Avian Physiology*, 5th ed. G.C. Whittow, ed. San Diego: Academic Press.

Chapple, R.P., Cuaron, J.A., and Easter, R.A. 1989a. Effect of glucocorticoids and limiting nursing on the carbohydrate digestive capacity and growth rate of piglets. *Journal of Animal Science* 67:2956–2973.

Chapple, R.P., Cuaron, J.A., and Easter, R.A. 1989b. Response of digestive carbohydrates and growth to graded doses and administration frequency of hydrocortisone and adrenocorticotropic hormone in nursing piglets. *Journal of Animal Science* 67:2974–2984.

Chapple, R.P., Cuaron, J.A., and Easter, R.A. 1989c. Temporal changes in carbohydrate digestive capacity and growth rate of piglets in response to glucocorticoid administration and weaning age. *Journal of Animal Science* 67:2985–2995.

Charlton, S.T., Cosgrove, J.R., Glimm, D.R., and Foxcroft, G.R. 1993. Ovarian and hepatic insulin-like growth factor-I gene expression and associated metabolic responses in prepubertal gilts subjected to feed restriction and refeeding. *Journal of Endocrinology* 139:143–152.

Chase, C.C., Kirby, C.J., Hammond, A.C., Olson, T.A., and Lucy, M.C. 1998. Patterns of ovarian growth and development in cattle with a growth hormone receptor deficiency. *Journal of Animal Science* 76:212–219.

Chen, W.Y., Wight, D.C., Wagner, T.E., and Kopchick, J.J. 1990. Expression of a mutated bovine growth hormone gene suppresses growth of transgenic mice. *Proceedings of the National Academy of Sciences* 6:598–606.

Christon, R. 1988. The effect of tropical ambient temperature on growth and metabolism in pigs. *Journal of Animal Science* 66:3112–3123.

Chung, C.S., and Etherton, T.D. 1980. Characterization of porcine growth hormone (pGH) binding to porcine liver microsomes: chronic administration of pGH induces pGH binding. *Endocrinology* 119:780–786.

Chung, C.S., Etherton, T.D., and Wiggins, J.P. 1985. Stimulation of swine growth by porcine growth hormone. *Journal of Animal Science* 60:118–130.

Clapper, J.A., Clark, T.M., and Rempel, L.A. 2000. Serum concentrations of IGF-I, estradiol-17b, testosterone, and relative amounts of IGF binding proteins (IGFBP) in growing boars, barrows, and gilts. *Journal of Animal Science* 78:2581–2588.

Clark, R.G., Mortensen, D., Reigsupreder, D., Mohler, M., Etchevery, T., and Mukkev, V. 1993. Recombinant human insulin-like growth factor binding protein 3: effects on the glycine and growth promotion activities of rhIGF-I in the rat. *Growth Regulation* 3:46–50.

Clemmons, D.R. 1999. Insulin-like growth factor binding proteins. In *Handbook of Physiology*. J.L. Kostyo, ed. New York and Oxford: Oxford University Press.

Cogburn, L.A., Liou, S.S., Rand, A.L., and McMurtry, J.P. 1989. Growth, metabolic and endocrine responses of broiler cockerels given a daily subcutaneous injection of natural or biosynthetic chicken growth hormone. *Journal of Nutrition* 119:1213–1222.

Coleman, M.E., and Etherton, T.D. 1991. Effects of exogenous porcine growth hormone on serum insulin-like growth factor-binding proteins in growing pigs. *Journal of Endocrinology* 128:175–180.

Coleman, M.E., and Etherton, T.D. 1994. Porcine insulin-like growth factor (IGF)-binding protein-3 elicits bi-phasic effects on IGF-I stimulated DNA synthesis in neonatal porcine skin fibroblasts. *Domestic Animal Endocrinology* 11:299–305.

Conover, C.A. 1990. Regulation of insulin-like growth factor (IGF)-binding protein synthesis by insulin and IGF-I in cultured bovine fibroblasts. *Endocrinology* 126:3139–3145.

Convey, E.M., Tucker, H.A., Smith, V.G., and Zolman, J. 1973. Bovine prolactin, growth hormone, thyroxine and corticoid response to thyrotropin-releasing hormone. *Endocrinology* 92:471–476.

Cooke, N.E., and Liebhaber, S.A. 1999. Regulation of growth hormone gene expression. In *Handbook of Physiology*. J.L. Kostyo, ed. New York and Oxford: Oxford University Press.

Cooke, P.S., and Nicoll, C.S. 1984. Role of insulin in the growth of fetal rat tissues. *Endocrinology* 114:638–643.

Corah, T.J., Tatum, J.D., Morgan, J.B., Mortimer, R.G., and Smith, G.C. 1995. Effects of a dexamethasone implant on deposition of intramuscular fat in genetically identical cattle. *Journal of Animal Science* 73:3310–3316.

Cowin, A.J., and Bidey, S.P. 1995. Porcine thyroid follicular cells in monolayer culture activate the iodide-responsive precursor form of transforming growth factor-β1. *Journal of Endocrinology* 144:67–73.

Cowin, A.J., Heaton, E.L., Cheshire, S.H., and Bidey, S.P. 1996. The proliferative responses of porcine thyroid follicular cells to epidermal growth factor and thyrotrophin reflect the autocrine production of transforming growth factor-β1. *Journal of Endocrinology* 148:87–94.

Cromwell, G.L., Sihombing, D.T.H., and Hays, V.W. 1975. Effects of iodine level on performance and thyroid traits of growing pigs. *Journal of Animal Science* 41:813–818.

Crooker, B.A., McGuire, M.A., Cohick, W.S., Harkins, M., Bauman, D.E., and Sejrsen, K. 1990. Effect of dose of bovine somatotropin on nutrient utilization in growing dairy heifers. *Journal of Nutrition* 120:1256–1263.

Cunningham, B.C., Ultsch, M., DeVos, A.M., Mulkerrin, M.G., Clauser, K.R., and Wells, J.A. 1991. Dimerization of the extracellular domain of the human growth hormone receptor by a single hormone molecule. *Science* 254:821–825.

Cynober, L., Aussel, C., Chatelain, P., Vaubourdolle, M., Agneray, J., and Ekindjian, O.G. 1985. Insulin-like growth factor I/somatomedin C action on 2-deoxyglucose and a-amino isobutyrate uptake in chick embryo fibroblasts. *Biochimie* 67:1185–1190.

Dalke, B.S., Roeder, R.A., Kasser, T.R., Veenhuizen, J.J., Hunt, C.W., Hinman, D.D., and Schelling, G.T. 1992. Dose-response effects of recombinant bovine somatotropin implants on feedlot performance in steers. *Journal of Animal Science* 70:2130–2137.

Danzmann, R.G., Van Der Kraak, G.J., Chen, T.T., and Powers, D.A. 1990. Metabolic effects of bovine growth hormone and genetically engineered rainbow trout growth hormone in rainbow trout (Oncorhynchus mykiss) reared at a high temperature. *Canadian Journal of Fisheries and Aquatic Sciences* 47:1291–1301.

Darras, V.M., Huybrechts, L.M., Kuhn, E.R., and Decuypere, E. 1990. Ontogeny of the effect of purified chicken growth hormone on the liver 5' monodeiodination activity in the chicken: reversal of the activity after hatching. *General and Comparative Endocrinology* 77:212–220.

Darras, V.M., Rudas, P., Hall, T.R., Huybrechts, L.M., Vanderpooten, A., Berghman, L.R., Decuypere, E., and Kuhn, E.R. 1993. Endogenous growth hormone controls high plasma levels of 3,3',5-triiodothyronine (T3) in growing chickens by decreasing the T3-degrading type III deiodinase activity. *Domestic Animal Endocrinology* 10:55–65.

Dasen, J.S., O'Connell, S.M., Flynn, S.E., Treier, M., Gleiberman, A.S., Szeto, D.P., Hooshmand, F., Aggarwal, A.K., and Rosenfeld, M.G. 1999. Reciprocal interactions of Pit1 and GATA2 mediate signaling gradient-induced determination of pituitary cell types. *Cell* 97:587–598.

Dauncey, M.J., Rudd, B.T., White, D.A., and Shakespear, R.A. 1993. Regulation of insulin-like growth factor binding proteins in young growing animals by alteration of energy status. *Growth Regulation* 3:198–207.

David, R.B., Blom, A.K., Sjaastad, Ø.V., and Harbitz, I. 2001. The porcine erythropoietin gene: cDNA sequence, genomic sequence and expression analyses in piglets. *Domestic Animal Endocrinology* 20:137–147.

Davis, M.E., and Simmen, R.C.M. 1997. Genetic parameter estimates for serum insulin-like growth factor I concentration and performance traits in Angus beef cattle. *Journal of Animal Science* 75:317–324.

Davis, S.L., Ohlson, D.L., Klindt, J., and Anfinson, M.S. 1978. Episodic patterns of prolactin and thyrotropin secretion in rams and wethers: influence of testosterone and diethylstilbestrol. *Journal of Animal Science* 46:1724–1729.

Davis, T.A., Fiorotto, M.L., Beckett, P.R., Burrin, D.G., Reeds, P.J., Wray-Cahen, D., and Nguyen, H.V. 2001. Differential effects of insulin on peripheral and visceral tissue protein synthesis in neonatal pigs. *American Journal of Physiology* 280:E770–E779.

Davison, T.F., Rea, J., and Rowell, J.G. 1983. Effects of dietary corticosterone on the growth and metabolism of immature Gallus domesticus. *General and Comparative Endocrinology* 50:463–468.

Dawe, S.R., Francis, G.L., McNamara, P.J., Wallace, J.C., and Ballard, F.J. 1988. Purification, partial sequences and properties of chicken insulin-like growth factors. *Journal of Endocrinology* 117:173–181.

de Pablo, F., Girbau, M., Gomez, J.A., Hernandez, E., and Roth, J. 1985. Insulin antibodies retard and insulin accelerates growth and differentiation in early embryos. *Diabetes* 34:1063–1067.

Desler, M.M., Jones, S.J., Smith, C.W., and Woods, T.L. 1996. Effects of dexamethasone and anabolic agents on proliferation and protein synthesis and degradation in C2C12 myogenic cells. *Journal of Animal Science* 74:1265–1273.

Dodson, M.V., Davis, S.L., Ohlson, D.L., and Ercanbrack, S.K. 1983. Temporal patterns of growth hormone, prolactin and thyrotropin secretion in Targhee rams selected for rate and efficiency of gain. *Journal of Animal Science* 57:338–342.

Donker, R.A., and Beuving, G. 1989. Effect of corticosterone infusion on plasma corticosterone concentration, antibody production, circulating leukocytes and growth in chicken lines selected for humoral immune responsiveness. *British Poultry Science* 30:361–369.

Donkin, S.S., Chiu, P.Y., Yin, D., Louveau, I., Swencki, B., Vockroth, J., Evock-Clover, C.M., Peters, J.L., and Etherton, T.D. 1996. Porcine somatotropin differentially down-regulates expression of the GLUT4 and fatty acid synthase genes in pig adipose tissue. *Journal of Nutrition* 126:2568–2577.

Doris, R.A., Thompson, G.E., Finley, E., Kilgour, E., Houslay, M.D., and Vernon, R.G. 1996. Chronic effects of somatotropin treatment on response of subcutaneous adipose tissue lipolysis to acutely acting factors in vivo and in vitro. *Journal of Animal Science* 74:562–568.

Down, N.E., Donaldson, E.M., Dye, H.M., Boone, T.C., Langley, K.E., and Souza, L.M. 1989. A potent analog of recombinant bovine somatotropin accelerates growth in juvenile coho salmon (Oncorhynchus kisutch). *Canadian Journal of Fisheries and Aquatic Sciences* 46:178–183.

Down, N.E., Donaldson, E.M., Dye, H.M., Langley, K., and Souza, L.M. 1988. Recombinant bovine somatotropin more than doubles the growth rate of coho salmon (Oncorhynchus kisutch) acclimated to seawater and ambient winter conditions. *Aquaculture* 68:141–155.

Drisko, J.E., Faidley, T.D., Chang, C.H., Zhang, D., Nicolich, S., Hora, D.F., McNamara, L., Rickes, E., Abribat, T., Smith, R.G., and Hickey, G.J.1998. Hypophyseal-portal concentrations of growth hormone-releasing factor and somatostatin in conscious pigs: relationship to production of spontaneous growth hormone pulses. *Proceedings of the Society for Experimental Biology and Medicine* 217:188–196.

Dubreuil, P., Lapierre, H., Pelletier, G., Petitclerc, D., Couture, Y., Gaudreau, P., Morisset, J., and Brazeau, P. 1988. Serum growth hormone release during a 60-hour period in growing pigs. *Domestic Animal Endocrinology* 5:157–164.

Ducy, P., Amling, M., Takeda, S., Priemel, M., Schilling, A.F., Beil, F.t., Shen, J., Vinson, C., Rueger, J.M., and Karsenty, G. 2000. Leptin inhibits bone formation through a hypothalamic relay: a central control of bone mass. *Cell* 100:197–207.

Duquette, P.F., Scanes, C.G., and Muir, L.A. 1984. Effects of ovine growth hormone and other anterior pituitary hormones on lipolysis of rat and ovine adipose tissue in vitro. *Journal of Animal Science* 58:1191–1204.

Early, R.J., McBride, B.W., and Ball, R.O. 1990a. Growth and metabolism in somatotropin-treated steers: I. Growth, serum chemistry and carcass weights. *Journal of Animal Science* 68:4134–4143.

Early, R.J., McBride, B.W., and Ball, R.O. 1990b. Growth and metabolism in somatotropin-treated steers: II. Carcass and noncarcass tissue components and chemical composition. *Journal of Animal Science* 68:4144–4152.

Eisemann, J.H., Hammond, A.C., Bauman, D.E., Reynolds, P.J., McCutcheon, S.N., Tyrrell, H.F., and Haaland, G.L. 1986b. Effect of bovine growth hormone administration on metabolism of growing Hereford heifers: protein and lipid metabolism and plasma concentrations of metabolites and hormones. *Journal of Nutrition* 116:2504–2515.

Eisemann, J.H., Hammond, A.C., Rumsey, T.S., and Bauman, D.E. 1989. Nitrogen and protein metabolism and metabolites in plasma and urine of beef steers treated with somatotropin. *Journal of Animal Science* 67:105–115.

Eisemann, J.H., Tyrrell, H.F., Hammond, A.C., Reynolds, P.J., Bauman, D.E., Haaland, G.L., McMurtry, J.P., and Varga, G.A. 1986a. Effect of bovine growth hormone administration on metabolism of growing Hereford heifers: dietary digestibility, energy and nitrogen balance. *Journal of Nutrition* 116:157–163.

Elliott, J.L., Oldham, J.M., Ambler, G.R., Bass, J.J., Spencer, G.S.G., Hodgkinson, S.C., Breier, B.H., Gluckman, P.D., and Suttie, J.M. 1992. Presence of insulin-like growth factor-I receptors and absence of growth hormone receptors in the antler tip. *Endocrinology* 130:2513–2520.

Ely, D.G., Boling, J.A., and Deweese, W.P. 1976. Dietary thyroprotein influence on lamb performance and blood constituents. *Journal of Animal Science* 42:1309–1315.

Engler, D., Pham, T., Fullerton, M.J., Ooi, G., Funder, J.W., and Clarke, I.J. 1989. Studies of the secretion of corticotropin-releasing factor and arginine vasopressin into the hypophysial portal circulation of the conscious sheep. I. Effect of an audiovisual stimulus and insulin-induced hypoglycemia. *Neuroendocrinology* 49:367–381.

Engster, H.M., Carew, L.B., Harvey, S., and Scanes, C.G. 1979. Growth hormone metabolism in essential fatty acid-deficient and pair-fed non-deficient chicks. *Journal of Nutrition* 109:330–338.

Enright, W.J., Quirke, J.F., Gluckman, P.D., Breier, B.H., Kennedy, L.G., Hart, I.C., Roche, J.F., Coert, A., and Allen, P. 1990. Effects of long-term administration of pituitary-derived bovine growth hormone and estradiol on growth in steers. *Journal of Animal Science* 68:2345–2356.

Estienne, M.J., Schillo, K.K., Hileman, S.M., Green, M.A., Hayes, S.H., and Boling, J.A. 1990. Effects of free fatty acids on luteinizing hormone and growth hormone secretion in ovariectomized lambs. *Endocrinology* 126:1934–1940.

Etherton, T.D., Wiggins, J.P., Chung, C.S., Evock, C.M., Rebhun, J.F., and Walton, P.E. 1986. Stimulation of pig growth performance by porcine growth hormone and growth hormone-releasing factor. *Journal of Animal Science* 63:1389–1399.

Fielder, P.J., Mortensen, D.L., Mallet, P., Carlsson, B., Baxter, R.C., and Clark, R.G. 1996. Differential long-term effects of insulin-like growth factor-I (IGF-I), growth hormone (GH), and IGF-I plus GH on body growth and IGF binding proteins in hypophysectomized rats. *Endocrinology* 137:1913–1920.

Finidori, J., and Kelly, P.A. 1995. Cytokine receptor signalling through two novel families of transducer molecules: Janus kinases, and signal transducers and activators of transcription. *Journal of Endocrinology* 147:11–23.

Fisher, J.W. 1997. Erythropoietin: physiologic and pharmacologic aspects. *Proceedings of the Society for Experimental Biology and Medicine* 216:358–369.

Fitzgerald, J., Michel, F., and Butler, W.R. 1982. Growth and sexual maturation in ewes: the role of photoperiod, diet and temperature on growth rate and the control of prolactin, thyroxine and luteinizing hormone secretion. *Journal of Animal Science* 55:1431–1440.

Fleming, J.S., Suttie, J.M., Montgomery, G.W., Gunn, J., Stuart, S.K., Littlejohn, R.P., and Gootwine, E. 1997. The effects of a duplication in the ovine growth hormone (GH) gene on GH expression in the pituitaries of ram lambs from lean and fat-selected sheep lines. *Domestic Animal Endocrinology* 14:17–24.

Ford, J.J., and Anderson, L.L. 1967. Growth in immature hypophysectomized pigs. *Journal of Endocrinology* 37:347–348.

Fowden, A.L., Mijovic, J., and Silver, M. 1993. The effects of cortisol on hepatic and renal gluconeogenic enzyme activities in the sheep fetus during late gestation. *Journal of Endocrinology* 137:213–222.

Francis, G.L., Upton, F.M., Ballard, F.J., McNeil, K.A., and Wallace, J.C. 1988. Insulin-like growth factors 1 and 2 in bovine colostrum. Sequences and biological activities compared with those of a potent truncated form. *Biochemical Journal* 251:95–103.

Freemark, M., Fleenor, D., Driscoll, P., Binart, N., and Kelly, P.A. 2001. Body Weight and Fat Deposition in Prolactin Reception-Deficient Mice. *Endocrinology* 142:532–537.

Frohman, L.A., and Kineman, R.D. 1999. Growth hormone-releasing hormone: discovery, regulation, and actions. In

Handbook of Physiology. J.L. Kostyo, ed. New York and Oxford: Oxford University Press.

Fulvio, M.D., Coleoni, A.H., Pellizas, C.G., and Masini-Repiso, A.M. 2000. Tri-iodothyronine induces proliferation in cultured bovine thyroid cells: evidence for the involvement of epidermal growth factor-associated tyrosine kinase activity. *Journal of Endocrinology* 166:173–182.

Garber, M.J., DeYonge, K.G., Byatt, J.C., Lellis, W.A., Honeyfield, D.C., Bull, R.C., Schelling, G.T., and Roeder, R.A. 1995. Dose-response effects of recombinant bovine somatotropin (Posilac) on growth performance and body composition of two-year-old rainbow trout (Oncorhynchus mykiss). *Journal of Animal Science* 73:3216–3222.

Gayrard, V., Alvinerie, M., and Toutain, P.L. 1996. Interspecies variations of corticosteroid-binding globulin parameters. *Domestic Animal Endocrinology* 13:35–45.

Gerfault, V., Louveau, I., and Mourot, J. 1999. The effect of GH and IGF-I on preadipocytes from Large White and Meishan pigs in primary culture. *General and Comparative Endocrinology* 114:396–404.

Girbau, M., Bassas, L., Roth, J., and de Pablo, F. 1989. Insulin reverses the growth retardation effect of phorbol ester in chicken embryos during organogenesis. *Life Sciences* 44:1971–1978.

Girbau, M., Gomez, J.A., Lesniak, M.A., and DePablo, F. 1987. Insulin and insulin-like growth factor I both stimulate metabolism, growth, and differentiation in the post-neurula chick embryo. *Endocrinology* 121:1477–1482.

Girbau, M., Lesniak, M.A., Gomez, J.A., and de Pablo, F. 1988. Insulin action in early embryonic life: anti-insulin receptor antibodies retard chicken embryo growth but not muscle differentiation in vivo. *Biochemical and Biophysical Research Communications* 153:142–148.

Gluckman, P.D., Butler, J.H., Comline, R., and Fowden, A. 1987. The effects of pancreatectomy on the plasma concentrations of insulin-like growth factors 1 and 2 in the sheep fetus. *Journal of Developmental Physiology* 9:79–88.

Goff, J.P., Caperna, T.J., and Steele, N.C. 1990. Effects of growth hormone administration on vitamin D metabolism and vitamin D receptors in the pig. *Domestic Animal Endocrinology* 7:425–435.

Gootwine, E., Sise, J.A., Penty, J., and Montgomery, G.W. 1993. The duplicated gene copy of the ovine growth hormone gene contains a Pvu II polymorphism in the second intron. *Animal Genetics* 24:319–321.

Gopinath, R., and Etherton, T.D. 1989a. Effects of porcine growth hormone on glucose metabolism of pigs: I. Acute and chronic effects on plasma glucose and insulin status. *Journal of Animal Science* 67:682–688.

Gopinath, R., and Etherton, T.D. 1989b. Effects of porcine growth hormone on glucose metabolism of pigs: II. Glucose tolerance, peripheral tissue insulin sensitivity and glucose kinetics. *Journal of Animal Science* 67:689–697.

Gross, W.B., Siegel, P.B., and DuBose, R.T. 1980. Some effects of feeding corticosterone to chickens. *Poultry Science* 59:516–522.

Gruppuso, P.A. 1989. Effects of fetal hypoinsulinemia on fetal hepatic insulin binding in the rat. *Biochimica Biophysica Acta* 1010:270–273.

Gruppuso, P.A., Boylan, J.M., Bienieki, T.C., and Curran, T.R. 1994. Evidence for a direct hepatotrophic role for insulin in the fetal rat: implications for the impaired hepatic growth seen in fetal growth retardation. *Endocrinology* 134:769–775.

Guillaume, V., Magnan, E., Cataldi, M., Dutour, A., Sauze, N., Renard, M., Razafindraibe, H., Conte-Devolx, B., Deghenghi, R., Lenaerts, V., and Oliver, C. 1994. Growth hormone (GH)-releasing hormone secretion is stimulated by a new GH-releasing hexapeptide in sheep. *Endocrinology* 135:1073–1076.

Hammond, A.C., Elsasser, T.H., and Olson, T.A. 1991. Endocrine characteristics of a miniature condition of Brahman cattle: circulating concentrations of some growth-related hormones. *Proceedings of the Society for Experimental Biology and Medicine* 197:450–457.

Hampson, R.K., and Rottman, F.M. 1987. Alternative processing of bovine growth hormone mRNA: nonsplicing of the final intron predicts a high molecular weight variant of bovine growth hormone. *Proceedings of the National Academy of Sciences* 84:2673–2677.

Harter, G.D., and Vetter, R.L. 1967. Feeder lamb response to cortisone acetate and diethylstilbestrol. *Journal of Animal Science* 26:1397–1403.

Harvey, S., and Scanes, C.G. 1978. Effect of adrenaline and adrenergic active drugs on growth hormone secretion in immature cockerels. *Experientia* 34:1096–1097.

Harvey, S., and Scanes, C.G. 1987. Opiate inhibition of growth hormone secretion in young chickens. *General and Comparative Endocrinology* 65:34–39.

Harvey, S., Scanes, C.G., Chadwick, A., and Bolton, N.J. 1978a. The effect of thyrotropin releasing hormone (TRH) and somatostatin (GHRIH) on growth hormone and prolactin secretion in vitro and in vivo in the domestic fowl (Gallus domesticus). *Neuroendocrinology* 26:249–260.

Harvey, S., Scanes, C.G., Chadwick, A., and Bolton, N.J. 1978b. Influence of fasting, glucose and insulin on the levels in the plasma of growth hormone and prolactin of the domestic fowl. *Journal of Endocrinology* 76:501–506.

Harvey, S., Scanes, C.G., and Howe, T. 1977. Growth hormone effects on in vitro metabolism of avian adipose and liver tissue. *General and Comparative Endocrinology* 33:322–328.

Harvey, S., Sterling, R.J., and Klandorf, H. 1983. Concentrations of triiodothyronine, growth hormone, and luteinizing hormone in the plasma of thyroidectomized fowl (Gallus domesticus). *General and Comparative Endocrinology* 50:275–286.

Hatch, R.H., Kercher, C.J., and Roehrkasse, G.P. 1972. Response of hyperthyroid, euthyroid and hypothyroid lambs to exogenous thyroxine. *Journal of Animal Science* 34:988–993.

Haynes, N.B., Kiser, T.E., Hafs, H.D., and Stellflug, J.N. 1978. Effect of intracarotid infusion of prostaglandin F2a on plasma prolactin and growth hormone in bulls. *Journal of Animal Science* 47:919–922.

Heap, D., Collier, R.J., Boyd, C.K., and Lucy, M.C. 1996. Expression of alternative growth hormone receptor messenger RNA in ovary and uterus of cattle. *Domestic Animal Endocrinology* 13:421–430.

Hembree, J.R., Pampusch, M.S., Yang, F., Causey, J.L., Hathaway, M.R., and Dayton, W.R. 1996. Cultured porcine myogenic cells produce insulin-like growth factor binding protein-3 (IGFBP-3) and transforming growth factor beta-1 stimulates IGFBP-3 production. *Journal of Animal Science* 74:1530–1540.

Hertelendy, F., and Kipnis, D.M. 1973. Studies on growth hormone secretion: V. Influence of plasma free fatty acid levels. *Endocrinology* 92:402–410.

Hertelendy, F., Machlin, L., and Kipnis, D.M. 1969. Further studies on the regulation of insulin and growth hormone secretion in the sheep. *Endocrinology* 84:192–199.

Hibbard, B., Peters, J.P., Shen, R.Y.W., and Chester, S.T. 1992. Effect of recombinant porcine somatotropin and dietary protein on pancreatic digestive enzymes in the pig. *Journal of Animal Science* 70:2188–2194.

Hickey, G.J., Drisko, J., Faidley, T., Chang, C., Anderson, L.L., Nicolich, S., McGuire, L., Rickes, E., Krupa, D., Feeney, W., Friscino, B., Cunningham, P., Frazier, E., Chen, H., Laroque, P., and Smith, R.G. 1996. Mediation by the central nervous system is critical to the in vivo activity of the GH secretagogue L-692,585. *Journal of Endocrinology* 148:371–380.

Higgs, D.A., Donaldson, E.M., Dye, H.M., and McBride, J.R. 1975. A preliminary investigation of the effect of bovine growth hormone on growth and muscle composition of Coho salmon (Oncorhynchus kisutch). *General and Comparative Endocrinology* 27:240–253.

Hintz, R.L. 1999. The somatomedin hypothesis of growth hormone action. In *Handbook of Physiology*. J.L. Kostyo, ed. New York and Oxford: Oxford University Press.

Hoggard, N., Hunter, L., Duncan, J.S., Williams, L.M., Trayhurn, P., and Mercer, J.G. 1997. Leptin and leptin receptor mRNA and protein expression in the murine fetus and placenta. *Proceedings National Academy of Science USA* 94:11073–11078.

Hooper, S.B., Bocking, A.D., White, S.E., Fraher, L.J., McDonald, T.J., and Han, V.K.M. 1994. Catecholamines stimulate the synthesis and release of insulin-like growth factor binding protein-1 (IGFBP-1) by fetal sheep liver in vivo. *Endocrinology* 134:1104–1112.

Hopkins, P.S., and Thorburn, G.D. 1972. The effects of fetal thyroidectomy on the development of the ovine fetus. *Journal of Endocrinology* 54:55–61.

Houseknecht, K.L., and Bauman, D.E. 1997. Regulation of lipolysis by somatotropin: functional alteration of adrenergic and adenosine signaling in bovine adipose tissue. *Journal of Endocrinology* 152:465–475.

Houseknecht, K.L., Bauman, D.E., Carey, G.B., and Mersmann, H.J. 1995b. Effect of bovine somatotropin and food deprivation of β-adrenergic and A1 adenosine receptor binding in adipose tissue of lactating cows. *Domestic Animal Endocrinology* 12:325–336.

Houseknecht, K.L., Dwyer, D.A., Lanna, D.P.D., and Bauman, D.E. 1995a. Effect of somatotropin on adipose tissue metabolism: ontogeny of the enhanced response to adrenergic challenge in the lactating cow. *Domestic Animal Endocrinology* 12:105–113.

Houston, B., and Goddard, C. 1988. Molecular forms of growth hormone in the chicken pituitary gland. *Journal of Endocrinology* 116:35–41.

Houston, B., and O'Neill, I.E. 1991. Insulin and growth hormone act synergistically to stimulate insulin-like growth factor-I production by cultured chicken hepatocytes. *Journal of Endocrinology* 128:389–393.

Howard, A.D., Feighner, S.D., Cully, D.F., Arena, J.P., Liberator, P.A., Rosenblum, C.I., Hamelin, M., Hreniuk, D.L., Palyha, O.C., Anderson, J., Paress, P.S., Diaz, C., Chou, M., Liu, K.K., McKee, K.K., Pong, S.S., Chaung, L.Y., Elbrecht, A., Dashkevicz, R., Heavens, R., Rigby, M., Sirinathsinghji, D.J.S., Dean, D.C., Melillo, D.G., Patchett, A.A., Nargund, R., Griffion, P.R., DeMartino, J.A., Gupta, S.K., Schaeffer, J.M., Smith, R.G., and Van der Ploeg, L.H.T. 1996. A receptor in pituitary and hypothalamus that functions in growth hormone release. *Science* 273:974–977.

Hsiung, H.M., Smith, D.P., Zhang, X., Bennett, T., Roseteck, P.R., and Lai, M. 1993. Structure and functional expression of a complementary DNA for porcine growth hormone-releasing hormone receptor. *Neuropeptides* 25:1–10.

Huang, N., Coghurn, L.A., Agarwal, S.K., Marks, H.L., and Burnside, J. 1993. Overexpression of a truncated growth hormone receptor in the sex-linked dwarf chicken: evidence for a splice mutation. *Molecular Endocrinology* 7:1391–1398.

Huff, G.R., Huff, W.E., Balog, J.M., and Rath, N.C. 1999. Sex differences in the resistance of turkeys to Escherichia coli challenge after immunosuppression with dexamethasone. *Poultry Science* 78:38–44.

Hurley, W.L., Convey, E.M., Edgerton, L.A., and Hemken, R.W. 1981. Bovine prolactin, TSH, T4 and T3 concentrations as affected by tall fescue summer toxicosis and temperature. *Journal of Animal Science* 51:374–379.

Huybrechts, L.M., King, D.B., Lauterio, T.J., Marsh, J., and Scanes, C.G. 1985. Plasma concentrations of somatomedin-C in hypophysectomized, dwarf and intact growing domestic fowl as determined by heterologous radioimmunoassay. *Journal of Endocrinology* 104:233–239.

Hylka, V.W., and Doneen, B.A. 1983. Ontogeny of embryonic chicken lung: effects of pituitary gland, corticosterone, and other hormones upon pulmonary growth and synthesis of surfactant phospholipids. *General and Comparative Endocrinology* 52:108–120.

Ihle, J.N., and Kerr, I.M. 1995. JAK5 and STAT5 in signaling by the cytokine receptor superfamily. *Trends in Genetics* 11:69–74.

Jelkman, W. 1992. Erythropoietin structure, control of production, and function. *Physiological Reviews* 72:449–489.

Johke, T. 1978. Effects of TRH on circulating growth hormone, prolactin and triiodothyronine levels in the bovine. *Endocrinologia Japonica* 25:19–26.

Johnson, R.J. 1988. Diminution of pulsatile growth hormone secretion in the domestic fowl (Gallus domesticus): evidence of sexual dimorphism. *Journal of Endocrinology* 119:101–109.

Johnsson, I.D., Hathorn, D.J., Wilde, R.M., Treacher, T.T., and Butler-Hogg, B.W. 1987. The effects of dose and method of administration of biosynthetic bovine somatotropin on live-weight gain, carcass composition and wool growth in young lambs. *Animal Production* 44:405–414.

Jozsa, R., Scanes, C.G., Vigh, S., and Mess, B. 1979. Functional differentiation of the embryonic chicken pituitary gland studies by immunohistological approach. *General and Comparative Endocrinology* 39:158–163.

Kafri, I., Rosebrough, R.W., McMurtry, J.P., and Steele, N.C. 1988. Corticosterone implants and supplemental dietary ascorbic acid effects on lipid metabolism in broiler chicks. *Poultry Science* 67:1356–1359.

Kahl, S., Rumsey, T.S., Elsasser, T.H., and Kozak, A.S. 1992. Plasma concentrations of thyroid hormone in steers treated with Synovex-S and 3,5,3'-triiodothyronine. *Journal of Animal Science* 70:3844–3850.

Kajimoto, Y., and Rotwein, P. 1989. Structure and expression of chicken insulin-like growth factor-I precursor. *Molecular Endocrinology* 3:1907–1914.

Kalliecharan, R., and Hall, B.K. 1974. A developmental study of the levels of progesterone, corticosterone, cortisol, and cortisone circulating in plasma of chick embryos. *General and Comparative Endocrinology* 24:364–372.

Kallincos, N.C., Wallace, J.C., Francis, G.L., and Ballard, F.J. 1990. Chemical and biological characterization of chicken insulin-like growth factor-II. *Journal of Endocrinology* 124:89–97.

Kampman, K.A., Ramsay, T.G., and White, M.E. 1993. Developmental changes in hepatic IGF-2 and IGFBP-2 mRNA levels in intrauterine growth-retarded and control swine. *Comparative Biochemistry and Physiology B.* 104:415-421.

Kawamura, K., Sato, N., Fukuda, J., Kodama, H., Kumagai, J., Tanikawa, H., Nakamura, A., and Tanaka, T. 2002. Leptin promotes the development of mouse preimplantation embryos in vitro. *Endocrinology* 143:1922–1931.

Kennedy, P.M., Young, B.A., and Christopherson, R.J. 1977. Studies on the relationship between thyroid function, cold acclimation and retention time of digesta in sheep. *Journal of Animal Science* 45:1084–1090.

King, D.B., and King, C.R. 1973. Thyroidal influence on early muscle growth of chickens. *General and Comparative Endocrinology* 21:517–529.

King, D.B., and King, C.R. 1976. Thyroidal influence on gastrocnemius and sartorius muscle growth of chickens. *General and Comparative Endocrinology* 29:473–479.

King, D.B., and Scanes, C.G. 1986. Effect of mammalian growth hormone and prolactin on the growth of hypophysectomized chickens. *Proceedings of the Society of Experimental Biology and Medicine* 182:201–207.

Kirchgessner, V.M., Roth, F.X., Schams, D., and Karg, H. 1987. Influence of exogenous growth hormone (GH) on performance and plasma GH concentrations of female veal calves. *Journal of Animal Physiology and Animal Nutrition* 58:50–59.

Klasing, K.C., Laurin, D.E., Peng, R.K., and Fry, D.M. 1987. Immunologically mediated growth depression in chicks: influence of feed intake, corticosterone and interleukin-1. *Journal of Nutrition* 117:1629–1637.

Klindt, J., Ohlson, D.L., Davis, S.L., and Schanbacher, B.D. 1985. Ontogeny of growth hormone, prolactin, luteinizing hormone, and testosterone secretory patterns in the ram. *Biology of Reproduction* 33:436–444.

Koenig, R.J. 1999. Thyroid hormone receptors. In *Handbook of Physiology*. J.L. Kostyo, ed. New York and Oxford: Oxford University Press.

Kojima, M., Hosoda, H., Date, Y., Nakazato, M., Matsuo, H., and Kangawa, K. 1999. Ghrelin is a growth-hormone–releasing acylated peptide from stomach. *Nature* 402:656–660.

Koury, S.T., Bondurant, M.C., Cairo, J., and Garber, S.E. 1989. Quantitation of erythropoietin-producing cells in kidneys of mice by in situ hybridization: Correlation with hematocrit, renal erythropoietin mRNA, and serum erythropoietin concentration. *Blood* 74:645–671.

Krett, N.L., Heaton, J.H., and Gelehrter, T.D. 1987. Mediation of insulin-like growth factor actions by the insulin receptor in H-35 rat hepatoma cells. *Endocrinology* 120:483–490.

Krick, B.J., Boyd, R.D., Roneker, K.R., Beermann, D.H., Bauman, D.E., Ross, D.A., and Meisinger, D.J. 1993. Porcine somatotropin affects the dietary lysine requirement and net lysine utilization for growing pigs. *Journal of Nutrition* 123:1913–1922.

Kurima, K., Weatherly, K.L., Sharova, L., and Wong, E.A. 1998. Synthesis of turkey Pit-1 mRNA variants by alternative splicing and transcription initiation. *DNA Cell Biology* 17:93–103.

Lacroix, M.C., Jammes, H., and Kahn, G. 1996. Occurrence of a growth hormone-releasing hormone-like messenger ribonucleic acid and immunoreactive peptide in the sheep placenta. *Reproduction Fertility and Development* 8:449–456.

Lanna, D.P.D., and Bauman, D.E. 1999. Effect of somatotropin, insulin, and glucocorticoid on lipolysis in chronic cultures of adipose tissue from lactating cows. *Journal of Dairy Science* 82:60–68.

Lascelles, A.K., and Setchell, B.P. 1959. Hypothyroidism in sheep. *Australian Journal of Biological Science* 12:445–465.

Latimer, A.M., Hausman, G.J., McCusker, R.H., and Buonomo, F.C. 1993. The effects of thyroxine on serum and tissue concentrations of insulin-like growth factors (IGF-I and -II) and IGF-binding proteins in the fetal pig. *Endocrinology* 133:1312–1319.

Lauterio, T.J., and Scanes, C.G. 1987. Hormonal responses to protein restriction in two strains of chickens with different growth characteristics. *Journal of Nutrition* 117:758–763.

Leach, R.M., and Rosselot, G.E. 1992. The use of avian epiphyseal chondrocytes for in vitro studies of skeletal metabolism. *Journal of Nutrition* 122:802–805.

Leakey, J., and Dutton, G.J. 1975. Precocious development in vivo of UDP-glucuronyltransferase and aniline hydroxylase by corticosteroids and ACTH, using a simple new "continuous flow" technique. *Biochemical and Biophysical Research Communications* 66:250–254.

Leaman, D.W., Simmen, F.A., Ramsay, T.G., and White, M.E. 1990. Insulin-like growth factor-I and -II messenger RNA expression in muscle, heart, and liver of streptozotocin-diabetic swine. *Endocrinology* 126:2850–2857.

Lee, H.-M., Wang, G., Englander, E.W., Kojima, M., and Greeley, G.H. 2002. Ghrelin, a new gastrointestinal endocrine peptide that stimulates insulin secretion: enteric distribution, ontogeny, influence of endocrine, and dietary manipulations. *Endocrinology* 143:185–190.

Lee, K.C., Azain, M.J., Hardin, M.D., and Williams, S.E. 1994. Effect of porcine somatotropin (pST) treatment and withdrawal on performance and adipose tissue cellularity in finishing swine. *Journal of Animal Science* 72:1702–1711.

Leshin, L.S., Barb, C.R., Kiser, T.E., Rampacek, G.B., and Kraeling, R.R. 1994. Growth hormone-releasing hormone and somatostatin neurons within the porcine and bovine hypothalamus. *Neuroendocrinology* 59:251–264.

Leung, F.C., Styles, W.J., Rosenblum, C.I., Lilburn, M.S., and Marsh, J.A. 1987. Diminished hepatic growth hormone receptor binding in sex-linked dwarf broiler and Leghorn chickens. *Proceedings of the Society for Experimental Biology and Medicine* 184:234–238.

Leung, F.C., Taylor, J.E., Wien, S., and Van Iderstine, A. 1986. Purified chicken growth hormone (GH) and a human pancreatic GH-releasing hormone body weight gain in chickens. *Endocrinology* 118:1961–1965.

Li, J., Saunders, J.C., Gilmour, R.S., Silver, M., and Fowden, A.L. 1993. Insulin-like growth factor-II messenger ribonucleic acid expression in fetal tissues of the sheep during late gestation: effects of cortisol. *Endocrinology* 132:2083–2089.

Liberti, J.P., Antoni, B.A., and Chlebowski, J.F. 1985. Naturally-occurring pituitary growth hormone is phosphorylated. *Biochemical and Biophysical Research Communications* 128:713–720.

Lin, J., Barb, C.R., Matteri, R.L., Kraeling, R.R., Chen, X., Meinersmann, R.J., and Rampacek, G.B. 2000. Long form leptin receptor mRNA expression in the brain, pituitary, and other tissues in the pig. *Domestic Animal Endocrinology* 19:53–61.

Listrat, A., Gerrard, D.E., Boulle, N., Groyer, A., and Robelin, J. 1994. In situ localization of muscle insulin-like growth factor-II mRNA in developing bovine fetuses. *Journal of Endocrinology* 140:179–187.

Liu, J., Boyd, C.K., Kobayashi, Y., Chase, C.C., Hammond, A.C., Olson, T.A., Elsasser, T.H., and Lucy, M.C. 1999. A novel phenotype for Laron dwarfism in miniature Bos indicus cattle suggests that the expression of growth hormone receptor 1A in liver is required for normal growth. *Domestic Animal Endocrinology* 17:421–437.

Liu, J., Carroll, J.A., Matteri, R.L., and Lucy, M.C. 2000. Expression of two variants of growth hormone receptor messenger ribonucleic acid in porcine liver. *Journal of Animal Science* 78:306–317.

Lord, A.P.D., Read, L.C., Owens, P.C., Martin, A.A., Walton, P.E., and Ballard, F.J. 1994. Rapid changes in plasma concentrations of insulin-like growth factor-I (IGF-I), IGF-II and IGF-binding proteins during anaesthesia in young sheep. *Journal of Endocrinology* 141:427–437.

Lucy, M.C., Hauser, S.D., Eppard, P.J., Krivi, G.G., Clark, J.H., Bauman, D.E., and Collier, R.J. 1993. Variants of somatotropin in cattle: gene frequencies in major dairy breeds and associated milk production. *Domestic Animal Endocrinology* 10:325–333.

Lucy, M.C., Hauser, S.D., Eppard, P.J., Krivi, G.G., and Collier, R.J. 1991. Genetic polymorphism within the bovine somatotropin (bST) gene detected by polymerase chain reaction and endonuclease digestion. *Journal of Dairy Science* 74:284.

Lund, P.K. 1999. Insulin-like growth factors: gene structure and regulation. In *Handbook of Physiology*. J.L. Kostyo, ed. New York and Oxford: Oxford University Press.

Lundström, K., Dahlberg, E., Nyberg, L., Snochowski, M., Standal, N., and Edqvist, L.-E. 1983. Glucocorticoid and androgen characteristics in two lines of pigs selected for rate of gain and thickness of backfat. *Journal of Animal Science* 56:401–409.

Machlin, D.J., Horino, M., Hertelendy, F., and Kipnis, D.M. 1968. Plasma growth hormone and insulin levels in the pig. *Endocrinology* 82:369–376.

Machlin, L.J. 1972. Effect of porcine growth hormone on growth and carcass composition of the pig. *Journal of Animal Science* 35:794–800.

Maddocks, S., Chandrasekhar, Y., and Setchell, B.P. 1985. Effects on wool growth of thyroxine replacement in thyroidectomized Merino rams. *Australian Journal of Biological Science* 38:405–410.

Marple, D.N., Cassens, R.G., Topel, D.G., and Christian, L.L. 1974. Porcine corticosteroid-binding globulin: binding properties and levels in stress-susceptible swine. *Journal of Animal Science* 38:1224–1228.

Marple, D.N., Nachreiner, R.F., Pritchett, J.F., Miles, R.J., Brown, H.R., and Noe, L.S. 1977. Thyroid and sarcoplasmic reticulum function in halothane-sensitive swine. *Journal of Animal Science* 45:1375–1381.

Marsh, J.A., Gause, W.C., Sandu, S., and Scanes, C.G. 1984a. Enhanced growth and immune development in dwarf chickens treated with mammalian growth hormone and thyroxine. *Proceedings of the Society for Experimental Biology and Medicine* 175:351–360.

Marsh, J.A., Lauterio, T.J., and Scanes, C.G. 1984b. Effects of triiodothyronine treatments on body and organ growth and development of immune function in dwarf chickens. *Proceedings of the Society for Experimental Biology and Medicine* 177:82–91.

Martin, R.J., Ramsay, T.G., and Harris, R.B.S. 1984. Central role of insulin in growth and development. *Domestic Animal Endocrinology* 1:89–104.

Martin, T.G., Mollett, T.A., Stewart, T.S., Erb, R.E., Malven, P.V., Veenhuizen, E.L. 1979. Comparison of four levels of protein supplementation with and without oral diethylstilbestrol on blood plasma concentrations of testosterone, growth hormone and insulin in young bulls. *Journal of Animal Science* 49:1489–1496.

Masuda, Y., Tanaka, T., Inomata, N., Ohnuma, N., Tanaka, S., Itsoh, Z., Hosoda, H., Kojima, M., and Kangawa, K.

2000. Ghrelin stimulates gastric acid secretion and motility in rats. *Biochemical Biophysical Research Communications* 276:905–908.

McAtee, J.W., and Trenkle, A. 1971. Effect of feeding, fasting and infusion of energy substrates on plasma growth hormone levels in cattle. *Journal of Animal Science* 33:612–616.

McCusker, R.H., Campion, D.R., Jones, W.K., and Clemmons, D.R. 1985. The insulin-like growth factor-binding proteins of porcine serum: endocrine and nutritional regulation. *Endocrinology* 125:501–509.

McGrath, J.A., and Goldspink, D.F. 1982. Glucocorticoid action on protein synthesis and protein breakdown in isolated skeletal muscles. *Biochemical Journal* 206:641–645.

McGuinness, M., and Cogburn, L., 1990. Measurement of developmental changes in plasma insulin-like growth factor-I levels of broiler chickens by radioreceptor assay and radioimmunoassay. *General and Comparative Endocrinology* 79:446–458.

McLaren, D.G., Bechtel, P.J., Grebner, G.L., Novakofski, J., McKeith, F.K., Jones, R.W., Dalrymple, R.H., and Easter, R.A. 1990. Dose response in growth of pigs injected daily with porcine somatotropin from 57 to 103 kilograms. *Journal of Animal Science* 68:640–651.

McLaughlin, C.L., Byatt, J.C., Curran, D.F., Veenhuizen, J.J., McGrath, M.F., Buonomo, F.C., Hintz, R.L., and Baile, C.A. 1997. Growth performance, endocrine, and metabolite responses of finishing hogs to porcine prolactin. *Journal of Animal Science* 75:959–67.

McLean, E., Donaldson, E.M., Dye, H.M., and Souza, L.M. 1990. Growth acceleration of coho salmon (Oncorhynchus kisutch) following oral administration of recombinant bovine somatotropin. *Aquaculture* 91:197.

McLellan, K.C., Hooper, S.B., Bocking, A.D., Delhanty, P.J.D., Phillips, I.D., Hill, D.J., and Han, V.K.M. 1992. Prolonged hypoxia induced by the reduction of maternal uterine blood flow alters insulin-like growth factor-binding protein-1 (IGFBP-1) and IGFBP-2 gene expression in the ovine fetus. *Endocrinology* 131:1619–1628.

McMahon, C.D., Radcliff, R.P., Lookingland, K.J., and Tucker, H.A. 2001. Neuroregulation of growth hormone secretion in domestic animals. *Domestic Animal Endocrinology* 20:65–87.

McMurtry, J.P., Francis, G.L., and Upton, Z. 1997. Insulin-like growth factors in poultry. *Domestic Animal Endocrinology* 14:199–229.

McMurtry, J.P., Francis, G.L., Upton, F.Z., Rosselot, G., and Brocht, D.M. 1994. Developmental changes in chicken and turkey insulin-like growth factor-I (IGF-I) studied with a homologous radioimmunoassay for chicken IGF-I. *Journal of Endocrinology* 142:225–234.

Menon, R.K., and Sperling, M.A. 1996. Insulin as a growth factor. *Endocrinology of Metabolism Clinic of North America* 25:633–647.

Mercer, J.G., Hoggard, N., Williams, L.M., Lawrence, C.B., Hannah, L.T., and Trayhurn, P. 1996. Localization of leptin receptor mRNA and the long form splice variant (Ob-Rb) in mouse hypothalamus and adjacent brain regions by in situ hybridization. *FEBS Letters* 387:113–116.

Messina, J.L. 1999. Insulin as a growth-promoting hormone. In *Handbook of Physiology*. J.L. Kostyo, ed. New York and Oxford: Oxford University Press.

Milley, J.R. 1986. The effect of chronic hyperinsulinemia on ovine fetal growth. *Growth* 50:390–401.

Moellers, R.F., and Cogburn, L.A. 1995. Chronic intravenous infusion of chicken growth hormone increases body fat content by young broiler chickens. *Comparative Biochemistry and Physiology* 110A:47–56.

Moore, G.E., Harvey, S., Klandorf, H., and Goldspink, G. 1984. Muscle development in thyroidectomized chicken (Gallus domesticus). *General and Comparative Endocrinology* 55:195–199.

Moritz, K., Butkus, A., Hantzis, V., Peers, A., Wintour, E.M., and Dodic, M. 2002. Prolonged low-dose dexamethasone, in early gestation, has no long-term deleterious effect on normal ovine fetuses. *Endocrinology* 143:1159–65.

Moseley, W.M., Krabill, L.F., and Olsen, R.F. 1982. Effect of bovine growth hormone administered in various patterns on nitrogen metabolism in the Holstein steer. *Journal of Animal Science* 55:1062–1070.

Muir, L.A., Wien, S., Duquette, P.F., Rickes, E.L., and Cordes, E.H. 1983. Effects of exogenous growth hormone and diethylstilbestrol on growth and carcass composition of growing lambs. *Journal of Animal Science* 56:1315–1323.

Nakazato, M., Murakami, N., Date, Y., Kojima, M., Matsuo, H., Kangawa, K., and Matsukura, S. 2001. A role for ghrelin in the central regulation of feeding. *Nature* 409:194–198.

Newby, D., Gertler, A., and Vernon, R.G. 2001. Effects of recombinant ovine leptin on in vitro lipolysis and lipogenesis in subcutaneous adipose tissue from lactating and nonlactating sheep. *Journal of Animal Science* 79:445–452.

Ohlson, D.L., Davis, S.L., Ferrell, C.L., and Jenkins, T.G. 1981. Plasma growth hormone, prolactin and thyrotropin secretory patterns in Hereford and Simmental calves. *Journal of Animal Science* 53:371–375.

Ohlsson, C., Lindahl, A., Isgaard, J., Nilsson, A., and Isaksson, O.G.P. 1999. The dual effector theory. In *Handbook of Physiology*. J.L. Kostyo, ed. New York and Oxford: Oxford University Press.

Ooi, G.T., Tseng, L.Y.-H., Tran, M.Q., and Rechler, M.M. 1992. Insulin rapidly decreases insulin–like growth factor–binding protein–1 gene transcription in streptozotocin–diabetic rats. *Molecular Endocrinology* 6:2219–2228.

Osborn, B.H., Fowlkes, J., Han, V.K.M., and Freemark, M. 1992. Nutritional regulation of insulin-like growth factor-binding protein gene expression in the ovine fetus and pregnant ewe. *Endocrinology* 131:1743–1750.

Owens, J.A., Kind, K.L., Carbone, F., Robinson, J.S., and Owens, P.C. 1994. Circulating insulin-like growth factors-I and -II and substrates in fetal sheep following restriction of placental growth. *Journal of Endocrinology* 140:5–13.

Pearson, P.L., Smith, T.P.L., Sonstegard, T.S., Klemcke, H.G., Christenson, R.K., and Vallet, J.L. 2000. Porcine erythropoietin receptor: molecular cloning and expression in embryonic and fetal liver. *Domestic Animal Endocrinology* 19:25–38.

Peebles, E.D., Burke, W.H., and Marks, H.L. 1988. Effects of recombinant chicken growth hormone in random bred meat-type chickens. *Growth, Development and Aging* 52:133–138.

Pell, J.M., Elcock, C., Harding, R.L., Morrell, D.J., Simmonds, A.D., and Wallis, M. 1990. Growth, body composition, hormonal and metabolic status in lambs treated long-term with growth hormone. British *Journal of Nutrition* 63:431–445.

Pelletier, G., Lanoë, J., Filion, M., and Dunnigan, J. 1983. Effect of age and glucocorticoid administration on the proteolytic activity of gastric mucosa: a comparative study in the young rat, calf and piglet. *Journal of Animal Science* 57:74–81.

Perez, F.M., Malamed, S., and Scanes, C.G. 1985. Biosynthetic human somatomedin C inhibits hpGRF (1–44) NH2-induced and TRH-induced GH release in a primary culture of chicken pituitary cells. *IRCS Medical Science* 13:871–872.

Pérez-Villamil, B., de la Rosa, E.J., Morales, A.V., and de Pablo, F. 1994. Developmentally regulated expression of the preproinsulin gene in the chicken embryo during gastrulation and neurulation. *Endocrinology* 135:2342–2350.

Plouzek, C.A., Molina, J.R., Hard, D.L., Vale, W.W., Rivier, J., Trenkle, A., and Anderson, L.L. 1988. Effects of growth hormone-releasing factor and somatostatin on growth hormone secretion in hypophysial stalk-transected beef calves. *Proceedings of the Society for Experimental Biology and Medicine* 189:158–167.

Porter, T.E., and Dean, K.J. 2001. Regulation of chicken embryonic growth hormone secretion by corticosterone and 3,5,3'-triiodothyronine: Evidence for a negative synergistic response. *Endocrine* 14:363–368.

Porter, T.E., Dean, C.E., Piper, M.M., Medvedev, K.L., Shavam, S., and Sandor, S. 2001. Growth hormone gene expression and secretagogue responses in somatotrophs induced to differentiate with glucocorticoids. *Journal of Endocrinology* 169:499–509.

Pralong, F.P., Roduit, R., Waeber, G., Castillo, E., Mosimann, F. Thorens, B., and Gaillard, R.C. 1998. Leptin inhibits directly glucocorticoid secretion by normal human and rat adrenal gland. *Endocrinology* 139:4264–4268.

Puvadolpirod, S., and Thaxton, J.P. 2000. Model of physiological stress in chickens 2. dosimetry of adrenocorticotropin. *Poultry Science* 79:370–376.

Rabii, J., Buonomo, F.C., and Scanes, C.G. 1981. The role of serotonin in the regulation of growth hormone and prolactin secretion in the domestic fowl. *Journal of Endocrinology* 90:355–358.

Radecki, S.V., Deaver, D.R., and Scanes, C.G. 1994. Triiodothyronine reduced growth hormone (GH) secretion and pituitary GH mRNA in the chicken in vivo and in vitro. *Proceedings of the Society for Experimental Biology and Medicine* 205:340–346.

Raheja, K.L., and Snedecor, J.G. 1970. Comparison of subnormal multiple doses of L-thyroxine and L-triiodothyro-

nine in propylthiouracil-fed and radiothyroidectomized chicks (Gallus domesticus). *Comparative Biochemistry and Physiology* 37:555–563.

Ramsay, T.G. 2001. Porcine leptin alters insulin inhibition of lipolysis in porcine adipocytes in vitro. *Journal of Animal Science* 79:653–657.

Ramsey, T.G., Wolverton, C.K., Hausman, G.J., Kraeling, R.R., and Martin, R.J. 1989. Alterations in adipogenic and mitogenic activity of porcine serum in response to hypophysectomy. *Endocrinology* 124:2268–2276.

Rasmussen, Å.K., Kayser, L., Bech, K., Feldt-Rasmussen, U., Perrild, H., and Bendtzen, K. 1990. Differential effects of interleukin 1α and 1β on cultured human and rat thyroid epithelial cells. *Acta Endocrinologica* 122:520–526.

Reed, D.K., Korytko, A.I., Hipkin, R.W., Wehrenberg, W.B., Schonbrunn, A., and Cuttler, L. 1999. Pituitary somatostatin receptor (sst)1-5 expression during rat development: age-dependent expression of sst2. *Endocrinology* 140:4739–4744.

Rhoads, R.P., Greenwood, P.L., Bell, A.W., and Boisclair, Y.R. 2000. Nutritional regulation of the genes encoding the acid-labile subunit and other components of the circulating insulin-like growth factor system in the sheep. *Journal of Animal Science* 78:2681-2689.

Richman, C., Baylink, D.J., Lang, K., Dony, C., and Mohan, S. 1999. Recombinant human insulin-like growth factor-binding protein-5 stimulates bone formation parameters in vitro and in vivo. *Endocrinology* 140:4699–4705.

Richman, R.A. 1999. The regulation of growth by insulin-like growth factor II. In *Handbook of Physiology*. J.L. Kostyo, ed. New York and Oxford: Oxford University Press.

Robcis, H.L., Caldes, T., and de Pablo, F. 1991. Insulin-like growth factor-I serum levels show a midembryogenesis peak in chicken that is absent in growth-retarded embryos cultured ex ovo. *Endocrinology* 128:1895–1901.

Romagnolo, D., Akers, R.M., Byatt, J.C., Wong, E.A., and Turner, J.D. 1994. IGF-I-induced IGFBP-3 potentiates the mitogenic actions of IGF-I in mammary epithelial MD-IGF-I cells. *Molecular and Cellular Endocrinology* 102:131–139.

Rosebrough, R., McMurtry, J., Proudman, J., and Steele, N. 1989. Comparison between constant-protein, calorie-restricted and protein-restricted, calorie-restricted diets on growth, in vitro lipogenesis and plasma growth hormone, thyroxine, triiodothyronine and somatomedin-C (Sm-C) of young chickens. *Comparative Biochemistry and Physiology* 93A:337–343.

Rosebrough, R., McMurtry, J., and Vasilatos-Younken, R. 1991. Effect of pulsatile or continuous administration of pituitary-derived chicken growth hormone (p-cGH) on lipid metabolism in broiler pullets. *Comparative Biochemistry and Physiology* 99:207–214.

Rosemberg, E., Thonney, M.L., and Butler, W.R. 1989. The effects of bovine growth hormone and thyroxine on growth rate and carcass measurements in lambs. *Journal of Animal Science* 67:3300–3312.

Rule, D.C., Beitz, D.C., de Boer, G., Lyle, R.R., Trenkle, A.H., and Young, J.W. 1985. Changes in hormone and metabolite concentrations in plasma of steers during a prolonged fast. *Journal of Animal Science* 61:868–875.

Rumsey, T.S., Bitman, J., and Tao, H. 1983. Changes in plasma concentrations of thyroxine, triiodothyronine, cholesterol and total lipid in beef steers fed ronnel. *Journal of Animal Science* 56:125–131.

Saadoun, A., Simon, J., and Leclercq, B. 1987. Effect of exogenous corticosterone in genetically fat and lean chickens. *British Poultry Science* 28:519–528.

Salmon, W.D., and Daughaday, W.H. 1957. A hormonally controlled serum factor which stimulates sulfate incorporation by cartilage in vitro. *Journal of Laboratory Clinical Medicine* 49:825–836.

Sarko, T.A., Bishop, M.D., and Davis, M.E. 1994. Relationship of air temperature, relative humidity, precipitation, photoperiod, wind speed and solar radiation with serum insulin-like growth factor I (IGF-I) concentration in Angus beef cattle. *Domestic Animal Endocrinology* 11:281–290.

Sartin, J.L., Cummins, K.A., Kemppainen, R.J., Carnes, R., McClary, D.G., and Williams, J.C. 1985b. Effect of propionate infusion on plasma glucagon, insulin and growth hormone concentrations in lactating dairy cows. *Acta Endocrinologica* 109:348–354.

Sartin, J.L., Cummins, K.A., Kemppainen, R.J., Marple, D.N., Rahe, C.H., and Williams, J.C. 1985a. Glucagon, insulin, and growth hormone responses to glucose infusion in lactating dairy cows. *American Journal of Physiology* 248:E108–E114.

Sasak, H., Bothner, B., Deli, A., and Fukuda, M. 1987. Carbohydrate structure of erythropoietin expressed in Chinese hamster ovary cells by a human erythropoietin cDNA. *Journal of Biological Chemistry* 262:12059–12076.

Sauerwein, H., Breier, B.H., Bass, J.J., and Gluckman, P.D. 1991. Chronic treatment with bovine growth hormone (bGH) up-regulates the high-affinity hepatic somatotrophic receptor in sheep. *Acta Endocrinologica* 124:307–313.

Scanes, C.G. 1992. Lipolytic and diabetogenic effects of native and biosynthetic growth hormone in the chicken: a re-evaluation. *Comparative Biochemistry and Physiology* 101A:871–878.

Scanes, C.G. 2000. Hormones and growth in domestic animals. In *Handbook of Physiology*. J.L. Kostyo, ed. New York & Oxford: Oxford University Press.

Scanes, C.G., Aust Peterla, T., Kantor, S., and Ricks, C.A. 1990. In vivo effects of biosynthetic chicken growth hormone in broiler-strain chickens. *Growth, Development and Aging* 54:95–101.

Scanes, C.G., Dunnington, E.A., Buonomo, F.C., Donoghue, D.J., and Siegel, P.B. 1989. Plasma concentrations of insulin-like growth factors (IGF)-I and IGF-II in dwarf and normal chickens of high and low weight selected lines. *Growth, Development and Aging* 53:151–157.

Scanes, C.G., Duyka, D.R., Lauterio, T.J., Bowen, S.J., Huybrechts, L.M., Bacon, W.L., and King, D.B. 1986. Effect of chicken growth hormone, triiodothyronine and hypophysectomy in growing domestic fowl. *Growth* 50:12–31.

Scanes, C.G., Griminger, P., and Buonomo, F.C. 1981. Effects of dietary protein restriction on circulating concentrations of growth hormone in growing domestic fowl (Gallus domesticus). *Proceeding of the Society for Experimental Biology and Medicine* 168, 334–337.

Scanes, C.G., and Harvey, S. 1989. Triiodothyronine (T3) inhibition of thyrotropin-releasing hormone (TRH) and growth hormone-releasing factor (GRF)-induced secretion of chicken growth hormone (GH) in vivo. *General and Comparative Endocrinology* 73:477–484.

Scanes, C.G., Marsh, J., Decuypere, E., and Rudas, P. 1983. Abnormalities in the plasma concentration of thyroxine, triiodothyronine and growth hormone in sex-linked dwarf and autosomal dwarf white leghorn domestic fowl (Gallus domesticus). *Journal of Endocrinology* 97:127–135.

Scanes, C.G., Thommes, R.C., Radecki, S.V., Buonomo, F.C., and Woods, J.E. 1997. Ontogenic changes in the circulating concentrations of insulin-like growth factor (IGF)-I, IGF-II, and IGF-binding proteins in the chicken embryo. *General and Comparative Endocrinology* 106:265–270.

Schulte, P.M., Down, N.E., Donaldson, E.M., and Souza, L.M. 1989. Experimental administration of recombinant bovine growth hormone to juvenile rainbow trout (Salmogairdneri) by injection or by immersion. *Aquaculture* 76:145–156.

Scott, T.R., Johnson, W.A., Satterlee, D.G., and Gildersleeve, R.P. 1981. Circulating levels of corticosterone in the serum of developing chick embryos and newly hatched chicks. *Poultry Science* 60:1314–1320.

Scully, K.M., and Rosenfeld, M.G. 2002. Pituitary development: regulatory codes in mammalian organogenesis. *Science* 295:2231-2235.

Seaman, J.S., Berg, E.P., Safranski, T.J., and Carroll, J. 2001. Effect of dexamethasone treatment on growth in neonatal swine. *Journal of Animal Science* 79Suppl1:30.

Sechen, S.J., Dunshea, F.R., and Bauman, D.E. 1990. Somatotropin in lactating cows: effect on response to epinephrine and insulin. *American Journal of Physiology* 258:E582–E588.

Serrano, J., Bevins, C., Young, S.W., and de Pablo, F. 1989. Insulin gene expression in chicken ontogeny: pancreatic, extrapancreatic, and prepancreatic. *Developmental Biology* 132:410–418.

Shaffer Tannebaum, G., and Epelbaum, J. 1999. Somatostatin. In *Handbook of Physiology*. J.L. Kostyo, ed. New York and Oxford: Oxford University Press.

Shen, W.-H., Yang, X., Boyle, D.W., Lee, W.H., and Liechty, E.A. 2001. Effects of intravenous insulin-like growth factor-I and insulin administration of insulin-like growth factor-binding proteins in the ovine fetus. *Journal of Endocrinology* 171:143–151.

Shipley, G.D., and Ham, R.G. 1983a. Control of entry of Swiss 3T3 cells into S phase by fibroblast growth factor under serum-free conditions. *Experimental Cell Research* 146:261–270.

Shipley, G.D., and Ham, R.G. 1983b. Multiplication of Swiss 3T3 cells in a serum-free medium. *Experimental Cell Research* 146:249–260.

Siegel, H.S., and Van Kampen, M. 1984. Energy relationships in growing chickens given daily injections of corticosterone. *British Poultry Science* 25:477–485.

Siegel, P.B., Gross, W.B., and Dunnington, E.A. 1989. Effects of dietary corticosterone in young Leghorn and meat-type cockerels. *British Poultry Science* 30:185–192.

Sierra-Honigmann, M.R., Nath, A.K., Murakami, C., Garcia-Cardena, G., Papapetroulos, A., Sessa, W.C., Madge, L.A., Schechner, J.S., Schwabb, M.B., Polverini, P., and Flores-Riveros, J.R. 1998. Biological action of leptin as an angiogenic factor. *Science* 281:1683–1686.

Sihombing, D.T.H., Cromwell, G.L., and Hays, V.W. 1974. Effects of protein source, goitrogens and iodine level on performance and thyroid status of pigs. *Journal of Animal Science* 39:1106–1109.

Silha, J.V., Gui, Y., Modric, T., Suwanichkul, A., Durham, S.K., Powell, D.R., and Murphy, L.J. 2001. Overexpression of the acid-labile subunit of the IGF ternary complex in transgenic mice. *Endocrinology* 142:4305–4313.

Silverman, B.L., Bettendorf, M., Kaplan, S.L., Grumbach, M.M., and Miller, W.L. 1989. Regulation of growth hormone (GH) secretion by GH-releasing factor, somatostatin, and insulin-like growth factor I in ovine fetal and neonatal pituitary cells in vitro. *Endocrinology* 124:84–89.

Silverman, B.L., Kaplan, S.L., Grumbach, M.M., and Miller, W.L. 1988. Hormonal regulation of growth hormone secretion and messenger ribonucleic acid accumulation in cultured bovine pituitary cells. *Endocrinology* 122:1236–1241.

Sornson, M.W., Wu, W., Dasen, J.S., Flynn, S.E., Norman, D.J., O'Connell, S.M., Gukovsky, I., Carriere, C., Ryan, A.K., and Miller, A.P. 1996. Pituitary lineage determination by the Prophet of Pit-1 homeodomain factor defective in Ames dwarfism. *Nature* 384:327–333.

Spencer, G.S.G., Hill, D.J., Garssen, G.J., Macdonald, A.A., and Colenbrander, B. 1983. Somatomedin activity and growth hormone levels in body fluids of the fetal pig: effect of chronic hyperinsulinaemia. *Journal of Endocrinology* 96:107–114.

Spurlock, G.M., and Clegg, M.T. 1962. Effect of cortisone acetate on carcass composition and wool characteristics of weaned lambs. *Journal of Animal Science* 21:494–500.

Takeuchi, S., Haneda, M., Teshigawara, K., and Takahashi, S. 2001. Identification of a novel GH isoform: a possible link between GH and melanocortin systems in the developing chicken eye. *Endocrinology* 142:5158–5166.

Tanaka, M., Yamamoto, I., Ohkubo, T., Wakita, M., Hoshino, S., and Nakashima, K. 1999. cDNA cloning and developmental alterations in gene expression of two Pit-1/GHF-1 transcription factors in the chicken pituitary. *General and Comparative Endocrinology* 114:441–448.

Tannebaum, G.S., and Epelbaum, J. 1999. Somatostatin. In *Handbook of Physiology*. J.L. Kostyo, ed. New York and Oxford: Oxford University Press.

Thue, T.D., and Schmutz, S.M. 1995. Localization of the somatostatin gene to bovine chromosome 1q23–q25 by in situ hybridization. *Mammalian Genome* 6:688–689.

Tixier-Boichard, M., Huybrechts, L.M., Decuypere, E., Kühn, E.R., Monvoisin, J.-L., Coquerelle, G., Charrier, J., and Simon, J. 1992. Effects of insulin-like growth factor-I (IGF-I) infusion and dietary tri-iodothyronine (T3) supplementation on growth, body composition and plasma hormone levels in sex-linked dwarf mutant and normal chickens. *Journal of Endocrinology* 133:101–110.

Tomas, F.M., Murray, A.J., and Jones, L.M. 1984. Modification of glucocorticoid-induced changes in myofibrillar protein turnover in rats by protein and energy deficiency as assessed by urinary excretion of Nτ-methyl-histidine. British *Journal of Nutrition* 51:323–337.

Tsuchiya, T., Shimizu, H., Horie, T., and Mori, M. 1999. Expression of leptin receptor in lung: leptin as a growth factor. *European Journal of Pharmacology* 365:273–279.

Tsuda, E., Kawanishi, G., Ueda, M., Masuda, S., and Sasaki, R. 1990. The role of carbohydrate in recombinant human erythropoietin. *European Journal of Biochemistry* 188:405–411.

Tsushima, T., Arai, M., Saji, M., Ohba, Y., Murakami, H., Ohmura, E., Sato, K., and Shizume, K. 1988. Effects of transforming growth factor-β on deoxyribonucleic acid synthesis and iodine metabolism in porcine thyroid cells in culture. *Endocrinology* 123:1187–1194.

Tuggle, C.K., and Trenkle, A. 1996. Control of growth hormone synthesis. *Domestic Animal Endocrinology* 13:1–33.

Tur, J., Esteban, S., Rayó, J.M., Moreno, M., Miralles, A., and Tur, J.A. 1989. Effect of glucocorticoids on gastrointestinal emptying in young broilers. *British Poultry Science* 30:693–698.

Upton, F.Z., Francis, G.L., Kita, K., Wallace, J.C., and Ballard, F.J. 1995. Production and characterization of recombinant chicken insulin-like growth factor-II from E.coli. *Journal of Molecular Endocrinology* 14:79–90.

Upton, F.Z., Szabo, L., Wallace, J.C., and Ballard, F.J. 1990. Characterization and cloning of bovine insulin-like growth factor binding protein. *Journal of Molecular Endocrinology* 5:77–84.

Valinsky, A., Shani, M., and Gootwine, E. 1990. Restriction fragment length polymorphism in sheep at the growth hormone locus is the result of variation in gene number. *Animal Biotechnology* 1:135–144.

Van As, P., Buys, N., Onagbesan, O.M., and Decuypere, E. 2000. Complementary DNA cloning and ontogenic expression of pituitary-specific transcription factor of chickens (Gallus domesticus) from the pituitary gland. *General and Comparative Endocrinology* 120:127–136.

van Buul-Offers, S.C., Reijen-Gresnigt, R., Bloemen, R.J., Hoogerbrugge, C.M., and Van den Brande, J.L. 1995. Coadministration of IGF-binding proteins-3 differentially inhibits the IGF-I induced total body and organ growth of Snell dwarf mice. *Progress in Growth Factor Research* 6:377–383.

van Buul-Offers, S.C., Ueda, I., and Van den Brande, J.L. 1986. Biosynthetic somatomedin-C (SM-C/IGF-I) increases the length and weight of Snell dwarf mice. *Pediatric Research* 20:825–827.

van Buul-Offers, S.C., Van Kleffens, M., Koster, J.G., Lindenbergh-Kortleve, D.J., Gresnigt, M.G., Drop, S.L.S.,

Hoogerbrugge, C.M., Bloemen, R.J., Koedam, J.A., and Van Neck, J.W. 2000. Human insulin-like growth factor (IGF) binding protein-1 inhibits IGF-I-stimulated body growth but stimulates growth of the kidney in Snell dwarf mice. *Endocrinology* 141:1493–1499.

Vanderpooten, A., Huybrechts, L.M., Decuypere, E., and Kuhn, E.R. 1991. Differences in hepatic growth hormone receptor binding during development of normal and dwarf chickens. *Reproduction, Nutrition et Development* 31:47–55.

Vann, R.C., Althen, T.G., Smith, W.K., Veenhuizen, J.J., and Smith, S.B. 1998. Recombinant bovine somatotropin (rbST) administration to creep-fed calves increases muscle mass but does not affect satellite cell number of concentration of myosin light chain-1f mRNA. *Journal of Animal Science* 76:1371–1379.

Vann, R.C., Althen, T.G., Solomon, M.B., Eastridge, J.S., Paroczay, E.W., and Veenhuizen, J.J. 2001. Recombinant bovine somatotropin (rbST) increases size and proportion of fast-glycolytic muscle fibers in semitendinosus muscle of creep-fed steers. *Journal of Animal Science* 79:108–114.

Varner, M.A., Davis, S.L., and Reeves, J.J. 1980. Temporal serum concentrations of growth hormone, thyrotropin, insulin, and glucagon in sheep immunized against somatostatin. *Endocrinology* 106:1027–1032.

Vasilatos, R., and Wangsness, P.J. 1980. Changes in concentrations of insulin, growth hormone and metabolites in plasma with spontaneous feeding in lactating dairy cows. *Journal of Nutrition* 110:1479–1487.

Vasilatos-Younken, R., Cravener, T.L., Cogburn, L.A., Mast, M.G., and Wellenreiter, R.H. 1988. Effect of pattern of administration on the response to exogenous pituitary-derived chicken growth hormone by broiler-strain pullets. *General and Comparative Endocrinology* 71:268–283.

Vasilatos-Younken, R., Tsao, P.H., Foster, D.N., Smiley, D.L., Bryant, H., and Heiman, M.L. 1992. Restoration of juvenile baseline growth hormone secretion with preservation of the ultradian growth-hormone rhythm by continuous delivery of growth hormone-releasing factor. *Journal of Endocrinology* 135:371–382.

Vasilatos-Younken, R., Wang, X.-H., Zhou, Y., Day, J.R., McMurtry, J.P., Rosebrough, R.W., Decuypere, E., Buys, N., Darras, V., and Beard, J.L. 1999. New insights into the mechanism and actions of growth hormone (GH) in poultry. *Domestic Animal Endocrinology* 17:181–190.

Veissier, I., van Reenen, C.G., Andanson, S., and Leushuis, I.E. 1999. Adrenocorticotropic hormone and cortisol in calves after corticotropin-releasing hormone. *Journal of Animal Science* 77:2047–2053.

Verde, L.S., and Trenkle, A. 1987. Concentrations of hormones in plasma from cattle with different growth potentials. *Journal of Animal Science* 64:42–432.

Vinter-Jensen, L., Juhl, C.O., Frystyk, J., Dajani, E.Z., Oksbjerg, N., and Glyvbjerg, A. 1996. The effect of epidermal growth factor on circulating levels of IGF and IGF-binding proteins in adult Goettingen minipigs. *Journal of Endocrinology* 151:401–407.

Walton, P.E., and Etherton, T.D. 1986. Stimulation of lipogenesis by insulin in swine adipose tissue: antagonism by porcine growth hormone. *Journal of Animal Science* 62:1584–1595.

Walton, P.E., and Etherton, T.D. 1989. Effects of porcine growth hormone and insulin-like growth factor-I (IGF-I) on immunoreactive IGF-binding protein concentration in pigs. *Journal of Endocrinology* 120:153–160.

Walton, P.E., Etherton, T.D., and Evock, C.M. 1986. Antagonism of insulin action in cultured pig adipose tissue by pituitary and recombinant porcine growth hormone: potentiation by hydrocortisone. *Endocrinology* 118:2577–2581.

Walton, P.E., Gopinath, R., Burleigh, B.D., and Etherton, T.D. 1989. Administration of recombinant human insulin-like growth factor I to pigs: determination of circulating half-lives and chromatographic profiles. *Hormone Research* 31:138–142.

Wangsness, P.J., Martin, R.J., and Gahagan, J.H. 1977. Insulin and growth hormone in lean and obese pigs. *American Journal of Physiology* 233:E104–E108.

Waterlow, J.C., Garlick, P.J., and Millward, D.J. 1978. *Protein turnovers in mammalian tissues and in the whole body.* Amsterdam: Elsevier/North-Holland Biomedical Press.

Waters, M.J. 1999. The growth hormone receptor. In *Handbook of Physiology.* J.L. Kostyo, ed. New York and Oxford: Oxford University Press.

Weaver, S.A., Aherene, F.X., Meaney, M.J., Schaefer, A.L., and Dixon, W.T. 2000a. Neonatal handling permanently alters hypothalamic-pituitary-adrenal axis function, behaviour, and body weight in boars. *Journal of Endocrinology* 164:349–359.

Weaver, S.A., Dixon, W.T., and Schaefer, A.L. 2000b. The effects of mutated skeletal ryanodine receptors on hypothalamic-pituitary-adrenal axis function in boars. *Journal of Animal Science* 78:1319–1330.

Wentworth, B.C., and Hussein, M.O. 1985. Serum corticosterone levels in embryos, newly hatched, and young turkey poults. *Poultry Science* 64:2195–2201.

Wheaton, J.E., Al-Raheem, S.N., Massri, Y.G., and Marcek, J.M. 1986. Twenty-four–hour growth hormone profiles in Angus steers. *Journal of Animal Science* 62:1267–1272.

Wilkie, R.S., O'Neill, I.E., Butterwith, S.C., Duclos, M.J., and Goddard, C. 1995. Regulation of chick muscle satellite cells by fibroblast growth factors: interaction with insulin-like growth factor-I and heparin. *Growth Regulation* 5:18–27.

Wintour, E.M., Butkus, A., Earnest, L., and Pompolo, S. 1996. The erythropoietin gene is expressed strongly in the mammalian mesonephric kidney. *Blood* 88:3349–3353.

Wishart, G.J., and Dutton, G.J. 1974. Precocious development of detoxicating enzymes following pituitary graft. *Nature* 252:408–410.

Wong, E.A., Silsby, J.L., and El Halawani, M.E. 1992. Complementary DNA cloning and expression of Pit-1/GHF-1 from the domestic turkey. *DNA Cell Biology* 11:651–660.

Wray-Cahen, D., Beckett, P.R., Nguyen, H.V., and Davis, T.A. 1997. Insulin-stimulated amino acid utilization during glucose and amino acid clamps decreases with development. *American Journal of Physiology* 273:E305–E314.

Wray-Cahen, D., Nguyen, H.V., Burrin, D.G., Beckett, P.R., Fiorotto, M.L., Reeds, P.J., Wester, T.J., and Davis, T.A. 1998. Response of skeletal muscle protein synthesis to insulin in suckling pigs decreases with development. *American Journal of Physiology* 275:E602–E609.

Wrutniak, C., Cabello, G., Charrier, J., Dulor, J.-P., Blanchard, M., and Barenton, B. 1987. Effects of TRH and GRF administration on GH, TSH, T4 and T3 secretion in the lamb. *Reproduction, Nutrition, Développement* 27:501–510.

Wu, S.-Y., Polk, D., Wong, S., Reviczky, A., Vu, R., and Fisher, D.A. 1992. Thyroxine sulfate is a major thyroid hormone metabolite and a potential intermediate in the monodeiodination pathways in fetal sheep. *Endocrinology* 131:1751–1756.

Yamashita, H., Shao, J., Ishizuka, T., Klepcyk, P.J., Muhlenkamp, P., Qiao, L., Hoggard, N., and Friedman, J.E. 2001. Leptin administration prevents spontaneous gestational diabetes in heterozygous Leprdb/+ mice: effects on placental leptin and fetal growth. *Endocrinology* 142:2888–2897.

Yen, J.T., and Pond, W.G. 1985. Plasma thyroid hormones, growth and carcass measurements of genetically obese and lean pigs as influenced by thyroprotein supplementation. *Journal of Animal Science* 61:566–572.

Young, I.R., Mesiano, S., Hintz, D.J., Ralph, M.M., Browne, C.A., and Thorburn, G.D. 1989. Growth hormone and testosterone can independently stimulate the growth of hypophysectomized prepubertal lambs without any alteration in circulating concentrations of insulin-like growth factor. *Journal of Endocrinology* 121:563–570.

Yu, T.-P., Sun, H.S., Wahls, S., Sanchez-Serrano, I., Rothschild, M.F., and Tuggle, C.K. 2001. Cloning of the full length pig pit-1 (POU1F1) CDNA and a novel alternative PIT1 transcript, and functional studies of their encoded proteins. *Animal Biotechnology* 12:1–19.

Yu, T.-P., Wang, L., Tuggle, C.K., and Rothschild, M.F. 1999. Mapping genes for fatness and growth on pig chromosome 13: a search in the region close to the pig PIT1 gene. *Journal of Animal Breeding and Genetics* 116:269–280.

Zackenfels, K., Oppenheim, R.W., and Rohrer, H. 1995. Evidence for an important role of IGF-I and IGF-II for the early development of chick sympathetic neurons. *Neuron* 14:731–741.

Zainur, A.S., Tassell, R., Kellaway, R.C., and Dodemaide, W.R. 1989. Recombinant growth hormone in growing lambs: effects on growth, feed utilization, body and carcass characteristics and on wool growth. *Australian Journal of Agricultural Research* 40:195–206.

Zapf, J., and Froesch, E.R. 1999. Insulin-like growth factor I actions on somatic growth. In *Handbook of Physiology*. J.L. Kostyo, ed. New York and Oxford: Oxford University Press.

Zhang, Y., Proenca, R., Maffei, M., Barone, M., Leopold, L., and Friedman, J.M. 1994. Positional cloning of the mouse obese gene and its human homologue. *Nature* 372:425–432.

6
Growth Factors

Colin G. Scanes

This chapter provides an overview of the numerous growth factors. Although these growth factors may be found in the circulation, they exert their effects predominantly at a local level, acting in a paracrine manner (on different but close/adjacent cells) and/or autocrine manner (on itself or close/adjacent cells) (see Figure 6.1). The aspects of the growth factors related to development and growth are covered. The growth factors are also intimately related to responses to foreign organisms (including immune functioning and inflammation) together with reproduction. These latter roles of the growth factors are outside the scope of this book. Some discussion of their involvement in the growth depression related to environment pathogens is included in Chapter 16.

EPIDERMAL GROWTH FACTOR (EGF) FAMILY

Members of the Epidermal Growth Factor (EGF) family are synthesized initially as pro-hormones that are membrane-bound. These can act either following proteolytic cleavage or by cell-to-cell interaction (reviewed Klonisch et al. 2001). Members of the EGF family include Epidermal Growth Factor (EGF), Transforming Growth Factor-α (TGF-α), Heparin-binding EGF (HB-EGF) together with amphiregulin, betacellulin (BTC), epiregulin, heregulin α and β (HRG α and β), and neuroregulin 2α and β (NRG2α and β), also called *neu* differentiation factor (NDF) (Jones et al. 1999; also reviewed Klonisch et al. 2001).

EGF Family Receptors

Members of the EGF family interact with tyrosine kinase type receptors of the *erbβ* gene family. The EGF receptors include *Erbβ1* (EGF receptor—EGFR), *Erbβ2*, *Erbβ3* and *Erbβ4*. The ligands of the EGF family show markedly different potencies in binding to the different receptors (Jones et al. 1999) (Table 6.1). EGF receptors are linked to tyrosine kinase. Activation of the tyrosine kinase requires binding to the ligand and receptor dimerization. Both homo- and heterodimers can be formed. For some ligands, for instance HRGα and β, there are marked increases in affinity when binding to a mixture of receptors resulting in heterodimer formation (Jones et al. 1999).

Epidermal Growth Factor (EGF)

EGF was first identified based on the ability of a polypeptide from the submaxillary salivary gland to affect the newborn mouse, inducing precocious eye opening and the eruption of the incisors (Cohen 1960, 1962). Moreover, EGF was named on the basis of its ability to induce keratinization of epidermal cells (Cohen and Elliott 1963). Since the discovery of EGF, numerous additional actions have been ascribed to it (see the section "Actions of EGF/TGFα" below).

Chemistry

The polypeptide EGF was initially purified from human urine and called urogastrone.

Transforming Growth Factorα (TGFα)

Transforming growth factorα (TGFα) is closely related to EGF. Both EGF and TGFα have similar actions, acting via a single receptor, the EGF receptor. Hence, both the receptor for EGF/TGFα and their biological activities are considered together.

EGF Receptor (EGFR)

The EGFR is the receptor for both EGF and TGFα. It is also the homolog of the avian erythroblastic viral (*v-erb-b*) oncogene.

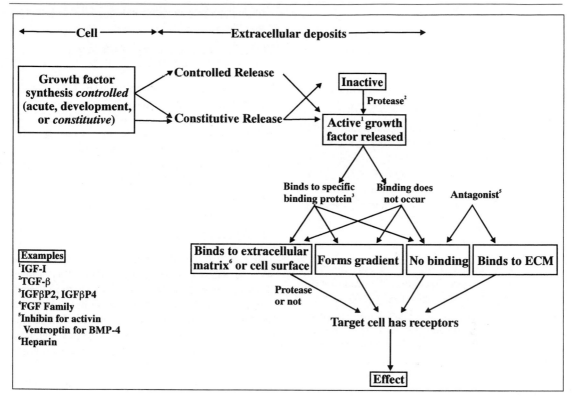

Figure 6.1. Interactions of growth factors with extracellular matrix, binding proteins, and cell receptors.

Table 6.1. Relative potencies[1] of members of EGF family—Epidermal Growth Factor (EGF), Transforming Growth Factor-α (TGF-α), Heparin-binding EGF (HB-EGF), heregulin α and β (HRG α and β), and neuroregulin 2α, 2β, and 3 (NRG2α, NRG2β, and NGF3)—as ligands for the various EGF receptors (based on Jones et al., 1999)

Ligand	Receptor		
	Erbβ1	Erbβ3	Erbβ4
EGF	74	<1	<1
TGFα	15	<1	<1
HB-EGF	20	<1	<1
BTC	100	<1	100
HRGα	<1	1	7
HRGβ	<1	100	<1
NRG2α	<1	<1	<1
NRG2β	<1	<1	6
NRG3	<1	<1	<1

[1]Highest affinity ligand is defined as 100%.

Actions of EGF/TGFα

Proliferation and differentiation of multiple tissues, including muscle and adipocytes, is influenced by EGF/TGFα.

EGF/TGFα and Muscle Development

There is a role for EGF/TGFα in muscle development, particularly precursor cell proliferation. EGF is a mitogen for porcine satellite cells (Doumit and Merkel 1992; Doumit et al. 1993) and fetal bovine myoblasts (Blachowski et al. 1993). EGF stimulates the proliferation of chick embryo heart mesenchymal (muscle progenitor) cells (Balk et al. 1982), an effect that is potentiated by IGF-I (Balk et al. 1984).

EGF/TGFα and Adipocytes

EGF and/or TGFα stimulate proliferation of preadipocytes and can either stimulate or inhibit differentiation. The mouse fibroblast line 3T3-L1 can differentiate into adipocytes. These cells express the EGF receptor and respond to EGF in a biphasic (developmental stage–dependent) manner. EGF inhibits differentiation of preadipocytes but promotes adipogenesis of differentiated mouse adipocytes (Adachi et al. 1994). In the chicken, EGF can stimulate the proliferation of preadipocytes (together with potentiating the effects of IGF-I, platelet-derived growth factor, and TGFβ) while blocking their differentiation (Butterwith et al. 1992). In pigs, EGF increases both DNA replication and differentiation of adipocyte precursors (reviewed Boone et al. 2000).

EGF/TGFα and the Gastrointestinal (GI) Tract

Both the growth/development and functioning of the gastrointestinal (GI) tract is influenced by EGF/TGFα. The administration of EGF enhances DNA synthesis throughout the GI tract (Scheving et al. 1979, 1980). Moreover, EGF increases stomach weight and stomach mucosal DNA (Dembinski and Johnson 1985) and small intestine dry weight (Oka et al. 1983). EGF administration to turkey embryos has been demonstrated to improve glucose absorption in the jejunum just prior to hatching (Croom et al. 1998). There are, also, EGF effects on GI peptide production. For instance, there are increases in the tissue content of neurotensin and peptide YY (PYY) in the intestines of TGFα overexpressing mice (Lee et al. 1999). Moreover, administration of EGF increases the circulating concentration of PYY in dogs (Lee et al. 1999). The proliferation of fetal and adult hepatocytes is increased by TGFα (Gruppuso et al. 1994).

EGF/TGFα and the Hypothalamic-Pituitary-GH-IGFI Axis

There are some interactions between EGF and the hypothalamic-pituitary-GH-IGF-I-growth axis that might be interpreted as EGF inhibiting the axis. For instance, there are marked changes in the GH-IGF-I axis with chronic EGF administration (increased circulating concentrations of IGFBP-1 and IGFBP-2 and decreased IGF-I and IGFBP-3 in pigs (Vinter-Jensen et al. 1996). Moreover, EGF administration reduces growth in rats (Oka et al. 1983).

EGF/TGFα and Other Tissues

Either EGF and/or TGFα can stimulate the proliferation of mammary alveolar cells (cattle: McGrath et al. 1991; sheep: Moorby et al. 1995), with EGF augmenting the effect of IGF-I (McGrath et al. 1991). Moreover, TGFα expression is observed in bovine mammary tissue in late pregnancy and lactation, supporting the involvement of TGFα in mammogenesis (Koff and Plaut 1995).

EGF/TGFα influences the proliferation and differentiation of various other tissues. TGFα stimulates the growth but not differentiation of metanephric mesenchymal cells and prevents their apoptosis (Barasch et al. 1997). TGFα and pituitary development/functioning TGFα may influence prolactin and/or GH release because TGFα has been found to co-localize in lactotrophs and possibly also somatotrophs in bovine pituitary glands (Kobrin et al. 1987). Not only does TGFα (and EGF) play a role in skin development, but also there is auto-induction (autocrine plus positive feedback) of TGFα expression with TGFα or EGF increasing TGFα expression in keratocytes (human) (Coffey et al. 1987):

$$EGF/TGF\alpha \Rightarrow Keratocyte\ TGF\alpha\ expression \Uparrow$$

EGF stimulates thyroid cell proliferation in, for instance, rats (Asmis et al. 1995), sheep (Westermark and Westermark 1982), and pigs (Tsushima et al. 1988; Cowin et al. 1996), and this effect is potentiated by TSH. There also appear to be effects of EGF on thyroid functioning, with chronic EGF administration increasing circulating concentrations of T_3 in pigs (Vinter-Jensen et al. 1996). This reflects either a paracrine effect or a pharmacological effect of EGF, circulating concentrations being very low.

FIBROBLAST GROWTH FACTOR (FGF) FAMILY

There are multiple members of the fibroblast growth factor (FGF) family, and these bind heparin. At least 23 have been identified and their nomenclature assigned according to the Human Gene Nomenclature Database (http://www.gene.ucl.ac.uk/cgi-bin/nomenclature/):

- FGF-1 acidic FGF, heparin-binding growth factor-1 (HBGF-1), FGFA, beta-endothelial cell growth factor (ECGF-beta)
- FGF-2 (basic or bFGF) heparin-binding growth factor-2 (HBGF-2)
- FGF-3 murine mammary tumor virus integration site (v-int-2) oncogene homolog
- FGF-4 heparin secretory transforming protein 1 (HSTF1), Kaposi sarcoma oncogene
- FGF-5 oncogene encoding fibroblast growth factor-related protein
- FGF-6 fibroblast growth factor-related gene, hst-2
- FGF-7 keratinocyte growth factor (KGF)
- FGF-8 androgen induced growth factor (AIGF)
- FGF-9 glia-activating factor (GAF)
- FGF-10 keratinocyte growth factor 2 (KGF-2)
- FGF-11 FGF homologous factor 3 (FHF-3)
- FGF-12 FGF homologous factor 1 (FHF-1)
- FGF-13 FGF homologous factor 2 (FHF-2)
- FGF-14 FGF homologous factor 4 (FHF-4)
- FGF-15–FGF-23

Chemistry

FGF-2 is a 146 amino-acid residue-containing protein. There is close homology between FGF-1 and FGF-2 and between other members of the family (reviewed Bikfalvi et al. 1997) (http://cytokine.medic.kumamoto-u.ac.jp/CFC/FGF/FGF-TREE.html).

Receptors

There are two classes of FGF receptors on cell membranes—high affinity receptors (e.g., FGFR 1–4) and low affinity binding proteins (e.g., heparin and heparin sulfate containing proteoglycans) (reviewed by Plotnikov et al. 1999). There are at least seven members of the FGF receptor (FGFR) gene family (http://www.gene.ucl.ac.uk/cgi-bin/nomenclature/):

- FGFR1 (fms-related tyrosine kinase 2)
- FGFR2

- FGFR3 [one isoform being the keratinocyte growth factor receptor (KGFR)]
- FGFR4
- FGFR6
- FGFRL1 (FGFR-like 1 or FGFR like embryonic kinase)
- FIBP (acidic FGF intracellular binding protein)

The FGF receptors consist of the ligand binding extracellular binding region, with three immunoglobulin (Ig-)-like domains (I, II, and III), a single transmembrane domain, and an intracellular domain/tyrosine kinase (reviewed Ornitz et al. 1996; Plotnikov et al. 1999). The FGFR1, FGFR2, and FGFR3 gene products can be alternatively spliced (tissue-dependent) in the Ig-like III domain. The resulting translated products are

- FGFR1IIIa, FGFR2IIIa, FGFR3IIIa (these are secreted with an unknown role)
- FGFR1IIIb, FGFR2IIIb, FGFR3IIIb (receptors)
- FGFR1IIIc, FGFR2IIIc, FGFR3IIIc (receptors)

These receptors (-b and -c) have different sequences of amino acid residues in the Ig-like domain III and different ligand binding properties (see Table 6.2). For instance, FGF-7 (keratinocyte growth factor) shows the highest activity with FGFR2IIIb (an alternatively spliced variant of the *bek* gene product—reviewed Ka et al. 2001); hence the latter is known as the keratinocyte growth factor receptor (KGFR).

The interaction of FGFs and their receptors has been recently characterized (Plotnikov et al. 1999). FGF binding to the receptor is insufficient to cause receptor dimerization and activation of the tyrosine kinase. Also required for receptor dimerization is the FGF acting in concert with soluble or cell surface heparin sulfate containing proteoglycans (reviewed Plotnikov et al. 1999). FGFs/FGF receptors act via tyrosine kinase (e.g. Johnson and Allen 1995).

Actions of FGFs

FGFs are released from cells and act very locally or are bound to extracellular proteins (FGFs binding to heparin and heparin-like proteins). FGFs are involved in the control of the following: cell differentiation and/or proliferation (e.g., adipocyte and chondrocyte), angiogenesis, organ formation (e.g., limb formation and lung budding during embryonic development), and differentiation and/or proliferation of multiple cells. FGF-11-14 (FHFs) are

Table 6.2. Relative ability of members of FGF family to bind to and activate FGF receptors/regulators (data from Ornitz et al., 1996)

	FGFR1IIIb	FGFR1IIIc	FGFR2IIIb	FGFR2c	FGFR3IIIb	FGFR3IIIc	FGFR4
FGF-1[a]	100	100	100	100	100	100	100
FGF-2	56	104	9	64	1	107	113
FGF-3	34	<1	45	4	1	1	6
FGF-4	16	102	15	94	1	69	108
FGF-5	4	59	5	25	1	12	7
FGF-6	5	55	5	61	1	9	79
FGF-7	6	<1	81	2	1	1	2
FGF-8	3	1	4	16	1	40	76
FGF-9	3	21	7	89	41	96	75

[a]FGF-1 is defined as a potency of 100.

nuclear localization signals (Smallwood et al. 1996).

FGF and Angiogenesis

Members of the FGF family induce angiogenesis, the proliferation of capillary endothelial cells (reviewed Bikfalvi et al. 1997). The mechanism for this includes other growth factors. For instance, FGF-2 induces vascular endothelial growth factor (VEGF) in endothelial cells (reviewed Reynolds and Redmer 1998).

FGF and Adipose Development

Not only can FGF-1 and FGF-2 stimulate proliferation of preadipocytes from the chicken (Butterwith et al. 1993) but FGF-2 is also expressed by chick adipocytes (Burt et al. 1992).

FGF and Muscle Growth

Members of the FGF family of growth factors affect satellite cell proliferation and muscle differentiation (for details, see Chapter 8). Skeletal muscle satellite cells express receptors to FGF-2 and can proliferate in response to FGF-2 (Johnson and Allen 1995). In addition, FGF-2 is involved in the control of smooth muscle cell differentiation and myogenesis (Bikfalvi et al. 1997). In contrast, based on studies with both chick and mouse embryos, FGF-5 inhibits skeletal muscle development through a mechanism that involves activated Ras and MAPK (Dorman and Johnson 1999; Clase et al. 2000).

FGF and Bone/Limb Growth

Four FGFs (FGF-2, FGF-4, FGF-8, and FGF-10) are important growth factors in the growth, pattern-

ing, and development of the limb bud based on studies with the chick embryo and "knock-out" mice (reviewed Smallwood et al. 1996; Hogan 1999). Three growth factors are critical to the development/patterning. These are produced sequentially: FGF-10 (from ectoderm), then FGF-18 (dependent on FGF-10), and finally FGF-4 and FGF-8. FGF-2 is also involved in the control of limb development and chondrogenesis (reviewed Bikfalvi et al. 1997). (See Figure 6.2.) FGF-2 (bFGF) is synthesized by osteoblasts and deposited in the matrix. This growth factor enhances proliferation of osteoprogenitor cells and osteoblast-like cells.

FGF and Early Embryonic Development

FGF is instrumental in the induction of mesoderm from ectodermal cells in very early embryonic development (Umbhauer et al. 2000). In early embryonic development, FGF-8 is expressed in the most caudal part of the segmentation plate (presomite cells) (reviewed Vasiliauskas and Stern 2001).

FGF and Lung Development

Based on studies in the mouse and rat, respectively, FGF-10 plays a critical role in bronchial branching during organogenesis of the lung, and FGF-7 induces surfactant synthesis and preparing the lung for functioning. Localized mesodermal production of FGF-10 regulates endodermal proliferation and bronchial bud outgrowth (Bellusci et al. 1997). Moreover, FGF-7 induces maturation of alveolar cells and their synthesis of the lung surfactant (Chelly et al. 2001).

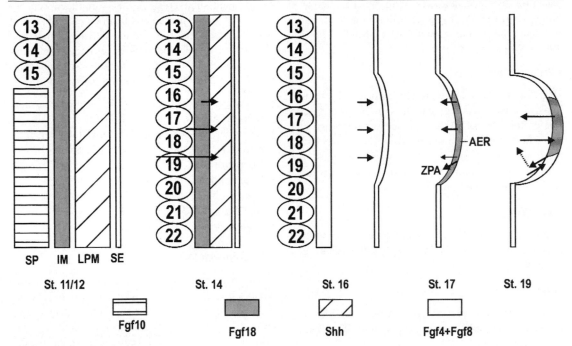

Figure 6.2. Role of FGF and Shh (Sonic hedgehog) in the development of the chick limb (wing bud) (Bikfalui et al. 1997).

FGF and Kidney Development

The growth factors FGF-2 and also FGF-9 stimulate the growth but not differentiation of metanephric mesenchymal cells and prevents apoptosis (Karavanova et al. 1996; Barasch et al. 1999). It might be noted that these metanephric mesenchymal cells also produce FGF-2 (Barasch et al. 1997). Moreover, based on studies with the FGF-7 null mouse, FGF-7 augments the growth of the ureteric bud that is critically important to kidney differentiation (see the section "Leukemia Inhibitory Factor (LIF)/IL-6 Family," later in this chapter) and increases the number of nephrons (Qiao et al. 1999).

FGF and Neural Development

FGF-2 is involved in the control of brain neural cell differentiation and survival (Bikfalvi et al. 1997). FGF-2 can stimulate the proliferation of neural crest cells (Murphy et al. 1994). Other FGFs affect neural development. For instance, FGF-9 stimulates proliferation of astrocytes (reviewed Smallwood et al. 1996), and FGF-8 appears to be involved in the induction of the midbrain (Crossley et al. 1996).

FGFs and Endocrine Tissue Development

FGFs influence the development of endocrine tissue. FGF-2 affects the development of the pancreatic endocrine progenitor cells into β cells, FGF-2 increasing proliferation while inhibiting differentiation (Lumelsky et al. 2001). In addition, FGF-2 affects the development of the anterior pituitary gland. FGF-2 stimulates the proliferation of the lactotrophs in the anterior pituitary gland. It is thought that TGF-β3 acts locally on foliculostellate cells to increase FGF-2 release, and this, in turn, increases the proliferation of the lactotrophs (Hentiges et al. 2000). Moreover, FGF-2 is produced by the thyroid and also stimulates thyroid cell proliferation (Logan et al. 1992).

HEPATIC GROWTH FACTOR(HGF)/SCATTER FACTOR(SF)

Hepatic growth factor (HGF) is a heparin-binding protein that has also been referred to as hepatopoietin A. HGF/scatter factors (SF) were initially identified based on different bioassays. With the characterization of their cDNA, it was determined that these are the same mitogenic growth factor (Naldini et al. 1991a; Weidner et al. 1991).

Chemistry

HGF/SF is a very large growth factor that binds to heparin sulfate proteoglycan. It is produced as inactive protein (90 KDa) that is processed (cleavage of a valine-arginine peptide bond) to an active heterodimer (α subunit 440 amino-acid residues; β subunit 234 amino-acid residues). The subunits are linked by disulfide bonds.

Receptor

The receptor for HGF/SF is the c-met-proto-oncogene tyrosine kinase (Naldini et al. 1991b; Clark et al. 1996).

Role

HGF/SF has multiple effects in growth and development. Examples of the effects of HGF/SF include the following:

- Stimulation of the proliferation of epithelial and endothelial cells is expressed in chondrocytes, hematopoietic cells, somites, squamous epithelium of the esophagus, and skin and bronchial epithelium in the developing rat (DeFrances et al. 1992).
- HGF/SF plays a critical role in liver development (Schmidt et al. 1995), increasing the proliferation of fetal hepatocytes (Gruppuso et al. 1994).
- HGF/SF is essential for skeletal muscle development, being released from satellite cells in an autocrine manner. HGF/SF activates satellite cells to enter the cell cycle (G_o to G_i) so that growth factors can stimulate proliferation (see Chapter 8 for details). HGF/SF also is a regulator of skeletogenesis, stimulating proliferation of chondrocytes, osteoblasts, and osteoclasts. HGF/SF can also stimulate angiogenesis (Grant et al. 1993).
- HGF/SF is involved in placentation—e.g., in horses.

NERVE GROWTH FACTOR (NGF) FAMILY

Nerve growth factor (NGF) was the first growth factor and identified by Stanley Cohen. The NGF was initially observed as an activity in mouse salivary glands (sub-submaxillary) that stimulated sensory and sympathetic nerve cells from chick embryos. It was later isolated from mouse salivary glands and shown to influence nervous development in mammals (Cohen 1960, 1962). There are several members of the NGF family including the following:

- Nerve growth factor, beta NGF, beta polypeptide (neurotropin 1), ligand for NTRK1
- Brain derived neurotropic factor (BDNF) (neurotropin 2), ligand for NTRK2 (TRKB)
- Neurotropin 3 (NT3)
- Neurotropin-4 (NT4), neurotropin 4/5, neurotropin-5, NT-4, NT-5, NT-4/5, ligand for NTRK2 (TRKB)
- Neurotropin-6A (NT6A)
- Neurotropin (NT6B)
- Neurotropin (NT6G)

The neurotropins are synthesized as larger precursors, pro-neurotropins, which are proteolytically cleaved (either intracellular or extracellular) to generate the biologically active neurotropin. There are also high affinity binding sites for pro-neurotropins (p75[NTR]), which can induce apoptosis. Thus, the pro-neurotropins may come to be recognized as distinct growth factors.

Nerve Growth Factor (NGF)

NGF is produced by the nervous system together with other tissues (e.g., salivary gland and ovary). It is required for the development of the sympathetic system and also plays a critical role in follicular development in the ovary.

Chemistry

NGF shows the closest homology with NT3 and then BDNF (http://cytokine.medic.kumamoto-u.ac.jp/CFC/NGF/NGF-TREE.html). NGF has ~120 amino-acid residues with three disulfide bridges (6 cysteines).

Receptor

NGF receptor is a member of the TNFR superfamily (the receptor has recently been designated as TNFRSF 16 by the Human Gene Nomenclature Database (http://www.gene.ucl.ac.uk/cgi-bin/nomenclature/). This receptor is unique in the TNFR superfamily in binding a ligand, NGF, which is not a member of the TNF superfamily (Locksley et al. 2001). In addition, NGF binds to low affinity neurotrophin receptor.

PLATELET-DERIVED GROWTH FACTOR (PDGF)/VASCULAR ENDOTHELIAL GROWTH FACTOR (VEGF) FAMILY

Th PDGF/VEGF family of growth factors include Platelet-Derived Growth Factor; Vascular Endothelial Growth Factors—VRGF-A, VEGF-B, VEGF-C, VEGF–D, and Placental growth factor-1 (PlGF-1), PlGF-2, and PlGF-3.

Platelet-Derived Growth Factor (PDGF)

PDGF has a number of mitogenic effects, which include enhancing the proliferation of the following cell types: smooth muscle cells, small intestine epithelial cells (Booth et al. 1995), adipocytes (chick: Butterwith and Goddard 1991). PDGF B and its receptor PDGF-Rβ are involved in kidney development. Mice lacking either show aberrant development of the glomerulus mesangial cells (Lindahl et al. 1998).

Vascular Endothelial Growth Factor A (VEGF)

Vascular Endothelial Growth Factor (VEGF) has multiple roles (reviewed Ferrara and Davis-Smyth 1997) related to the following: angiogenesis, adipogenesis, myogenesis, and bone development.

Chemistry

VEGF is a homodimeric glycoprotein. VEGF-1 exists in several forms (VEGF$_{121}$; VEGF$_{165}$; VEGF$_{189}$; VEGF$_{206}$ containing respectively 121, 165, 189, and 206 amino-acid residues) due to alternative splicing of the RNA. The major form is a heparin-binding glycoprotein based on VEGF$_{165}$ (reviewed Ferrara and Davis-Smyth 1997).

Receptors

The VEGF receptors are tyrosine kinases that bind homo- or heterodimers of the VEGF family. The receptors (reviewed Fraser and Lunn 2001) include VEGF receptor 1 (VEGFR1) (*fms* like tyrosine kinase, Flt-1), VEGFR2 (kinase insert domain-containing region, FDR), and VEGFR3. These have different ligand binding characteristics: VEGF receptor 1 (VEGFR1) binds VEGF-A, VEGF-2, and PlGF; VEGFR2 (found in the liver) binds VEGF-A, VEGF-B, and VEGF-D; and VEGFR3 binds VEFG-C and VEGF-D.

Actions of VEGF—Angiogenesis

VEGF affects angiogenesis-enhancing endothelial cell proliferation. VEGF is expressed in highly vascular tissues. Knock-out mice lacking VEGF receptor show much reduced blood vessel formation. Similarly, antisera to VEGF blocks angiogenesis (reviewed Frasier and Lunn 2001). One isoform, VEGF$_{165}$, has been demonstrated to increase both angiogenesis and vasculogenesis in cultured embryonic quail hearts (Yue and Tomanek 2001).

VEGF and Skeletal Development

VEGF is involved in skeletal development. It is expressed in osteoblasts, with its expression increased by FGF-2, TGFβ2, and TGFβ3. VEGF has a possible role on osteoblast differentiation. VEGF also influences pituitary functioning, being released from follicular-stellate cells.

TRANSFORMING GROWTH FACTOR-β SUPERFAMILY

The TGF superfamily growth factors are active as dimers—usually homodimers but in some cases, heterodimers (e.g., inhibins) (reviewed Massaqué et al. 2000). Members of the TGFβ superfamily include the following (based on http://www.gene. ucl.ac.uk/cgi-bin/nomenclature/):

- Transforming Growth Factor-β (TGFβ)
- Activin and the ligand antagonist, Inhibin
- Bone Morphogenic Proteins (BMP-1–5)
- Bone Morphogenic Protein 6 (BMP-6) or VGR-1
- Bone Morphogenic Protein 7 (BMP-7) or osteogenic protein-1 (OP-1),OP3,BMPa
- Bone Morphogenic Protein 8 (BMP-8) or osteogenic protein-2 (OP-2)
- Bone Morphogenic Protein 15 (BMP-15) or GDF-9B
- Müllerian hormone (AMH) or Müllerian inhibitory substance (MIS)
- Growth differentiation or development factor (GDF)-1 (GDF-1) or embryonic growth factor
- GDF-2 or BMP-9
- GDF-3–7
- GDF-8 or myostatin
- GDF-9
- GDF-10 or BMP-3B
- GDF-11 or BMP-11
- Glial cell line derived neurotropic factor (GDNF)
- Vegital hemisphere protein (Vg1) from Xenopus frog
- Mouse protein nodal
- Chicken dorsalin-1 (dsl-1)

Chemistry/Phylogeny

The members of the superfamily show varying degrees of homology, with TGF-β1 and TGF-β2 being closely related as are, for instance, inhibin βA and βB and BMP 5, 6, 7, and 8 (http://cytokine. medic.kumamoto-u.ac.jp/CFC/TGF/TGFB-TREE.html).

Mechanism of Members of the TGF-β Family

TGF-β and related growth factors act by assembling a receptor complex, bringing together a specific type I and type II receptor (both serine/threonine kinases). The type II receptor phosphorylates the type I receptor, which, in turn, phosphorylates/activates the appropriate Smad transcription factor (reviewed Massagué et al. 2000).

Transforming Growth Factor-β (TGF)

Several TGFβs exist (http://cytokine.medic. kumamoto-u.ac.jp): TGFβ1; TGFβ2 [BSC-1 cell growth inhibitor]; TGFβ3; TGF-β4 [Lefty preproprotein, Stra3 protein, left-right determination factor A (lefty A), LEFTA, Endometrial bleeding associated factor (EBAF), LEFTY1, BETA-4, LEFTY2, left-right determination factor B (LEFTB)]; and TGF-β5.

Chemistry

TGFβs are synthesized as precursor (~400 amino-acid residues). The TGFβs are homodimers of the C-terminal polypeptide1 (~112 amino-acid residues) of the precursor, linked together by disulfide bonds (Lawrence et al. 1985).

Binding Protein and Receptors

The pro-peptide of the TGFβ (latency associated protein) binds TGFβ, and this prevents binding to the receptor. There are three TGFβ receptor isoforms: TGFβ receptor typeI TGFβRI, TGFβRII, and TGFβRIII. TGFβ2 binds poorly to the TGFβRII. (For signal transduction, see Figure 6.3.)

Actions

In general, TGFβs inhibit growth of epithelial cells and stimulate proliferation of mesenchymal cells (Morris et al. 1988):

- TGFβ-1 stimulates the synthesis of IGFBP-3 by porcine myogenic/myoblast cells in vitro (Hembree et al. 1996).

- TGFβ1 is produced by growth plate chondrocytes in a latent form.
- TGFβ1 inhibits the proliferation of myogenic cells from sheep fetuses and of satellite cells from newborn sheep (Hathaway et al. 1994).
- TGFβ1 stimulates proliferation of fibroblasts (Hathaway et al. 1994).
- TGFβ1 also inhibits cortisol production by adrenocortical cells (Le Roy et al. 2000).
- TGFβ1 inhibits proliferation of lactotrophs. However, TGFβ3 stimulates proliferation of lactotrophs; TGFβ3 acts on folliculostellate cells to increase FGF2 release (Hentges et al. 2000).
- TGF β1 stimulates proliferation of preadipocytes and blocks differentiation (chicken: Butterwith and Gilroy 1991; Butterwith and Goddard 1991; differentiation in pigs: Richardson et al. 1989).
- TGFβ inhibits differentiation of chondrocytes (chick: O'Keefe et al. 1988).

TGFβ1 and Cartilage Development

TGFβ1 is produced by growth plate chondrocytes in a latent form and decreases differentiation of chondrocytes. There is some evidence of a link between TGF-β1 and tibial dyschondroplasia in chickens. TGF-β1 immunoreactivity is observed in chondrocytes and in the matrix in the growth plate. There is considerably more immunoreactivity in the matrix adjacent to collapsed cartilage canals in lines of broiler chickens with low incidence of dyschondroplasia than there is in chickens with high incidence of dyschondroplasia (Ling et al. 2000) (also see Table 6.3 and Chapter 9).

TGFβ1 and Thyroid Development

TGFβ-1 inhibits thyroid follicular cell proliferation induced by EGF or TSH or iodide or plasmin (sheep and pigs: Yusa et al. 1992; Cowin and Bidey 1995; Cowin et al. 1996). TGFβ's anti-proliferative effect may be mediated by IGF-I; TGFβ inhibits IGF-I release from these cells (Beere et al. 1991). TGFβ-1 also inhibits thyroid functioning, reducing TSH-induced iodide uptake (Tsushima et al. 1988).

Activins/Inhibins

Chemistry

Activin is a homodimer of one or the other of the βsubunits of inhibin (βA:βA or βB:βB) or heterodimer (βA and βB). Inhibin is a heterodimer (α:βA or α:βB) containing two subunits: α and either βA or βB. These are linked by disulfide

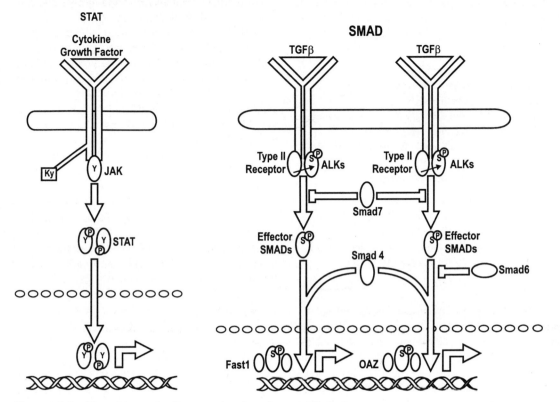

Figure 6.3. Signal transduction mechanism for growth factors.

Table 6.3. Comparison of TGFβ1 immunoreactivity in growth plates of broiler chickens from lines with low and high incidence of dyschondroplasia (data from Ling et al., 2000)

	TGFβ1 Immunoreactivity	
	Low Dyschondroplasia Line	High Dyschondroplasia line
Low proliferative zone		
Chondrocytes	65	64
Matrix	0	0
Prehypertroxic zone		
Chondrocytes	60	61
Matrix	2	2
Hypertrophic zone		
Chondrocytes	32	32
Matrix between canals	10	11
Matrix adjacent to the collapsed cartilage canals	23	7[*]

[*]Difference between lines $p<0.01$.

bridges. These are separate gene products encoded by different genes for each of the three subunits (reviewed Ying 1988). Precursor expression, translation, and processing involve the following:

- Propeptide-α subunit mRNA⇒
  Propeptide-α subunit⇒cleavage⇒αsubunit
- Propeptide-βA subunit mRNA⇒
  Propeptide-βA subunit⇒cleavage⇒βA subunit
- Propeptide-βB subunit mRNA⇒
  Propeptide-βB subunit⇒cleavage⇒βB subunit

Binding Protein and Receptors

Activin activity is opposed by a high affinity binding protein, follistatin. Activin can be bound by follistatin and hence sequestered. Follistatin is structurally unrelated to the TGFβ superfamily. Activin acts by binding to the activin type II receptor (ActRIIA).

Actions

The major roles of activins/inhibins are related to reproductive functioning. Activins stimulate the release of follicle stimulating hormone (FSH); inhibins have the opposite effect (reviewed Ying 1988). In addition, activins/inhibins exert intra-gonadal actions (reviewed Knight and Glister 2001). Other activities of activin include increasing apoptosis by hepatocytes and hence reducing liver mass.

Bone Morphogenic Proteins (BMP)

Bone Morphogenic Proteins (BMPs) influence the differentiation of bone and other tissues (see the section "Actions," below).

Chemistry

BMP-1 is a metalloprotease encoded by the *Bmp* 1 gene which is related to the *Drosophila tolloid* (Suzuki et al. 1996). Most BMPs are either homo- or heterodimers with the heterodimer being more active (Kawakami et al. 1996).

BMP Receptors

At least three BMP receptors exist (based on http://www.gene.ucl.ac.uk/cgi-bin/nomenclature/): BMP receptor, type IA (BMPR1A); BMP receptor, type IB (BMPR1B); and BMP receptor, type II serine/threonine kinase (BMPR2).

Actions

BMP-1 is a secreted metalloprotease that cleaves pro-collagen. Studies with knock-out mice indicate there is little effect on embryonic growth except

abnormalities of collagen and a failure/lesion of the ventral body wall (Suzuki et al. 1996).

BMP-2 and BMP-7 are involved in limb formation. They are expressed in overlapping regions of the limb bud leading to the possibility of the production of the more active heterodimer. Both BMP-2 and -7, together with the heterodimer, stimulate bone formation (Kawakami et al. 1996). BMP-7 induces osteoclast cell differentiation and IGF-BP5 synthesis. Based on chick embryo studies, BMP-2 and -4 are involved in the apoptosis in the limb buds that leads digit formation. BMP-2 and -4 induce interdigital apoptosis. Blocking these leads to webbed feet (Yokouchi et al. 1996; Zou and Niswander 1996). BMP-4 also induces the differentiation/development of the cartilage of the vertebrae (Monsoro-Burg et al. 1996).

BMP-2 and BMP-4 are expressed at the time of visceral (primitive gut) endoderm differentiation. They act via the BMP receptor IB; blocking this prevents both differentiation (expression of the visceral endoderm marker *Hnf* 4) and cavitation (formation of the gut cavity by apoptosis) (Coucouvanis and Martin 1999). BMP-4 causes apoptosis in the hindbrain of the chick embryo (Graham et al. 1994). The retina also expresses ventropin, an antagonist for BMP-4, in a gradient pattern (Sakuta et al. 2001).

Anti-Müllerian Hormone (AMH)

Anti-Müllerian hormone (AMH) or Müllerian inhibitory substance (MIS) is produced by the testes of the male fetus and specifically by the Sertoli cells.

Receptor

Anti-Müllerian hormone (AMH) binds to receptor AMHRII on mesenchymal cells adjacent to the Müllerian epithelium.

Action

AMH causes regression of the Müllerian ducts (which would go on to form the oviduct, uterus, cervix and anterior vagina). In birds, AMH (produced by the ovary) induces the regression of the right oviduct.

GDF8/Myostatin

Myostatin is expressed by skeletal muscle and acts to reduce muscle mass based on studies with knock-out mice. GDF8/myostatin null mice are larger and have considerably more muscling than wild-type mice (see Table 6.4) (McPherron et al. 1997). The double muscling in some breeds of cattle (e.g., Belgian blues) is thought to be related to myostatin/GDF7 (see also Chapter 2):

Table 6.4. Effect of myostatin (GDF8) on growth and muscling in mice (data from McPherron et al., 1997)

	Wild-Type	Myostatin Null	(% of Wild-Type)
Body weight (g)	30.3	40.9	(135%)
Muscles			
Pectoralis (g)	0.178	0.467	(262%)
Soleum (g)	0.006	0.012	(200%)

- Double muscling is a single allelic trait most prevalently found in Piedmontese and Belgian Blue breeds of cattle (Fahrenkrug et al. 1999).
- The trait increases muscling and hence meat by ~7% (Casas et al. 1999).
- Double muscling is due to at least two different mutations in the myostatin gene (MSTN) (Kambadur et al. 1997; McPherron and Lee 1997); Grobet et al. 1998):
  - Belgian Blue cattle with double muscling show an 11-base pair deletion causing premature termination of translation.
  - Piedmontese cattle with double muscling have a single nucleotide change leading to a substitution of cysteine by a tyrosine residue.

TUMOR NECROSIS FACTOR SUPERFAMILY (TGFSF)

There are presently 17 ligands and 23 receptors identified in the TGFSF superfamily of cytokines and are designated as TNFRSF 1-18 and TNFRSF 1-19 by the Human Gene Nomenclature Database (http://www.gene.ucl.ac.uk/cgi-bin/nomenclature/) (also see Table 6.5). Most play critical roles in immune functioning (reviewed Locksley et al. 2001). Another member of the TNF family is BAFF (B cell activation factor) (also known as TALL-1, THINK, bLyS, and zTNF4). BAFF binds to three receptors: BCMA, TAC1, and BAFF-R (Thompson et al. 2001). Only two ligands (TNFSF 2 and TNFSF 11) and three receptors (TNFRSF 1A, TNFRSF 11, and TNFRSF 16) are considered in this book because of their roles in growth and development. TNF receptors are type 1 transmembrane proteins (Locksley et al. 2001).

TGFSF 2—Tumor Necrosis Factor (TNFα)

Tumor necrosis factor (TNFα), alternatively known as cachectin, is produced by a number of cell types, including lymphocytes and macrophages. It causes fever and wasting (reviewed Locksley et al. 2001).

Chemistry

Although there is obviously homology between TNF and other members of the TNF superfamily, TNF shows the closest homology with Lymphotoxin (LT) and close homology with TNFSF 15 (see Table 6.5) (http://cytokine.medic.kumamoto-u.ac.jp/CFC/TNF/TNF-TREE.html).

Receptor

The TNF receptor is TNFR1A (see Table 6.5).

Actions

Tumor necrosis factor induces lysis, apoptosis, and programmed cell death in a number of cell types including tumors, osteoblasts, etc. In addition, TNFα has a role in mammary development: stimulating branching of the lobulo-alveolar ducts in mammary development, and modulating lactogenesis (Shea-Eaton et al. 2001).

TGFSF11—Osteoprotegerin-Ligand (OPGL)

Osteoprotegerin-ligand (OPGL) is also known as osteoclast differentiation factor (ODF) (Yasuda et al. 1998), tumor necrosis factor related activation cytokine (TRANCE) (Wong et al. 1997) and RANKL (RANK ligand). This protein plays a critical role in the development of bone, together with the mammary gland, and has marked effects on the immune system. OPGL is expressed by osteoblasts in lymph nodes (Wong et al. 1997); in activated but not resting T-cells (Kong et al. 1999); in dentritic cells (Anderson et al. 1997); and those mammary epithelial cells that are the progenitors for the alveolus, but only during late pregnancy (Fata et al.

Table 6.5. Nomenclature of the members of the tumor necrosis factor (TNF)/TNF receptor (TNFR) superfamily (based on Locksley et al., 2001 and http://www.gene.UCL.ac.uk/cgi-bin/nomenclature/search gene[a])

Standardized Names	Other Names	Probable Actions		Interacting Receptors
		Immune	Other	
Ligands Tumor Necrosis Factor Superfamily (TNFSF)				
TNFSF1	Lymphotoxin (LTα), TNFB	√		TNFRSF1A,1B
TNFSF2	TNF, cachectin, TNFA	√		TNFRSF1A
TNFSF3	LTβ, TNFC, p 33	√		TNFRSF3
TNFSF4	OX4OL, tax-transcriptionally activated glycoprotein 1, (gp 34), glycoprotein (TXGP1)	√		TNFRSF4
TNFSF5	CD4OL, IMO3, HIGMl, TRAP, CO154, gp 39	√		TNFRSF5
TNFSF6	FasL, APT1LG1	√		TNFRSF6,6A
TNFSF7	CD27L	√		
TNFSF8	CD3OL	√		TNFRSF8
TNFSF9	4-1 BBL	√		TNFRSF9
TNFSF10	TRAIL, Apo-2LTL2	√		TNFRSF10
TNFSF11	RANKL, TRANCE, OPGL, ODF	√	Mammary gland and osteoclast differentiation	TNFRSF11A (receptor) TNFRSF11B (decoy)
TNFSF12	TWEAK, DR3LAPO3L	√		TNFRSF12
TNFSF13	APRIL	√		TNFRSF17
TNFSF13β	BLYS, BAFF, THANK, TALL1	√		TNFRSF17
TNFSF14	LIGHT, LT, HVEM-L			
TNFSF15	VEGI	—		
TNFRSF18	AITRL, TL6, hGITRL	√	Angiogenesis inhibitor	TNFRSF18
Receptor (Tumor Necrosis Factor Receptor Super-family TNFRSF)				*Interacting ligand*
TNFRSF1A	TRFRI, CD12Oa, p55-R, TNFAR, TRFR60, TNF-R-I	√		TNFSF1,2
TNFRSF1B	CD120a, p 75, TNFBR, TNFR8O, TNF-R-II	√		TNFSF1

Standardized Names	Other Names	Probable Actions		Interacting Receptors
		Immune	Other	
TNFRSF3	LTβR, TNFR-2-RP, TNFCR, TNF-R-III	√		TNFSF3,4
TNFRSF4	OX40, CD134, ACT35, TXGP1L	√		TNFSF4
TNFRSF5	CD40, p50, Bp50	√		TNFSF5
TNFRSF6	FAS, CD95, APO-1, APT1	√		TNFSF6
TNFRSF6B (decoy)	DcR3			TNFSF6,14
TNFRSF7	CD27, Tp55, S152	√		
TNFRSF8	CD30, Ki-1, DISI66E			TNFSF8
TNFRSF9	4-1BB, CD137, ILA	√		TNFSF9
TNFRSF10A	DR4, Apo2, TRAILR-1	√		TNFSF10
TNFRSF10B	DR5, KILLER, TRICK2A, TRAIL-R2, TRICKB	√		TNFSF10
TNFRSF10C[b] decoy	DcR1, TRAILR3, LIT, TRID	√		TNFSF10
TNFRSF10D[c] decoy	DcR2, TRUNDD, TRAILR4 TRFSF10	√		
TNFRSF11A[d]	RANK, TRANCE-R	√	Mammary gland and osteoclast differentiation	TNFSF11
TNFRSF11B	OPG, OC1F, TR1, osteoprotegerin	√		TNFSF11
TNFRSF12	DR3, translocating chain-associated membrane protein (TRAMP), WSL-1, LARD, WSL-LR, DOR3, TR3, APO-3			TNFSF12
TNFRSF12L	TNFRSF 12 like			
TNFRSF14	Herpes virus entry mediator (HveA), HVEM, ATAR, TR2, LIGHTR	√		TNFSF14
TNFRSF16	NGFR, p75		Sensory neurons	NGF[e]
TNFRSF17	BCMA			TNFSF13
TNFRSF18	AITR, GITR	√		TNFSF18
TNFRSF19	Troy, Taj	-	Hair follicles	

[a]For cytogenetic localization in human genome, see Web site.
[b]Decoy without an intracellular domain.
[c]Decoy with truncated death domain.
[d]Activator of NFKB.
[e]*Note:* NGF is not a member of the TNF/TNFR superfamily.

2000). OPGL is found in the cell membrane of osteoblasts (Yasuda et al. 1998).

Chemistry

OPGL is a type II transmembrane protein (316 amino-acid residues) in the TNF cytokine family (Anderson et al. 1997; Wong et al. 1997).

Receptor (RANK) and Binding Protein (OPG)

OPGL binds to its receptor, RANK (receptor activator of NFβB, a member of the nuclear factor family of transcription factors). RANK is a type I transmembrane protein and a member of the TNF receptor (TNFR) family (Anderson et al. 1997; Hsu et al. 1999). RANK is ubiquitously expressed, and is found in muscle, thymus, liver, small intestine, adrenal gland, colon, etc. (Anderson et al. 1997), osteoclasts (Lacey et al. 1998), and mammary cells (Fata et al. 2000). In addition, OPGL binds to osteoprogerin (OPG) (also known as osteoclastogenesis inhibitory factor). This is a soluble binding protein or decoy receptor, which blocks the effect of OPGL (Kong et al. 1999).

RANK is expressed and found in the cell membrane of chondrocytes, osteoclasts, and progenitor cells (Hsu et al. 1999). OPGL is the critical factor stimulating osteoclast differentiation and activation and hence bone resorption (breakdown), thereby mobilizing calcium and facilitating bone remodeling. OPGL/RANK mediates the effect of factors that influence bone resorption via the osteoclasts including glucocorticoids and PTHrP (parathyroid related peptide) (Li et al. 2000). For instance, it has been observed that RANK nullizygous mice (RANK-/-) do not show increased circulating concentrations of ionized calcium in response to OPGL or PTH or 1,25 (OH)2 vitamin D3, but wild-type mice do (Li et al. 2000). OPGL is also required for mammary development and the initiation of lactation in late pregnancy (Fata et al. 2000).

OTHER CYTOKINES

Cytokines are produced by monocytes and by cells in other tissues. They are often small proteins (8–10kDa). Although their major roles are related to defense mechanisms of an animal, they may also play a role in development. Hence their role as growth factors are considered in this section.

Colony Stimulating Factor-1 (CSF-1)

Colony stimulating factor-1 (CSF-1) is produced by osteoblastic cells; these are terminally differentiated multinucleated cells derived from monocyte/macrophage that reabsorb bone.

Interleukins

The interleukin cytokines have critical roles related to the immune system and defence mechanisms. In addition they can have important roles related to the endocrine system and/or development. This section considers, albeit briefly, only the endocrine and/or developmental roles of interleukins. The inflammatory cytokines can depress growth (reviewed Johnson 1997) (also see Chapter 16).

Interleukin-1 (IL-1)

Interleukin-1α and β (IL-1α and IL-1β) have respectively 159 and 151 amino-acid residues (March et al. 1985). IL-1β, but not IL-1α, influences cell proliferation—for instance, inhibiting the proliferation of thyroid follicular epithelial cells (Rasmussen et al. 1990) and stimulating the proliferation of cells from the immediate lobe of the pituitary gland (Stepien et al. 1994).

Interleukin-6 (IL-6)

Interleukin-6 (IL-6) is produced by testis Sertoli cells where it exerts local effects. Another action of IL-6 is to stimulate the release of GH and other pituitary hormones (LH, FSH, prolactin, and ACTH). In this case, IL-6 is produced by follicostellate cells that are adjacent to the hormone producing cells. Interleukin-6 acts via the IL-6 receptor. This is a heterodimeric receptor with IL-6 specific binding subunit.

Interleukin-8 (IL-8)

Interleukin-8 (IL-8) is produced by macrophages, neutrophils, endothelial cells, and osteoclasts, and has effects on the immune system and bone.

Interleukin-11 (IL-11)

Interleukin-11 (IL-11) acts via a similar receptor and signal transduction mechanism to IL-6, LIF, ciliary neurotropic factor (CNTF). The IL-11 receptor is expressed by pituitary cells, including those cells that produce GH and ACTH. IL-11 stimulates ACTH release and POMC expression and the proliferation of both follicular-stellate cells and somatomammotrophs. IL-11 increases release of VEGF from follicular-stellate cells

Interleukin-20 (IL-20)

Interleukin-20 (IL-20) is closely related to IL-10 and is involved in epidermal differentiation

(Blumberg et al. 2001). IL-20 acts via two cytokine class II receptor subunits; IL-20Rα and IL-20Rβ (Blumberg et al. 2001).

Leukemia Inhibitory Factor (LIF)/IL-6 Family

Members of the LIF/IL-6 family include IL-6, Leukemia inhibitory factor (LIF), or differentiation-stimulating factor, and oncostatin (OSM).

Leukemia Inhibitory Factor (LIF)

LIF influences the differentiation and proliferation of a number of cell types, including hemopoietic cells (reviewed Auernhammer and Melmed 2000). The LIF receptor is heterodimeric consisting of the LIF specific binding subunit and the Gp130 receptor subunit; the latter is also the receptor for IL-6, oncostatin, and IL-11.

LIF has multiple actions related to growth and development. In a manner similar to IL-6, LIF is also secreted by the follicostellate cells of the pituitary gland and affects the release of ACTH and also inhibits angiogenesis. The embryonic ureteric bud cells produce LIF (Barasch et al. 1997). This, in turn, induces the differentiation (epithelialization) of the metanephric mesenchymal cells (Barasch et al. 1999). LIF can induce differentiation of neural crest cells (Murphy et al. 1994). LIF is produced by testis Sertoli cells and affects testes function. Chick blastodermal cells proliferate without differentiation in the presence of LIF (reviewed Etches et al. 1997).

Ciliary Neurotropic Factor (CNTF)

Ciliary Neurotropic Factor (CNTF) stimulates proliferation of both follicular-stellate cells and somatomammotrophs. CNTF increases the release of VEGF from follicular-stellate cells and both GH and prolactin from somatomammotrophs. The CNTF receptor expressed by pituitary cells.

OTHER PEPTIDES

Adrenomedullin (ADM)

Adrenomedullin (ADM) is a member of the calcitonin-gene–related peptide family. It inhibits proliferation of vascular smooth muscle and stimulates proliferation of adrenal cortical zona glomerulosa cells (which produce aldosterone).

Amylin

Amylin is a 37 amino-acid residue peptide that is produced by pancreatic β cells and co-secreted with insulin. Central nervous administration of amylin inhibits food intake.

Neuropeptide Y (NPY) and Peptide YY (PYY)

Neuropeptide Y (NPY) is a 36 amino-acid residue peptide related to Pancreatic Polypeptide (PP) and Peptide YY. NPY stimulates food intake (appetite) and hence body weight gain. Hypothalamic levels of NPY increase with food deprivation. Growth of chicks has been observed to be improved following the administration of peptide YY (PYY) in ovo (Coles et al. 1999). This may be due to effect of PYY on improving nutrient absorption following hatch, at least in young turkeys (Croom et al. 1998). NPY and PPY acts via NPY receptors (Y1, Y3, Y4, Y5, and Y6). NPYR Y5 is the putative receptor involved in food intake.

Glucose-Dependent Insulinotropic Peptide (GIP)

Glucose-dependent Insulinotropic Peptide (GIP) affects osteoblast derived cells and osteocytes with increased collagen synthesis. GIP receptors are found on osteoblasts.

GIP acts via cAMP.

PROSTAGLANDINS

There is evidence that prostaglandins are involved in the control of growth. Heifers actively immunized against prostaglandin $F_{2\alpha}$ show a slight (~9.6%) but significant decrease in growth rate compared to controls (immunized against human serum albumin) (Crowe et al. 1995). Prostaglandins (particularly prostaglandin E_2) are also produced by osteoblasts and stimulate bone resorption. Prostaglandin E_2 induces osteoclast formation via PGE receptor EP4 and partially EP2 (there being 4 sub-classes of PGE receptors) by increasing cAMP and osteoclast differentiation factor.

RETINOIDS

The retinoids are a family of lipids (alcohols, aldehydes, acids; cis and trans forms) with different biological activities. The dietary sources of retinoid precursors are carotenoids (e.g., β-carotene) and fatty acid retinyl esters.

The biologically active retinoid, retinoic acid (RA) and retinaldehyde are synthesized from the precursor, retinol (vitamin A alcohol). Biologically active retinoids act by binding to members of the nuclear receptor superfamily, which in turn bind to specific sequences of DNA and thus influence gene expression. These biologically active retinoids can be considered as a retinoid hormonal system (reviewed Vieira et al. 1995). Retinoic acid (RA) is one of the hormonal active forms of vitamin A, and it plays a critical role in development.

Binding Proteins and Receptors

Retinol is transported in the blood bound to retinol-binding protein alone or linked to serum protein transthyretin. There are multiple genes in the two classes of nuclear receptors of retinoids that are ligand dependent transcription factors: RAR retinoic acid receptor (e.g., RARα, β, γ) and RXR retinoid X receptor. The RAR binds both trans-retinoic acid and 9-cis RA, and RXR binds 9-RA. The RAR receptors function as either homodimers or heterodimers (RAR and RXR). The RXR can also function as a heterodimer with the vitamin D receptor or the thyroid hormone triiodothyronine receptor (reviewed Vieira et al. 1995).

The RAR genes are in the IB subfamily for nuclear receptors. RARα, RARβ, and RARγ are the trivial names for nuclear receptor/B1 (NR1B1), NR1B2 and NR1B3, respectively. The RXR genes are in the 2B subfamily. RXRA, RXRB, and RXRG are, respectively, NR2B1, NR2B2, and NR2B3 under the unified nomenclature for the nuclear receptor superfamily. Retinoic acid exerts its effect by binding to the retinoic acid receptor (RAR) and/or to the retinoid X receptor (RXR); both are members of the superfamily of steroid hormone receptors. The ligand bound receptors act as transcription factors either as heterodimers (RAR-RXR) or homodimers (RXR-RXR) (Mangelsdorf and Evans 1995).

Actions

Retinoic acid plays a critical role patterning the embryonic axis in early development. For instance, retinoic acid regulates the expression of *Hox* genes (homeobox containing transcription factors) (reviewed Vasiliauskas and Stern 2001). Retinoic acid stimulates the differentiation of chick embryo blastodermal cells in culture (reviewed Etches et al. 1997). Retinoic acid inhibits differentiation of porcine preadipocytes (Suryawan and Hu 1997).

CALCITRIOL/1,25 DIHYDROXYVITAMIN D3 [1,25(OH)$_2$D$_3$]

1,25 dihydroxyvitamin D3 [1,25(OH)$_2$D$_3$] has two roles. The major physiological role of 1,25(OH)$_2$D$_3$ is control of circulating concentrations of calcium. 1,25(OH)$_2$D$_3$ is also a growth factor, influencing cellular proliferation (depressing) and differentiation (accelerating). For instance, 1,25(OH)$_2$D$_3$ reduces proliferation of chondrocytes but enhances differentiation (Gerstenfeld et al. 1990; Farquharson et al. 1996).

REFERENCES

Adachi, H., Kurachi, H., Homma, H., Adachi, K., Imai, T., Morishige, K.-I., Matsuzawa, Y., and Miyake, A. 1994. Epidermal growth factor promotes adipogenesis of 3T3-L1 cell in vitro. *Endocrinology* 135:1824–1830.

Anderson, D.M., Maraskovsky, E., Billingsley, W.L., Dougall, W.C., Tometsko, M.E., Roux, E.R., Teepe, M.C., DuBose, R.F., Cosman, D., and Galibert, L. 1997. A homologue of the TNF receptor and its ligand enhance T-cell growth and dendritic-cell function. *Nature* 390:175–179.

Asmis, L.M., Gerber, H., Kaempf, J., and Studer, H. 1995. Epidermal growth factor stimulates cell proliferation and inhibits iodide uptake of FRTL-5 cells in vitro. *Journal of Endocrinology* 145:513–520.

Auernhammer, C.J., and Melmed, S. 2000. Leukemia-inhibitory factor-neuroimmune modular of endocrine function. *Endocrine Reviews* 21:313–345.

Balk, S.D., Morisi, A., Gunther, H.S., Svoboda, M.F., van Wyk, J.J., Nissley, S.P., and Scanes, C.G. 1984. Somatomedins (insulin-like growth factors), but not growth hormone are mitogenic for chicken heart mesenchymal cells and act synergistically with epidermal growth factor. *Life Science* 35:335–346.

Balk, S.D., Shiu, R.P.C., LaFleur, M.M., and Young, L.L. 1982. Epidermal growth factor and insulin cause normal chicken heart mesenchymal cells to proliferate like their Rous sarcoma virus-infected counterparts. *Proceedings of the National Academy of Sciences of the U.S.A.* 79:1154–1157.

Barasch, J., Qiao, J., McWilliams, G., Chen, D., Oliver, J.A., and Herzlinger, D. 1997. Ureteric bud cells secrete multiple factors, including bFGF, which rescue renal progenitors from apoptosis. *American Journal of Physiology* 273:F757–F767.

Barasch, J., Yang, J., Ware, C.B., Taga, T., Yoshida, K., Erdjument-Bromage, H., Tempst, P., Parravicini, E., Malach, S., Aranoff, T., and Oliver, J.A. 1999. Mesenchymal to epithelial conversion in rat metanephros is induced by LIF. *Cell* 99:377–386.

Beere, H.M., Soden, J., Tomlinson, S., and Bidey, S.P. 1991. Insulin-like growth factor-I production and action in porcine thyroid follicular cells in monoculture: regulation by transforming growth factor-β. *Journal of Endocrinology* 130:3–9.

Bellusci, S., Grindley, J., Emoto, H., Itoh, N., and Hogan, B.L.M. 1997. Fibroblast growth factor 10 (FGF10) and branching morphogenesis in the embryonic mouse lung. *Development* 124:4867–4878.

Bikfalvi, A., Klein, S., Pintucci, G., and Rifken, D.B. 1997. Biological roles of fibroblast growth factor-2. *Endocrine Reviews* 18:26–45.

Blachowski, S., Motyl, T., Orzechowski, A., Grzelkowska, K., and Interewicz, B. 1993. Comparison of metabolic effects of EGF, TGF-alpha and TGF-beta 1 in primary culture of fetal bovine myoblasts and rat L6 myoblasts. *International Journal of Biochemistry* 25:15171–11577.

Blumberg, H., Conklin, D., Xu, W.-F., Grossmann, A., Brender, T., Carollo, S., Eagan, M., Foster, D., Haldeman, B.A., Hammond, A., Haugen, H., Jelinek, L., Kelly, J.D., Madden, K., Maurer, M.F., Parrish-Novak, J., Prunkard, D., Sexson, S., Sprecher, C., Waggie, K., West, J., Whitmore, T.E., Yao, L., Kuechle, M.K., Dale, B.A., and Chandrasekher, Y.A. 2001. Interleukin 20: discovery, receptor identification, and role in epidermal function. *Cell* 104:9–19.

Boone, C., Mourot, J., Gregoire, F., and Remacle, C. 2000. The adipose conversion process: regulation by extracellular and intracellular factors. *Reproduction, Nutrition et Developpement* 40:325–58.

Booth, C., Evans, G.S., and Potten, C.S. 1995. Growth factor regulation of proliferation in primary cultures of small intestinal epithelium. *In Vitro Cell and Developmental Biology* 31:234–243.

Burt, D.W., Boswell, J.M., Paton, I.R., and Butterwith, S.C. 1992 Multiple growth factor mRNAs are expressed by chicken adipocyte precursor cells. *Biochemical Biophysical Research Commununication* 187:1298–1305.

Butterwith, S.C., and Gilroy, M. 1991. Effects of transforming growth factor b1 and basic fibroblast growth factor on lipoprotein lipase activity in primary cultures of chicken (Gallus domesticus) adipocyte precursors. *Comparative Biochemistry and Physiology* 100A:473–476.

Butterwith, S.C., and Goddard, C. 1991. Regulation of DNA synthesis of chicken adipocyte precursor cells by insulin-like growth factors, platelet-derived growth factor and transforming growth factor-b. *Journal of Endocrinology* 130: 203–209.

Butterwith, S.C., Peddie, C.D., and Goddard, C. 1992. Effects of transforming growth factor-b on chicken adipocyte precursor cells in vitro. *Journal of Endocrinology* 134:163–168.

Butterwith, S.C., Peddie, C.D., and Goddard, C. 1993. Regulation of adipocyte precursor DNA synthesis by acid and basic fibroblast growth factors: Interaction with heparin and other growth factors. *Journal of Endocrinology* 137:369–374.

Casas, E., Keele, J.W., Fahrenkrug, S.C., Smith, T.P.L., Cundiff, L.V., and Stone, R.T. 1999. Quantitative analysis of birth, weaning and yearling weights and calving ease in Piedmontese crossbreds segregating an inactive myostatin allele. *Journal of Animal Science* 77:1686–1692.

Chelly, N., Henrion, A., Pinteur, C., Chailley-Heu, B., and Bourbon, J.R. 2001. Role of keratinocyte growth factor in the control of surfactant synthesis by fetal lung mesenchyme. *Endocrinology* 142:1814–1819.

Clark, D.E., Smith, S.K., Sharkey, A.M., Sowter, H.M., and Charnock-Jones, D.S. 1996. Hepatocyte growth factor/scatter factor and its receptor c-met: localisation and expression in the human placenta throughout pregnancy. *Journal of Endocrinology* 151:459–467.

Clase, K.L., Mitchell, P.J., Ward, P.J., Dorman, C.M., Johnson, S.E., and Hannon, K. 2000. FGF5 stimulates expansion of connective tissue fibroblasts and inhibits skeletal muscle development in the limb. *Developmental Dynamics* 219:368–380.

Coffey, R.J., Derynck, R., Wilcox, J.N., Bringman, T.S., Goustin, A.S., Moses, H.L., and Pittelkow, M.R. 1987. Production and auto-induction of transforming growth factor-a in human keratinocytes. *Nature* 328:817–820.

Cohen, S. 1960. Purification of a nerve growth promoting protein from the mouse salivary gland and its neurocytotoxic antiserum. *Proceedings of the National Academy of Sciences of the USA* 46:302–311.

Cohen, S. 1962. Isolation of a mouse submaxillary gland protein accelerating incisor eruption and eyelid opening in the new-born animal. *Journal of Biological Chemistry* 237:1555–1562.

Cohen, S., and Elliott, G.A. 1963. The stimulation of epidermal keratinization by a protein isolated from the submaxillary gland of the mouse. *Journal of Investigation of Dermatology* 40:1.

Coles, B.A., Croom, W.J., Brake, J., Daniel, L.R., Christensen, V.L., Phelps, C.P., Gore, A., and Taylor, I.L. 1999. In Ovo peptide YY administration improves growth and feed conversion ratios in week-old broiler chicks. *Poultry Science* 78:1320–1322.

Coucouvanis, E., and Martin, G.R. 1999. BMP signalling plays a role in visceral endoderm differentiation and cavitation in the early mouse embryo. *Development* 126:535–546.

Cowin, A.J., and Bidey, S.P. 1995. Porcine thyroid follicular cells in monolayer culture activate the iodide-responsive precursor form of transforming growth factor-β1. *Journal of Endocrinology* 144:67–73.

Cowin, A.J., Heaton, E.L., Cheshire, S.H., and Bidey, S.P. 1996. The proliferative responses of porcine thyroid follicular cells to epidermal growth factor and thyrotrophin reflect the autocrine production of transforming growth factor-β1. *Journal of Endocrinology* 148:87–94.

Croom, W.J., McBride, B., Bird, A.R., Fan, Y.-K., Odle, J., Froetschel, M., and Taylor, I.L. 1998. Regulation of intestinal glucose absorption: A new issue in animal science. *Canadian Journal of Animal Science* 78:1–13.

Crossley, P.H., Martinez, S., and Martin, G.R. 1996. Midbrain development induced by FGF8 in the chick embryo. *Nature* 380:66–68.

Crowe, M.A., Enright, W.J., Swift, P., and Roche, J.F. 1995. Growth and estrous behavior of heifers actively immunized against prostaglandin $F_{2\alpha}$. *Journal of Animal Science* 73:345–352.

DeFrances, M.C., Wolf, H.K., Michalopoulos, G.K., and Zarnegar, R. 1992. The presence of hepatocyte growth factor in the developing rat. *Development* 116:387–395.

Dembinski, A.B., and Johnson, L.R. 1985. Effect of epidermal growth factor on the development of rat gastric mucosa. *Endocrinology* 116:90–94.

Dorman, C.M., and Johnson, S.E. 1999. Activated Raf inhibits avian myogenesis through a MAPK-dependent mechanism. *Oncogene* 18:5167–5176.

Doumit, M.E., Cook, D.R., and Merkel, R.A. 1993. Fibroblast growth factor, epidermal growth factor, insulin-like growth factors, and platelet-derived growth factor-B

stimulate proliferation of clonally derived porcine myogenic satellite cells. *Journal of Cell Physiology*
157:326–32.

Doumit, M.E., and Merkel, R.A. 1992. Isolation and culture
of porcine myogenic satellite cells. *Tissue and Cell*
24:253–262.

Etches, R.J., Clark, M.E., Zajchowski, L., Speksnijder, G.,
Verrinder Gibbins, A.M., Kino, K., Pain, B., and Samarut,
J. 1997. Manipulation of blastodermal cells. *Poultry
Science* 76:1075–1083.

Fahrenkrug, S.C., Casas, E., Keele, J.W., and Smith, T.P.L.
1999. Direct genotyping of the double-muscling locus
(mh) in Piedmontese and Belgian Blue Cattle by fluorescent PCR. *Journal of Animal Science* 77:2028–2030.

Farquharson, C., Rennie, J.S., Loveridge, N., and
Whitehead, C.C. 1996. In vivo and in vitro effect of 1,25-
dihydroxyvitamin D3 and 1,25-dihydroxy-16-ene-23-yne-
vitamin D3 on the proliferation and differentiation of
avian chondrocytes: their role in tibial dyschondroplasia.
Journal of Endocrinology 148:465–474.

Fata, J.E., Kong, Y.-Y., Li, J., Sasaki, T., Irie-Sasaki, J.,
Moorehead, R.A., Elliott, R., Scully, S., Voura, E.B.,
Lacey, D.L., Boyle, W.J., Khokha, R., and Penninger,
J.M. 2000. The osteoclast differentiation factor osteopro-
tegerin-ligand is essential for mammary gland develop-
ment. *Cell* 103:41–50.

Ferrara, N., and Davis-Smyth, T. 1997. The biology of vascular endothelial growth factor. *Endocrine Reviews*
18:9–25.

Fraser, H.M., and Lunn, S.F. 2001. Regulation and manipulation of angiogenesis in the primate corpus luteum.
Reproduction 121:355–362.

Gerstenfeld, L.C., Kelly, C.M., Von Deck, M., and Lian, J.B.
1990. Effect of 1,25-hydroxyvitamin D3 on induction of
chondrocyte maturation in culture: extracellular matrix
gene expression and morphology. *Endocrinology*
126:1599–1609.

Graham, A., Francis-West, P., Brickell, P., and Lumsden, A.
1994. The signalling molecule BMP 4 mediates apoptosis
in the rhombencephalic neural crest. *Nature* 372:684–686.

Grant, D.S., Kleinman, H.K., Goldberg, I.D., Bhargava,
M.M., Nickoloff, B.J., Kinsella, J.L., Polverini, P., and
Rosen, E.M. 1993. Scatter factor induces blood vessel
formation in vivo. *Proceedings of the National Academy
of Sciences of the USA* 90:1937–1941.

Grobet, L., Poncelet, D., Royo, L. J., Brouwers, B., Pirottin,
D., Michaux, C., Ménissier, F., Zanotti, M., Dunner, S.,
and Georges, M. 1998. Molecular definition of an allelic
series of mutations disrupting the myostatin function and
causing double-muscling in cattle. *Mammalian Genome*
9:210–213.

Gruppuso, P.A., Boylan, J.M., Bienieki, T.C., and Curran,
T.R. 1994. Evidence for a direct hepatotrophic role for
insulin in the fetal rat: implications for the impaired
hepatic growth seen in fetal growth retardation.
Endocrinology. 134: 769–775.

Hathaway, M.R., Pampusch, M.S., Hembree, J.R., and
Dayton W.R. 1994. Transforming growth factor beta-1
facilitates establishing clonal populations of ovine muscle
satellite cells. *Journal of Animal Science* 72:2001–2007.

Hembree, J.R., Pampusch, M.S., Yang, F., Causey, J.L.,
Hathaway, M.R., and Dayton, W.R. 1996. Cultured
porcine myogenic cells produce insulin-like growth factor
binding protein-3 (IGFBP-3) and transforming growth
factor beta-1 stimulates IGFBP-3 production. *Journal of
Animal Science* 74:1530–1540.

Hentges, S., Pastorcic, M., De, A., Boyadjieva, N., and
Sarkar, D.K. 2000. Opposing actions of two transforming
growth factor-β isoforms on pituitary lactotropic cell proliferation. *Endocrinology* 141:1528–1535.

Hogan, B.L.M. 1999. Morphogenesis. *Cell* 96:225–233.

Hsu, H., Lacey, D.L., Dunstan, C.R., Solovyev, I.,
Colombero, A., Timms, E., Tan, H.L., Elliott, G., Kelley,
M.J., Sarosi, I., Wang, L., Xia, X.-Z., Elliott, R., Chiu, L.,
Black, T., Scully, S., Capperelli, C., Morony, S.,
Shimamoto, G., Bass, M.B., and Boyle, W.J. 1999. Tumor
necrosis factor receptor family member RANK mediates
osteoclast differentiation and activation induced by osteoprotegerin ligand. *Proceedings of the National Academy
of Science, USA* 96:3540–3545.

Johnson, R.W. 1997. Inhibition of growth by pro-inflamma-
tory cytokines: an integrated view. *Journal of Animal
Science* 75: 1244–1255.

Johnson, S.E., and Allen, R.E. 1995. Activation of skeletal
muscle satellite cells and the role of fibroblast growth factor receptors. *Experimental Cell Research* 219:449–453.

Jones, J.T., Akita, R.W., and Sliwkowski, M.X. 1999.
Binding specificities and affinities of egf domains for
ErbB receptors. *FEBS Letters* 447:227–231.

Ka, H., Jaeger, L.A., Johnson, G.A., Spencer, T.E., and
Bazer, F.W. 2001. Keratinocyte growth factor is up-regulated by estrogen in the porcine uterine endometrium and
functions in trophectoderm cell proliferation and differentiation. *Endocrinology* 142:2303–2310.

Kambadur, R., Sharma, M., Smith, T.P.L., and Bass, J.J. 1997.
Mutations in myostatin (GDF8) in double-muscled Belgian
Blue and Piedmontese cattle. *Genome Research* 7:910–915.

Karavanova, I.D., Dove, L.F., Resau, J.H., and Perantoni,
A.O. 1996. Conditioned medium from a rat ureteric bud
cell line in combination with bFGF induces complete differentiation of isolated metanephric mesenchyme.
Development 122:4159–4167.

Kawakami, Y., Ishikawa, T., Shimabura, M., Tanda, N.,
Enomoto-Iwamoto, M., Iwamoto, M., Kawana, T., Ueki,
A., Noji, S., and Nohno, T. 1996. BMP signalling during
bone pattern determination in the developing limb.
Development 122:3557–3566.

Klonisch, T., Wolf, P., Hombach-Klonisch, S., Vogt, S.,
Kuechenhoff, A., Tetens, F., and Fischer, B. 2001.
Epidermal growth factor-like ligands and erbB genes in
the peri-implantation rabbit uterus and blastocyst. *Biology
of Reproduction* 64:1835–1844.

Knight, P.G., and Glister, C. 2001. Potential local regulatory
functions of inhibins, activins and follistatin in the ovary.
Reproduction 121:503–512.

Kobrin, M.S., Asa, S.L., Samsoondar, J., and Kudlow, J.E.
1987. α-Transforming growth factor in the bovine anteri-
or pituitary gland: Secretion by dispersed cells and
immunohistochemical localization. *Endocrinology*
121:1412–1416.

Koff, M.D., and Plaut, K. (1995) Expression of transforming growth factor-α like transcripts by bovine mammary gland. *Journal of Dairy Science* 78:1903–1908.

Kong, Y.Y., Yoshida, H., Sarosi, I., Tan, H.L., Timms, E., Capparelli, C., Morony, S., Oliveira-dos-Santos, A.J., Van, G., Itie, A., Khoo, W., Wakeham, A., Dunstan, C.R., Lacy, D.L., Mak, T.W., Boyle, W.J., and Pennington, J.M. 1999. OPGL is a key regulator of osteoclastogenesis, lymphocyte development and lymph-node organogenesis. *Nature* 397:315–323.

Lacey, D.L., Timms, E., Tan, H.L., Kelley, M.J., Dunstan, C.R., Burgess, T., Elliott, R., Colombero, A., Elliott, G., Scully, S., Hsu, H., Sullivan, J., Hawkins, N., Davy, E., Capparelli, C., Eli, A., Qian, Y.X., Kaufman, S., Sarosi, I., Shalhoub, V., Senaldi, G., Gou, J., Delaney, J., and Boyle, W.J. 1998. Osteoprotegerin ligand is a cytokine that regulates osteoclast differentiation and activation. *Cell* 93:165–176.

Lawrence, D.A., Pircher, R., and Jullien, P. 1985. Conversion of a high molecular weight latent β TGF from chicken embryo fibroblasts into a low molecular weight active β-TGF under acidic conditions. *Biochemical and Biophysical Research Communications* 133:1026–1034.

Lee, H.-M., Udupi, V., Englander, E.W., Rajaraman, S., Coffey, R.J., and Greeley, G.H. 1999. Stimulatory actions of insulin-like growth factor-I and transforming growth factor-a on intestinal neurotensin and peptide YY. *Endocrinology* 140:4065–4069.

Le Roy, C., Li, J.Y., Stocco, D.M., Langlois, D., and Saez, J.M. 2000. Regulation by adrenocorticotropin (ACTH), angiotensin II, transforming growth factor-β, and insulin-like growth factor I of bovine adrenal cell steroidogenic capacity and expression of ACTH receptor, steroidogenic acute regulatory protein, cytochrome P450c17, and 3b-hydroxysteroid dehydrogenase. *Endocrinology* 141:1599–1607.

Li, J., Sarosi, I., Yan, X.Q., Morony, S., Capparelli, C., Tan, H.L., McCabe, S., Elliott, R., Scully, S., Van, G., Kaufman, S., Juan, S.-C., Sun, Y., Tarpley, J., Martin, L., Christensen, K., McCabe, J., Kostenuik, P., Hsu, H., Fletcher, F., Dunstan, C.R., Lacey, D.L., and Boyle, W.J. 2000. RANK is the intrinsic hematopoietic cell surface receptor that controls osteoclastogenesis and regulation of bone mass and calcium metabolism. *Proceedings of National Academy of Science, USA* 97:1566–1571.

Lindahl, P., Hellstrom, M., Kalen, M., Karlsson, L., Pekny, M., Lekna, M., Soriano, P., and Betsholtz, C. 1998. Paracrine PDGF-B/PDGF-Rβ signaling controls mesangial cell development in kidney glomeruli. *Development* 125:3313–3322.

Ling, J., Kincaid, S.A., McDaniel, G.R., and Waegell, W. 2000. Immunolocalization analysis of transforming growth factor-b1 in the growth plates of broiler chickens with high and low incidences of tibial dyschondroplasia. *Poultry Science* 79:1172–1178.

Locksley, R.M., Killeen, N., and Lenardo, M.J. 2001. The TNF and TNF receptor superfamilies: integrating mammalian biology. *Cell* 104:487–501.

Logan, A., Black, E.G., Gonzalez, A.-M., Buscaglia, M., and Sheppard, M.C. 1992. Basic fibroblast growth factor: an autocrine mitogen of rat thyroid follicular cells? *Endocrinology* 130:2363–2372.

Lumelsky, N., Blondel, O., Laeng, P., Velasco, I., Ravin, R., and McKay, R. 2001. Differentiation of embryonic stem cells to insulin-secreting structures similar to pancreatic islets. *Science* 292:1389–1394.

Mangelsdorf, D.J., and Evans, R.M. 1995. The RXR heterodimers and orphan receptors. *Cell* 83:841–850.

March, C.J., Mosley, B., Larsen, A., Ceretti, D.P., Braedt, G., Price, V., Gillis, S., Henney, C.S., Kronheim, S.R., Grabstein, H., Conlon, P.J., Hopp, T.P., and Cosman, D. 1985. Cloning, sequence and expression of two distinct human interleukin-1 complementary DNAs. *Nature* 315:641–647.

Massagué, J., Blain, S.W., and Lo, R.S. 2000. TGFβ signaling in growth control, cancer, and heritable disorders. *Cell* 103: 295–309.

McGrath, M.F., Collier, R.J., Clemmons, D.R., Busby, W.H., Sweeney, C.A., and Krivi, G.G. 1991. The direct in vitro effect of insulin-like growth factors (IGFs) on normal bovine mammary cell proliferation and production of IGF binding proteins. *Endocrinology* 129:671–678.

McPherron, A.C., Lawler, A.M., and Lee, S.-J. 1997. Regulation of skeletal muscle mass in mice by a new TGF-β superfamily member. *Nature* 387:83–90.

McPherron, A.C., and Lee, S.-J. 1997. Double muscling in cattle due to mutations in the myostatin gene. *Proceedings of the National Academy of Science, USA* 94:12457–12461.

Monsoro-Burg, A.-H., Duprez, D., Watanabe, Y., Bontoux, M., Vincent, C., Brickell, P., and LeDouarin, N. 1996. The role of bone morphogenetic proteins in vertebrate development. *Development* 122:3607–3616.

Moorby, C.D., Taylor, J.A., and Forsyth, I.A. 1995. Transforming growth factor-alpha: receptor binding and action on DNA synthesis in the sheep mammary gland. *Journal of Endocrinology* 144:165–171.

Morris, J.C., Ranganathan, G., Hay, I.D., Nelson, R.E., and Jiang, N.-S. 1988. The effects of transforming growth factor-b on growth and differentiation of the continuous rat thyroid follicular cell line, FTRL-5. *Endocrinology* 123:1385–1394.

Murphy, M., Reid, K., Ford, M., Furness, J.B., and Bartlett, P.F. 1994. FGF-2 regulates proliferation of neural crest cells, with subsequent neuronal differentiation regulated by LIF or related factors. *Development* 120:3519–3528.

Nakamura, T., Nishizawa, T., Hagiya, M., Seki, T., Shimonishi, M., Sugimura, A., Tashiro, K., and Shimizu, S. 1989. Molecular cloning and expression of human hepatocyte growth factor. *Nature* 342:440–443.

Naldini, L., Vigna, E., Narsimhan, R.P., Gaudino, G., Zarnegar, R., Michalopoulos, G.K., and Comoglio, P.M. 1991b. Hepatocyte growth factor (HGF) stimulates the tyrosine kinase activity of the receptor encoded by the proto-oncogene c-MET. *Oncogene* 6:501–504.

Naldini, L., Weidner, K.M., Vigna, E., Gaudino, G., Bardelli, A., Ponzetto, C., Narsimhan, R.P., Hartmann, G., Zarnegar, R., Michalopoulos, G.K., Birchmeier, W., and Comoglio, P.M. 1991a. Scatter factor and hepatocyte growth factor are indistinguishable ligands for the c-met receptor. *EMBO Journal* 10:2867–2878.

Oka, Y., Ghishan, F.K., Greene, H.L., and Orth, D.N. 1983. Effect of mouse epidermal growth factor/urogastrone on the functional maturation of rat intestine. *Endocrinology* 112:940–944.

O'Keefe, R.J., Puzas, J.E., Brand, J.S., and Rosier, R.N. 1988. Effect of transforming growth-factor-b on DNA synthesis by growth plate chondrocytes: Modulation by factors present in serum. *Calcified Tissue International* 43:352–358.

Ornitz, D.M., Xu, J., Colvin, J.S., McEwen, D.G., MacArthur, C.A., Coulier, F., Gao, G., and Goldfarb, M. 1996. Receptor specificity of the fibroblast growth factor family. *Journal of Biological Chemistry* 271:15292–15297.

Plotnikov, A.N., Schlessinger, J., Hubbard, S.R., and Mohammadi, M. 1999. Structural basis for FGF receptor dimerization and activation. *Cell* 98:641–650.

Qiao, J., Uzzo, R., Obara-Ishihara, T., Degenstein, L., Fuchs, E., and Doris, H. 1999. FGF-7 modulates ureteric bud growth and nephron number in the developing kidney. *Development* 126:547–554.

Rasmussen, Å.K., Kayser, L., Bech, K., Feldt-Rasmussen, U., Perrild, H., and Bendtzen, K. 1990. Differential effects of interleukin 1α and 1β on cultured human and rat thyroid epithelial cells. *Acta Endocrinologica* 122:520–526.

Reynolds, L.P., and Redmer, D.A. 1998. Expression of the angiogenic factors, basic fibroblast growth factor and vascular endothelial growth factor, in the ovary. *Journal of Animal Science* 76:1671–1681.

Richardson, R.L., Campion, D.R., Hausman, G.J., and Wright, J.T. 1989. Transforming growth factor type β (TGF-β) and adipogenesis in pigs. *Journal of Animal Science* 67:2171–2180.

Sakuta, H., Suzuki, R., Takahashi, H., Kato, A., Shintani, T., Iemura, S.-I., Yamamoto, T.S., Ueno, N., and Noda, M. 2001. Ventroptin: A BMP-4 antagonist expressed in a double-gradient pattern in the retina. *Science* 293:111–115.

Scheving, L.A., Yeh, Y.C., Tsai, T.H., and Scheving, L.E. 1979. Circadian phase-dependent stimulatory effects of epidermal growth factor on deoxyribonucleic acid synthesis in the tongue, esophagus, and stomach of the adult male mouse. *Endocrinology* 105:1475–1480.

Scheving, L.A., Yeh, Y.C., Tsai, T.H., and Scheving, L.E. 1980. Circadian phase-dependent stimulatory effects of epidermal growth factor on deoxyribonucleic acid synthesis in the duodenum, jejunum, ileum, caecum, colon, and rectum of the adult male mouse. *Endocrinology* 106:1498–1503.

Schmidt, C., Bladt, F., Goedecke, S., Brinkmann, V., Zschiesche, W., Sharpe, M., Gherardi, E., and Birchmeier, C. 1995. Scatter factor/hepatocyte growth factor is essential for liver development. *Nature* 373:699–702.

Shea-Eaton, W.K., Lee, P.-P.H., and Ip, M.M. 2001. Regulation of milk protein gene expression in normal mammary epithelial cells by tumor necrosis factor. *Endocrinology* 142:2558–2568.

Smallwood, P.M., Munoz-Sanjuan, I., Tong, P., Macke, J.P., Hendry, S.H.C., Gilbert, D.J., Copeland, N.G., Jenkins, N.A., and Nathans, J. 1996. Fibroblast growth factor (FGF) homologous factors: new members of the FGF

family implicated in nervous system development. *Proceedings of the National Academy of Sciences of the USA* 93:9850–9857.

Stepien, H., Zerek-Meten, G., Mucha, S., Winczyk, K., and Fryczak, J. 1994. Interleukin-1 beta stimulates cell proliferation in the intermediate lobe of the rat pituitary gland. *Journal of Endocrinology* 140:337–341.

Suryawan, A., and Hu, C.Y. 1997. Effect of retinoic acid on differentiation of cultured pig preadipocytes. *Journal of Animal Science* 75:112–117.

Suzuki, N., Labosky, P.A., Furuhide, Y., Hargett, L., Dunn, R., Fogo, A.B., Takahara, K., Peters, D.M.P., Greenspan, D.S., and Hogan, B.L.M. 1996. Failure of ventral body wall closure in mouse embryos lacking a procollagen C-proteinase encoded by Bmp 1, a mammalian gene related to Drosophila tolloid. *Development* 122:3587–3595.

Thompson, J.S., Bixler, S.A., Qian, F., Vora, K., Scott, M.L., Cachero, T.G., Hession, C., Schneider, P., Sizing, I.D., Mullen, C., Struch, K., Zafari, M., Benjamin, C.D., Tschopp, J., Browning, J.J., and Ambrose, C. 2001. BAFF-R, a newly identified TNF receptor that specifically interacts with BAFF. *Science* 293:2108–2111.

Tsushima, T., Arai, M., Saji, M., Ohba, Y., Murakami, H., Ohmura, E., Sato, K., and Shizume, K. 1988. Effects of transforming growth factor-β on deoxyribonucleic acid synthesis and iodine metabolism in porcine thyroid cells in culture. *Endocrinology* 123:1187–1194.

Umbhauer, M., Penzo-Mendez, A., Clavilier, L., Boucaut, J., and Riou, J. 2000. Signaling specificities of fibroblast growth factor receptors in early Xenopus embryo. *Journal of Cell Science* 113:2865–2875.

Vasiliauskas, D., and Stern, C.D. 2001. Patterning of the embryonic axis: FGF signaling and how vertebrate embryos measure time. *Cell* 106:133–136.

Vieira, A.V., Schneider, W.J., and Vieira, P.M. 1995. Retinoids: transport, metabolism, and mechanisms of action. *Journal of Endocrinology* 146:201–207.

Vinter-Jensen, L., Orloff Juhl, C., Frystyk, J., Dajani, E.Z., Oksbjerg, N., and Flyvbjerg, A. 1996. The effect of epidermal growth factor on circulating levels of IGF and IGF-binding proteins in adult Goettingen minipigs. *Journal of Endocrinology* 151:401–407.

Weidner, K.M., Arakaki, N., Hartmann, G., Vande Kercklove, J., Weingart, S., Rieder, H., Fanatsch, C., Tsubouchi, H., Hishida, T., Daikuhara, Y., and Birchmeier, W. 1991. Evidence for the identity of human scatter factor and human hepatocyte growth factor. *Proceedings of the National Academy of Sciences of the USA* 88:7001–7005.

Westermark, K., and Westermark, B. 1982. Mitogenic effect of epidermal growth factor on sheep thyroid cells in culture. *Experimental Cell Research* 138:47–55.

Wong, B.R., Rho, J. Arron, J., Robinson, E., Orlinick, J., Chao, M., Kalachikov, S., Cayani, E., Bartlett, F.S., Frankel, W.N., Lee, S.Y., and Choi, Y. 1997. TRANCE is a novel ligand of the tumor necrosis factor receptor family that activates c-Jun N-terminal kinase in T cells. *Journal of Biological Chemistry* 272:25190–25194.

Yasuda, H., Shima, N., Nakagawa, N., Yamaguchi, K., Kinosaki, M., Mochizuki, S., Tomoyasu, A., Yano, K.,

Goto, M., Murakami, A., Tsuda, E., Morinaga, T., Higashio, K., Udagawa, N., Takahashi, N., and Suda, T. 1998. Osteoclast differentiation factor is a ligand for osteoprotegerin/osteoclastogenesis-inhibitory factor and is identical to TRANCE/RANKL. *Proceedings of National Academy of Science, USA* 95:3597–3602.

Ying, S. 1988. Inhibins, activins and follistatins: gonadal proteins modulating the secretion of follicle-stimulating hormone. *Endocrine Reviews* 9:267–293.

Yokouchi, Y., Sakiyama, J., Kameda, T., Iba, H., Suzuki, A., Ueno, N., and Kuroiwa, A. 1996. BMP-2/-4 mediate programmed cell death in chicken limb buds. *Development* 122: 3725–3734.

Yuasa, R., Eggo, M.C., Meinkoth, J., Dillmann, W.H., and Burrow, G.N. 1992. Iodide induces transforming growth factor beta-1 (TGF-β1) mRNA in sheep thyroid cells. *Thyroid* 2:141–145.

Yue, X., and Tomanek, R.J. 2001. Effects of VEGF(165) and VEGF(121) on vasculogenesis and angiogenesis in cultured embryonic quail hearts. *American Journal of Physiology* 280:H2240–2247.

Zou, H., and Niswander, L. 1996. Requirement for BMP signalling in interdigital apoptosis and scale development. *Science* 272:738–741.

7

Extracellular Matrix and Growth

Sandra G. Velleman

HISTORICAL PERSPECTIVE OF THE EXTRACELLULAR MATRIX

The extracellular matrix is defined to include all secreted molecules that are immobilized outside cells. The major macromolecular components of the extracellular matrix include collagens, proteoglycans, and noncollagenous glycoproteins. Until the recent advent of molecular biology, the extracellular matrix was viewed as a passive ground substance in that the cells were merely embedded and upon extraction formed a gluelike substance. This view of the extracellular matrix largely stems from the physical methods used to extract the extracellular matrix and the cell theory in which the cells were deemed to be the fundamental component necessary for sustaining life.

During the past 20 years, the complexity and diversity of the extracellular matrix has been elucidated. Figure 7.1 illustrates a general schematic of a cellular environment being surrounding by an extracellular matrix containing collagen fibrils that are

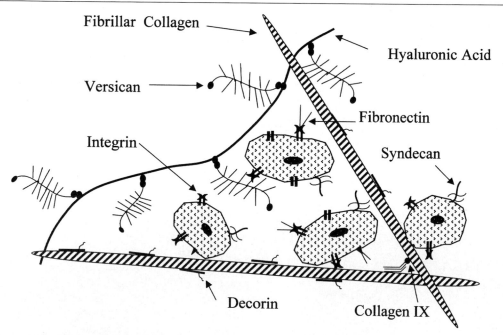

Figure 7.1. Generalized schematic of an extracellular matrix surrounding cells.

linked together by fibril-associated collagens (e.g., collagen type IX). Two different functional classes of proteoglycans are illustrated in Figure 7.1. The aggregating class of proteoglycans, of which versican is a member, binds to hyaluronic acid and is involved in water-holding capacity by ionically interacting with water. Nonaggregating proteoglycans, such as decorin or syndecan, interacts with other extracellular matrix macromolecules or directly with the cells. The extracellular matrix functions by largely communicating information back to the cells through cellular transmembrane receptors called integrins. Frequently, fibronectin in the extracellular matrix will bind to the integrin receptor. This communication or signaling between the extracellular matrix and cell results in the modulation of cellular characteristics critical in tissue development and function, including—but not limited to—cell migration, cell death or survival, and growth factor responsiveness. In contrast to earlier views of the extracellular matrix not being an important functional component in tissue formation and function, it is now thought to play a pivotal role.

The complexity of the extracellular matrix is further augmented by its diverse composition. Different tissues have unique extracellular matrices that change as an animal ages. With the advent of molecular biology, the number of detected extracellular matrix macromolecules has dramatically increased. For example, it wasn't until the late 1960s that the presence of more than one type of collagen was identified. Until 1971, only the fibrillar collagens type I, II, and III were known. Currently, there are at least 19 different collagens, which are the products of unique genes. It is not unreasonable to expect, as we proceed further into the 21st century, that the functions and diversity of the extracellular matrix will continue to grow.

This chapter gives an overview of several of the key macromolecular components of the extracellular matrix. Emphasis is then placed on extracellular matrix proteoglycans due to their emerging roles in tissue formation and growth factor regulation.

MACROMOLECULAR COMPONENTS OF THE EXTRACELLULAR MATRIX

Collagens

Extracellular matrix collagens form an extracellular supramolecular scaffold necessary for mechanical support and to provide the architecture necessary for cell migration, adhesion, and differentiation.

Collagens are characterized by a triple helical domain containing the amino acid repeat glycine-X-Y, where X and Y can be any amino acid but are frequently proline or lysine. There are at least 19 different vertebrate collagens (types I through XIX) with tissue-specific distributions and unique functional properties. These unique collagen types can be subdivided into the following classes based on function or size: fibrillar, fibril-associated, network forming, filamentous, short chain, and long chain collagens (for review, see van der Rest and Garrone 1991).

The fibrillar collagens include types I, II, III, V, and XI. These collagens exhibit a tissue-specific distribution. For example, cartilage contains type II collagen, whereas bone is composed of type I collagen. These collagens contain a single triple-helical domain consisting of three α polypeptide chains with over 300 repeats of glycine-X-Y. Many of the proline and lysine residues are posttranslationally hydroxylated. The hydroxylation of proline and lysine residues results in the formation of a stable triple helical structure at 37° C. After the collagen triple helices are secreted from the cell into the extracellular space, they align into a quarter-stagger array forming collagen fibrils, which are necessary for the structure of the extracellular matrix, and through interactions with the cell and other matrix macromolecules influence cell migration and differentiation during embryonic tissue formation. The collagen fibrils are stabilized by the formation of crosslinks between the collagen fibrils. When collagen crosslinking is initiated between individual fibrils, larger diameter fibrils will form. Crosslinking between and among collagen molecules is a major element in modulating the tensile strength of the collagen fibril network.

The fibril-associated collagens or FACIT collagens contain collagen triple helical domains interrupted by non-triple helical regions. These collagens are thought to link fibrillar collagens to other extracellular matrix macromolecules. Type IX collagen is the most widely studied of the FACIT collagens. It was originally thought to be specific to cartilage, but through alternative splicing a smaller form has been identified in the corneal stroma (Svoboda et al. 1988; Nishimura et al. 1989). During cornea formation in the eye, the primary corneal stroma swells permitting mesenchymal cell migration. Type IX collagen is detected just prior to the swelling of the stroma (Fitch et al. 1988) and may function in maintaining the extracellular matrix in a compact state (Linsenmeyer 1991).

Type X collagen is a short chain collagen found only in hypertrophic cartilage. During the formation of bone, there is a transition from a cartilage to a bone extracellular matrix. The cartilage extracellular matrix is mainly composed of type II collagen, which resists swelling that results in increased collagen fiber tension and enables the cartilage to support load-bearing stress. Bone requires a mineralized rigid matrix that is able to support weight. During the transition from a cartilage to a bone matrix, the chondrocytes in the central portion of the developing bone enlarge and produce a unique noncartilaginous extracellular matrix. The cells are now termed hypertrophic chondrocytes and secrete a matrix containing type X collagen (Schmid and Linsenmeyer 1985). Type X collagen is critical in the process of mineralization (Schmid and Linsenmeyer, 1987).

Tibial dyschondroplasia (TD) is a skeletal disease common to rapidly growing commercial poultry stocks. The disease is caused by the formation of an avascular cartilaginous lesion extending from the epiphyseal growth plate into the bone metaphysis (Leach and Nesheim 1965). Birds with TD are prone to fractures at the processing plant. In birds with TD, type X collagen is not secreted into the extracellular matrix space and remains intracellular. Thus, type X collagen does not interact with the existing extracellular matrix architecture, which may result in an extracellular matrix that does not have the appropriate organization to permit vascularization necessary for bone formation.

Fibronectin

Fibronectin is a multifunctional extracellular matrix macromolecule secreted as a dimer held together by disulfide bonds at the C-terminus of the molecule. Each subunit of fibronectin has a molecular weight in the range of 235,000–270,000 daltons. The fibronectin molecule contains distinct binding sites for heparin, fibrin, collagen, and cells. The cellular binding domain is characterized by the amino acid sequence arginine-glycine-aspartate (RGD), which is the target sequence for integrin binding. This cell-matrix interaction between fibronectin and integrins permits cell substrate adhesion and migration.

Fibronectin exists in multiple forms due to alternative splicing of the fibronectin mRNA (for review, see Ffrench-Constant 1995). Fibronectin is composed of three types of homologous repeating modules: types I, II, and III. The modules form domains with distinctive functions. The type I modules bind to heparin, fibrin, and collagen. Type II modules are found in the collagen binding domain. There are two cell binding domains, with one in the type III module and the other in the type III connecting segment. Alternative splicing can occur at the EIIIA and EIIIB sites in the type III module and at the type III connecting segment. The process of alternative splicing can result in either nucleotide insertions or deletions resulting in a large number of fibronectin variants in the cell binding domains. Different cell types will synthesize different forms of fibronectin, and different fibronectin variants are thought to be produced at specific developmental periods. Although little is known about the developmental regulation of fibronectin alternative splice forms, it is likely that the different variants play instructive roles in modulating cell adhesion to the extracellular matrix and cell migration to a specific target.

Proteoglycans

Extracellular matrix proteoglycans are proteins that contain carbohydrates called glycosaminoglycans, which are covalently attached to a central core protein. Based on this definition, the proteoglycans are a diverse family of macromolecules that exhibit both developmental and tissue specificity in terms of their expression. Unlike the collagens with a unique triple helical domain, there is no common structural feature associated with proteoglycans. The proteoglycan central core protein varies greatly in size from approximately 40,000 to greater than 350,000 daltons (Iozzo and Murdoch 1996). The glycosaminoglycans are polymers of disaccharide repeats that are highly sulfated and are, therefore, negative in charge. The negative charge permits ionic interactions with molecules such as water. Typical glycosaminoglycans attached to the proteoglycan central core protein include chondroitin/dermatan sulfate, heparan sulfate, and keratan sulfate. Chondroitin sulfate is composed of repeats of glucuronic acid and N-acetylglucosamine with sulfate groups in the 4- or 6-position of the amino sugar. Heparan sulfate consists of repeats of glucuronic acid and N-acetylglucosamine. Keratan sulfate contains disaccharide repeats of galactose and N-acetylglucosamine with the sulfate at the 6-position of the amino sugar. Hyaluronic acid is an unsulfated glycosaminoglycan of glucuronic acid and N-acetylglucosamine that ionically interacts with only certain proteoglycan core proteins (for review, see Carrino et al. 1999). Figure 7.2 contains diagrammatic representations of the proteoglycans decorin, syndecan, glypican, and versican.

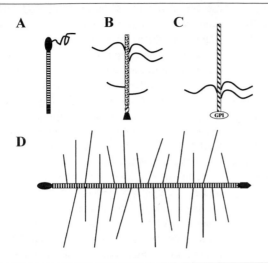

Figure 7.2. Diagrammatic representation of the proteoglycans: (A) decorin, (B) syndecan, (C) glypican, and (D) versican. GPI = glycosylphosphatidylinositol linkage.

Decorin (Figure 7.2A) is a chondroitin/dermatan sulfate proteoglycan that associates with both types I and II collagen (Vogel et al. 1984; Vogel and Trotter 1987; Scott 1988). Decorin has been identified in a number of tissues and localized in the extracellular environment surrounding the cells. Decorin is a multifunctional proteoglycan that has been shown to play roles in collagen fibril organization (Vogel et al. 1984; Vogel and Trotter 1987; Scott 1988), cell proliferation and differentiation (Yamaguchi and Ruoslahti 1988; Santra et al. 1995; Moscatello et al. 1998), growth factor regulation (Yamaguchi et al. 1990), and collagen binding to lipids during the formation of atherosclerotic plaques (Pentikäinen et al. 1997).

The proteoglycans, syndecan (Figure 7.2B) and glypican (Figure 7.2C) are cell surface heparan sulfate containing marcomolecules that are ubiquitous to most tissues. A variety of functions have been ascribed to the heparan sulfate class of cell surface proteoglycans, including playing roles in extracellular matrix organization, and cell adhesion and differentiation. The syndecan family of proteoglycans contains four members, syndecan-1 through -4. The syndecans are transmembrane proteoglycans with an ectodomain containing around three heparan sulfate side chains, but often the heparan sulfate is substituted with another glycosaminoglycan-like chondroitin sulfate, a transmembrane domain, and cytoplasmic domain. Unlike the syndecans, the glypicans are not transmembrane proteoglycans but

are linked to the cell surface by a glycosylphosphatidylinositol link. There are six known glypican family members, glypican-1 through -6. Therefore, the glypicans have an extremely large extracellular domain, which contains just attached heparan sulfate chains.

Versican (Figure 7.2D) is a large extracellular chondroitin sulfate containing proteoglycan with a total molecular weight of greater than 1,000,000 daltons. Versican contains a hyaluronic acid binding domain at the N-terminus of the core protein. Similar to the cartilage aggrecan proteoglycan, versican can form aggregates with hyaluronic acid (for review, see Carrino et al. 1999). The high affinity of versican for hyaluronic acid suggests that this interaction is likely of biological significance. The large number of attached chondroitin sulfate chains gives this proteoglycan a high negative charge density that results in ionic interactions with positively charged molecules like water, which is important in tissue hydration and creating pathways for cell migration.

ROLE OF THE EXTRACELLULAR MATRIX IN TISSUE FORMATION

The formation of tissues requires the migration of cells to the appropriate site and then the attachment of cells to one another. For cells to migrate, they must attach and spread across the extracellular matrix substrate. Therefore, appropriate expression of extracellular matrix marcomolecules and interactions between these molecules is essential for cells to assemble into and maintain a functional tissue.

Cell adhesion to the extracellular matrix is mediated by cell surface receptors called integrins binding to the fibronectin RGD cell attachment domain. The integrins are a widely expressed family of heterodimeric cell surface glycoprotein receptors containing α- and β-subunits that link the extracellular matrix to the cellular cytoskeleton. The α-subunits are homologous to each other and the β-subunits form their own homologous group. The α- and β-subunits contain cytoplasmic, transmembrane, and extracellular domains (for review, see Schwartz 2001). There are numerous isoforms of each integrin subunit with tissue-specific distributions and unique functional properties. In addition to integrins linking the cell to the extracellular matrix, this interaction results in the formation of an association of the external extracellular matrix to the internal cellular cytoskeleton. The interaction of integrins with the extracellular matrix is not a passive mechanical association but activates focal adhesion kinase and growth factor signaling pathways (Ruoslahti 1997) modulating cell proliferation and differentiation. The integrin receptors are not randomly located across the plasma membrane but form focal adhesion clusters regulating cell shape. Chen et al. (1997) showed the binding of integrins to the extracellular matrix substrate caused the cells to extend over a large surface area, whereas rounded cells exhibited a loss of extracellular matrix contact and had reduced survival and proliferation. Figure 7.3 illustrates a cell with an extended morphological shape and attachment to the extracellular matrix substrate. This type of attachment and morphological appearance is thought to promote cell survival and growth. In contrast, rounded cells are likely to exhibit a reduction in survival and induce the process of programmed cell death or apoptosis. Figure 7.4 illustrates a cell with reduced extracellular matrix contact and forming a rounded morphology resulting in apoptosis.

Apoptosis differs from cell death resulting from necrosis. Apoptosis is part of a normal physiological state in which the cell participates in its own death. Apoptotic cells will have membrane blebbing with no loss in integrity, shrinkage of the cytoplasm, condensation of the nucleus, and fragmentation of the cell into smaller membrane bound apoptotic bodies. In contrast, necrotic cells lose membrane integrity, swell, and undergo lysis with disintegration of the cellular organelles. Biochemically, apoptosis is characterized by the degradation of chromatin into fragments of 50–300 Kb (Oberhammer et al. 1993). Apoptosis is induced by the activation of cysteine proteases called caspases. When the caspases are activated, the cell begins to autodigest. Caspase activation is prevented in vertebrates by the expression of mitochondrial protein Bcl-2, which inserts itself into the outer mitochondrial membrane.

Apoptosis is necessary for normal tissue formation to occur and essential for life. During development, apoptosis is necessary for the elimination of transient tissues and tissue remodeling. For example, during vertebrate limb formation, if apoptosis is not activated the digits will remain joined (Saunders and Fallon 1966).

Integrin mediated cell adhesion to the extracellular matrix is requisite for cell migration, tissue formation, and preventing apoptosis. During skeletal muscle formation, myoblasts will migrate, align, and then fuse to form multinucleated myotubes.

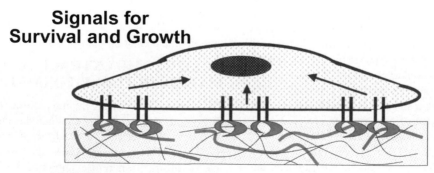

Figure 7.3. Cell with maximal extracellular matrix contact promoting signals for survival and growth.

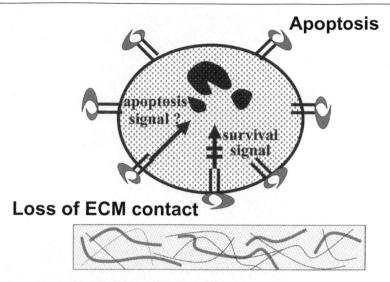

Figure 7.4. Cell with reduced extracellular matrix contact leading to apoptosis.

Cell migration involves a series of complex steps, including cell extension at the leading edge, formation of stable contacts between the cell and extracellular matrix, contraction of the cellular cytoskeleton, translocation of the cell, and release of the cell-extracellular matrix contact at the rear of the cell. Boettiger et al. (1995) have shown by blocking the α5β1 integrin that both cell migration and myotube morphogenesis are inhibited. The α5β1 integrin elevates the expression of Bcl-2 and hence has anti-apoptotic properties (Zhang et al. 1995).

When cell migration is complete, the newly migrated cells begin to interact with one another and reorganize into a functional tissue. Appropriate expression of the extracellular matrix and interaction of extracellular matrix macromolecules with each other plays a pivotal role in the formation and maintenance of tissues. For example, considerable experimental data suggest that a specific functional interaction occurs between decorin and collagen. Molecular modeling studies have predicted that the decorin core protein binds to fibrillar collagen in the gap zone between adjacent collagen molecules (Weber et al. 1996). In a mouse targeted decorin gene disruption, collagen fibrils were irregular in size and diameter (Danielson et al. 1997). Although the mice were viable, their skins were extremely fragile and would tear with applied force. These data are suggestive of decorin influencing the maturation of collagen fibrils into larger fibrils and fiber

networks. Thus, if the organization of fibrillar collagen is modified, tissue functional properties such as elasticity and tensile strength are likely to be altered.

The chicken Low Score Normal (LSN) genetic muscle weakness is characterized by subnormal muscle development and function. Prior to 20 days of embryonic development, LSN glycosaminoglycan and proteoglycan levels do not vary significantly from amounts expressed in normal muscle (Velleman et al. 1996); however, at 20 days of embryonic development there is a dramatic increase in decorin proteoglycan concentration. Subsequent to the increase in decorin, LSN collagen crosslink levels are elevated nearly 200% by 6-week posthatch. Although collagen crosslinking was modified, collagen concentration remains unaffected. By transmission electron microscopy, collagen fibril organization was examined at 6 weeks posthatch (Velleman et al. 1997). At 6 weeks posthatch, there was a significant parallel alignment of collagen fibrils in the LSN pectoral muscle which was not observed in the normal pectoral muscle (Figures 7.5A and 7.5B). This change in LSN collagen fibril organization is likely caused by the change in decorin-collagen interactions resulting in an increase in collagen crosslinking. In terms of skeletal muscle function, the LSN birds exhibit decreased pectoral muscle function as measured by an exhaustion score test. An exhaustion score test

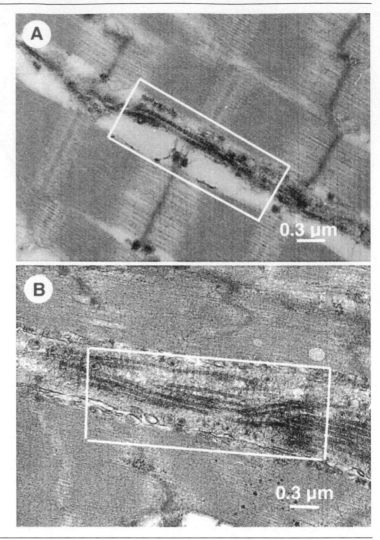

Figure 7.5. Morphological characteristics of 6-week eliminate posthatch normal and Low Score Normal (LSN) collagen fibers. Representative transmission electron micrographs of (A) normal and (B) LSN collagen fibers are shown. A box has been placed around the collagen fibers.

measures the number of times a bird can right itself when repeatedly placed on its back. Low Score Normal birds have an intermediate level of physical strength between normal and muscular dystrophy birds (Velleman et al. 1993). The decrease in physical performance of the LSN birds is, in part, due to the increase in collagen crosslinking. Highly crosslinked collagen is less elastic, and skeletal muscle would have a decreased ability to stretch.

The LSN chicken is an excellent model system to study how changes in extracellular matrix organization affect muscle formation. During muscle development, myoblasts migrate across the extracellular matrix substrate and then align to form multinucleated myotubes leading to the formation of the sar-

comere contractile unit. Transmission electron microscopy studies showed by 6 week posthatch that LSN sarcomere organization was modified. At 6 week posthatch, the normal sacromeres showed a regular pattern with distinct Z banding and myosin-actin overlaps (Figure 7.6A). In contrast, in the LSN pectoral muscle at 6 week posthatch, sarcomere organization was irregular (Figure 7.6B) and this phenotype was termed LSN moderate. The 6 week posthatch LSN pectoral muscle also contained a more severe phenotype characterized by complete sarcomere disorganization, and abnormal mitochondria shape and enlargement (Figure 7.6C). This extreme LSN phenotype was termed LSN severe. The modifications in the LSN extracellular matrix

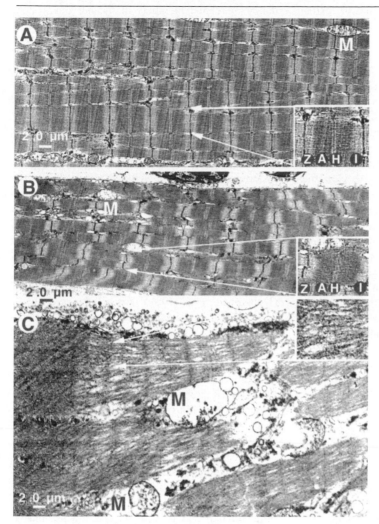

Figure 7.6. Morphological characteristics of 6-week posthatch normal and Low Score Normal (LSN) pectoral muscle sarcomeres. Representative transmission electron micrographs of (A) normal sarcomere phenotype, (B) LSN moderate sarcomere phenotype, and (C) LSN severe sarcomere phenotype. Enlargements of normal and LSN sarcomeres are shown in (A), (B), and (C) with Z, A, H, and I regions labeled. Mitochondria are labeled with an M.

may be associated with changes in signal transduction from the extracellular matrix to the cellular integrin receptors.

The β1 integrin has been shown to be important in myoblast fusion (Rosen et al. 1992) and is located at sites of adhesion and migration (Jaffredo et al., 1988; Lakonishok et al. 1992), myotendon junctions (Bozyczko et al. 1989; Syfrig et al. 1991), and neuromuscular junctions (Bozyczko et al. 1989). During LSN muscle differentiation, the β1 integrin is down-regulated in its expression (Velleman et al. 2000). It is likely that the decrease in integrin expression will alter LSN muscle cell migration. During the differentiation period, cell migration is occurring at a high rate, which requires a high

degree of integrin expression to adhere the muscle cells to the extracellular matrix and create an environment permission for cellular migration. It is still unclear as to why the LSN defect alters both decorin and β1 integrin expression, but preliminary studies indicate a potential link to the expression of transforming growth factor-beta (TGF-β). Heino et al. (1989) and Kagami et al. (1996) showed integrin expression and assembly to be regulated by TGF-β. In LSN muscle, TGF-β expression is elevated late in embryonic development through 1 week posthatch (Velleman and Coy 1998). Although more research is required in determining how β1 integrin expression is regulated by TGF-β, modulation of β1 integrin expression by TGF-β could be a pivotal factor in signaling between the cell and the extracellular matrix, and cell migration and adhesion processes critical in tissue formation.

In addition to extracellular matrix proteoglycans playing a critical role in cell migration and tissue formation, proteoglycans may take part in nervous system development. The steps in nervous system development include the migration of neural precursor cells, neurite outgrowth, pathfinding of neurons, and the formation and stabilization of synapses. The nervous system has been reported to contain at least 25 different proteoglycan core proteins (Herndon and Lander 1990) and the diversity is further enhanced by differences in the attached glycosaminoglycan side chains. Therefore, the number of different proteoglycans found in the nervous system is immense. Typical proteoglycans identified in the nervous system include but are not limited to the following: aggrecan, versican, neurocan, decorin, biglycan, syndecans 1 through 4, perlecan, and glypicans 1 through 6. Many of these proteoglycans have specific temporal and spatial expression patterns. For example, glypican-2 is expressed in the developing nervous system and is mainly localized in the fiber tracts of the brain and spinal cord during neurite outgrowth, but after the neurites reach their targets glypican-2 is no longer expressed (Stipp et al. 1994).

Determining a specific in vivo function for each of the neuronal proteoglycans has been largely approached by transgenic knockouts of specific proteoglycan genes. However, many of these experiments have not resulted in phenotypes being able to be correlated to neuronal function or expected function based on in vitro studies (for review, see Hartmann and Maurer 2001). It is possible that some of the neuronal proteoglycans may function in a redundant fashion by substituting for one if it is absent. This type of functional redundancy has been shown for other pivotal developmental regulators like the MyoD family of muscle transcriptional regulatory factors (Rudnicki et al. 1993), which includes Myf-5, myogenin, and MRF4. MyoD is the primary activator of skeletal muscle gene expression, but in knockout mice lacking MyoD, Myf-5 is expressed at a 3.5-fold increase and displays no obvious skeletal muscle defects (Rudnicki et al. 1992). Unlike the MyoD family of skeletal muscle transcriptional regulators, the proteoglycans are a diverse and large group of macromolecules, so it becomes difficult to determine which ones are coordinately expressed. Hence, making appropriate transgenic knockouts to test for functional redundancy of related members of the nervous system proteoglycans is a formidable task.

EXTRACELLULAR MATRIX REGULATION OF GROWTH FACTOR ACTIVITY

Controlling the onset of proliferation and differentiation is, in part, regulated by the extracellular matrix environment. Proliferation is the division of cells to increase cell number whereas differentiation is the generation of cellular diversity. Skeletal muscle proliferation and differentiation are particularly sensitive to growth factor activity. For example, growth factors like fibroblast growth factor (FGF) and TGF-β either stimulate or inhibit skeletal muscle proliferation and differentiation.

Basic FGF is a potent stimulator of muscle cell proliferation and an inhibitor of differentiation (Dollenmeier et al. 1981). The cellular response to basic FGF is modulated by heparan sulfate containing proteoglycans such as syndecan and glypican which act as co-receptors for basic FGF (Larraín et al. 1998). If heparan sulfate is removed, basic FGF no longer functions as an inhibitor of muscle differentiation (Rapraeger et al. 1991). Therefore, the presence of heparan sulfate proteoglycans is necessary for skeletal muscle formation.

Although both syndecan and glypican are co-receptors for basic FGF, their expression has been shown to be differentially regulated during skeletal muscle differentiation (Brandan et al. 1996; Larraín et al. 1997). Syndecan expression is high early in skeletal muscle differentiation and is subsequently down-regulated, whereas glypican expression is the reverse of that observed for syndecan (Brandan et al. 1996; Larraín et al. 1997). It is unclear as to why these two proteoglycans, which are both co-receptors for basic FGF, are expressed in such opposite manners. Brandan and Larraín (1998) have postulated that syndecan may function as a presenter of basic FGF during myoblast proliferation and glypican may function as a sequester of basic FGF during differentiation to prevent the inhibitory effects of basic FGF. Figure 7.7 shows a possible model for this interaction during muscle cell proliferation where syndecan expression is higher than that for glypican, and syndecan is presenting basic FGF to its receptor. In contrast, during the formation of multinucleated myotubes, glypican levels are higher and glypican functions by preventing basic FGF from binding to its receptor, providing a permissive environment for differentiation.

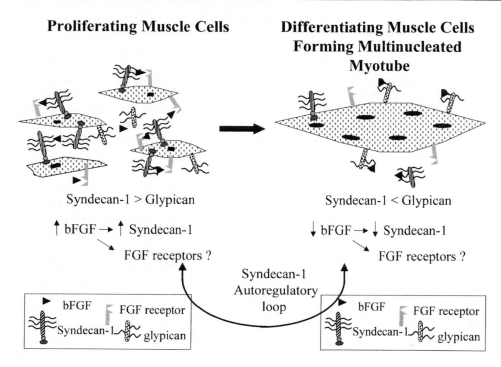

Figure 7.7. Model for heparan sulfate proteoglycan regulation of muscle development. In this model, syndecan-1 stimulates proliferation by presenting basic fibroblast growth factor (bFGF) to its receptor, and glypican permits differentiation by sequestering bFGF. The possibility of an autoregulatory loop with bFGF regulating syndecan-1 expression is also illustrated.

In support of a proteoglycan functioning as a sequester of a growth factor, decorin has been shown to function in this mode for TGF-β. Transforming growth factor-beta binds to decorin at its core protein (Schönherr et al. 1998) and is a potent inhibitor of both proliferation and differentiation (Moscatello et al. 1998; Iozzo et al. 1999). When TGF-β is bound to the decorin core protein its activity is suppressed (Yamaguchi et al. 1990). Transfection studies reducing decorin expression during myogenesis decreased muscle cell responsiveness to TGF-β and accelerated muscle differentiation (Riquelme et al. 2001).

As well as proteoglycans regulating cellular responsiveness to growth factors, growth factors may also exert regulatory roles on the expression of proteoglycans. Recent evidence with mouse mesenchymal cells indicates that an autoregulatory loop exists between basic FGF and syndecan expression (Jaakkola et al. 1997; Jaakkola and Jalkanen 2000). Thus, in response to increases in basic FGF, synde-

can expression is up-regulated. Although an autoregulatory loop involving basic FGF regulation of syndecan expression has not been shown to date for skeletal muscle, Figure 7.7 depicts this possible interaction. In this model, syndecan expression is directly associated with basic FGF expression. How this regulation of syndecan by basic FGF affects the expression of receptors for FGF remains to be determined.

WHY IS THE EXTRACELLULAR MATRIX IMPORTANT FOR DOMESTIC ANIMAL INDUSTRIES?

Developing a comprehensive understanding of tissue formation and growth is important to the improvement and maintenance of domestic animals. The extracellular matrix environment as discussed in this chapter plays important roles in cell adhesion, migration, proliferation, differentiation, water-holding capacity, and growth factor regulation. The domestic animal industries have largely selected animals based on growth rate and muscling. In the case of skeletal muscle, this type of selection regime will alter muscle fiber proportions (Dransfield and Sosnicki 1999). As well as muscle fiber proportions being modified, it is likely that the degree of extracellular matrix space surrounding the muscle fibers and its composition will be changed. Both the swine and turkey industries are experiencing a meat quality problem termed pale, soft, and exudative (PSE) meat. When cooked, meat from animals with the PSE condition has a softer texture, poor meat binding, poor juiciness due to reduced water-holding, and increased yield losses. The extracellular matrix proteoglycan component is a major determinant in tissue water-holding capacity, but it has not been studied to date with regard to PSE. The proteoglycan glycosaminoglycans are highly sulfated and have a negative charge density. The negative charge draws water into the tissue and creates a water compartment. The versican proteoglycan is highly substituted with chondroitin sulfate chains and is a likely candidate to function in this manner in skeletal muscle. If the amount of proteoglycan has been reduced in animals selected for growth rate and muscling, the reduced degree of water-holding capacity would directly impact the juiciness and drip loss. Therefore, the domestic animal industries should consider how the extracellular matrix is affected by genetic selection, and the effect on both antemortem and postmortem skeletal muscle properties.

Because certain proteoglycans are regulators of growth factors like basic FGF and TGF-β, which are potent mitogens affecting skeletal muscle proliferation and differentiation, it may be beneficial to include in the selection process screening of the expression of key proteoglycans, such as syndecan, glypican, and decorin. For example, selection for growth rate has been shown to delay myogenesis by prolonging the period of proliferation (Summers and Medrano 1997). Basic fibroblast growth factor is a strong stimulator of muscle cell proliferation, and the prolonged period of proliferation may be associated with increased basic FGF responsiveness and syndecan expression. However, issues like this one must be resolved in order to develop selection strategies that optimize growth properties while maintaining animal quality.

Changes induced in the extracellular matrix by selection strategies can alter meat quality. The muscle foods industry comprises a significant part of the agricultural economy. Tenderness is the single most important factor by which consumers judge muscle food quality and is influenced by skeletal muscle extracellular matrix collagens and proteoglycans. Research studies evaluating the effect of the extracellular matrix on meat tenderness have largely focused on differences in the fibrillar collagens. Skeletal muscle is primarily composed of types I and III collagen. With age and maturation, there is a progressive increase from type III to more type I collagen and an increase in crosslinking in skeletal muscle. These developmental changes in skeletal muscle contribute to meat toughening (McCormick 1994, 1999). Investigations evaluating meat tenderness have been largely limited to measurements of collagen concentration, heat solubility, and more recently collagen crosslink concentration and phenotype proportionality between types I and III collagen. Attempts to establish correlations between collagen solubility, phenotype, and crosslink profile have been unsuccessful because precise relationships between collagen phenotype variability, collagen fibril composition and crosslinking have not yet been elucidated (McCormick 1994, 1999). Furthermore, tissues like skeletal muscle containing both types I and III collagen forms fibrils that are heteropolymers of both types of collagen, which will affect the physical properties of collagen (Henkel and Glanville 1982; Fleischmajer et al. 1990; Kuypers et al. 1994).

To complicate the situation further with how the extracellular matrix influences meat tenderness, only a few limited investigations have examined how proteoglycans affect meat tenderness. Proteoglycans can play a role in tenderness by influencing collagen fibril organization and water-holding capacity. In a recent study by Pedersen et al. (2001), the amount of decorin contained in the tougher bovine *M. semitendinosus* was higher than that in the tender *M. psoas major* at both the protein and mRNA levels. How this difference in decorin expression is correlated to tenderness is still an enigma. But several studies have shown a functional interaction to occur between fibrillar collagen and decorin that affects collagen fibril diameter (Vogel et al. 1984; Vogel and Trotter 1987; Danielson et al. 1997) and may modify collagen crosslinking (Velleman et al. 1996). Future research in this area will need to address the interaction of fibrillar collagens with other extracellular matrix macromolecules like decorin to determine the effect on meat tenderness properties.

CONCLUSIONS

The macromolecular components of the extracellular matrix are expressed in a tissue-specific and dynamic fashion during development. Regulation of both proteoglycan synthesis and spatial distribution may play a pivotal role in tissue morphogenesis in terms of growth factor responsiveness, cellular growth, and extracellular matrix architecture. The heparan sulfate family of proteoglycans is crucial in regulating the cellular response to basic FGF. Proteoglycans like decorin are multifunctional and are critical in modulating TGF-β, cellular growth properties, and collagen fibril organization. How each type of extracellular matrix macromolecule influences tissue formation and growth still remains somewhat of an enigma, but the expression of the individual extracellular matrix components must also be examined as to how their expression affects extracellular matrix organization and signal transduction from the extracellular matrix to the cell.

REFERENCES

Boettiger, D., Enomoto-Iwamot, M., Yoon, H.Y., Hofer, U., Menklo, A.S., and Chiquet-Ehrismann, R. 1995. Regulation of integrin α5β1 affinity during myogenic differentiation. *Developmental Biology* 169:261–272.

Bozyczko, D., Decker, C., Muschler, J., and Horwitz, A.F. 1989. Integrin on developing and adult skeletal muscle. *Experimental Cell Research* 183:72–91.

Brandan, E., Carey, D.J., Larraín, J., Melo, F., and Campos, A. 1996. Synthesis and processing of glypican during differentiation of skeletal muscle cells. *European Journal of Cell Biology* 71:170–176.

Brandan, E., and Larraín, J. 1998. Heparan sulfate proteoglycans during terminal skeletal muscle cell differentiation: Possible functions and regulation of their expression. *Basic and Applied Myology* 8:107–114.

Carrino, D.A., Sorrell, J.M., and Caplan, A.I. 1999. Dynamic expression of proteoglycans during chicken skeletal muscle development and maturation. *Poultry Science* 78:769–777.

Chen, C.S., Mrksich, M., Huang, S., Whitesides, G.M., and Ingber, D.E. 1997. Geometric control of cell life and death. *Science* 276:1425–1428.

Danielson, K.G., Baribault, H., Holmes, D.F., Graham, H., Kadler, K.E., and Iozzo, R.V. 1997. Targeted disruption of decorin leads to abnormal collagen fibril morphology and skin fragility. *Journal of Cell Biology* 136:729–743.

Dollenmeier, P., Turner, D.C., and Eppendberger, H.M. 1981. Proliferation and differentiation of chick skeletal muscle cells cultured in a chemically defined medium. *Experimental Cell Research* 135:47–61.

Dransfield, E., and Sosnicki, A.A. 1999. Relationship between muscle growth and poultry meat quality. *Poultry Science* 78:743–746.

Ffrench-Constant, C. 1995. Alternative splicing of fibronectin—many different proteins but few different functions. *Experimental Cell Research* 221:261–271.

Fitch, J.M., Mentzer, A., Mayne, R., and Linsenmayer, T.F. 1988. Acquisition of type IX collagen by the developing avian primary corneal stroma and vitreous. *Developmental Biology* 128:396–405.

Fleischmajer, R., Perlish, J.S., Burgeson, R.E., Shaikh-Bahai, F., and Timpl, R. 1990. Type I and type III collagen interactions during fibrillogenesis. *Annals of the New York Academy of Science* 586:161–175.

Hartmann, U., and Maurer, P. 2001. Proteoglycans in the nervous system—the quest for functional roles in vivo. *Matrix Biology* 20:23–35.

Heino, J., Ignotz, R.A., Hemler, M.E., Crouse, C., and Massagué, J. 1989. Regulation of cell adhesion receptors by transforming growth factor-β. *Journal of Biological Chemistry* 264:380–388.

Henkel, W., and Glanville, R.W. 1982. Covalent crosslinking between molecules of type I and type III collagen. *European Journal of Biochemistry* 05:213.

Herndon, M.E., and Lander, A.D. 1990. A diverse set of developmentally regulated proteoglycans is expressed in the rat central nervous system. *Neuron* 4:949–961.

Iozzo, R.V., Moscatello, D.K., McQuillan, D.J., and Eichstetter, I. 1999. Decorin is a biological ligand for the epidermal growth factor receptor. *Journal of Biological Chemistry* 274:4489–4492.

Iozzo, R.V., and Murdoch, A.D. 1996. Proteoglycans of the extracellular environment: clues from the gene and protein side offer novel perspectives in molecular diversity and function. *The FASEB Journal* 10:598–614.

Jaakkola, P., and Jalkanen, M. 2000. Transcriptional regulation of syndecan-1 expression by growth factors. *Progress in Nucleic Acid Research and Molecular Biology* 63:109–137.

Jaakkola, P., Vihinen, T., Määttä, A., and Jalkanen, M. 1997. Activation of an enhancer on the syndecan-1 gene is restricted to fibroblast growth factor family members in mesenchymal cells. *Molecular and Cellular Biology* 17:3210–3219.

Jaffredo, T., Horwitz, A.F., Buck, C.A., Rong, P.M., and Dieterlan, L.F. 1988. Myoblast migration specifically inhibited in the chick embryo by grafted CSAT hybridoma cells secreting an anti-integrin antibody. *Development* 103:431–446.

Kagami, S., Kuhara, T., Yasutomo, K., Okada, K., Löster, K., Reutter, W., and Kuroda, Y. 1996. Transforming growth factor-β (TGF-β) stimulates the expression of β1 integrins and adhesion by rat mesangial cells. *Experimental Cell Research* 229:1–6.

Kuypers, R., Tyler, M., Kurth, L.M., and Horgan, D.J. 1994. The molecular location of Ehrlich chromogen and pyridinoline crosslinks in bovine perimysial collagen. *Meat Science* 37:67–89.

Lakonishok, M., Muschler, J., and Horwitz, A.F. 1992. The α5β1 integrin associates with a dystrophin-containing lattice during muscle development. *Developmental Biology* 152:209–220.

Larraín, J., Carey, D.J., and Brandan, E. 1998. Syndecan-1 expression inhibits myoblast differentiation through a basic fibroblast growth factor-dependent mechanism. *Journal of Biological Chemistry* 273:32288–32296.

Larraín, J., Cizmeci-Smith, G., Troncoso, V., Stahl, R.C., Carey, D.J., and Brandan, E. 1997. Syndecan-1 expression is down-regulated during myoblast terminal differentiation. Modulation by growth factors and retinoic acid. *Journal of Biological Chemistry* 272:18418–18424.

Leach, R.M., Jr., and Nesheim, M.C. 1965. Nutritional, genetic and morphological studies of an abnormal cartilage formation in young chickens. *Journal of Nutrition* 86:236–244.

Linsenmeyer, T.F. 1991. Collagen. In *Cell Biology of Extracellular Matrix*. Elizabeth D. Hay, ed. New York: Plenum Press.

McCormick, R.J. 1994. The flexibility of the collagen compartment of muscle. *Meat Science* 36:79–91.

McCormick, R.J. 1999. Extracellular modifications to muscle collagen: Implications for meat quality. *Poultry Science* 78: 778–784.

Moscatello, D.K., Santra, M., Mann, D.M., McQuillan, D.J., Wong, A.J., and Iozzo, R.V. 1998. Decorin suppresses tumor cell growth by activating the epidermal growth factor receptor. *Journal of Clinical Investigation* 101:406–412.

Nishimura, I., Muragaki, Y., and Olsen, B.R. 1989. Tissue-specific forms of type IX collagen-proteoglycan arise from the use of two widely separated promoters. *Journal of Biological Chemistry* 264:20033–20041.

Oberhammer, F., Wilson, J.W., Dive, C., Morris, I.D., Hickman, J.A., Wakeling, A.E., Walker, P.R., and Sikorska, M. 1993. Apoptotic death in epithelial cells: cleavage of DNA to 300 and/or 50 kb fragments prior to or in the absence of internucleosomal fragmentation. *EMBO Journal* 12:3679–3684.

Pedersen, M.E., Kulseth, M-A., Kolset, S.O., Velleman, S., and Eggen, K.H. 2001. Decorin and fibromodulin expression in two bovine muscles (M.semitendinosus and M.psoas major) differing in texture. *Journal of Muscle Foods* 12:1–17.

Pentikäinen, M.O, Öörni, K., Lassia, R., and Kovanen, P.T. 1997. The proteoglycan decorin links low density lipoproteins with collagen type I. *Journal of Biological Chemistry* 272:7633–7638.

Rapraeger, A.C., Krufka, A., and Olwin, B.B. 1991. Requirement of heparan sulfate for bFGF-mediated fibroblast growth and myoblast differentiation. *Science* 252:1705–1708.

Riquelme, C., Larraín, J., Schönherr, E., Henriquez, J.P., Kresse, H., and Brandan, E. 2001. Antisense inhibition of decorin expression in myoblasts decreases cell responsiveness to transforming growth factor β and accelerates skeletal muscle differentiation. *Journal of Biological Chemistry* 276:3589–3596.

Rosen, G.D., Sanes, J.R., LaChance, R., Cunningham, J.M., Roman, J., and Dean, D.C. 1992. Roles for the integrin VLA-4 and its counter receptor VCAM-β1 in myogenesis. *Cell* 69:1107–1119.

Rudnicki, M.A., Braun, T., Hinuma, S., and Jaenisch, R. 1992. Inactivation of MyoD in mice leads to up-regulation of the myogenic HLH gene Myf-5 and results in apparently normal muscle development. *Cell* 71:383–390.

Rudnicki, M.A., Schnegelsberg, P.N.J., Stead, R.H., Braun, T., Arnold, H-H., and Jaenisch, R. 1993. MyoD or Myf-5 is required for the formation of skeletal muscle. *Cell* 75:1351–1359.

Ruoslahti, E. 1997. Stretching is good for a cell. *Science* 276:1345–1346.

Santra, M., Skorski, T., Calabretta, B., Lattime, E.C., and Iozzo, R.V. 1995. De novo decorin gene expression suppresses the malignant phenotype in human colon cancer cells. *Proceedings of the National Academy of Sciences USA* 92:7016–7020.

Saunders, J.W., Jr., and Fallon, J.F. 1966. Cell death and morphogenesis. In *Major Problems of Developmental Biology*. M. Locke, ed. New York: Academic Press.

Schmid, T.M., and Linsenmeyer, T.F. 1985. Immunohistochemical localization of short chain collagen (type X) in avian tissues. *Journal of Cell Biology* 100:598–605.

Schmid, T.M., and Linsenmeyer, T.F. 1987. Immunohistochemical localization of short chain collagen (type X) in avian tissues. *Journal of Cell Biology* 100:598–605.

Schönherr, E., Broszat, M., Brandan, E., Bruckner, P., and Kresse, H. 1998. Decorin core protein fragment Leu155-Val260 interacts with TGF-β but does not compete for decorin binding to type I collagen. *Archives of Biochemistry and Biophysics* 355:241–248.

Schwartz, M.A. 2001. Integrin signaling revisited. *Trends in Cell Biology* 11:466–470.

Scott, J.E. 1988. Proteoglycan-fibrillar collagen interactions. *Journal of Biochemistry* 252:313–323.

Stipp, C.S., Litwack, E.D., and Lander, A.D. 1994. Cerebroglycan: an integral membrane heparan sulfate proteoglycan that is unique to the developing nervous system and expressed specifically during neuronal differentiation. *Journal of Cell Biology* 124:149–160.

Summers, P.J., and Medrano, J.F. 1997. Delayed myogenesis associated with muscle fiber hyperplasia in high-growth mice. *Proceedings of the Society of Experimental Biology and Medicine* 214:380–385.

Svoboda, K.K., Nishimura, I., Sugrue, S.P., Ninomiya, Y., and Olsen, B.R. 1988. Embryonic chicken cornea and cartilage synthesize type IX collagen molecules with amino-terminal domains. *Proceedings of the National Academy of Sciences USA* 85:7496–7500.

Syfrig, J., Mann, K., and Paullson, M. 1991. An abundant chick gizzard integrin is the avian α5β1 integrin heterodimer and functions as divalent cation dependent collagen IV receptor. *Experimental Cell Research* 194:165–173.

van der Rest, M., and Garrone, R. 1991. Collagen family of proteins. *The FASEB Journal* 6:2639–2645.

Velleman, S.G., Brown, S.M., Gustafson, S.K., Faustman, C., Beaurang, P.A., Craft, F., and Hausman, R.E. 1993. Partial characterization of a novel avian defect affecting adult muscle function. *Muscle and Nerve* 16:881.

Velleman, S.G., and Coy, C.S. 1998. Transforming growth factor-β gene expression in avian low score normal pectoral muscle. *Poultry Science* 77:464–467.

Velleman, S.G., Coy, C.S., Gannon, L.S., Wick, M., and McFarland, D.C. 2000. β1 integrin expression during normal and low score normal avian myogenesis. *Poultry Science* 79:1179–1182.

Velleman, S.G., McFarland, D.C., Li, Z., Ferrin, N.H., Whitmoyer, R., and Dennis, J.E., 1997. Alterations in sarcomere structure, collagen organization, mitochondrial activity, and protein metabolism in the avian low score normal muscle weakness. *Development Growth and Differentiation* 39:563–570.

Velleman, S.G., Yeager, J.D., Krider, H., Carrino, D.A., Zimmerman, S.D., and McCormick, R.J. 1996. The avian low score normal muscle weakness alters decorin expression and collagen crosslinking. *Connective Tissue Research* 34:33–39.

Vogel, K.G., Paulsson, M., and Heinegård, D. 1984. Specific inhibition of type I and type II collagen fibrillogenesis by the small proteoglycan of tendon. *Journal of Biochemistry* 223:587–597.

Vogel, K.G., and Trotter, J.A. 1987. The effects of proteoglycans on the morphology of collagen fibrils formed in vitro. *Collagen and Related Research* 7:105–114.

Weber, I.T., Harrison, R.W., and Iozzo, R.V. 1996. Model structure of decorin and implications for collagen fibrillogenesis. *Journal of Biological Chemistry* 271:31767–31770.

Yamaguchi, Y., Mann, D.M., and Ruoslahti, E. 1990. Negative regulation of transforming growth factor-β by the proteoglycan decorin. *Nature* 346:281–284.

Yamaguchi, Y., and Ruoslahti, E. 1988. Expression of human proteoglycan in Chinese hamster ovary cells inhibits cell proliferation. *Nature* 336:244–246.

Zhang, Z., Vuori, K., Reed, J.C., and Ruoslahti, E. 1995. The α5β1 integrin supports survival of cells on fibronectin and up-regulates Bcl-2 expression. *Proceedings of the National Academy of Sciences USA* 92:6161–6165.

8

Cellular and Developmental Biology of Skeletal Muscle as Related to Muscle Growth

Ronald E. Allen and Darrel E. Goll

Skeletal muscle comprises a greater proportion of animal mass than any other single tissue or organ does. From an agricultural perspective, this is fortunate because muscle is the major food product derived from domestic animals and is a rich source of vitamins, minerals, and high-quality protein. From a biological perspective, however, muscle exists for the purpose of animal mobility (muscle contraction) and as an important reservoir of amino acids when the animal is in an energy-deficient state. Contractile functions of muscle are diverse, and three types of muscle can be distinguished both structurally and physiologically (Table 8.1; see Goll et al. 1984, for a summary of muscle properties). Contraction of two of these muscle types, smooth muscle and cardiac muscle, is controlled without conscious thought (thankfully for cardiac muscle, because forgetfulness would be fatal). Skeletal muscle is the type of interest to muscle growth. Contraction of the diaphragm muscle, a striated skeletal muscle, is initiated from the phrenic motor neuron rather than from the cerebrospinal nervous system (Table 8.1), and also occurs automatically and at a regular pace as animals breathe; this con-

Table 8.1. Three types of muscle tissue in vertebrates

Muscle Tissue Type	Characteristics
Skeletal muscle	Voluntary nerve control, innervated by the cerebrospinal nervous system; cross-striated appearance in the phase-contrast microscope with alternating light and dark bands; most abundant in terms of mass of the three types of muscle tissue.
Cardiac muscle	Involuntary nerve control, innervated with an intrinsic nervous system for generating rhythmic contractions; also cross-striated in appearance in the phase-contrast microscope with alternating light and dark bands, but contains structures such as intercalated disks that skeletal muscles do not have; exists only in the heart.
Smooth muscle	Involuntary nerve control, innervated by the autonomic nervous system; no cross-striated appearance; widely distributed in different tissues, such as walls of blood vessels, lining of the intestinal tract, uterine wall, and walls of the respiratory passages from the trachea to the alveolar ducts, but not present in large amounts in any one tissue, such as skeletal muscle is. Slow contractile velocity but sustained for long periods of time.

tractile activity is controlled differently than the contractile activity of many large muscles that function only intermittently as the body moves. Other muscles function in subtle ways that we seldom consider because we do not associate them with movement. These muscles are required to maintain posture; they contract on a continuous, repetitive basis as we stand or walk. Specific muscles or groups of muscles have evolved to meet unique roles, but the fundamental cellular structure and mechanisms of muscle fiber formation and growth discussed in this chapter are shared by all skeletal muscles.

This chapter first briefly describes the composition and structure of striated muscle, starting at the whole muscle level and then proceeding to the molecular thick and thin filament structure and contraction of the myofibril first described by Huxley and Hanson nearly 40 years ago. A short summary of muscle fiber types and physiology follows, and the events that occur during prenatal muscle development (embryonic growth) are then described. These sections are followed by a description of myogenesis (muscle fiber formation) and then postnatal muscle growth, with a section on the role of satellite cells in postnatal muscle growth. The discussion then progresses from the cellular aspects of muscle growth to close with a description of muscle fiber hypertrophy and modulation of muscle mass.

MUSCLE COMPOSITION AND STRUCTURE

Muscle Composition

Skeletal muscle can be grouped into three categories based on solubility of the muscle proteins (Table 8.2). The major fraction is the myofibrillar proteins, which constitute the fraction that contains the contractile proteins together with the proteins needed to regulate contraction and to maintain the myofibrillar structure. The myofibrillar protein fraction is also responsible for most of the differences in the culinary properties of meat, such as texture. Research during the past 20 years has shown that the stroma protein fraction—which contains the extracellular matrix proteins in addition to membrane proteins, including hormone receptors—has important effects on skeletal muscle growth. Hormones and growth factors, however, are discussed in separate chapters in this book, which also contains a chapter devoted to extracellular matrix proteins. Consequently, this chapter focuses on the

myofibrillar protein fraction, with only brief references to the sarcoplasmic protein fraction.

Muscle Structure

An entire muscle (top, Figure 8.1) is surrounded by a sheath of connective tissue called the *epimysium* (Figure 8.2) that separates individual muscles from each other. These epimysial sheaths, which contain Type I collagen fibers, often contain areas of large fat deposits in obese animals. Within each muscle, bundles of muscle cells (fibers) are grouped together in structures called *fasciculi* (Figure 8.2). The connective tissue sheaths dividing different fasciculi are called the *perimysium* (Figure 8.2). Fasciculi can be seen without the aid of a microscope. The diameters of fasciculi in muscles are responsible for what is often called "muscle texture; the larger the fasciculi, the coarser the texture. Muscles that perform large motions, such as arm and leg muscles, generally have larger fasciculi and therefore coarser texture. Each fasciculus contains a number (usually between 50 to 200–300) of muscle fibers (muscle cells) that are separated from each other by a finer connective tissue layer called the *endomysium* (Figure 8.2). Between the endomysial connective tissue and the plasma membrane of the muscle cell, which is called the *sarcolemma* in skeletal muscle cells, is an amorphous layer of small connective tissue fibers containing collagen Types III and IV and a matrix of different proteoglycans (discussed in Chapter 7). This amorphous layer is called the basement membrane or basal lamina. Although the epimysial, perimysial, and endomysial connective tissue layers are often discussed as separate entities, they are interconnected within the muscle and all join together at the myotendinous junction (Figure 8.2). This network of strong connective tissue layers forms a scaffolding that transmits force generated by the myofibrils inside muscle cells to the skeleton.

The muscle cell has a long, cylindrical, tubular shape with tapering conical ends; muscle cells are not perfectly round in cross-section (Figure 8.2). Because of their shape, muscle cells are often referred to as "muscle fibers." Skeletal muscle cells are large, ranging from 1 mm to sometimes, many centimeters in length with an average length of 20–30 mm, and from 10–100μm in diameter. Skeletal muscle cells are unique in that they are one of only a few cell types that are multinucleated, containing 100 or more nuclei per cell. The nuclei, sometimes called myonuclei, are located just beneath the sarcolemma and are oriented parallel

Table 8.2. Protein composition of mammalian muscles[a]

Protein Class	Properties
Sarcoplasmic proteins	Soluble at ionic strengths of 0.1 or less at neutral pH. Constitutes 30–35% of total protein, by weight, in skeletal muscle and slightly more in cardiac muscle; contains at least 200–300 different proteins, including the glycolytic enzymes and other metabolic enzymes, enzymes involved in protein synthesis, and other soluble proteins; called cytoplasmic proteins in nonmuscle cells.
Myofibrillar proteins[b]	Constitute the myofibril; are 52–65% of total muscle protein, by weight, in skeletal muscle but less than this (45–50%) in cardiac muscle. Ionic strengths above 0.3 are generally required to solubilize myofibrillar proteins (that is, to disrupt the myofibril), but many of the myofibrillar proteins (e.g., G-actin; α-actinin, troponin, some of the minor Z-disk proteins such as CapZ) are soluble at low ionic strength after they have been extracted from the myofibril.
Stroma proteins	Insoluble in neutral aqueous solvents. Constitute 10–15% of total muscle protein, by weight, in skeletal muscle and slightly more than this in cardiac muscle; includes extracellular proteins such as collagen (a major component; may make up 40–60% of total stroma protein in some muscles), elastin (may make up 10–15% in some muscles), proteins from the extracellular matrix; and proteins from the plasma membrane (the sarcolemma in skeletal muscle) including some hormone receptors and proteins, such as dystrophin, the protein missing in Duchenne muscular dystrophy.

[a]Muscle tissue is defined as muscle cells (fibers) plus the associated extracellular tissue that would be found in an intact muscle.

[b]Cytoskeletal proteins—such as talin, vinculin, desmin, and spectrin—are partly, but usually not completely, extracted with the myofibrillar proteins. These proteins in total constitute a small proportion of total muscle protein, and may be extracted with the sarcoplasmic proteins or left with the stroma protein fraction, depending on extraction conditions.

with the long axis of the muscle cell in skeletal muscle (second panel from top, Figure 8.1).

The sarcolemma or plasma membrane of the skeletal muscle cell is a lipid bilayer, similar to the plasma membranes of other cells, but it is specialized in skeletal muscle cells to enable it to conduct action potentials from a nerve impulse to the contractile machinery in the cell. The sarcolemma has two unique features: the motor endplate or neuromuscular junction, and the transverse tubule system.

The motor endplate is a specialized region that interacts with the terminal ends of the axon of a motoneuron. The sarcolemma in this region forms synaptic clefts, which are closely positioned adjacent to the terminal ends of the axon. Acetylcholine is released from the axon into these clefts and binds to the acetylcholine receptors on the surface of the sarcolemma. This binding alters permeability of the sarcolemma to ions and initiates an action potential that

is propagated along the sarcolemma to trigger muscle contraction. A second specialized part of this area of the sarcolemma is the enzyme, acetylcholinesterase, which is associated with the synaptic clefts in this region of the sarcolemma. Acetylcholinesterase cleaves acetylcholine and terminates the action potential and the contractile signal.

The second unique feature of the sarcolemma, the transverse tubule system, consists of a series of invaginations of the sarcolemma into the muscle cell at regular intervals along the length of the cell (Figure 8.3); these invaginations occur at the level of every Z-disk (one invagination per sarcomere, usually in slow-contracting muscles) or at every A/I-band junction (two invaginations per sarcomere, usually in fast-contracting muscles). The T-tubules run in a direction perpendicular to the long axis of the muscle cell (Figure 8.3) and surround the myofibril at every Z-disk or A/I junction. Because

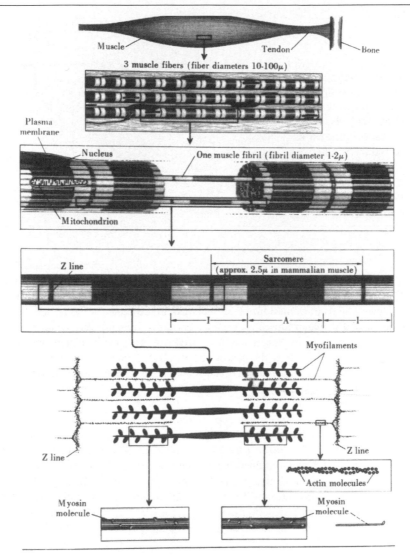

Figure 8.1. Diagram of a mature vertebrate skeletal muscle, such as the *biceps femoris* or *semitendinosus*, at different levels of organization ranging from an entire muscle, shown in this diagram as a fusiform muscle with tendon attachments (top panel), to the molecular thick and thin filament structure of the myofibril at the bottom. Three muscle cells or fibers are shown in the second panel, which also shows the cross-striated appearance of the myofibril and the peripheral location of a nucleus just beneath the sarcolemma. Small, longitudinal lines represent mitochondria. The third panel shows a single muscle cell (fiber) and its myofibrils together with a nucleus and a mitochondrion. This would be a structure observed at an intermediate light microscope level. The fourth panel shows the structure of a myofibril as it would be seen as a high light microscope level. What appear to be fine filaments within the myofibril at this level of magnification are seen in the fifth panel as an interdigitating array of thick and thin filaments when observed at a high electron microscope magnification (and with very thin sections to prevent interference from the layer of thick and thin filaments that lie in the plane immediately under the plane shown). Schematic diagrams of the double stranded F-actin filament and the myosin molecule with a globular head at one end of a rod-shaped coiled coil are shown in the bottom right of the figure. From Novikoff and Holtzman, 1984, reprinted with permission of H.E. Huxley.

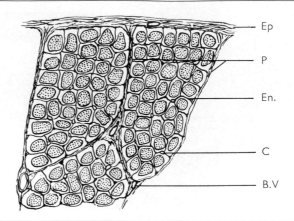

Figure 8.2. Diagrammatic representation of a cross section through an entire muscle, such as the *semitendinosus*, showing the connective tissue framework associated with muscles and muscle cells. Ep, epimysium; P, perimysium; En, endomysium; C, capillary; BV, blood vessel (Gould 1973).

the T-tubules are invaginations of the sarcolemma, the lumen of the T-tubule is extracellular. The T-tubule system allows rapid transmission of the action potential initiated at the neuromuscular junction to the interior of all parts of the large muscle cell, so the area of the muscle fiber near the neuromuscular junction doesn't initiate contraction before the action potential reaches areas of the muscle fiber distal to the neuromuscular junction.

The contractile properties of muscle cells are due to the presence of structures called myofibrils in striated muscle cells (Figure 8.1, third panel). Myofibrils are protein threads (1–3 μm in diameter, so ~10–50 myofibrils per muscle cell) that extend uninterrupted from one end of the muscle fiber to the other. Myofibrils are not surrounded by membranes, but exist as structural entities in muscle cells because the proteins constituting the myofibrils are insoluble at the ionic strengths that are present in muscle cells. Myofibrils occupy approximately 75% of the volume of a skeletal muscle cell, and myofibrillar proteins constitute 52–65% of total muscle protein (Table 8.2). In contrast to the 100–200 or more proteins in the sarcoplasmic protein fraction (Table 8.2), the myofibrillar protein fraction contains a relatively limited number of proteins (Table 8.3). Myosin is a major protein in skeletal muscle and alone constitutes ~25% of all protein in skeletal muscle. When viewed in a light (phase) microscope, myofibrils are cross-striated containing alternating light and dark bands (Figure 8.1, panels 3 and 4). Because the light and dark bands of adjacent myofibrils are in register, skeletal and cardiac muscle cells are also cross-striated (hence, the name, *striated muscle*). The light bands are called the I-

band (for isotropic); the dark bands are called the A-band (for anisotropic or birefringent); and the dark disk in the center of the I-band that can be observed at higher magnification and with a good quality light microscope is called the Z-disk (Figure 8.1, panels 2, 3, and 4). The distance from one Z-disk to another is called a *sarcomere*, and is the smallest contractile unit of a myofibril.

It was observed early that width of the I-band and the distance from Z-disk to Z-disk (i.e., sarcomere length) decreased when the muscle shortened or contracted. It wasn't until a combination of electron microscopy and thin sections was used, however, that it was learned that myofibrils contained interdigitating thick and thin filaments (Figure 8.1, panel 5; Figure 8.4), and that muscle contraction was accomplished by a sliding of the thick and thin filaments past one another. In mammalian skeletal muscle, thick filaments are 14–16 nm in diameter and 1.5 μm long, whereas thin filaments are 6–8 nm in diameter and 1.0 μm long. A great deal of work has shown that thick filaments contain all the myosin and that thin filaments contain all the actin in the myofibril. The myosin molecule consists of a long rod-like "tail" that is ~135–145 nm in length and a globular "head" region, called the S1 domain (bottom right in Figure 8.1). Most of the rod-like myosin tail assembles in an overlapping side-to-side arrangement to form the shaft of the thick filament (Figure 8.1). The S1 domain represents the N-terminal part of the myosin molecule, and this domain plus a small part of the rod form the myosin cross-bridges that protrude out from the shaft of the thick filament (Figure 8.1, panel 5; Figure 8.4). The S1 domain binds ATP, has all the ATPase activity of the

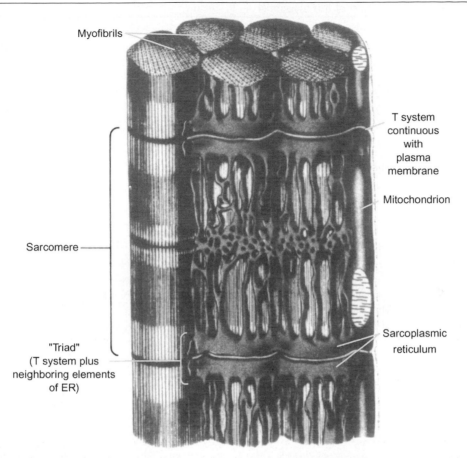

Myofibrils

T system
continuous
with
plasma
membrane

Mitochondrion

Sarcomere

Sarcoplasmic
reticulum

"Triad"
(T system plus
neighboring elements
of ER)

Figure 8.3. Diagram of the T-tubule and sarcoplasmic reticular system in skeletal muscle. T-tubules in this diagram are shown at the level of every Z-disk; T-tubules in fast-glycolytic muscles would be at the level of every A/I junction, so there would be two T-tubules for every sarcomere. The sarcoplasmic reticulum is shown as an extensive, three-dimensional, membranous network running parallel with the long axis of the muscle fiber, and completely surrounding the fiber. The "sacs" on either side of the T-tubule where the sarcoplasmic reticular membranes coalesce are called lateral cisternae, and together with the T-tubule, they constitute a structure called the triad. ER is endoplasmic reticulum. A mitochondrion is shown lying just underneath the sarcolemma. Reprinted with permission from Peachey and Fawcett, 1970, modified from *Journal of Cell Biology* 25, 209–231 (1965).

myosin molecule, and is the domain that binds to the thin actin filament. These are properties that the cross-bridges would be expected to have. The rod-like myosin tail can assemble without the head portion to form thick filaments that have no cross-bridges. The gap in the middle of the sarcomere where actin filaments from opposing Z-disks do not exist is called the psuedo H-zone (Figure 8.4); the M-line, which is seen only in electron micrographs of striated muscle, consists of a series of lines (three shown in Figure 8.4) that result from an end-on

view of cross sections of short filaments that connect thick filaments at their centers and keep them in register. One other myofibrillar protein not shown in the schematic diagrams in Figures 8.1 and 8.4 is the titin filament, which is a long, thin filament (smaller than the thin filament) that extends all the way from the Z-disk to the M-line and serves to connect the Z-disk to proteins in the thick filament and the M-line. It seems likely that titin filaments have a role in assembling myofibrils in developing muscle, serving as a scaffold for positioning newly

Table 8.3. Protein composition of the myofibril[a]

Protein Name	Location	Mass (daltons) and Number of Subunits/ Molecule[b]	% of Myofibril (w/w)
Myosin	Thick filament	516,000 (six) (two-220,000) (one-20,700) (two-19,050) (one-16,508)	44 %
Actin	Thin filament	41,785 (one)	22%
Titin	Length of sarcomere	~3,000,000 (one)	10%
Nebulin	Length of thin filament	600,000 to 800,000 (one)	5%
Tropomyosin	Thin filament	68,000 (two)[c]	5%
Troponin	Thin filament	69,000 (three) (one-30,503-TN-T) (one-20,864-TN-I) (one-17,846-TN-C)	5%
C-protein	Thick filament	140,000(one)	2%
Myomesin	M-line	165,000 (one)	2%
α-actinin	Z-disk	206,000 (two)[c]	2%
Creatine kinase	M-line	84,000 (two)[c]	<1%
Desmin	Z-disk-periphery	55,000 (one)	<1%
Filamin	Z-disk-periphery	500,000 (two)[c]	<1%
H-protein	Thick filament–M-line end	74,000 (one)	<1%
I-protein	Thick filament–A/I junction	100,000 (two)[c]	<1%
Synemin	Z-disk-periphery	460,000 (two)[c]	<1%

[a]The myofibril contains small amounts of proteins in addition to those listed. Some of these are in the Z-disk and some are associated with the thin filament (e.g., tropomodulin) and other areas of the myofibril.

[b]Subunit molecular masses of many of the myofibrillar proteins differ among slow-twitch, oxidative; fast-twitch, oxidative-glycolytic; and fast-twitch, glycolytic muscle fibers. Figures are for fast-twitch, glycolytic muscle fibers where the differences are known. The derived amino acid sequence is known for all of the myofibrillar proteins except H-protein and I-protein, although not all isoforms of each protein have been sequenced.

[c]Where number of subunits is indicated as two but the separate subunits are not listed, the molecules are homodimers.

synthesized myosin molecules. Other ultrastructural features of the myofibril are not discussed here because they are not critical to understanding muscle growth and development (see Goll et al. 1984, for more details on muscle structure).

Muscle Contraction

Muscle contraction commences when the myosin cross-bridges attach to the thin actin filaments, ATP is hydrolyzed, and the cross-bridges tilt or swivel to push the actin filaments toward the center of the sarcomere. This increases the degree of overlap between the thick and thin filaments, decreases the distance between opposing Z-disks, and shortens the sarcomere. Hence, the sliding filament mechanism

of muscle contraction directly explains the decrease in sarcomere length and the narrowing of the I-band observed years earlier in the light microscope. Length of the thick and thin filaments themselves does not change during muscle contraction, consistent with the previous light microscope observations that width of the A-band did not change during muscle contraction. Observations during the past 15 years have shown that the energy in ATP is used to "cock" the myosin cross-bridge and that hydrolysis of ATP itself results in little change in free energy. The cocked cross-bridge pushes the actin filaments toward the center of the sarcomere, and then detaches from the actin filament. Note that the cross-bridges in Figure 8.1 are in the cocked state, where-

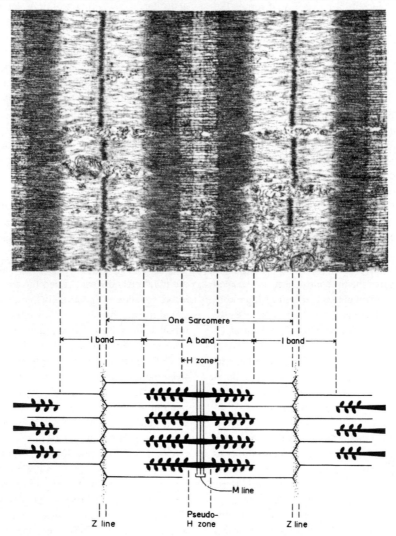

One Sarcomere

I band — A band — I band

H zone

M line

Pseudo-H zone

Z line   Z line

Figure 8.4. Electron micrograph of a longitudinal section of a mammalian skeletal muscle (top), and a diagram of a longitudinal view of the interdigitating thick and thin filament structure of the myofibril (bottom). The diagram is arranged so the thick and thin filaments are aligned with their locations in the electron micrograph. The M-line in the electron micrograph is very faint, as often occurs in electron micrographs, because the M-line is the end-on view of filaments running perpendicular to the long axis of the myofibril. The pseudo-H-zone, however, is clearly seen in this micrograph. Sarcomere length of the myofibril is ~2.5 μm, which is the normal sarcomere length for resting mammalian skeletal muscle. Elements of the sarcoplasmic reticulum can be seen in the I-band region between the myofibrils in the lower part of the micrograph. Electron micrograph is ~x28,000.

as the cross-bridges in Figure 8.4 are at the end of the contractile stroke (the "rigor" state). The hydrolyzed ATP, ADP, is then released, so the cross-bridge can bind another ATP, re-cock and undergo another cycle of binding to the thin filament, swiveling, and releasing from the thin filament.

Contraction can occur as long as ATP is available and all living cells have a number of mechanisms to maintain ATP availability for a variety of intracellular purposes; hence, contraction must be regulated to prevent continual contractile cycles in cells. In skeletal and cardiac muscle, this regulation is due to the presence of tropomyosin and troponin on the thin filament. In other contractile systems, such as smooth muscle, the regulation is due to the myosin S1 itself. The association between actin and myosin is ultimately responsible for contraction in skeletal, cardiac, and smooth muscle, and in all nonmuscle cells. Different isoforms of myosin and actin exist in these different cells, and the filaments formed by these different isoforms are not the same as the thick and thin filaments in Figures 8.1 and 8.4. Also, smooth muscle cells and nonmuscle cells do not contain troponin and have a tropomyosin isoform that is different from the one in skeletal muscle. These two differences together with a different myosin isoform result in contraction in striated muscle fibers being regulated differently than contraction in smooth muscle or nonmuscle cells. Nonmuscle contraction, or perhaps more accurately, nonmuscle motility, is mediated by one of several nonmuscle myosin isoforms and by actin filaments and is responsible for a wide variety of cellular functions, including cytokinesis following mitosis, alterations in cell shape, and movement of subcellular particles within cells.

Actin is a small, globular protein (Table 8.3) that aggregates in the presence of salt concentrations as low as 100 mM (ionic strength in skeletal muscle cells is ~150 mM) to form F-actin filaments; these filaments are the backbone of the thin filament in skeletal muscle. F-actin filaments resemble two strings of beads that are twisted around each other (bottom, Figure 8.1). In skeletal muscle thin filaments, the long rod-shaped tropomyosin molecules lie end-to-end in the grooves that are formed by the two strands of actin. The tropomyosin rods can be in either of two positions in the groove of the actin helix; if they are located in the outer edges of the groove, they block access of the myosin cross-bridge to actin and myosin cannot bind. Hence, there is no contraction when tropomyosin is in this position. If they move to the center of the groove, the myosin-binding site is exposed and contraction is initiated.

The position of tropomyosin in the grooves of the double-stranded actin helix is regulated by troponin. One troponin molecule has three different subunits (Table 8.3); troponin T is the subunit that binds to tropomyosin; troponin I is the subunit that binds to actin and to the other troponin subunits and influences tropomyosin's position in the actin helix; troponin C binds Ca^{2+}. Ca^{2+}-binding to TN-C alters the affinity of TN-I for actin, and results in movement of the tropomyosin "block" into the groove of the actin helix so the myosin cross-bridge can bind. Hence, initiation of contraction in skeletal muscle is regulated by binding of Ca^{2+} to the TN-C subunit of troponin. Because smooth muscle and nonmuscle motile systems do not contain troponin, they are regulated in an entirely different manner than contraction in skeletal muscle is.

TN-C binds Ca^{2+} whenever the intracellular Ca^{2+} concentrations increase to a level that allows binding by the TN-C molecule. What then regulates Ca^{2+} concentration in the skeletal muscle cell? The T-tubule system formed by invaginations of the sarcolemma was discussed earlier. An extensive three-dimensional, membranous network, called the *sarcoplasmic reticulum,* extends longitudinally parallel with and surrounding the myofibril from either side of the T-tubule (Figure 8.3). The sarcoplasmic reticular membranes contain a number of different proteins: among these is one that uses the energy of ATP to pump Ca^{2+} from the muscle cell cytoplasm into the lumen of the sarcoplasmic reticulum (SR), and another that binds large numbers of Ca^{2+} atoms in the lumen of the sarcoplasmic reticulum. Intracellular Ca^{2+} concentrations in skeletal muscle cells are maintained at 0.05–0.10 µM by this Ca^{2+} ATP pump. These concentrations are too low to allow binding of Ca^{2+} by TN-C. Depolarization of the sarcolemma and the T-tubule caused by release of acetylcholine at the neuromuscular junction initiates a signal in the SR that results in release of Ca^{2+} into the muscle cell cytoplasm. The intracellular Ca^{2+} concentrations in skeletal muscle cells may increase as much as tenfold, up to 0.5–1.0 µM. TN-C can bind Ca^{2+} at this concentration, triggering the movement of TN-I and tropomyosin and initiating muscle contraction. After the wave of depolarization passes, the intracellular Ca^{2+} is pumped back into the SR, the tropomyosin block is restored, and contraction ceases. This is a thumbnail sketch of the contraction/relaxation cycle in skeletal muscle and the proteins and membrane system involved. See Gordon et al. (2000) for a more detailed description of the events accompanying muscle contraction.

Muscle Fiber Types

Although the basic events accompanying contraction and relaxation are common to all skeletal muscles, some muscle fibers have adapted in subtle ways to meet specific needs. Some muscles may need to contract more rapidly than others; some may not need to contract rapidly but need to sustain contractile activity over long periods of time without rest. To meet these specific needs, muscle cells have developed metabolic and contractile properties that are suited to perform the tasks required of them.

Skeletal muscles in domestic animals (and other mammals including the human) contain three basic types of fibers (Table 8.4; Schiaffino and Reggiani 1996). A number of different systems of nomenclature have evolved to distinguish these different fiber types. In general, these systems distinguish the fiber types on the basis of their contractile speed as fast or slow, or on the basis of the predominant metabolic pathways used to provide energy for the muscle's activity. The three types and the names that will be used in this chapter are

- Slow-twitch, oxidative (SO)
- Fast-twitch, glycolytic (FG)
- Fast-twitch, oxidative/glycolytic (FOG)

Some other common names used for these types are

- SO = Type I = red = beta red
- FG = Type IIB = white = alpha white
- FOG = Type IIA = intermediate = alpha red

Fibers in the major skeletal muscles in domestic animals are all twitch fibers, but due to expression of specific isoforms of myosin and some other contractile proteins (the troponin subunits are expressed in a number of different isoforms), the contractile speed of different muscles may vary widely. Those fibers that are controlled by the same motor neuron, meaning that they are all part of the same motor unit, all have the same contractile speed and fiber type. Light microscopy and histochemical analysis of myosin ATPase has been widely used to distinguish between fast- and slow-contracting fibers. The three fiber types distinguished in this chapter differ with regard to contractile protein isoform expressed; they also differ metabolically and structurally.

Metabolically, the primary path for ATP synthesis for fibers classified as oxidative (SO and FOG) is aerobic, whereas the primary path for ATP synthesis for FG fibers is anaerobic (Table 8.4). Consequently, SO and FOG fibers are able to degrade glycogen via the citric acid (Krebs) cycle to produce CO_2 and H_2O. Oxidative fibers can also use fatty acids to generate ATP through β-oxidation and

the citric acid cycle. As a result, oxidative fibers have higher fatty acid content, succinate dehydrogenase content, and NADH dehydrogenase content than glycolytic fibers (Table 8.4). Because oxidative phosphorylation and electron transport generate ATP in the mitochondria, oxidative fibers also have a high mitochondria content (Table 8.4). In contrast, glycolytic fibers do not depend on oxidation of metabolites to CO_2 and H_2O, but use conversion of glycogen to lactic acid through glycolysis. The lactic acid is subsequently removed from the muscle and sent to the liver for further metabolism. This process generates less ATP, but is rapid and does not require oxygen. Hence, the rate of fatigue is rapid in FG fibers and is slow in FOG and SO fibers. The dependency on oxidative metabolism and high mitochondria content also requires that oxidative fibers have a high myoglobin content to ensure a supply of oxygen. Myoglobin is a red pigmented iron-carrying protein, and the high myoglobin content is the reason that oxidative fibers are redder in color than glycolytic fibers (Table 8.4). Indeed, muscles rich in oxidative or in glycolytic fibers are often simply referred to as "red" or "white" muscles, respectively. A good example of this is the glycolytic breast muscle and the oxidative leg muscles of the chicken.

There are also structural differences between oxidative and glycolytic fibers. SO fibers are generally smaller in diameter than glycolytic fibers, probably to facilitate rapid diffusion of O_2 into the middle of the fiber. Oxidative fibers have higher nuclei:cytoplasm ratios than glycolytic fibers, possibly because oxidative fibers contract more frequently and for longer periods of time than glycolytic fibers, which may result in a greater demand for protein synthesis in the oxidative fibers. Some of the other differences between oxidative and glycolytic fibers are listed in Table 8.4; in general, the differences between the fibers are logical considering their different physiological roles. A basic feature of glycolytic fibers is that they have the "fast" myosin and troponin isoforms. Fast myosin hydolyzes ATP at a faster rate than the "slow" myosin isoform, and the fast troponin isoforms also support a more rapid conversion of the "off" and "on" forms of the thin filament.

The physiological demands placed on a muscle can result in a switch in the myosin isoform synthesized and in the muscle fiber type. In general, SO fibers do not undergo a switch in muscle fiber type, but FG fibers can be transformed to FOG fibers in

Table 8.4. Some functional and structural properties of different muscle fiber types

Fiber Type	Fast-Twitch, Glycolytic; FG	Slow-Twitch, Oxidative; SO	Fast-Twitch, Oxidative-Glycolytic; FOG
Structural Characteristics			
Color	White	Red	Pink
Fiber diameter	Large	Small	Medium to small
Mitochondria	Few	Many	Many
Nuclei density	Low	High	Intermediate
Satellite cell density	Low	High	Intermediate
Capillary density	Sparse	Rich	Rich
Metabolic characteristics			
Twitch rate	Fast	Slow	Fast
Rate of fatigue	Fast	Slow	Intermediate
Myosin ATPase activity	Fast	Slow	Fast
Myoglobin content	Low	High	High
Primary pathway for ATP synthesis	Anaerobic	Aerobic	Aerobic
Contractile speed	Fast	Slow	Fast
Histochemistry			
Glycogen content	High	Low	Intermediate
Neutral fat content	Low	High	Intermediate
ATPase, pH 9.4	High	Low	High
ATPase, pH 4.3	Low	High	Low
Succinic dehydrogenase	Low	High	Medium to high
NADH dehydrogenase	Low	High	Medium to high

response to repeated, chronic demands for sustained activity, such as endurance running. This is physiologically reasonable, because endurance running requires muscles to maintain activity over extended periods of time, which would require oxidative metabolism. In contrast, activities that require expenditure of strength for short periods of time would best be accomplished by FG fibers, which are larger and therefore stronger than FOG fibers. Weight training or similar activities enhance the size of FG fibers and may shift FOG fibers to FG fibers. That muscle fiber types can shift from FOG to FG or vice versa has implications for animal agriculture, because a shift in fiber type can change the muscle mass without changing muscle fiber number. Certain growth promoters may preferentially act on specific muscle fiber types. It also seems likely that selective breeding pressure has resulted in an increase in the proportion of FG fibers in the muscles of domestic animals because such fiber types would result in larger muscles.

PRENATAL MUSCLE DEVELOPMENT

The cells that ultimately form muscle fibers originate from the mesodermal layer of the embryo. Cells of the mesoderm segregate into different regions, and the region of greatest interest to a discussion of muscle development is the somite. Somites are ball-like clusters of mesodermal cells that form on each side of the neural tube of the developing embryo. The dorsomedial domain generates muscles of the back, and the ventrolateral region of the somite gives rise to limb, abdominal, and intercostal muscles. The exquisitely coordinated process of cell proliferation, migration, and differentiation is mediated through the interplay of specific growth factors, cell surface receptors, and transcription factors.

A cascade of gene transcriptional transitions leads cells to become specific muscles in specific locations. Using the limb as an example, the transcription factor, Pax-3, is expressed in somite cells that migrate from the lateral edge of the somite into the forming limb bud. A specific growth factor receptor, c-met, is also expressed in these cells, which regulates the migration of these cells in response to the *hepatocyte growth factor (HGF)*. Therefore, synthesis of HGF in the developing limb bud attracts the future muscle cells into that region. When in the limb region, Pax-3 expression is turned off and expression of members of the muscle-specific transcription factor family is turned on. This important family of transcription factors known as the MyoD family regulates the expression of many muscle protein genes and the formation of multinucleated muscle fibers. In the mouse, premuscle masses are found in the limb by day 13 post coitum, and the initial muscle fibers are formed. This corresponds roughly to about 45–50 days in the human. In the human, the first immature muscle fibers are seen by 45 days, and by 50 days the basic organizational pattern for major muscles and bones is essentially complete. After the initial period of pattern formation, different muscles and even regions within a given muscle develop at different rates (see Hawke and Garry 2001; Ordahl 1999, for more details).

Not all muscle fibers within a muscle are formed simultaneously. "Primary fibers" are formed relatively early in development. These fibers have centrally located nuclei and contain myofibrils. Furthermore, they are surrounded by many mononucleated myogenic cells that will continue to divide and differentiate to form the remainder of the fibers, referred to as "secondary fibers." Secondary fibers actually form alongside the primary fibers and appear to use the primary fiber to assist in orientation. In the human *gastrocnemius* muscle, for example, well-developed primary myofibers are present by 62 days, but the majority of cells are still mononucleated muscle precursor cells. The percentage of mononucleated cells decreases to approximately 50% by day 72 and further diminishes to 20% by day 95. By day 146, only a small percentage of the cells are mononucleated and the remainder have formed multinucleated muscle fibers. In most animals, including man, fiber formation is essentially complete at the time of birth. Therefore, beyond birth or the neonatal period, muscle fiber number remains virtually constant. The exceptions to this statement are animals that are born in very immature states, such as mice or marsupials. In these animals, formation of new fibers persists for a period beyond birth. This is a very important concept, because it implies that growth of muscle postnatally must be due to enlargement of existing muscle fibers and not by the addition of new fibers.

One of the fundamental questions of developmental biology centers on the differentiation of cells and the role that changes in gene expression plays in determining the ultimate fate of cells. Cells destined to become muscle descend from common precursor cells in the mesoderm, but they do not immediately turn into muscle cells in just one generation. It appears that there is a myogenic lineage through which all muscle cells descend during the course of several generations, and as in all families, unique characteristics and capabilities develop within branches of the family tree through this process.

Several branches of the myogenic family tree have been defined or at least postulated to exist. The primary fibers formed early in development are the product of one branch of the lineage referred to as "early" myogenic cells. There may be several branches within this group that lead to fibers with slightly different contractile properties. The second major branch is responsible for forming secondary fibers, and these cells are referred to as "late" myogenic cells. These cells do not arise from the early myogenic cell class. They have different growth requirements and characteristics, including the dependence on innervation for secondary fiber formation. A third major branch of the myogenic family tree contains *satellite cells*. These cells function in postnatal muscle to assist in muscle growth and to regenerate new fibers following injury. As with early myogenic cells, the late myogenic cells and satellite cells may have subgroups that form fibers with different contractile speeds and energy metabolism preferences. Therefore, the formation of primary fibers, secondary fibers, or postnatal satellite cells is not a random process of differentiation or proliferation from a common pool of identical precursor cells. Rather, it is a carefully orchestrated series of divisions and alterations in gene expression that allows various subpopulations of cells to acquire unique characteristics that will guide their subsequent interactions and functions.

MYOGENESIS

The previous section has described the gross changes that take place in developing muscle and has indicated that these events are the result of transitions in gene expression, controlled by specific transcription factors. Although every step is critical to the formation of functional muscle, the final steps in muscle fiber formation have received the most attention. The discovery of the MyoD family of muscle-specific transcription factors was made in this context. This gene family is composed of four closely related proteins that are expressed sequentially during muscle cell differentiation. MyoD and myf5 are found in proliferating myogenic precursors followed by the expression of myogenin immediately before the final differentiation step. Finally, MRF4 is expressed at terminal differentiation (see Buckingham 2001, for more details).

Little is known of the properties of myogenic precursor cells from early in the lineage. Obviously, these cells are capable of division and are programmed to generate progeny that will ultimately differentiate into muscle. The last cell type in the myogenic lineage, immediately preceding the terminally differentiated phenotype, is referred to as a *myoblast*. These are the cells that express the MyoD family of transcription factors, and they are capable of differentiating only into muscle fibers. Studies conducted with cultured myogenic cells have shown that when myoblasts are cultured at very low densities (clonal density) so that colonies arise from individual cells, all cells in these colonies have the ability to divide and to differentiate into muscle fibers. Consequently, it is clear that myoblasts are proliferative cells that express unique proteins and that myoblasts can differentiate in one "step" to form the terminally differentiated cell type.

In its initial state, the terminally differentiated muscle cell is a spindle-shaped mononucleated cell called a *myocyte*. The myocyte has biosynthetic capabilities that are not possessed by the myoblast. For the first time, these cells are able to synthesize a large variety of proteins that are found only in the terminally differentiated muscle fiber. These include the myofibrillar proteins, acetylcholine receptors, sarcoplasmic reticulum proteins, and metabolic enzymes that are responsible for maintaining constant ATP concentrations in contracting muscle cells. The myocyte state is rather short-lived in most situations because among the hosts of new proteins being synthesized are those responsible for recognition of other myocytes and for fusion with other myocytes to form multinucleated cells.

The multinucleated cells that are formed initially are called *myotubes* because of their centrally located nuclei that are surrounded by developing myofibrils. As mentioned previously, histological cross-sections of these cells look like tubes. During the myotube stage, the contractile machinery is being assembled, and the unique sarcoplasmic reticular and T-tubule membrane systems are being formed. Innervation also takes place during this phase of maturation. As myotubes assemble myofibrils and become innervated, they begin to contract, and the contractile activity and increased accumulation of myofibrils probably results in displacement of nuclei to the subsarcolemmal location that is characteristic of mature muscle fibers. At this point, the cell has the appearance of a muscle fiber and is no longer referred to as a myotube. In reality, a myotube and a *myofiber* are not different cell types nor do they represent different states of differentiation, but they can be considered to be at different stages of maturation.

There are two important points to remember about prenatal muscle development and muscle fiber formation. One point of crucial importance in understanding muscle development and growth is the fact that nuclei in myocytes, myotubes, and myofibers do not replicate their DNA or divide. Therefore, the only dividing cells are myoblasts or their precursors; this concept has very important implications for postnatal muscle growth. The second point is that prenatal events that govern the extent of muscle precursor cell proliferation and the timing of differentiation determine the number of fibers a muscle will contain in postnatal life. Perhaps the most dramatic examples of this is found in the muscle hypertrophy seen in "double muscle" cattle which have more muscle fibers than their normal counterparts (McPherron et al. 1997). In general, genetic differences in muscularity between and within breeds of livestock are manifested during the embryonic and fetal stages of prenatal development when the pattern is being set.

POSTNATAL MUSCLE GROWTH

In general, cells in most tissues proliferate and differentiate during prenatal life, and during postnatal development, cells increase in size. The terms *hyperplasia* and *hypertrophy* refer to these two aspects of growth, increases in cell number and increases in cell size, respectively. During the early years of this century, histologists and anatomists found this generalization to be true for skeletal muscle of most mammals and birds. As discussed in the previous section, myogenic precursor cells are actively dividing and differentiating during embryonic and fetal life. However, the formation of new fibers comes to a halt shortly before or shortly after birth. In others words, the number of fibers that will exist in the mature muscle is essentially the same as the number found in the very young animal. There are exceptions to this rule, particularly in species in which parturition takes place at a relatively early stage in development. In mice and rats, for example, some fiber formation is still occurring for a couple of days after birth. The marsupials probably represent the most extreme example. In man and domestic animals, however, the rule holds, and fiber number is fixed at birth.

Even though muscle fiber number is fixed during the perinatal period, the number of nuclei in skeletal muscle continues to increase throughout the postnatal growth period. This has been demonstrated in mice, rats, chickens, sheep, cattle, and swine. In many muscles of mature animals, as much as 90% of the DNA in the muscle is synthesized during postnatal life. Clearly, this amount is too great to attribute to nonmuscle cells, such as connective tissue cells or cells in the vasculature. In fact, the majority of these nuclei are in muscle fibers.

But why must new nuclei be recruited? It has actually been demonstrated that each nucleus in a muscle fiber has a certain domain within the fiber for which it provides protein. These domains are not clearly delineated as if nuclei resided in individual cells, because proteins and other macromolecules can diffuse away from the site of synthesis, at least until they are incorporated into a subcellular organelle such as the myofibril. The size of these nuclear domains is dictated by the rate at which a nucleus can produce the various RNA species required to support protein synthesis and the rate at which protein is being degraded in that region of the fiber (Allen et al. 1999). The continual degradation and resynthesis of protein in the fiber is a common feature of all cells (Tipton and Wolfe 2001); therefore, there is a constant demand for protein synthesis in order to maintain constant muscle mass, even in mature muscle. By continual addition of nuclei to fibers during growth, fibers can maintain a nuclear:cytoplasmic ratio that permits efficient production and utilization of protein (Allen et al. 1979). In other words, the relatively small number of nuclei that may have formed the original myotube in the fetus could not be expected to direct the synthesis of all the proteins required by a large muscle fiber in a

mature animal. Because fiber formation is finished at birth and nuclei within muscle fibers do not divide, new nuclei must come from an outside source.

Satellite Cells

In 1961, Alexander Mauro reported on a previously undescribed cell type in skeletal muscle. These cells had very little cytoplasm and were found wedged between the basement membrane that surrounded the muscle fiber and the sarcolemma of the fiber (see Allen et al. 1998; Hawke and Garry 2001, for a more detailed description of satellite cells). He referred to these cells as "satellite cells" and predicted that they served as a reserve source of myogenic cells. It was demonstrated later that these cells had the ability to replicate DNA, divide, and fuse with the adjacent fiber (Figure 8.5). Through this process, new nuclei are added to muscle fibers during growth. In addition, it has been demonstrated that satellite cells are stimulated to add nuclei to muscle fibers during work-induced muscle hypertrophy. Furthermore, satellite cells are responsible for muscle regeneration. When a muscle is injured and muscle fibers die, satellite cells are stimulated to divide until a large number of mononucleated myogenic cells are generated, and then these cells begin to fuse to form new muscle fibers. These fibers generally form within the existing basement membrane tube that once encased the original muscle fiber. It is also noteworthy that a reserve population of satellite cells is retained after regeneration.

In very young animals, satellite cells may account for up to 10% of the nuclei associated with muscle fibers. This percentage, however, drops as the animal matures and finally stabilizes at about 3–6%. In some species, it has been shown that the fall in percentage of satellite cells is due to a net loss in satellite cells through differentiation and fusion. In other animals, such as the pig, the total number of satellite cells actually increases during growth even though the percentage of satellite cells to total muscle cells declines. The percentage depends to some extent on muscle fiber type; slow-twitch oxidative fibers generally have a higher percentage of satellite cells than fast-twitch fibers. When maturity is reached, the percentage declines very little.

Because there is very little DNA accretion taking place beyond maturity, there is very little satellite cell activity. Consequently, satellite cells spend most of their life in a quiescent or dormant state. Satellite cells in this state have only a thin rim of cytoplasm, and their nuclei appear to be inactive.

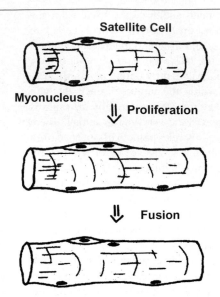

Figure 8.5. Satellite cell function in skeletal muscle growth. Satellite cells reside in close association with muscle fibers and are normally found in a dormant state. During muscle growth, satellite cells receive signals to divide and differentiate. Following division, it is thought that one daughter cell fuses with the fiber adjacent to it, and the other daughter cell remains a satellite cell.

Table 8.5. Protein growth factors that affect satellite cells

Growth Factors	Activation	Proliferation	Differentiation
Hepatocyte growth factor	Stimulates	Stimulates	Inhibits
Fibroblast growth factor (FGF)	No effect	Stimulates	Inhibits
Insulin-like growth factors (IGF)	No effect	Stimulates	Stimulates
Transforming growth factor β (TGF-β)	No effect	Inhibits	Inhibits
Myostatin	No effect	Inhibits	Inhibits

Few ribosomes or other intracellular organelles can be seen in quiescent satellite cells. Even in growing animals, satellite cells may not be dividing constantly. They may go through the cell cycle and exit mitosis into a protracted G_1 state, often referred to as G_0. Consequently, one important aspect of muscle growth regulation is the activation of satellite cells from their dormant state and the regulation of their proliferation and differentiation.

Satellite cell proliferation, differentiation, and quiescence are regulated directly by growth factors (Allen and Rankin 1990; Florini and Magri 1989). Although all of the details are not yet available, it is likely that many of the factor(s) are generated and stored within the muscle tissue. Many growth factors can be found in the basement membrane that surrounds muscle fibers and are therefore available for a rapid response to changes in muscle, such as stress or injury. For example, hepatocyte growth factor is thought to be responsible for activating quiescent satellite cells and stimulating their division. HGF has been shown to be released from its binding in the extracellular matrix of muscle when muscle is stretched or injured. Many other growth factors can be found in association with proteoglycans such as heparan sulfate proteoglycans outside muscle fibers.

Certain growth factors have been shown to affect satellite cell activation, proliferation, and differentiation, and these factors can be synthesized in the tissue itself. Most of the information available on growth factor effects has been derived from cell culture experiments (Allen et al. 1998), but these effects have recently been demonstrated in living muscle tissue. The growth factors listed in Table 8.5 currently represent the best candidates for satellite cell regulation.

The first factor noted to stimulate satellite cell division was fibroblast growth factor (FGF); this protein was originally isolated from brain tissue but has subsequently been found in many other tissues, including skeletal muscle. There are now about twenty members of the FGF gene family, and satellite cells have been shown to proliferate in response to several of these, including FGF2 (basic FGF), which is present in the extracellular matrix of muscle fibers.

Another family of protein growth factors that stimulate satellite cell division and differentiation is the insulin-like growth factor (IGF) family. IGF-I or somatomedin C was originally discovered by Daughaday in the late 1950s because of its relationship to growth hormone. It was demonstrated that somatomedin C mediated the action of growth hormone (somatotropin) at the cellular level—hence its name. Another group of investigators discovered the same protein in the course of their research on the action of insulin. They found a set of proteins that could stimulate some of the activities of insulin, but these proteins were not insulin. It was soon learned that the proteins, IGF-I and IGF-II, are very closely related to insulin and have many amino acid sequences in common, so they were named insulin-like growth factors. As investigators accumulated more information on the nature of IGF-I and somatomedin C, it became apparent that these two proteins were one and the same. IGFs can be found in the circulation in association with binding proteins that modify their activity, and they can be found in tissue. The importance of the IGFs to muscle growth has been demonstrated in experiments that artificially increased production of IGF-I in muscle by introduction of an IGF-I gene. Overexpresssing IGF-I in muscle of mice and pigs increased muscle growth in these species.

The IGFs stimulate proliferation and differentiation of embryonic myogenic cells and satellite cells. The particular activity that is stimulated, however, may depend on the presence of other growth factors, such as FGF. For example, if FGF is present, IGF may preferentially stimulate proliferation. IGF alone, however, will stimulate cultured satellite cells to differentiate and form myotubes. Consequently, the regulation of satellite cells may be more complex than one hormone or growth factor acting on a cell to stimulate a single response.

Finally, a third family of growth factors have been shown to have dramatic effects on myoblasts of embryonic origin as well as satellite cells. These are the transforming growth factors of the beta class (TGF-β). TGF-β1 and TGF-β2 are both very potent inhibitors of differentiation; not even IGF-I can stimulate differentiation if TGF-β is present. The factors can also inhibit satellite cell division in cells from bovine, rat, and porcine muscle; this property may be more variable, however. For example, division of ovine cells apparently is not inhibited by TGF-β, and satellite cell proliferation proceeds even in the presence of TGF-β if FGF is present. So again, the interactions of growth factors may determine the activity of satellite cells. TGF-β may be particularly interesting because it is present in very high quantities in blood platelets and is released when these platelets become activated. This happens when tissue is injured; therefore, TGF-β would be expected to be present in injured muscle and could play a role in regulating satellite cells during regeneration. It has recently been shown that a new member of the TGFβ super-family of genes, myostatin, is the gene whose mutation is the cause of the double muscle condition. When this gene was mutated in mice or cattle, it resulted in a loss of inhibition of myoblast proliferation and differentiation which caused more muscle fibers and increased muscle size.

As satellite cells are exposed to different growth factors or combinations of growth factors, they can be expected to either divide, differentiate, or become quiescent. Currently, an important area of growth biology research centers around the regulation of growth factor production and action in muscle tissue and the manner in which endocrinology, nutrition, and exercise influence these events.

Hypertrophy of Muscle Fibers and Muscle Protein Degradation

The preceding two sections have discussed the formation of muscle fibers during prenatal life and have shown how satellite cells add nuclei to fibers during postnatal development. This section reviews how the cellular framework established during postnatal development accumulates muscle proteins and grows. This process is referred to as muscle fiber hypertrophy. As mentioned in the previous section, all cells are constantly synthesizing and degrading protein, and the balance between these two processes determines whether protein content increases, decreases, or remains constant. For example, if the rate of protein synthesis is equal to the rate of protein degradation, there is no net change in muscle protein content. During growth, however, the rate of protein synthesis must be greater than the rate of protein degradation in order to accumulate protein in a cell (Tipton and Wolfe 2001). Finally, in a cell that is decreasing in size and protein content, the rate of degradation must exceed the rate of protein synthesis. This is a simple mathematical concept, but it is central to a discussion of muscle fiber hypertrophy.

If contractile proteins are continually synthesized and degraded in muscle fibers, mechanisms must exist for inserting and removing proteins from the highly organized myofibril. For years this was a perplexing problem because entire sarcomeres or myofibrils were not found in states of assembly or degradation in normal muscle when examined with the electron microscope. Today, it has come to be appreciated that myofibrils are not rigid permanent structural entities, but they are very dynamic structures.

Increases in myofibril length and diameter occur as muscle fibers grow. Only after extensive ultrastructural examination was it discovered that growth in myofibril length does not occur by extending the length of individual sarcomeres, nor does growth in length occur by inserting new sarcomeres at random along the myofibril. Myofibrils grow in length by adding new sarcomeres at the ends of myofibrils. This process maintains the integrity of the myofibril while permitting the length of the myofibril to increase as the muscle fiber increases in length.

Myofibrils increase in diameter by adding new thick and thin filaments to the periphery of existing myofibrils. The very nature of myofibrillar proteins drives these proteins to aggregate in very specific ways to form filaments. Consequently, as proteins such as myosin and actin are synthesized on polyribosomes, they assemble into new filaments, and these new filaments associate with existing filaments in myofibrils. Therefore, the new filaments are added to the surface of myofibrils, and they are integrated into the structure.

The logical extension of this process would result in a relatively small number of very large myofibrils within each muscle fiber, but this is not the case. Within muscle fibers, myofibrils increase in length, diameter, and number. The mechanism that enables myofibrils to increase in number is myofibril splitting. When myofibrils reach a certain diameter, it is thought that the force generated by contraction facilitates longitudinal splitting of the myofibril, resulting in two smaller myofibrils. The precise regulation of myofibril splitting has not been established, and it may be common even in myofibrils that are not increasing in diameter. One theory on myofibril growth and assembly suggests that

myofibrils are dynamic structures that may split and possibly fuse continuously. This suggestion is based on ultrastructural evidence of myofibril splitting. The dynamic nature of myofibrils may also be an important aspect of muscle protein degradation. As indicated before, new myofilaments are added to the periphery of existing myofibrils, and degradation of myofilaments also may occur preferentially in this region. Therefore, myofibril fission would expose myofilaments that had been in the interior of myofibrils, thus subjecting these myofilaments to degradation.

Degradation of muscle proteins is one of the most critical but possibly least understood aspects of muscle growth. As described previously, this process occurs continuously and is highly regulated and balanced with protein synthesis. The factors responsible for muscle protein degradation and how rate of degradation is regulated are not well understood, however. It is clear that degradation of intracellular proteins must be mediated by proteolytic enzymes and that these proteolytic enzymes must be located intracellularly (Sugden and Fuller 1991). There are three classes of intracellular proteolytic enzymes that are present in quantities sufficient to sustain the level of proteolysis needed to turnover muscle proteins (Table 8.6) (the caspases, which degrade proteins during apoptosis, have substantial proteolytic capability, but are not involved in muscle growth and are active only in response to an apoptotic signal). In classical cell biology, the lysosome has been assigned the role of intracellular protein degradation, but lysosomes are difficult to identify ultrastructurally in skeletal muscle. The sarcoplasmic reticulum may also serve as lysosomes in skeletal muscle, because lysosomal enzymes have been found in this structure. However, large myofibril fragments have not been observed in membrane-bound vesicles that resemble lysosomes, and lysosomes have not been observed in association with myofibrils. Moreover, the proteolytic enzymes in lysosomes, the cathepsins, are not active at the neutral pH values in muscle cell cytoplasm, so any lysosomal degradation of myofibrils would need to occur inside the lysosome. Therefore, other mechanisms for degradation of myofibrillar proteins must exist.

The most likely mechanism for myofibrillar protein degradation would require proteases that are located in the cytoplasm and that selectively cleave those proteins in the myofibril that would lead to disassembly of the filaments around the edges of the myofibril. Individual proteins or released filaments

Table 8.6. Three major intracellular proteolytic systems that may be involved in skeletal muscle growth

Proteolytic System	Characteristics
Lysosomal system	Enzymes are localized in lysosomal structures that have very acidic interior pH (intralysosomal pH is 3–5); a number of lysosomal proteases, cathepsins, have been identified and are numbered cathepsin A through cathepsin S, cathepsin X, etc.; a major function of lysosomes is to degrade endocytosed proteins, including some hormone receptors, but because there is very little endocytosis in muscle cells (fibers), muscle cells have relatively few lysosomes and hence relatively low cathepsin activity; not all the cathepsins that have been identified are found in muscle lysosomes; the major cathepsins in muscle cells are cathepsin B, cathepsin D, and cathepsin L; *lysosomes cannot engulf intact myofibrils, and thick and thin filaments have never been observed in lysosomal structures*; because the lysosomal cathepsins are inactive at the cytoplasmic pH of living cells (pH 7.0–7.5), they cannot degrade the myofibrillar proteins outside the myofibril; *hence, lysosomal cathepsins likely have a minimal role in the normal metabolic turnover of myofibrillar proteins.*
Proteasome	Major enzyme system responsible for intracellular protein degradation; analogous to the ribosome in protein synthesis; large (1,500 kDa; 26 S) multisubunit structure shaped like a barrel with the active site of the proteases in the central cavity of the barrel; has at least four different kinds of proteolytic activities in one structure; will degrade polypeptide chains to peptides of 6–12 amino acids in a single pass through the center cavity; present in every organism from bacteria to mammals; located in the cell cytoplasm and optimally active at pH 7.0–8.0, so its activity is regulated by access to the central cavity of the barrel to prevent indiscriminate protein degradation; because the entrance to the central cavity is 10–13 Å, *the proteasome cannot degrade myofibrillar proteins until they have been removed from the myofibril*; the proteasome likely has the major role in degrading sarcoplasmic proteins and in degrading myofibrillar proteins *after they have been removed from the myofibril.*
Calpain system	Consists of three well-characterized proteins in muscle cells; two proteolytic enzymes; μ-calpain, a Ca^{2+}-dependent protease that requires 3–50 μM Ca^{2+} for half-maximal activity, and m-calpain, a Ca^{2+}-dependent protease that requires 300–500 μM Ca^{2+} for half-maximal proteolytic activity; and calpastatin, a protein whose only known function is to inhibit the activity of the two calpains; other calpains have been identified as mRNAs, including one specific to skeletal muscle (calpain 3a), but they have not been isolated in protein form and their functions are unknown; the calpains are maximally active at pH 7.2–7.8, and are located in the cell cytoplasm; their activity is regulated by some as yet unknown factor in cells; the calpains do not degrade proteins to amino acids, but they do degrade those proteins in the myofibril that are involved in assembly of the myofibrillar structure; titin and nebulin are degraded at the point where they enter the Z-disk and desmin and troponin and tropomyosin are degraded; the *evidence indicates that the calpains are responsible for disassembly of myofibrillar proteins to release them from the surface of the myofibril* and make them available for subsequent degradation by the proteasome (or lysosomal cathepsins).

may then be attacked by other proteolytic systems that would degrade the released proteins to peptides and eventually to amino acids (Goll et al. 1992).

As in most metabolic processes, the initial steps in myofibrillar protein turnover may be the key to regulation. The most likely candidates for initiating myofibrillar protein turnover are the calpains, μ- and m-calpain (Table 8.6). These two closely related proteinases are activated by calcium ions, as are many other important biochemical regulatory events, and they are also subject to inhibition by a specific protein inhibitor, calpastatin. The precise biochemical details of calpain regulation have not been firmly established; however, these enzymes are elevated in muscle tissue under conditions expected to result in greater degradation of protein. Moreover, calpastatin activities are increased in conditions where muscle protein turnover is decreased. Finally, the calpains selectively cleave many of the key proteins responsible for keeping the myofibrillar proteins assembled in the myofibrillar structure (Goll et al. 1992, 1998). The calpains were discovered because of their ability to rapidly remove Z-lines from myofibrils. Subsequently, the calpains were demonstrated to cleave desmin, a protein that connects Z-disks in adjacent myofibrils and attaches Z-disks to the sarcolemma; to degrade titin and nebulin at the points where they enter the Z-disk, thereby severing the connections of the Z-disk to the remainder of the sarcomere; and to degrade C-protein, tropomyosin, and troponin (Table 8.6), proteins that act to keep the myosin molecules assembled in thick filaments (C-protein) and actin molecules assembled in thin filaments (tropomyosin and troponin). It is interesting to note that calpains are localized in the cytoplasm but appear to be found in highest concentration at the Z-disk region of the myofibril.

The proteasome is the third cytoplasmic proteolytic system found in skeletal muscle (Table 8.6; see Attaix et al. 1998; Glickman and Cienchanover 2002, for recent reviews on the proteasome). A large amount of evidence obtained during the last 10 years has shown that the proteasome is the major proteolytic system responsible for intracellular protein degradation, not only in skeletal muscle cells but in all cells from bacteria to mammals. The proteasome is a large protein complex that can be seen in the electron microscope and that is composed of 28 subunit polypeptides assembled in the form of a large hollow cylinder or barrel-like structure approximately 11–12 nm in diameter and 14–17 nm long. The proteasome has four different proteolytic activities; the active sites of all four activities are in the hollow center of the cylinder. The proteasome is present in large amounts in the cell cytoplasm, so its activity must be carefully regulated to prevent unwanted and indiscriminate degradation of intra-

cellular proteins. Current evidence indicates that activity of the proteasome is regulated in at least two ways:

- The proteasome prefentially degrades polypeptides that have been ubiquitinated, so the polypeptides must be tagged with ubiquitin before they are readily degraded by the proteasome.
- The entrance to the central hole of the proteasome containing the catalytically active sites is 1–1.3 nm in diameter, so large protein complexes such as thick or thin filaments (14–16 nm and 6–8 nm in diameter, respectively) physically cannot enter the central cavity of the proteasome until they have been dissembled to their polypeptides.

Moreover, entrance to the central cavity of the proteasome is regulated by a group of proteins that are attached to either end of the cylindrical proteasome structure and that serve as "gatekeepers" to the entrance. Entrance of ubiquitinated polypeptides is favored, and it is unlikely that the myofibrillar proteins could be ubiquitinated until they are disassembled from the myofibril. Hence, although the proteasome can degrade polypeptide chains to peptides of 6–12 amino acids in a single pass, it cannot degrade the myofibrillar proteins until they have been disassembled from the myofibril. It presently seems, therefore, that the calpains and the proteasome act in concert to degrade myofibrillar proteins (Hasselgren 1999). The proteasome is present in large amounts in cells, and the rate of substrate ubiquitination is the rate-limited step in proteasome-mediated proteolysis. Several recent studies have shown that expression of ubiquitinating enzymes specific for skeletal muscle is up-regulated in several models of muscle wasting. That these enzymes are likely to be rate-limiting in proteasome-mediated degradation of muscle proteins suggests that the proteasome has an important role in muscle protein turnover. Finally, it should be indicated explicitly that the proteasome can degrade the sarcoplasmic proteins directly because they do not need to be disassembled from a larger structure.

Modulation of Muscle Mass

Muscle mass can be increased or decreased in adult or growing animals by several physiological conditions. The obvious conditions that decrease muscle mass are injury, starvation, disuse, and aging. On the positive side are factors such as work-induced hypertrophy and certain drug or hormone treatments. These last two factors are not discussed in this chapter, but some of these modulating conditions will be presented in order to demonstrate how all these changes can be explained in the context of the previous discussions of mechanisms of muscle growth (see Cameron-Smith 2002; Goldspink 1996, 1998, for a more detailed discussion of factors affecting skeletal muscle growth).

Muscle mass can be increased by exercise, as is commonly found in athletic training. The type of exercise determines whether muscle size increases. For instance, small workloads over a long time period, as in the case of endurance training, result in a relatively small change in muscle mass when compared to the increased mass that results from heavy workloads over a short time, such as weight lifting. The actual increase in muscle mass that results from work-induced hypertrophy is due to an increase in myofibrillar protein content, which leads to fiber hypertrophy. Hypertrophy also appears to be fiber-type–specific, with fast-twitch fibers responding preferentially.

Although work-induced hypertrophy is often attributed to increased protein synthesis, satellite cells have also been shown to become activated under these conditions. Activation of satellite cells leads to the addition of nuclei to fibers, and in extreme cases, to the formation of new fibers. Stretch-induced hypertrophy, a form of hypertrophy that may be closely related to work-induced hypertrophy, is accompanied by increased satellite cell activity and the addition of nuclei to fibers. The specific mechanisms responsible for satellite cell activation in work-induced hypertrophy may be the same regulatory mechanisms that control muscle regeneration following injury.

Fortunately, muscle is one of the tissues in the body that possesses amazing regenerative abilities. In the case of large animals, this property of muscle becomes important during certain phases of production when confinement and transportation lead to crowding and increased incidence of bruising. Another common cause of muscle damage is injection of antibiotics, vaccines, and local anesthetics. A significant amount of money is lost every year due to abscess or scar tissue formation at injection sites; in other words, when normal muscle regeneration fails, there are important economic consequences. Interestingly, application of a local anesthetic has been used extensively as an experimental model for studying muscle degeneration and regeneration.

Muscle regeneration can also be induced following extreme exercise training, as in the case of race training in horses.

Mild injuries can result in segmental damage to muscle fibers, where a small region is damaged but the entire fiber does not die. In the case of segmental damage, the sarcolemma on each side of the damaged region seals off, and satellite cells migrate to the region. Satellite cells proliferate, differentiate, and fuse with the sealed ends of the fiber on each side of the damaged area. Fusion of satellite cells results in bridging between the sealed ends to reconnect the fiber as a contiguous cell.

In cases of severe injury, entire fibers may die and must be replaced. Following damage to the muscle, the affected fibers die and the organelles and contractile machinery begin to be degraded. The sarcolemma is also disrupted, but the basal lamina remains intact. Initial degradation of intracellular constituents results from the liberation and activation of intracellular proteases and nucleases; however, with the dissolution of the sarcolemma, macrophages invade the area and remove the remainder of the cellular debris. The next step in the regenerative process is activation of satellite cells. Maximum proliferation is often observed approximately three days post-injury. These cells proliferate to form a large population of myogenic cells which subsequently fuse to create new myofibers. Proliferation and differentiation of satellite cells proceeds in a fashion similar to that found in embryonic muscle development. The newly formed myofibers contain centrally located myonuclei, a distinguishing feature in regenerated myofibers, but the myonuclei migrate to the periphery of the fiber as the fiber matures. In addition, quiescent satellite cells are maintained as in uninjured muscle and await another activation stimulus.

In damaged muscle, repair must include not only myogenesis but the generation of new blood vessels to supply the regenerated muscle fibers and the formation of new nerve connections. The process of formation of a new vascular network in damaged muscle is called angiogenesis and must be coordinated with new muscle fiber formation. New nerve connections, re-innervation, of the myofibers occurs later. Nerves arise from regrowth of existing axons from the motor neurons or from the branching, or sprouting, of neighboring nerves. The nerve axons form functional neuromuscular junctions by making contact with basal lamina in areas of previous junction sites. The regeneration of the fiber is now complete, and the fiber will mature and become essentially indistinguishable from nondamaged fibers (for more details on muscle injury, see Carlson and Faulkner 1983).

Muscle atrophy in livestock is generally caused by malnutrition, aging, disuse or dennervation. In the case of malnutrition, the decrease in muscle mass is the result of a decrease in muscle fiber diameter. This also holds true for atrophy due to disuse; as might be expected, fast-twitch fibers are affected to greater extent than slow-twitch fibers. Aging can lead to decreased fiber diameter, and in some muscles, the loss of fibers. The end result of muscle atrophy is a decrease in muscle mass, which in turn leads to a decrease in muscle performance.

SUMMARY

This chapter summarizes some elementary background on the structure and function of skeletal muscle. The treatment of the subject has not been intended to be comprehensive or detailed; only enough information to facilitate the subsequent discussion of muscle development and growth has been presented. Muscle growth and development can be viewed as the interplay between the cellular aspects of development and the protein metabolism and growth of differentiated fibers. Cellular aspects of muscle development occupy center stage prenatally as myogenic cells proliferate and differentiate to form fibers; however, this process continues during postnatal life through the activities of satellite cells. These events provide a cellular framework for muscle hypertrophy. Muscle hypertrophy, or muscle fiber growth, is a function of protein synthesis and protein degradation; the balance between the positive and negative sides of this cycle of protein turnover determines the net increase or decrease in muscle mass. Many factors affect these basic processes, foremost of which are genetically programmed developmental patterns, nutritional background, and level/type of muscle activity. In summary, efficient and profitable growth and development of skeletal muscle in meat animals is dependent on wise animal husbandry and breeding practices.

ACKNOWLEDGMENTS

We thank Janet Christner for help in preparing and formating the manuscript, and Valery Thompson for preparing Figures 8.4 and 8.5. The authors' research programs have been supported by grants from the Muscular Dystrophy Association; the American Heart Association, Arizona Affiliate; the NIH; and the National Research Initiative Competitive Grants Program, Nos. 2001-35503-10776, 2002-35206-11630, and 95040-74.

REFERENCES

Allen, D.L., Roy, R.R., Edgerton, V.R., and Edgerton, V.R. 1999. Myonuclear domains in muscle adaptation and disease. *Muscle & Nerve* 22:1350–1360.

Allen, R.E., Merkel, R.A., and Young, R.B. 1979. Cellular aspects of muscle growth: myogenic cell proliferation. *Journal of Animal Science* 49:115–127.

Allen, R.E., and Rankin, L.L. 1990. Regulation of satellite cells during skeletal muscle development. *Proceedings of the Society of Experimental Biology and Medicine* 194:81–86.

Allen, R.E., Temm-Grove, C.J., Sheehan, S.M., and Rice, G. 1998. Skeletal muscle satellite cell cultures. *Methods in Cellular Biology* 52:155–176.

Attaix, D., Aurousseau, E., Combaret, L., Kee, A., Larbaud, D., Ralliere, C., Souweine, B., Taillandier, D., and Tilignac, T. 1998. Ubiquitin-proteasome-dependent proteolysis in skeletal muscle. *Reproduction, Nutrition et Development* 38:153–165.

Buckingham, M. Skeletal muscle formation in vertebrates. 2001. *Current Opinions in the Genetics of Development* 11:440–448.

Cameron-Smith, D. 2002. Exercise and skeletal muscle gene expression. *Clinical Experimental Pharmacology and Physiology* 29:209–213.

Carlson, B.M., and Faulkner, J.A. 1983. The regeneration of skeletal muscle fibers following injury: a review. *Medical Science of Sports Exercise* 15:187–198.

Florini, J.R., and K.A. Magri. 1989. Effects of growth factors on myogenic differentiation. *American Journal of Physiology* 256:C701–C711.

Glickman, M.H., and Cienchanover, A. 2002. The ubiquitin-proteasome proteolytic pathway: destruction for the sake of construction. *Physiological Reviews* 82:373–428.

Goldspink, G. 1996. Muscle growth and muscle function: a molecular biological perspective. *Research in Veterinary Science* 60:193–204.

Goldspink, G. 1998. Cellular and molecular aspects of muscle growth, adaptation, and ageing. *Gerodontology* 15:35–43.

Goll, D.E., Robson, R.M., and Stromer, M.H. 1984. Skeletal muscle, nervous system, temperature regulation, and special senses. In *Dukes Physiology of Domestic Animals*, 10th ed. M.J. Swenson, ed. Ithaca, New York: Cornell University Press.

Goll, D.E., Thompson, V.F., Taylor, R.G., and Christiansen, J.A. 1992. Role of the calpain system in muscle growth. *Biochimie* 74:225–237.

Goll, D.E., Thompson, V.F., Taylor, R.G., and Ouali, A. 1998. The calpain system and skeletal muscle growth. *Canadian Journal of Animal Science* 78:503–512.

Gordon, A.M., Homsher, E., and Regnier, M. 2000. Regulation of contraction in striated muscle. *Physiological Reviews* 80:853–924.

Gould, R.P. 1973. *The Structure and Function of Muscle*, 2nd ed. vol. 2. G.H. Bourne, ed. New York: Academic Press.

Grant, A.L., and Gerrard, D.E. 1998. Cellular and molecular approaches for altering muscle growth and development. *Canadian Journal of Animal Science* 78:493–502.

Hasselgren, P-O. 1999. Pathways of muscle protein breakdown in injury and sepsis. *Current Opinions in Clinical Nutrition and Metabolic Care* 2:155–160.

Hawke, T.J., and Garry, D.J. 2001. Myogenic satellite cells: physiology to molecular biology. *Journal of Applied Physiology* 91:534–551.

McPherron, A.C., Lawler, A.M., and Lee, S-J. 1997. Regulation of skeletal muscle mass in mice by a new TGF-β superfamily member. *Nature* 387:83–90.

Novikoff, A.B., and Holtzman, E. 1984. *Cells and Organelles*. New York: Holt, Rinehart, and Winston.

Ordahl, C.P. 1999. Myogenic shape-shifters. *Journal of Cell Biology* 147:695–697.

Peachey, L.D., and Fawcett, D.W. 1970. Cells and Organelles. New York: Holt, Reinhart, and Winston. Modified from *Journal of Cell Biology* 25: 209–231 (1965).

Schiaffino, S., and Reggiani, C. 1996. Molecular diversity of myofibrillar proteins: gene regulation and functional significance. *Physiological Review* 76:371–423.

Sugden, P.H., and Fuller, S.J. 1991. Regulation of protein turnover in skeletal and cardiac muscle. *Biochemical Journal* 273:21–37.

Tipton, K.D., and Wolfe, R.R. 2001. Exercise, protein metabolism, and muscle growth. *International Journal of Sports Nutritional Exercise Metabolism* 11:109–132.

Wolfe, R.R. 2002. Regulation of muscle protein by amino acids. *Journal of Nutrition* 132:3219S–3224S.

9
Bone Growth

Colin Farquharson

Bone is a complex tissue made up of living cells enmeshed in a mineralized collagenous rich matrix. The inorganic mineral provides strength and resists compression, whereas the organic collagen fibers withstand tension and torsion. Bone has three main functions:

- To provide a supportive framework for the body including attachment points for muscle, which are essential for locomotion
- To serve as a store for calcium and phosphorus that can be made available during disturbances in mineral homeostasis
- To protect internal organs, such as the brain (skull) and heart and lungs (ribs)

Bones grow in two directions: through a cartilage template to increase its length (longitudinal or endochondral growth), and through the formation of new bone on the outer surfaces of existing bone to increase its width (appositional growth). This chapter focuses on the endochondral process as it provides for the elongation of most of the skeletal mass during growth and is ultimately connected with overall body growth. For completeness, however, a brief description of the appositional growth process is given.

The mechanisms of long bone growth are similar across many animal species. There are, however, major variations in the growth rate between similar bones of different species, bones of an individual animal and the two growing regions (growth plates) of the same bone. Similarly, diverse rates of appositional growth also occur, and these variations are a consequence of differences in the activities of the cartilage forming chondrocyte and the bone-forming osteoblast. To fully appreciate the bone growth process, a thorough understanding of the diverse range of cell and matrix associated events is required. A description of these forms the basis of this chapter.

HISTORICAL REVIEW

An understanding of how long bones grow was first obtained by Stephen Hales in 1727. He positioned pins into the proximal and distal bone shaft (diaphysis) of the tibia of young chickens and after several weeks in which the tibia had grown in length he noted that the distance between the marker pins had remained unchanged. This pioneering work provided clear evidence that long bones, like trees, grow in length from the active growth regions at their ends. It was not, however, until the next century in 1836 that the basic mechanism of endochondral ossification, was first described. This was followed 9 years later by the first complete description of the growth plate by Todd and Bowmann (Trueta 1968). Since these early studies, further investigations have revealed the fine anatomical structure of the growth plate and the underlying molecular control of chondrocyte function. Such studies have substantiated the pivotal role of the growth plate in longitudinal bone growth.

EMBRYONIC BONE

Embryonic bone formation occurs through two distinct processes. Intramembranous growth results in the formation of flat bones—such as the cranium, mandible, and scapula—whereas the process of endochondral growth accounts for the formation of long bones—such as the tibia, femur, and humerous. Both mechanisms result in bone formation, but the endochondral growth process and the activities of cartilaginous growth plate are responsible for bone growth. This chapter confines itself to this latter process.

Long bones of the skeleton first appear as limb buds, and the earliest observable morphological event in this process (between 10.5 and 12.5 days postcoitum in the embryonic mouse) is the aggregation of committed, undifferentiated mesenchymal cells into structures known as precartilage condensations. These cells differentiate into chondrocytes and secrete extracellular matrix, resulting in the formation of a cartilaginous template of the future bone. Concomitant with this, other mesenchymal cells at the periphery of the template differentiate to form a perichondrial sheath. The proliferating chondrocytes within the cartilage template eventually hypertrophy and this is accompanied by the expression of markers of the terminally differentiated chondrocyte—alkaline phosphatase (ALP) activity and collagen type X. Perichondrial cells around the mid-diaphyseal region of the cartilage model differentiate into osteoblasts and begin to lay down a bony collar. This primary bone collar is penetrated by blood vessels that gain access to the underlying cartilage template, bringing elements that will form the bone marrow together with osteoclasts that erode the internal calcified cartilage (Howell and Dean 1992). Osteoclastic resorption continues toward both ends of the template forming the primary ossification center, with osteoblasts replacing the eroded cartilage with new lamellar bone. At about birth in mammals, a secondary ossification center develops in the cartilage of the epiphyseal region, and a transverse flat disc of cartilage situated between the two centers of ossification forms the epiphyseal growth plate (Figure 9.1). This assumes the specialized function of elongation and growth during postnatal bone formation.

POSTNATAL BONE GROWTH

General Principles

The growth plate cartilage comprises both chondrocytes and their extracellular matrix where proteoglycans and collagen type II predominate. A characteristic of endochondral bone growth is the precise temporal and spatial organization of chondrocytes within the growth plate where they differentiate through a series of maturational stages while remaining in a spatially fixed location throughout its existence (Hunziker et al. 1987, Figure 9.2). The time taken for a chondrocyte to differentiate from a proliferative to a hypertrophic phenotype is species-dependent and is approximately 21 hours in the meat-type chicken and 2 days in the rat (Thorp 1988; Kember and Sissons 1976). Undifferentiated progenitors within the reserve stem cell zone differentiate into chondrocytes and progress through a proliferative phase. In the proliferative zone, the

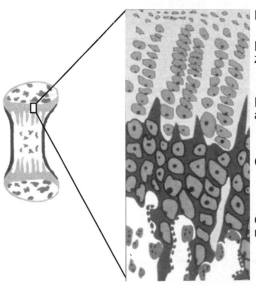

Resting layer

Proliferative zone

Differentiation and Hypertrophy

Calcification

Osteoclastic resorption

Figure 9.1. Schematic representation of the position of the growth plate at the ends of a long bone. The cellular zones of the growth plate that are comprised of chondrocytes at various stages of differentiation are also illustrated.

cells have a flattened, oblate shape and the percentage of dividing chondrocytes within the rat and chicken growth plate has been estimated at 12% and 24%, respectively (Farquharson and Loveridge 1990; Farquharson et al. 1992, Figure 9.3). Immediately after the cessation of cell division, the cells change to a spherical prolate form and undergo terminal differentiation into hypertrophic chondrocytes (Breur et al. 1994) where the chondrocytes become more voluminous with increases in rough endoplasmic reticulum and Golgi apparatus, reflecting increased matrix production (Buckwalter et al. 1986). Associated with this hypertrophic phenotype are increased membrane ALP activity and expression of collagen type X, chondrocalcin, osteonectin and osteopontin, and the down regulation of collagen type II expression. The volume of hypertrophic chondrocytes is approximately 10 times larger than the volume of proliferative chondrocytes, and chondrocyte height increases up to fivefold (in the direction of growth) between the proliferative and hypertrophic zones (Hunziker et al. 1987). Consequently,

the growth plate can be divided into several distinct zones containing resting, proliferating, maturing, and terminally differentiated hypertrophic chondrocytes (Figure 9.1).

Histologically, the chondrocytes are arranged in columns that parallel the longitudinal axis of the bone. Each column and each chondrocyte within a column are respectively separated by longitudinal and transverse septa made up of a collagenous and proteoglycan rich extracellular matrix (Figure 9.4). Although a smooth transition exists between each maturational zone, the cells of each region are distinguished by differences in their rate of proliferation, morphology, and biosynthetic ability of matrix proteins (Hunziker and Schenk 1989; Breur et al. 1994; Buckwalter et al. 1986; Hunziker et al. 1987; Farnum and Wilsman 1987, 1993). During terminal differentiation, mineralization of the matrix surrounding the hypertrophic chondrocytes occurs; this, however, is limited to the longitudinal septa, and no mineralization is observed in the transverse septa. Functionally, the matrix changes to an envi-

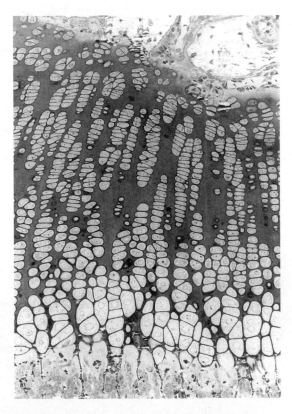

Figure 9.2. The histological architecture of the growth plate in the distal tibia of a 28-day-old Long-Evans rat. (Reprinted with permission from Wilsman et al., 1996a.)

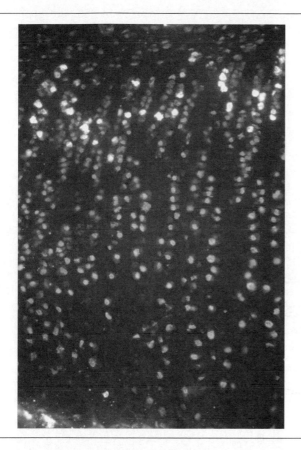

Figure 9.3. Photomicrograph of a metatarsal growth plate from a 21-day-old Hooded Lister rat showing the distribution of dividing cells as demonstrated by the BrdU technique. Chondrocyte proliferation was limited to the proliferating zone.

ronment allowing vascular invasion (Buckwalter 1983), and this results in the complete osteoclastic resorption of the transverse septa, terminal chondrocytes, and 60% of the longitudinal septa. The remaining calcified septa become the scaffold for new bone formation by first being thickened by the deposition of unmineralized bone matrix (osteoid) by osteoblasts. The osteoid is subsequently mineralized forming the primary spongiosa, and due to further remodeling, it is itself replaced by secondary spongiosa, which is made up of lammelar bone (Howell and Dean 1992).

Although chondrocyte dynamics and cartilage mineralization, and its replacement by bone, are coupled physiologically it is only the activities of the chondrocytes that result in "true" bone growth. However, both processes are described in this chapter, because endochondral growth is classically recognized to represent the culmination of a sequence of changes in chondrocytes and their associated matrix.

Regulation of Bone Growth: The Role of the Chondrocyte

The contribution of individual growth plates to the growth rates of long bones varies enormously. In the domestic fowl (*Gallus domesticus*), one of the fastest growing bone tips is the proximal tibia that grows at 0.86 mm/day (Kirkwood et al. 1989). Growth rates at the same growth plates in the rat and rabbit are 0.22 and 0.39 mm/day, respectively (Kember 1983, 1985) and reflect the slower bone growth rates in these species and mammals as a whole. Human bones grow extremely slowly and the growth rate of the distal femur has been estimated at 0.04 mm/day, whereas deer antlers, which grow by mechanisms similar to that of long bones, have a very rapid growth rate of 17.5 mm/day.

In growth plates, with a normal columnar chondrocyte arrangement, it has been established that the final hypertrophic volume and the accompanying changes in incremental vertical height in the direction of

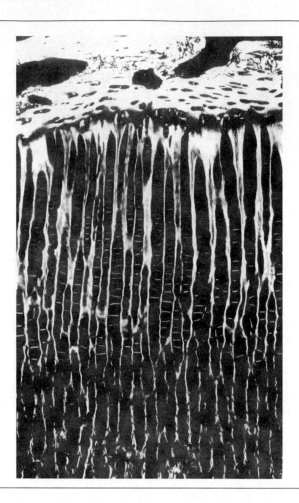

Figure 9.4. Polarization microscopy of a Sirius red-stained section from a distal radial growth plate of a 17-week-old Scottish deerhound. Birefringent material (collagen) is oriented either parallel (longitudinal septa) or perpendicular (transverse septa) to the long axis of the bone. The absence of the thin transverse septa marks the chondro-osseous junction within the metaphysis. (Reprinted with permission from Breur et al., 1992. Copyright is owned by *The Journal of Bone and Joint Surgery, Inc.*)

growth of the hypertrophic chondrocyte are strongly correlated with the rate of growth. In a study of 16 growth plates spread among 4 locations and two species at two different ages, a strong correlation (rat = 0.98, pig = 0.83) and a positive linear relationship between the volume of the hypertrophic chondrocyte and the rate of bone growth was found (Breur et al. 1991). This variation in hypertrophic cell volume accounts for the different growth rates between species and also the different growth rates that occur at the proximal and distal ends within the same long bone (Hunziker et al. 1987). Growth plates of birds, however, do not show a columnar chondrocyte arrangement, and analysis of such a nonparallel growth system have also been undertaken (Kember and Kirkwood 1987). Simplistically, the growth plates elongating at the fastest rate have the largest hypertrophic chondrocytes. The chondrocyte proliferation rate and the size of the proliferative pool also correlate

positively with growth rates. A study (Wilsman et al. 1996a), which focussed on four different rat growth plates with growth rates ranging from 50–400 μm per day, showed that there was a correspondingly large difference in cell cycle time (30.9–76.3h and this range in cell cycle times was attributable to significant differences in the length of the G1 phase (23.6–66.6h). It is now accepted that the rate of bone growth attributed to a specific growth plate in any given period of time is determined by a complex interplay of proliferative kinetics, matrix production in the transverse septa, and hypertrophic chondrocyte enlargement (Breur et al. 1991). The individual contribution, however, of each variable to bone growth differs with the rate of bone growth and is not uniform for all bones. In the proliferative zone, cell duplication is more significant at faster rates of growth, whereas matrix synthesis is more significant at slower rates of growth. During hypertrophy, chondrocyte enlarge-

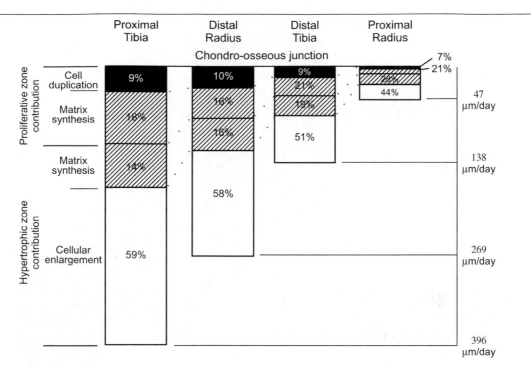

Figure 9.5. Relative contributions to daily total elongation at the chondro-osseous junction in four growth plates from 28-day-old Long-Evans rats. (Reprinted with permission from Wilsman et al., 1996b.)

ment is the major contributor to growth, and its contribution is more significant at faster rates of growth (Wilsman et al. 1996b; Figure 9.5).

Matrix Proteins

Collagen type II is the principal structural protein of the growth plate matrix (Figure 9.6A). It interacts with collagen types IX and XI to form heterotypic fibrils that are distributed throughout the cartilage matrix (Mwale et al. 2002). During chondrocyte maturation, collagen type II gene expression decreases and the hypertrophic chondrocytes initiate the synthesis of collagen type X—a protein unique to this cell type (Schmid and Linsenmayer 1985; Figure 9.6B). This collagen type is a nonfibrillar, short chain collagen and is thought to provide a structural role in maintaining the organization and mechanical properties of the matrix (Chan and Jacenko 1998). There are also a number of proteoglycans, of which aggrecan predominates, and noncollagenous proteins such as osteopontin and osteonectin within the growth plate matrix (Pacifici

ct al. 1990; Byers et al. 1992). As chondrocytes differentiate, and hypertrophy, concomitant changes also occur within the extracellular matrix; evidence suggests that chondrocytes must provide the correct extracellular network and establish cell-matrix interactions to allow progressive differentiation. This observation is consistent with a change from aggrecan to decorin and biglycan synthesis during normal chondrocyte maturation (Bianco et al. 1990).

Programmed Cell Death

The fate of the terminally differentiated hypertrophic chondrocyte is unclear. It is accepted however, that in order to compensate for the rapid chondrocyte proliferation and hypertrophy rates, the differentiated chondrocyte must be removed to maintain the steady-state thickness of the growth plate. In growing rats it has been calculated that eight hypertrophic chondrocytes (including their associated matrices) are eliminated from each column of cells every day (Hunziker et al. 1987). It was long considered that the terminally differentiated chondrocyte died through necrosis,

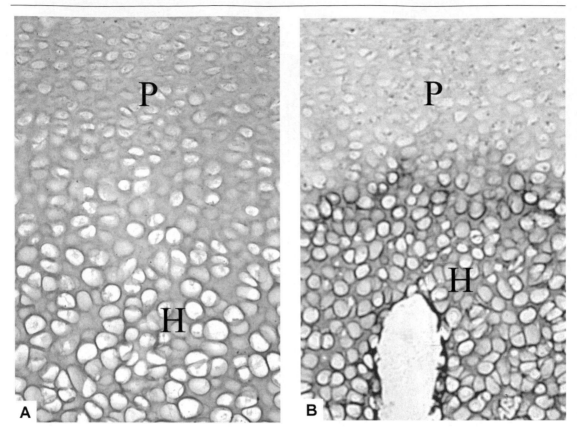

Figure 9.6. Immunoperoxidase staining of (A) collagen type II and (B) collagen type X within the growth plate of the proximal tibiotarsus of a 21-day-old chicken. Collagen type II is distributed throughout the entire matrix of the growth plate, whereas collagen type X is restricted to the matrix surrounding the more differentiated hypertrophic chondrocytes.

but this interpretation was based on artifactual ultrastructural morphology. Authorities now contend that terminally differentiated chondrocytes either redifferentiate into bone cells (Cancedda et al. 1995), proliferate with one daughter chondrocyte dying and the other becoming an osteoblast (Roach et al. 1995), or undergo the widely accepted route of programmed cell death (Farnum and Wilsman 1987; Gibson et al. 1995; Hatori et al. 1995).

Matrix Mineralization

Cartilage mineralization is required before vascular invasion of the growth plate can occur. Mineralization of cartilage and bone occurs by a series of complex physio-chemical and biochemical processes that together facilitate the deposition of a solid phase in specific extracellular areas of the organic matrix (Anderson 1995). In the first phase, calcium and phosphorus are complexed together to form the first small insoluble solid particles within matrix vesicles. These amorphous calcium phosphate particles are transformed via intermediates to form true hydroxyapatite. Phase 2 of the mineralization process begins with the penetration of the matrix vesicle membrane by the hydroxyapatite crystals and their exposure to the extracellular fluid. The rate of mineral crystal formation from this point onward is governed by the concentrations of $Ca2+$ and PO_4^{3-} in the extracellular fluid, the pH, and the concentration of matrix components such as proteoglycans that might promote or impair the mineralization process (Mwale et al. 2002).

A minimum concentration of Ca^{2+} and PO_4^{3-} has to be reached before precipitation and crystalization takes place. Their concentration in extracellular fluids is 1.25 mM Ca^{2+} and 1 mM PO_4^{3-} and is insufficient to initiate de novo apapatite crystal formation; therefore, local concentrations of both ions within matrix vesicles have to be raised. The attraction of Ca^{2+} into the matrix vesicle is through Ca^{2+} ion channels and their affinity for Ca^{2+} binding lipids and proteins. This is accompanied by the cleavage of phosphate-containing substrates by membrane-bound phosphatases and the release of inorganic phosphate (Robison 1923). These actions raise the concentration of Ca^{2+} and PO_4^{3-}, and the initial deposition of $CaPo_4$ near the vesicle membrane occurs. The generation of high concentrations of inorganic phosphate has traditionally been attributed to the actions of the bone/liver/kidney form of ALP, which is preferentially localized to the matrix vesicle membrane.

Vascularization

Proteolytic degradation of the collagen-rich extracellular matrix is a key feature in the development and growth of the skeleton, and this is of particular importance at the chondro-osseous junction where vascular invasion of the mineralized matrix occurs. Matrix metalloproteinases (MMPs), which includes collagenases and gelatinases, are a family of enzymes capable of performing this function, whereas tissue inhibitors of MMPs (TIMPs) are believed to play an important role in regulating their activity (Blair et al. 1989; Lee et al. 1999). Degradation of matrix components facilitates blood vessel penetration into the growth plate, and thereafter the vasculature provides a conduit for the recruitment of hematopoietic osteoclast precursor cells and perivascular osteoblast progenitors for the further resorption of cartilage and replacement by bone. The growth of new blood vessels—angiogenesis—is initiated by the migration and replication of vascular endothelial cells from the existing capillary network within the bone metaphysis. Although a number of angiogenic factors (as well as antiangiogenic factors) are expressed by chondrocytes, most attention has centered on the family of vascular endothelial growth factors (VEGF) that can promote angiogenesis in vivo. The VEGF family is comprised of five structurally related proteins (VEGF-A, -B, -C, and -D, and placental growth factor). VEGF-A gene and protein are highly expressed by hypertrophic chondrocytes of mice, rat, and chick growth plates, but are not expressed by the less mature proliferating chondrocytes. The receptors for VEGF (VEGFR-1, -2, and -3) have been shown to be localized mainly in

endothelial cells (Ferrara and Davis-Smyth 1997), and this evidence suggests that VEGF is actively responsible for hypertrophic cartilage neovascularization through the paracrine release by chondrocytes, with invading endothelial cells as the target. When chondrocyte hypertrophy is inhibited, angiogenesis and subsequent endochondral ossification is blocked (Karaplis et al. 1994). The colocalization of VEGFR-2 to hypertrophic chondrocytes (Carlevaro et al. 2000) also suggests that the role of VEGF family members in the growth plate is not confined to the stimulation of vascularization but may also involve an autocrine/paracrine loop functioning within the growth plate itself. In mice in which VEGF activity was sequestered, there was suppressed blood vessel invasion of the growth plate, reduced femur lengthening, and an expansion of the hypertrophic chondrocyte zone that appeared to be due to delayed chondrocyte apoptosis and cartilage resorption (Gerber et al. 1999). This study provides direct evidence that blood vessels provide not only nutrients to the growth plate but also pro-apoptotic signals and cells required for matrix remodeling.

ENDOGENOUS MEDIATORS OF BONE GROWTH

The rate of longitudinal bone growth is controlled by numerous systemic and local growth mediators that interact to regulate the activities of the growth plate chondrocytes. The factors that regulate the behavior and activities of chondrocytes are as varied as they are numerous. They can be divided into two broad groups, those with a systemic action, such as growth hormone (GH), and those that act in a local autocrine/paracrine manner, such as transforming growth factor-β (TGF-β).

Growth Hormone and Insulin-Like Growth Factor-I

It has long been established that GH is one of the principal endocrine factors that controls postnatal longitudinal bone growth. In 1957, Salmon and Daughaday postulated the somatomedin—the old name for insulin-like growth factors (IGF)—hypothesis in which the growth plate chondrocytes response to GH was mediated through the hepatic production of somatomedins and its release into the circulation. From there, IGF-I reaches its target tissues (cartilage and bone) and interacts with its receptors, which convey a growth signal to the cell. This hypothesis is compatible with an endocrine action of IGF-I and was based on experimental evidence that the addition of GH to cartilage fragments in culture had little effect, whereas the addition of serum stimulated cellular processes associated with chondrocyte proliferation and differentiation. However, serum from hypophysectomized animals had a lesser effect and subsequent GH therapy resulted in a serum with normal growth promoting activities. The somatomedin hypothesis has been questioned by other experiments showing that low concentrations of GH directly infused into the growth plate showed stimulated longitudinal growth in comparison to the contralateral limb (Isaksson et al, 1982). These and similar studies have led to an alternative hypothesis of GH action in which GH has a direct effect on bone and other peripheral tissues (nonhepatic) resulting in the local production of IGF-I (D'Ercole et al. 1984). This hypothesis was supported by the observation that GH was found to increase IGF-I mRNA expression in growth plate chondrocytes and that the growth promoting effects of locally administered GH were eliminated when an IGF-I antiserum was coinfused with GH (Schlechter et al. 1986). This data is compatible with the idea that under the influence of GH, IGF-I produced by chondrocytes within all maturational zones mediates chondrocyte maturation and longitudinal bone growth in an autocrine/paracrine manner. According to the dual effector theory, another level of control may exist in the germinal stem cells where GH, independently of IGF-I, directly promotes the differentiation of stem cells into IGF-responsive proliferating chondrocytes (Zezulak and Green 1986). One of the remaining unanswered questions is the relative contribution of the direct and indirect actions of GH on bone growth.

Parathyroid Hormone-Related Peptide

Parathyroid hormone (PTH) has long been recognized together with 1,25 dihydroxyvitamin D_3 (1,25-D) to be an essential regulator of the circulating levels of calcium and phosphate by modulating the activities of cells in the intestine, kidney, and bone. Recently, a second member of the PTH family, parathyroid hormone-related peptide (PTHrP) has been discovered. In humans, the amino acid sequence of PTHrP is homologous with the amino terminus region of PTH, where 8 of the 13 amino acids are identical. Beyond this region, little sequence homology exists. The homologous domain is a critical region because it is required for binding and activation of the common PTH/PTHrP receptor. Like PTH, PTHrP also causes hypercalcemia and hypophosphatemia, but as its normal circulating levels are significantly lower than PTH levels; it is thought unlikely that PTHrP has any major role in maintaining calcium homeostasis. The physiological roles for PTHrP are now recognized to be numerous and complex, because recent data has shown that PTHrP is expressed by a wide variety of embryonic and adult tissues. This suggests that during normal cell growth and differentiation, PTHrP functions mainly as an autocrine/paracrine factor, acting through the common receptor. This local control of cellular function extends to cells of the skeleton and in particular to the growth plate chondrocytes.

Mice missing the PTH/PTHrP receptor gene have a growth plate morphology similar to that of mice that are homozygous for the ablation of the PTHrP gene (Lanske et al. 1996). There is widespread accelerated differentiation of chondrocytes and premature mineralization resulting in a narrow growth plate. In contrast, the phenotype of mice in which the PTHrP gene is overexpressed is characterized by a dramatic slowing down of the differentiation of chondrocytes and a wider growth plate (Weir et al. 1996). These and other experiments have led to the acceptance that PTHrP, together with the morphogen Indian hedgehog (Ihh), is one of the major influences on the endochondral growth process, and a model for the molecular regulation of chondrocyte terminal differentiation in embryonic tissue has been proposed. In this model, Ihh is produced by prehypertrophic chondrocytes committed to hypertrophy and acting through its receptor, patched within the perichondrium, increases the expression of PTHrP in the periarticular region. PTHrP then binds to PTH/PTHrP receptors expressed on prehypertrophic chondrocytes—i.e., prior to their conversion to Ihh expressing cells—and blocks their further differentiation. As the population of committed cells progresses to the hypertrophic phenotype, they stop expressing Ihh, thereby attenuating the negative feedback loop and allowing the further differentiation of uncommitted prehypertrophic cells (Figure 9.7). A similar pathway for controlling growth in postnatal growth plates is also likely to exist, but the presence within the growth plate of functional components of the PTHrP-Ihh pathway suggests that local mechanisms intrinsic to the growth plate control the rate of endochondral ossification (Farquharson et al. 2001).

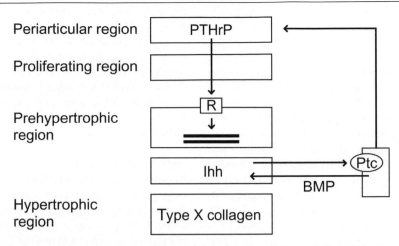

Figure 9.7. Schematic demonstration of the coordinated regulation of chondrocyte differentiation by PTHrP and Ihh in the embryonic growth plate.

Transforming Growth Factor-β Superfamily

The members of the TGF-β superfamily comprise a large number of structurally related gene products, which have been classified into several distinct groups. The members of the superfamily that are known to effect bone growth are TGF-β1–4, of which only TGF-β4 is found in chicken, and the bone morphogenetic proteins (BMPs).

TGF-β exert their biological effects through binding with specific TGF-β receptors (TβRI and TβRII), and the TGF-β receptor complex is known to interact with members of the Smad family, which are mediators of TGF-β signalling. These molecules translocate to the nucleus where they activate gene transcription. Within the chick growth plate TGF-β1, -β2 and, -β3 have been immunolocalized primarily to the prehypertrophic and hypertrophic chondrocytes with little or no staining observed in the resting or proliferating chondrocytes (Thorp et al. 1992). Similar observations have been observed in mammalian growth plates. TGF-β has very complex effects on chondrocyte physiology, depending, for example, on the concentration of factor, site of action, and differentiation status of chondrocytes. In summary, the bulk of published evidence supports a role for TGF-β as a stimulator of growth plate chondrocyte proliferation and inhibitor of differentiation

and mineralization (O'Keefe et al. 1988; Battegay et al. 1990; Ballock et al. 1993; Bohme et al. 1995). It is possible that TGF-β and PTHrP interact in a common signal cascade to regulate endochondral bone formation. In experiments with mouse embryonic metatarsal bone rudiments, TGF-β1 was found to act upstream of PTHrP to regulate the rate of hypertrophic differentiation (Serra et al. 1999). The importance of TGF-β signaling in endochondral bone growth has been unequivocally demonstrated in TGF-β1 knock-out mice (TGF-β1 -/-). In comparison to normal mice, the TGF-β1 -/- mice had narrower growth plates (23%) and a reduction in bone growth rate (63%) and tibial length (12%). In addition, the height of the hypertrophic chondrocytes was also decreased (24%), which might explain the observed slower growth rates (Geiser et al. 1998). Similar observations on long bone growth have been observed in TGF-β2 knock-out mice (Sanford et al. 1997).

The BMPs are a family of growth factors that were originally isolated from demineralized bone. In a similar way to TGF-β isoforms, BMPs also interact with either type I (BMP receptor 1A or BMP receptor 1B) or type II (BMP receptor II) receptor that is a prerequisite for signal transduction. Signal transduction is mediated by Smads 1 and 5, which have been specifically implicated in BMP signaling. To date, 15 distinct BMPs have been identified. The hallmark of BMPs is their ability to induce de novo bone formation in nonskeletal tissue, of which the initial stages are characterized by the stimulation of collagen type II and the formation of a cartilaginous matrix (Urist 1965). Recent data has indicated that BMPs can regulate the complete cascade of events in cartilage formation, which includes the differentiation of the committed mesenchymal stem cells to the chondrocyte phenotype, their terminal differentiation, and the mineralization of the cartilage matrix. More specifically, BMP4 and BMP6 have been implicated in mediating the effects of PTHrP in regulating the pace of chondrocyte differentiation (Grimsrud et al. 1999; Farquharson et al. 2001).

FIBROBLAST GROWTH FACTOR.   The fibroblast growth factor (FGF) family is known to consist of at least nine members and share up to 50% amino acid sequence homology. FGF signaling is critical for chondrocyte maturation and skeletal development during postnatal bone growth, and the specific functions of FGF-1 (acidic) and FGF-2 (basic) in these events have been studied widely. As expected for structurally related molecules, both acidic and basic FGF have similar biological effects and interact with members of the FGF receptor family of transmembrane tyrosine kinases to elicit their biological response. Up-regulation of FGF receptor signaling results in bone abnormalities during endochondral growth, and is the basis of several genetic forms of human dwarfism.

Both FGF-1 and FGF-2 are expressed by growth plate chondrocytes and have been immunolocalized to the proliferative and hypertrophic chondrocytes. In rabbits, injection of basic FGF into the growth plate accelerates vascularization and mineralization of the cartilage, whereas in culture, FGF-2 is a powerful mitogen for growth plate chondrocytes and an inhibitor of their terminal differentiation and mineralization (Wroblewski and Edwal-Arvidsson 1995). While these properties are similar to those observed with PTHrP notable differences in their actions have been observed. Chondrocytes are responsive to PTHrP throughout all developmental stages, whereas the responsiveness to FGF-2 is greater at the early stages of maturation.

Vitamin D.   The major active metabolite of vitamin D_3, 1,25-D, has a significant role in chondrocyte metabolism and appears to be essential for normal bone formation. The actions of this vitamin are mediated through its interaction with its nuclear receptor (VDR) that binds its ligand with high affinity. VDR is a phosphoprotein that regulates gene expression by heterodimerizing with the retinoid X receptor and associating with the vitamin D response elements on target genes. Vitamin D deficiency, or mutations in the enzyme, that converts 25-D to 1,25-D (25-hydroxyvitamin D-1 α-hydroxylase) or the VDR gene results in rickets within the growth plate. A similar phenotype is observed in the VDR knock-out mouse.

Receptors for 1,25-D have been located on growth plate chondrocytes, suggesting a direct role for this metabolite in chondrocyte metabolism and bone growth with a higher expression of the VDR noted in the hypertrophic chondrocytes (Berry et al. 1996). 1,25-D has direct effects on chondrocyte proliferation and differentiation and cartilage matrix synthesis under defined culture conditions, and a stimulation of chondrocyte differentiation in vivo has been shown (Farquharson et al. 1993). This is in broad agreement with the accumulated evidence on other cell types where 1,25-D causes an inhibition of growth and an induction of differentiation. Old data suggests that 24,25 dihydroxyvitamin D_3 (24,25-D) is the major vitamin D metabolite in promoting cartilage maturation, differentiation, and mineralization (Ornoy et al. 1978). Although this has been disputed, more recent evidence has clearly indicated that growth plate chondrocytes also bind and respond to 24,25-D. The response of chondrocytes to 1,25-D and 24,25-D is dependent on the maturation state of the responding cells. 1,25-D primarily affects cells in the growth zone, whereas 24,25-D primarily affects cells in the resting zone. The differential response to 1,25-D and 24,25-D is mediated by separate membrane receptors, which in turn mediate their physiological effects through protein kinase C (Schwartz et al. 1988).

DISORDERS OF BONE GROWTH

Growth plate chondrocyte activities and matrix mineralization and replacement with bone generally proceed normally in the growth and development of long bones. There are, however, a number of common growth plate disorders found in several domestic species, and these are often the result of dietary nutrient imbalances or genetic selection for rapid growth.

Osteochondrosis

This is a generalized skeletal disease, which is common in growing pigs and is characterized by impaired endochondral ossification in the growth plate and the articular-epiphyseal growth cartilages. This results in areas of retained cartilage extending into the subchondral bone (Reiland 1978). In pigs, osteochondrotic lesions are observed as early as 25 days of age, and the lesion may heal spontaneously or lead to secondary degenerative changes, such as osteoarthrosis and osteoarthritis and subsequent clinical manifestations. The consensus of opinion is that porcine osteochondrosis is a result of incomplete chondrocyte differentiation, but the underlying causes are unknown (Ekman and Heinegard 1992).

Dyschondroplasia

This common growth plate disorder is common in poultry and is associated with rapidly growing growth plates, such as the proximal tibiotarsus. It is characterized by a mass of noncalcified avascular opaque cartilage situated below the growth plate and extending into the metaphysis (Farquharson and Jefferies 2000; Figure 9.8). Dyschondroplasia was first described by Leach and Nesheim (1965) as a spontaneously occurring cartilage abnormality. It is now known that both nutrition and selective breed-

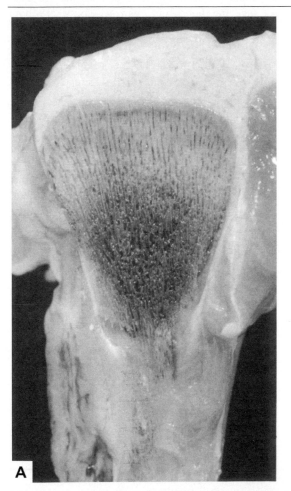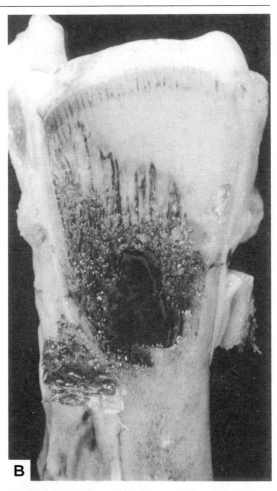

Figure 9.8. Comparison of (A) normal and (B) dyschondroplastic growth plates of the proximal tibiotarsus of a 21-day-old chicken. The dyschondroplastic lesion is opaque and avascular and occupies a large area of the metaphysis under the growth plate. (Reprinted with permission from Farquharson and Jefferies, 2000.)

ing can affect its incidence. The size of the TD lesion is variable. It can exist as a small cartilaginous mass within a discrete area under the growth plate, or can occupy the metaphysis under the entire width of the growth plate. The small lesions are likely to be subclinical, whereas the larger lesions have been shown to lead to significant bone deformities and lameness in broilers. Abnormal, nonuniform bone growth within the area of the lesion leads to increased tibial plateau angle and tibial bowing (Lynch et al. 1992). The precise underlying cellular defect that occurs in TD remains unclear. It is now generally accepted, however, that the observed impaired vascularization, altered rates of chondrocyte apoptosis, abnormal cartilage matrix structure, and the failure of osteoclastic cartilage resorption (Farquharson and Jefferies 2000) are secondary to the inability of the maturing chondrocytes to undergo terminal differentiation, which normally leads to hypertrophy, vascularization, and mineralization.

Rickets

Rickets is characterized by thickened and irregular growth plates and is associated with a lack of calcium, phosphorus, or vitamin D, or an imbalance between the two minerals. In poultry, hypocalcemic rickets results in a thickening of the proliferating chondrocytes zone due to an accumulation of randomly orientated chondrocytes, whereas phosphorus deficiency results in widening of the hypertrophic chondrocyte zone. Both types of rickets have decreased amounts of calcified cartilage. Hypocalcemic rickets is regarded to be a result of delayed chondrocyte hypertrophy; hypophosphatemic rickets is caused by a decreased rate of cartilage resorption at the chondro-osseous junction (Lacey and Huffer 1982). Widening of the hypertrophic zone is characteristic of rickets observed in mammals.

Pseudoachondroplasia

The pseudoachondroplastic dog is distinguished by a bone growth rate that is 65% of that in normal animals. The diameters of both proliferating and hypertrophic chondrocytes are altered in this disorder. Due to irregular, thickened longitudinal septa within the growth plate, the usual shape of the hypertrophic chondrocyte is not maintained by the matrix. Therefore, the increase in cellular volume of the hypertrophic chondrocytes occurs in an indiscriminate manner and is not directed toward growth (Breur et al. 1992).

APPOSITIONAL GROWTH

In order for a bone to withstand the pressures of loading due to increased body weight, the bone must increase its width and thereby increase the cross sectional moment of inertia. In most animal species, the width of weight-bearing long bones such as the tibia are highly correlated to the weight of the animal. Bone diaphyseal width increases as a result of the activities of the osteoblasts within the outer covering of bone (periosteum) where bone is deposited in a successive laminar pattern to form the outer circumferential lamellae. This process does not occur in isolation but is coupled to bone resorption by osteoclasts within the internal covering of bone (endosteum). As periosteal bone is added, endosteal cortical bone is eroded and the net result is that the bone and marrow cavity are both increased in diameter. Due to differential osteoblast activity on the periosteal surface, longitudinal depressions entrap blood vessels and periosteal elements. These hollow depressions become covered by bone and primary osteons are formed. The internalized bone-forming cells are now referred to as endosteal elements and lay down sheets of concentric lamellae during the infilling period. The osteon is regarded as the structural unit of bone, and although osteonal remodeling is essential for replacing old lamellar bone with new bone this process is not associated with growth. In the adult, when appositional growth has ceased, the periosteum is required for the maintenance of the bone surface.

ACKNOWLEDGMENTS

The author is grateful to the Biotechnology and Biological Sciences Research Council for financial support.

REFERENCES

Anderson, H.C. 1995. Molecular-biology of matrix vesicles. *Clinical Orthopaedics and Related Research* 314:266–280.

Ballock, R.T., Heydemann, A., Wakefield, L.M., Flanders, K.C., Roberts, A.B., and Sporn, M.B. 1993. TGF-beta-1 prevents hypertrophy of epiphyseal chondrocytes—regulation of gene-expression for cartilage matrix proteins and metalloproteases. *Developmental Biology* 158:414–429.

Battegay, E.J., Raines, E.W., Seifert, R.A., Bowenpope, D.F., and Ross, R. 1990. TGF-beta induces bimodal proliferation of connective-tissue cells via complex control of an autocrine PDGF loop. *Cell* 63:515–524.

Berry, J.L., Farquharson, C., Whitehead, C.C., and Mawer, E.B. 1996. Growth plate chondrocyte vitamin D receptor number and affinity are reduced in avian tibial dyschondroplastic lesions. *Bone* 19:197–203.

Bianco, P., Fisher, L.W., Young, M.F., Termine, J.D., and Robey, P.G. 1990. Expression and localization of the 2 small proteoglycans biglycan and decorin in developing human skeletal and nonskeletal tissues. *Journal of Histochemistry & Cytochemistry* 38:1549–1563.

Blair, H.C., Dean, D.D., Howell, D.S., Teitelbaum, S.L., and Jeffrey, J.J. 1989. Hypertrophic produce immunoreactive collagenase in vivo. *Connective Tissue Research* 23:65–73.

Bohme, K., Winterhalter, K.H., and Bruckner, P. 1995. Terminal differentiation of chondrocytes in culture is a spontaneous process and is arrested by transforming growth-factor-beta-2 and basic fibroblast growth-factor in synergy. *Experimental Cell Research* 216:191–198.

Breur G.J., Turgai, J., Vanenkevort, B.A., Farnum, C.E., and Wilsman N.J. 1994. Stereological and serial section analysis of chondrocytic enlargement in the proximal tibial growth-plate of the rat. *Anatomical Record* 239:255–268.

Breur, G.J., Vanenkevort, B.A., Farnum, C.E., and Wilsman, N.J. 1991. Linear relationship between the volume of hypertrophic chondrocytes and the rate of longitudinal bone-growth growth plates. *Journal of Orthopaedic Research* 9:348–359.

Breur, J.J., Farnum, C.E., Padgett, G.A., and Wilsman, N.J. 1992. Cellular basis of decreased rate of longitudinal growth of bone in pseudoachondroplastic dogs. *Journal of Bone and Joint Surgery—American Volume* 74A:516–528.

Buckwalter, J.A. 1983. Proteoglycan structure in calcifying cartilage. *Clinical Orthopaedics and Related Research* 172:207–232.

Buckwalter, J.A., Mower, D., Ungar, R., Schaeffer, J., and Ginsberg, B. 1986. Morphometric analysis of chondrocyte hypertrophy. *Journal of Bone and Joint Surgery—American Volume* 68A:243–255.

Byers, S., Caterson, B., Hopwood, J.J., and Foster, B.K. 1992. Immunolocation analysis of glycosaminoglycans in the human growth plate. *Journal of Histochemistry & Cytochemistry* 40 275–282.

Cancedda, R., Cancedda, F.D., and Castagnola, P. 1995. Chondrocyte differentiation. *International Review of Cytology* 159:265–358.

Carlevaro, M.F., Cermelli, S., Cancedda, R., and Cancedda, F.D. 2000. Vascular endothelial growth factor (VEGF) in cartilage neovascularization and chondrocyte differentiation: auto- paracrine role during endochondral bone formation. *Journal of Cell Science* 113: 59–69.

Chan, D., and Jacenko, O. 1998. Phenotypic and biochemical consequences of collagen X mutations in mice and humans, *Matrix Biology* 17:169–184.

D'Ercole, A.J., Stiles, A.D., and Underwood, L.E. 1984. Tissue concentrations of somatomedin-C—further evidence for multiple sites of synthesis and paracrine or autocrine mechanisms of action. *Proceedings of the National Academy of Sciences of the United States of America* 81:935–939.

Ekman, S., and Heinegard, D. 2002. Immunohistochemical localization of matrix proteins in the femoral joint cartilage of growing commercial pigs. *Veterinary Pathology* 29:514–520.

Farnum, C.E., and Wilsman, N.J. 1987. Morphological stages of the terminal hypertrophic chondrocyte of growth plate cartilage. *Anatomical Record* 219:221–232.

Farnum, C.E., and Wilsman, N.J. 1993. Determination of proliferative characteristics of growth plate chondrocytes by labeling with bromodeoxyuridine. *Calcified Tissue International* 52: 110–119.

Farquharson, C., and Jefferies, D. 2000. Chondrocytes and longitudinal bone growth: The development of tibial dyschondroplasia. *Poultry Science* 79:994–1004.

Farquharson, C., Jefferies, D., Seawright, E., and Houston, B. 2001. Regulation of chondrocyte terminal differentiation in the postembryonic growth plate: The role of the PTHrP-Indian hedgehog axis. *Endocrinology* 142:4131–4140.

Farquharson, C., and Loveridge, N. 1990. Cell-proliferation within the growth plate of long bones assessed by bromodeoxyuridine uptake and its relationship to glucose-6-phosphate-dehydrogenase activity. *Bone and Mineral* 10:121–130.

Farquharson, C., Whitehead, C.C., Rennie, J.S., and Loveridge, N. 1993. In-vivo effect of 1,25-dihydroxycholecalciferol on the proliferation and differentiation of avian chondrocytes. *Journal of Bone and Mineral Research* 8:1081–1088.

Farquharson, C., Whitehead, C.C., Rennie, J.S., Thorp, B., and and Loveridge, N. 1992. Cell-proliferation and enzyme-activities associated with the development of avian tibial dyschondroplasia—an insitu biochemical-study. *Bone* 13:59–67.

Ferrara, N., and Davis-Smyth, T. 1997. The biology of vascular endothelial growth factor. *Endocrine Reviews* 18:4–25.

Geiser, A.G., Zeng, Q.Q., Sato, M., Helvering, L.M., Hirano, T., and Turner, C.H. 1998. Decreased bone mass and bone elasticity in mice lacking the transforming growth factor-beta 1 gene. *Bone* 23:87–93.

Gerber, H.P., Vu, T.H., Ryan, A.M., Kowalski, J., Werb, Z., and Ferrara, N. 1999. VEGF couples hypertrophic cartilage remodeling, ossification and angiogenesis during endochondral bone formation. *Nature Medicine* 5:623–628.

Gibson, G.J., Kohler, W.J., and Schaffler, M.B. 1995. Chondrocyte apoptosis in endochondral ossification of chick sterna. *Developmental Dynamics* 203:468–476.

Grimsrud, C.D., Romano, P.R., D'Souza, M., Puzas, J.E., Reynolds, P.R., Rosier, R.N., and O'Keefe, R.J. 1999. BMP-6 is an autocrine stimulator of chondrocyte differentiation. *Journal of Bone and Mineral Research* 14:475–482.

Hatori, M., Klatte, K.J., Teixeira, C.C., and Shapiro, I.M. 1995. End labeling studies of fragmented dna in the avian growth-plate—evidence of apoptosis in terminally differentiated chondrocytes. *Journal of Bone and Mineral Research* 10:1960–1968.

Howell, D.S., and Dean, D.D. 1992. The biology, chemistry, and biochemistry of the mammalian growth plate. In *Disorders of Bone and Mineral Metabolism*, F.L. Coe and M.J. Favus, eds. New York: Raven Press.

Hunziker, E.B., and Schenk, R.K. 1989. Physiological-mechanisms adopted by chondrocytes in regulating longitudinal bone-growth in rats. *Journal of Physiology-London* 414:55–71.

Hunziker, E.B., and Schenk, R.K., and Cruzorive L.M. 1987. Quantitation of chondrocyte performance in growth-plate cartilage during longitudinal bone-growth. *Journal of Bone and Joint Surgery-American Volume* 69A:162–173.

Isaksson, O.G.P., Jansson, J.O., and Gause, I.A.M. 1982. Growth-hormone stimulates longitudinal bone-growth directly. *Science* 216:1237–1239.

Karaplis, A.C., Luz, A., Glowacki, J., Bronson, R.T., Tybulewicz, V.L.J., Kronenberg, H.M., and Mulligan, R.C. 1994. Lethal skeletal dysplasia from targeted disruption of the parathyroid hormone-related peptide gene. *Genes & Development* 8:277–289.

Kember, N.F. 1983. Cell kinetics of cartilage. In *Cartilage*, vol. 1. R.K. Hall, ed. New York: Academic Press.

Kember, N.F. 1985. Comparative patterns of cell-division in epiphyseal cartilage plates in the rabbit. *Journal of Anatomy* 142:185–190.

Kember, N.F., and Kirkwood, J.K. 1987. Cell kinetics and longitudinal bone growth in birds, *Cell and Tissue Kinetics* 20:625–629.

Kember, N.F., and Sissons, H.A. 1976. Quantitative histology of the human growth plate. *Journal of Bone and Joint Surgery-British Volume* 68B:425–435.

Kirkwood, J.K., Spratt, D.M.J., Duignan, P.J., and Kember, N.F. 1989. Patterns of cell-proliferation and growth-rate in limb bones of the domestic-fowl (*Gallus-domesticus*). *Research in Veterinary Science* 47:139–147.

Lacey, D.L., and Huffer, W.E. 1982. Studies on the pathogenesis of avian rickets. 1. Changes in epiphyseal and metaphyseal vessels in hypocalcemic and hypophosphatemic rickets. *American Journal of Pathology* 109:288–301.

Lanske, B., Karaplis, A.C., Lee, K., Luz, A., Vortkamp, A., Pirro, A., Karperien, M., Defize, L.H.K., Ho, C., Mulligan, R.C., AbouSamra, A.B., Juppner, H., Segre, G.V., and Kronenberg, H.M.. 1996. PTH/PTHrP receptor in early development and Indian hedgehog-regulated bone growth. *Science* 273:663–666.

Leach, R.M., and Nesheim, M. 1965. Nutritional, genetic and morphological studies on an abnormal cartilage formation in young chicks. *Journal of Nutrition* 86:236–244.

Lee, E.R., Murphy, G., El Alfy, M., Davoli, M.A., Lamplugh, L., Docherty, A.J., and Leblond, C.P. 1999. Active gelatinase B is identified by histozymography in the cartilage resorption sites of developing long bones. *Developmental Dynamics* 215:190–205.

Lynch, M., Thorp, B.H., and Whitehead, C.C. 1992. Avian tibial dyschondroplasia as a cause of bone deformity. *Avian Pathology* 21:275–285.

Mwale, F., Tchetina, E., Wu, C.W., and Poole, A.R. 2002. The assembly and remodeling of the extracellular matrix in the growth plate in relationship to mineral deposition and cellular hypertrophy: An in situ study of collagens II and IX and proteoglycan. *Journal of Bone and Mineral Research* 17:275–283.

O'Keefe, R.J., Puzas, J.E., Brand, J.S., and Rosier, R.N. 1988. Effect of transforming growth factor-beta on dna-synthesis by growth plate chondrocytes—modulation by factors present in serum. *Calcified Tissue International* 43:352–358.

Ornoy A., Goodwin, D., Noff, D., and Edelstein, S. 1978. 24,25-dihydroxyvitamin D is a metabolite of vitamin D essential for bone formation, *Nature* 276: 517–519.

Pacifici, M., Oshima, O., Fisher, L.W., Young, M.F., Shapiro, I.M., and Leboy, P.S. 1990. Changes in osteonectin distribution and levels are associated with mineralization of the chicken tibial growth cartilage. *Calcified Tissue International* 47:51–61.

Reiland, S. 1978. Growth and skeletal development of the pig. *Acta Radiologica Supplement* 358: 15–22.

Roach, H.I., Erenpreisa, J., and Aigner, T. 1995. Osteogenic differentiation of hypertrophic chondrocytes involves asymmetric cell divisions and apoptosis. *Journal of Cell Biology* 131:483–494.

Robison, R. 1923. The possible significance of hexophosphoric esters in ossification. *Biochemical Journal* 24:1927–1941.

Salmon, W.D.J., and Daughaday, W.H. 1957. A hormonally controlled serum factor which stimulates sulfate incorporation by cartilage in vitro. *Journal of Laboratory and Clinical Medicine* 49:825–836.

Sanford, L.P., Ormsby I., GittenbergerdeGroot A.C., Sariola H., Friedman R., Boivin G.P., Cardell E.L., and Doetschman T. 1997. TGF beta 2 knockout mice have multiple developmental defects that are nonoverlapping with other TGF beta knockout phenotypes. *Development* 124:2659–2670.

Schlechter, N.L., Russell, S.M., Spencer, E.M., and Nicoll, C.S. 1986. Evidence suggesting that the direct growth-promoting effect of growth-hormone on cartilage invivo is mediated by local production of somatomedin. *Proceedings of the National Academy of Sciences of the United States of America* 83:7932–7934.

Schmid, T.M., and Linsenmayer, T.F. 1985. Immunohistochemical localization of short chain cartilage collagen (type-X) in avian-tissues. *Journal of Cell Biology* 100:598–605.

Schwartz, Z., Schlader, D.L., Swain, L.D., and Boyan, B.D. 1988. Direct effects of 1,25-dihydroxyvitamin D3 and 24,25-dihydroxyvitamin D3 on growth zone and resting zone chondrocyte alkaline phosphatase and phospholipase-A2 specific activities. 123:2878–2884.

Serra R., Karaplis, A., and Sohn, P. 1999. Parathyroid hormone-related peptide (PTHrP)-dependent and -independent effects of transforming growth factor beta (TGF-beta) on endochondral bone formation. *Journal of Cell Biology* 145:783–794.

Thorp, B.H. 1988. Relationship between the rate of longitudinal bone-growth and physeal thickness in the growing fowl. *Research in Veterinary Science* 45: 83–85.

Thorp, B.H., Anderson, I., and Jakowlew, S.B. 1992. Transforming growth factor-beta-1, factor-beta-2 and factor-beta-3 in cartilage and bone-cells during endochondral ossification in the chick. *Development* 114:907–911.

Trueta, J. ed. 1968. From gel to bone. In *Studies of the Development and Decay of the Human Frame*. London: Heinemann Medical.

Urist, M.R. 1965. Bone: formation by autoinduction. *Science* 150:893–899.

Weir E.C., Philbrick, W.M., Amling, M., Neff, L.A., Baron, R., and Broadus, A.E. 1996. Targeted overexpression of parathyroid hormone-related peptide in chondrocytes caus-es chondrodysplasia and delayed endochondral bone formation. *Proceedings of the National Academy of Sciences of the United States of America* 93:10240–10245.

Wilsman, N.J., Farnum, C.E., Green, E.M., Lieferman, E.M., and Clayton, M.K. 1996a. Cell cycle analysis of proliferative zone chondrocytes in growth plates elongating at different rates. *Journal of Orthopaedic Research* 14:562–572.

Wilsman, N.J., Farnum, C.E., Lieferman, E.M., Fry, M., and Barreto, C. 1996b. Differential growth by growth plates as a function of multiple parameters of chondrocytic kinetics. *Journal of Orthopaedic Research* 14:927–936.

Wroblewski, J., and Edwal-Arvidsson, C. 1995. Inhibitory effects of basic fibroblast growth-factor on chondrocyte differentiation. *Journal of Bone and Mineral Research* 10:735–742.

Zezulak, K.M., and Green, H. 1986. The generation of insulin-like growth factor-I–sensitive cells by growth-hormone action. *Science* 233:551–553.

10
Adipose Growth

Colin G. Scanes

Adipose tissue predominantly contains mature adipocytes. During development/growth, there are increases in both adipocyte number and size, the latter being due to the accumulation of lipid, predominantly triglyceride. During development and the early phase of growth, there are major increases in adipocyte number (see Figure 10.1). This is due to the proliferation of adipocyte precursors, differentiated adipocytes not being capable of cell division. Thus growth of adipose is a mix of hyperplasia and hypertrophy, with the latter becoming progressively more important later in growth.

During fetal development and the early phase of postnatal growth, adipogenesis occurs. Adipocytes are recruited from uncommitted mesenchymal cells with cell proliferation and subsequent differentiation (see Figure 10.1). The recruitment occurs predominantly during fetal development and growth. Even mature adipose tissue contains adipocyte precursor cells. These are at various levels of maturity, with stromal-vascular cells being the less differentiated precursor cells (reviewed Minguell et al. 2001).

During postnatal growth and particularly its later stages, adipose tissue increases in volume/weight due predominantly to adipocytes increasing in volume (due to lipid accumulation) but there is some increase in adipose cell number. The accumulation

Figure 10.1. Idealized schematic of adipocyte precursor recruitment, proliferation, differentiation and maturation.

$\Leftarrow \quad \Leftarrow \quad \Leftarrow$
$\Downarrow \qquad \qquad \Uparrow$

Adipocyte precursor cells –
pluripotent mesenchymal cells $\Rightarrow$ *Proliferating*
(stem cells)

Recruitment
$\Downarrow$

Preadipocytes $\Rightarrow$ *Proliferating*
OR
$\Downarrow$

(Cell proliferation arrested at G_1/S stage)

$\Downarrow \quad$ *Differentiating*

Adipocytes *Non-Proliferating*

$\Downarrow \quad$ *Net lipid filling [triglyceride formation*
$\Downarrow \quad$ *from fatty acids) less lipolysis]*

Mature lipid filled adipocyte

of lipid (triglyceride) is the result of fatty acid esterification exceeding lipolysis (breakdown of triglycerides to glycerol and fatty acids). The fatty acids are derived from the diet or synthesized either in the adipocyte in cattle, sheep, and pigs or in the liver in chickens (Goodridge 1968a; Yeh and Leveille 1971).

The bone marrow contains uncommitted stem cells that, it is thought, can migrate to distant tissues. These mesenchymal stem cells from the bone marrow can be adipocyte precursors. This recruitment is stimulated by leukemia inhibitory factor (LIF) and precluded by either 1,25 (OH)$_2$ vitamin D$_3$ or leptin (reviewed Minguell et al. 2001) (also see Chapters 5 and 6).

PROLIFERATION OF ADIPOCYTE PRECURSORS

There is both basal and stimulated proliferation of adipose-precursor cells. The proliferation of preadipocytes can increase greatly in the presence of growth factors. Table 10.1 summarizes the effect of growth factors on the proliferation of chicken preadipocytes.

ADIPOCYTE DIFFERENTIATION

Hormones and Differentiation

Adipogenesis or adipocyte differentiation can be induced by a "cocktail" of hormones (glucocorticoids and insulin/IGF-I). Adipocyte differentiation is not fully understood. Based on studies with rodent models and cell lines, it is clear that adipogenesis is under the control of several transcription factors, of which the two major ones are CCAAT/ enhancer binding protein α (C/EBPα) and peroxisome proliferator-activated receptorγ (PPARγ). For instance, expression of the adipocyte-specific fatty acid binding protein (aP2) is controlled by both these transcription factors. The aP^2 gene has promoter sites for both C/EBPα and PPARγ (reviewed Lowell 1999).

Adipocytes are derived from mesenchymal cells via a mechanism involving peroxisome proliferator-activated receptor (PPARγ).

Pluripotent mesenchymal cells $\Rightarrow$ C/EBPβ and
C/EBPδ $\Rightarrow$ Early Adipocyte differentiation

PPARγ is a member of the nuclear receptor superfamily of transcription factors (Braissant et al. 1996). It is not clear what the natural ligand is for PPARγ, although various prostaglandins including deoxy-delta 12, 14-prostaglandin J$_2$ have been proposed (Forman et al. 1995; Kliewer et al. 1997). PPARγ forms a heterodimer with another member of the RXR superfamily, which is the receptor for 9-cis retinoic acid receptor. The heterodimer binds to PPAR responsive elements in the promoters of target genes (Glass and Rosenfeld 2000).

Expression of C/EBPα is "turned on" during differentiation prior to the expression of many adipocyte-specific genes; the latter contain C/EBPα response elements (reviewed Lowell 1999). C/EBPα does not appear to be required for adipogenesis, but it is essential for the development of a mature adipocyte capable of lipid accumulation.

Early differentiated adipocyte $\rightarrow$
C/EBPα $\Rightarrow$ Mature adipocyte

Adipocytes express two other transcription factors prior to C/EBPα. These, C/EBPβ and C/EBPδ,

Table 10.1. Stimulation of the proliferation of chicken adipocyte precursors by growth factors and their interactions (data from Butterwith and Goddard, 1991; Butterwith et al., 1992, 1993)

	0	IGF-I	TGF-α	FGF-1	FGF-2	PDGF
0	0					
IGF-I	+					
TGF-α	++					
FGF-1	++	+++	+++			
FGF-2	+	++	++	+		
PDGF	+++	+++	++++	++++	+++	
TGF-β1	+	++	+++	++	++	++

+1.5–5.0-fold increase.
++5.1–10.0-fold increase.
+++10.1–80-fold increase.
++++>80-fold increase.

are expressed prior to C/EBPα and are involved in the early stages of differentiation. Knock-out of both C/EBPβ and C/EBPδ reduces adipose tissue but does not affect expression of C/EBPα or PPARγ (reviewed Lowell 1999).

Expression of transcription factors is induced by adipogenic hormones. For instance, dexamethasone (glucocorticoid) and insulin (in the presence of methylisobutylxanthine) increases expression of both C/EBPβ and C/EBPδ in 3T3-L1 cells (Cao et al. 1991).

Indices of Differentiation

There are indices of terminal differentiation of adipocytes (reviewed Minguell et al. 2001). These include the appearance of molecular markers:

- Peroxisome proliferator-activated receptorγ (PPARγ2) (or mRNA for PPARγ2)
- CCAAT/enhancer binding protein β (C/EBPβ) (or mRNA for C/EBPβ)
- Adipocyte-specific fatty acid binding protein (aP2) (or mRNA for aP2)
- Leptin (or mRNA for leptin)
- Lipoprotein lipase (or mRNA for lipoprotein lipase) (*an early marker for adipocyte differentiation*)
- Adipsin (or mRNA for adipsin)
- Glycerol-3-phosphate dehydrogenase (GPDH) (*a late marker for adipocyte differentiation*)

An additional cytoplasmic marker of terminal adipocyte differentiation is the appearance/accumulation of lipid droplets that stain with oil red.

PROLIFERATION AND DIFFERENTIATION OF LIVESTOCK ADIPOCYTES

Porcine Preadipocytes Proliferation and Differentiation

There has been considerable attention placed on the proliferation and differentiation of porcine preadipocytes (stromal-vascular cells).

Growth Factors and Hormones

The effects of growth factors on the proliferation and differentiation of porcine preadipocytes is summarized in Table 10.2. Among the factors required for differentiation of porcine preadipocytes are IGF-I, insulin, and the glucocorticoid cortisol Glucocorticoids induce differentiation (as indicated by lipogenesis and the activities of adipose enzymes— e.g., lipoprotein lipase and SN-glycerol-3-phosphate dehydrogenase) in vitro of preadipocytes from some adipose stores (from the ham and shoulder but not perirenal region) (Ramsey et al. 1989b; Richardson et al. 1992). Although glucocorticoid appeared to stimulate proliferation, as indicated by increases in the number of adipocytes in a cell cluster, this appeared to be due to differentiation of more cells in the available pool of precursors because no changes in the ^{3}H-thymidine incorporation by preadipocytes were observed (Ramsey et al. 1989b). Insulin stimulates differentiation of preadipocytes (Ramsey et al. 1989b). Some synergistic effect of glucocorticoid and insulin on adipocyte differentiation has been observed (Ramsey et al. 1989b). It would appear that under at least some circumstance both glucocorticoid and insulin are required for adipocyte differentiation (Hausman and Richardson 1998) (see Table 10.3). IGF-I stimulates both proliferation and differentiation (adipose enzyme activities: lipoprotein lipase and SN-glycerol-3-phosphate dehydrogenase) of porcine adipocytes (Ramsey et al. 1989a). Not only does IGF-I increase both proliferation and differentiation but also porcine preadipocytes release IGF-I and IGF-binding proteins (IGF-BPs) (Chen et al. 1996) with IGF-I capable of exerting an autocrine/ paracrine role. Moreover, the release of IGF-I and IGF-BPs from cultured preadipocytes is influenced by the presence of hormones (see Table 10.4). In vitro differentiation of porcine preadipocytes is inhibited by GH but not by IGF-I, but both depress their proliferation (Gerfault et al. 1999).

A number of growth factors influence preadipocyte proliferation and differentiation. These effects include the following:

- EGF increases both proliferation (DNA replication) in pig adipocyte precursors and differentiation as indicated by lipoprotein lipase activity (Boone et al. 2000).
- TGF-β inhibits differentiation as indicated by the reduced number of cells filling with lipid in primary cultures of newborn pig stromal vascular cells (Richardson et al. 1989).
- Retinoic acid inhibits differentiation of porcine preadipocytes (Suryawan and Hu 1997).

Table 10.2. Effects of growth factors and hormones in the proliferation and differentiation of preadipocytes in the pig

Growth Factor	Proliferation	Differentiation	Reference
IGF-I	+	+	Ramsay et al., 1989a; Richardson et al., 1992; Wright and Hausman, 1995
EGF, TGFα	+	+	Boone et al., 2000
TGFβ	+	−	Richardson et al., 1989, 1992
TNF-α	+	−	Boone et al., 2000
Insulin			
Glucocorticoids	0/+	+	Ramsey et al., 1989b
Retinoic acid		−	Suryawan and Hu, 1997

Table 10.3. Possible requirement for both insulin and glucocorticoid for the differentiation of porcine-adipose precursors (data from Hausman and Richardson, 1998)

GPDH[2]	Activity
O[1]	100[a]
Dexamethasone	96±4[a]
Insulin	100[a]
Insulin + Dexamethasone	166±16[b]

[a,b]Different letters indicate different $p<0.05$.
[1]Preadipocytes were cultured in a serum-free medium containing transferin + selenium.
[2]Glycerol-3-phosphate dehydrogenase—a marker for adipocyte differentiation.

Table 10.4. Effect of hormones on IGF-I release from porcine preadipocytes in culture (data from Chen et al., 1996)

	IGF-I (pg/ml)	IGF-BP-1	IGF-BP-2	IGF-BP-3	IGF-BP-4
Control[1]	100±4.3[c]	100[a]	100[a]	100[a]	100[a]
GH	154±1.5[a]	147±5[b]	146±10[b]	170±13[b]	149±6[b]
Dexamethasone	65±3.6[c]	50±5[c]	59±5[c]	71±11[c]	62±6[c]
T4	153±10[b]	191±18[b]	180±16[b]	174±6[b]	363±48[c]

[a,b,c]Different letters indicate different $p<0.05$.
[1]Control IGF-I release 845 pg/ml.

- In vitro differentiation does not appear to require triiodothyronine (T_3) (Suryawan et al. 1997), but there are effects of the thyroid hormone, thyroxine (T_4) on differentiation in vivo in hypophysectomized fetal pigs (Hausman and Yu 1998).

Transcription Factors

During differentiation, porcine adipocytes have been shown to express C/EBPα, C/EBPβ, and C/EBPδ (Yu and Hausman 1998). Based on an in vitro study in which preadipocytes were treated with either fetal bovine serum alone or with the glucocorticoid dexamethasone, it would appear that glucocorticoid can induce C/EBPα expression/translation (Hausman 2000).

Extracellular Matrix

Preadipocyte recruitment, proliferation, and differentiation has been demonstrated to be affected by the extracellular matrix (Hausman et al. 1996). For an example of a study, see Table 10.5.

Table 10.5. Effect of extracellular matrix on proliferation and differentiation of porcine adipose precursor cells (based on Hausman et al., 1996)

	Control	Extracellular Matrix[1]
Adipocytes number per unit area	106 ± 48^a	414 ± 48^b
Adipocyte volume ($\mu^2 \times 100^2$)	17 ± 1^a	83 ± 1^b

[a,b]Different letters indicate different $p<0.05$.
[1]Extract of Engelbeth-Holm-Swarm tumor cells.

Chicken Preadipocyte Proliferation and Differentiation

There are profound effects of growth factors on the preadipocyte proliferation and adipocyte differentiation in chickens. These are summarized in Tables 10.1 and 10.6. Not only do FGF-2, IGF-I, and TGF-βs (TGF-β1) stimulate proliferation of preadipocytes but also FGF-2, IGF-I, and TGF-βs (TGF-β2, TGF-β3, and TGF-β4) are expressed by chicken adipocyte precursors (Burt et al. 1992).

Based on in vitro studies, there is a markedly lower rate of preadipocyte proliferation in layer- than broiler-type chickens (Donnelly et al. 1993). These breeds exhibit relatively low and high adipose accumulation, respectively.

ADIPOSE GROWTH IN LIVESTOCK (ADIPOCYTE NUMBER AND VOLUME)

There is considerable information on the characteristics of adipocytes during growth of livestock. Adipose tissue grows by a mix of hyperplasia (increase in cell number) and hypertrophy (increase in the volume of individual cells). The majority of quantitative studies on the changes in number and volume of adipocytes have employed the techniques of fixing the adipose tissue with osmium tetroxide, separation of the cells, and then both sizing and counting the cells in a Coulter counter (Hirsch and Gallian 1968). The approach has the advantage of great precision but will provide an underestimate of the number of cells in an adipose depot as it misses cells with a diameter of less than 25μ. Another approach is measurement of adipose DNA. This overestimates the number of adipocytes because adipose tissue also contains endothelial cells, fibroblasts, macrophages, mast cells, etc., which account for ~50% DNA (Rodbell 1964).

Adipose Growth in Cattle

Changes in adipocyte characteristics during growth of cattle are summarized in Tables 10.7, 10.8, and 10.9. In cattle, adipose tissue growth occurs by a mix of increases in adipocyte number (hyperplasia) and the average volume/size of the adipocytes (hypertrophy). The latter is quantitatively considerably more important. Increases in the average volume of adipocytes account for ~85% of growth between 15 and 25% of mature body weight, ~93% of growth between 35 and 45% of mature body weight, and >95% of growth between 55 and 65% of mature body weight (calculated from Robelin 1981) (Table 10.7). Although adipocyte size (diameter) increases progressively between 11 and 19 months of age, there is little change in adipocyte number (Cianzio et al. 1985) (Table 10.8 and 10.9 and Figure 10.2).

Table 10.6. Effects of growth factors on the proliferation and differentiation of chicken preadipocytes (based on Butterwith and Gilroy, 1991; Butterwith and Goddard, 1991; Butterwith et al., 1992, 1993)

Growth Factor	Proliferation	Adipocyte Differentiation
IGF-I, IGF-II	+	
EGF/ TGFα	+	–
FGF-2	+	
PDGF	+	
TGFβ	+	–

Table 10.7. Effect of age on adipocyte volume characteristics in cattle

A. *In Hereford cattle (data from Hood and Allen, 1973)*

	Age (Months)	
	8	14
Carcass weight (kg)	111	168
Perirenal adipocyte volume (pL)[2]	104	258
Subcutaneous adipocyte volume (pL)[1]	146	206

B. *In Charolais and Friesian bulls (data from Robelin, 1981)*

	4.2	7.7	10.2	13	16.3	20.2
% mature weight	15	25	35	45	55	65
Adipose tissue (kg)	6.8	19	38	56	76	101
Adipocyte volume[1] (pL)	47	156	344	540	556	695
Total Adipocyte number (# $\times 10^{10}$)	5.6	6.6	6.6	7.1	10.8	10.2
Number of small[2] adipocytes (# $\times 10^8$)	546	456	212	216	343	210
Number of medium[2] adipocytes (# $\times 10^8$)	11	207	444	462	675	711
Number of large[2] adipocyte (# $\times 10^8$)	0	0	5	30	60	98

[1]Volume = 4/3 Π r^3 or 1/6 Π D^3 where r = radius and D = diameter.
[2]Small 25–63 μm; medium 63–125 μm; large > 125 μm.

Table 10.8. Increases in the diameter of adipocytes in six fat depots during growth in steers (data from Cianzio et al., 1985)[a]

	Age at Slaughter (Months)				
	11	13	15	17	19
Fat Depot	Adipocyte diameter (μm)				
Subcutaneous	95 ± 5[b]	120 ± 3[c]	122 ± 3[c]	138 ± 6[c]	122 ± 6[c]
Intermuscular	93 ± 4[b]	112 ± 3[b,c]	119 ± 4[c]	133 ± 4[c]	123 ± 6[c]
Intramuscular	73 ± 3[b]	86 ± 3[b,c]	96 ± 3[c,d]	107 ± 3[d]	97 ± 3[c,d]
Mesenteric	103 ± 3[b]	117 ± 3[b,c]	145 ± 9[c]	149 ± 6[c]	137 ± 7[c]
Kidney	93 ± 4[b]	122 ± 5[b,d]	148 ± 10[b,c]	183 ± 10[c]	175 ± 9[c,d]
Brisket	74 ± 6[b]	96 ± 4[b,c]	117 ± 4[c]	116 ± 8[c]	103 ± 3[c]

[a]Values are means ± SE of eight steers/slaughter group.
[b,c,d] Different superscripts in a row indicate different p<.05.

Table 10.9. Increases in the number of adipocytes in five fat depots during growth in steers (data from Cianzio et al., 1985)

	Age at Slaughter (Months)				
	11	13	15	17	19
Depot	*Adipocyte Number × 109*				
Subcutaneous	15.5[a]	12.5[b]	15.1[a]	16.3[a]	14.3[a,b]
Intermuscular	29.7[a]	28.3[a]	30.8[a,b]	33.2[b]	29.5[a]
Brisket (external)	1.2[a]	1.4[a]	1.2[a]	1.8[b]	2.0[b]
Kidney	5.6[a]	4.9[c]	3.9[a,b]	2.8[b]	3.7[b,c]
Mesenteric	4.0[a,b]	5.7[a,c]	3.5[b]	4.2[a,b]	6.0[c]
Total	56.1[a,c]	52.8[b]	54.5[a,b]	58.3[c]	55.5[b,c]

[a,b,c]Different superscripts indicate different p<.05.

Adipocyte size does not appear to follow a normal distribution. Robelin (1981) examined the changes in the number of adipocytes in three arbitrarily defined size groupings (Table 10.7). During growth, there were increases in medium and particularly large adipocytes, but a steady number of small adipocytes starting from approximately 10 months of age and thereafter.

Adipose Depot

There are some differences in the average adipocyte volume in the various adipose depots but these are manifest only at certain ages (see Tables 10.8 and 10.9).

Breed

Although there is only very limited information available, it would appear that substantial differences in

adipocyte characteristics exist between different breeds of cattle (Hood and Allen 1973) (Table 10.10).

Adipose Growth in Pigs

The changes in adipocyte characteristics during growth of pigs have received detailed consideration (e.g., Anderson and Kauffman 1973; Mersmann et al. 1975; Hood and Allen 1977; Steffan et al. 1979). There is strong unanimity between the studies (see Table 10.11). Growth of the adipose tissue of pigs involves both hyperplasia (increase in cell numbers) and hypertrophy, with the former making a greater contribution earlier in growth. Increases in adipocyte number account for the following proportion of adipose growth: 97% (1–2 months old); 41% (2–3.9 months old, and 35% between 5–6.5 months old (calculated from data in Table 10.11).

Table 10.10. Effect of breed and adipose depot on adipose tissue characteristics in (14-month) cattle (data from Hood and Allen, 1973)

	Holstein	Hereford × Angus	Hereford
Perirenal adipose tissue			
Cell volume (nL)	1.16[a]	1.68[b]	0.26[c]
Subcutaneous adipose tissue			
Cell volume (nL)	0.92[a]	1.50[b]	0.21[c]
Thickness of fat (cm)	0.36[a]	1.22[b]	0.23[c]

[a,b,c]Different superscript letters indicate breed different p<0.05.

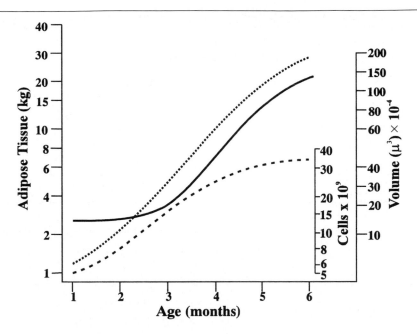

Figure 10.2A. Changes in adipose tissue, adipocyte volume, and volume during growth of pigs (adapted from Anderson and Kauffman, 1973).

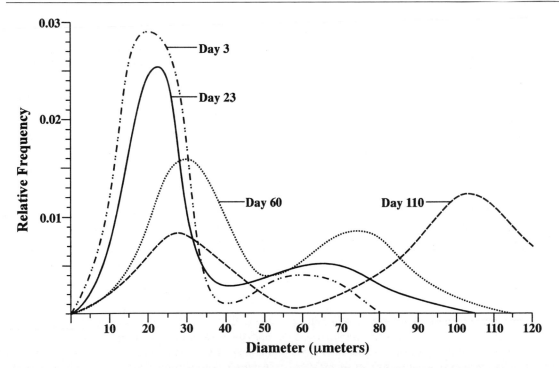

Figure 10.2B. Changes in the size of adipocytes during growth of pigs (adapted from Mersman et al., 1975).

Table 10.11. Changes in adipocyte numbers and volume during growth in pig

A. *Changes in adipose tissue characteristics together with adipocyte cell number and volume in castrate male Chester White Pigs (barrows) (data from Anderson and Kauffman, 1973)*

	Age (Months)				
Parameter	1	2	3.5	5	6.5
Body weight (kg)	8	16	43	73	106
Adipose weight (kg)	1.2	2.1	6.9	18	31
Cell volume (pL)	150	155	298	838	1515
Adipocyte number per animal (# $\times 10^9$)	5	8.2	20	31	35

B. *Changes in adipocyte characteristics during growth on Hampshire $\times$ Yorkshire barrows (Hood and Allen, 1977)*

Parameter	2.7	3.9	5.6
Body weight (kg)	28	54	109
Cell volume (pL)	171	340	485
Cells # $\times 10^6$			
extramuscular	25	33	64
perirenal	1.1	1.7	4.4

C. *Changes in adipocyte characteristics during growth based on bimodel distribution of adipocyte size in back fat from crossbred (Chester White $\times$ Hampshire) pigs (data from Mersmann et al., 1975)*

	Age (Days)						
Parameter	3	9	23	40	60	110	160
Cells per g tissue ($\times 10^6$)	7.5	11.8	11.1	4.9	5.8	1.9	2.5
Small Adipocytes							
Average volume (pL)	10	14.7	10.4	9.1	24.1	20.8	6.2
Small cells as a percentage of cells in adipose tissue	91	75	69	88	56	31	32
Small cells as a percentage of adipose volume	47	22	10	3	10	1	0
Large Adipocytes							
Average volume (pL)	111	158	205	181	262	655	621
Large cells as a percentage of cells in adipose tissue	9	25	31	62	44	69	68
Large cells as a percentage of adipose volume	52	78	90	97	90	99	100

Adipocyte size shows a clear bimodal distribution and hence adipocytes can be classified into two size categories: small and large (Mersman et al. 1975). The small adipocytes make up <10% of the volume of the adipose tissue (from 23 days of age), but more than 30% of adipocytes (Table 10.11). During growth, there are major increases in size and the number of the large adipocytes due respectively to accumulation of triglyceride and recruitment. (See Figure 10.2.)

Growth-Related Changes in Adipocyte Triglyceride and Triglyceride Biosynthetic Enzymes

Table 10.12 shows changes during growth in adipocyte triglyceride and the activities of key enzymes critical to triglyceride synthesis. During growth, the triglyceride proportion of adipose tissue increases, with concomitant reductions in protein (Steffen et al. 1979) (see Table 10.12 for details) and water. The biosynthetic apparatus for triglyceride synthesis is fully established in very young pigs (Table 10.12).

There is a progressive decline in the activities of the triglyceride biosynthetic enzymes during growth (Steffen et al. 1979) (see Table 10.12 for details). Although this decline in the activities of the triglyceride biosynthetic enzymes partially reflects adipocyte enlargement and engorgement with triglyceride, there is also a change in adipocyte biosynthetic capability with age/stage of growth. There are marked differences in lipogenesis (fatty acid synthesis) and glyceryl synthesis (reflecting glycolysis and triglyceride formation) from ^{14}C-glucose with stage of growth and adipocyte size (Etherton et al. 1981) (for details see Table 10.13). These include the following:

- Irrespective of age/stage of growth, rates (per cell) of lipogenesis and, to a somewhat less extent, glyceryl synthesis increase with adipocyte size (Table 10.13)
- Irrespective of adipocyte size, rates (per cell) of lipogenesis and glyceryl synthesis decrease with age/stage of growth (Table 10.13).

Table 10.12. Changes in adipose tissue composition and triglyceride biosynthetic enzyme activities (data from or calculated from Steffen et al., 1979)

Parameter	Age (Days)				
	3	25	45	75	155
Triglyceride (mg/g)	297	494	544	621	791
Protein (mg/g)	3.2	0.9	1.3	0.9	0.8
Acyl-CoA-*sn*-glycerol-3-phosphate acyl transferase	79	46	68	41	22
Phosphatidate phosphohydrolase	112	32	38	22	16
1,2-diglyceride-*o*-acyl transferase	5.5	5.5	7.5	7.8	4.5

Table 10.13. Effect of age/stage of growth and cell size on biosynthetic capacity of pig adipocytes (adapted from Etherton et al., 1981)

	Age (Days)		
	111	155	201
C^{14}-*Glucose* → *Glyceryl*			
Small adipocytes[1]	58[a]	44[b]	17[c]
Medium adipocytes[1]	94[a]	102[a]	65[b]
Large adipocytes[1]	141[a]	108[a]	72[b]
C^{14}-*glucose* → *fatty acids*			
Small adipocytes[1]	511[a]	402[b]	70[c]
Medium adipocytes[1]	1055[a]	1019[a]	380[b]
Large adipocytes[1]	1337[a]	1149[a]	369[b]

[a,b,c]Different superscript letters indicate age different $p<0.05$.
[1]Cell sizes: small adipocytes—diameter 20–63 μm; medium adipocytes—63–102 μm; large adipocytes—102–153 μm.

Breed Differences

There are substantial differences in body fat with breed and within a breed genetic background. Hood and Allen (1977) examined breed differences in adipocyte characteristics. In this study, the fatter breed had substantially larger adipocytes in at least three adipose depots (Table 10.14) but a tendency for fewer adipocytes.

Adipose Growth in Chickens

Pattern of Growth

The changes in adipose tissue size/weight/composition during growth and development of chickens are well described.

Embryonic Adipose Development/Growth

The weight of subcutaneous adipose tissue increases during embryonic development (Table 10.15)

with a decreases in the proportion of water and increases in adipose lipid (Langslow and Lewis 1974). This increase in adipose weight consists of both *hyperplasia* and *hypertrophy*. Hyperplasia (increase in adipocytes number) is reflected by the 3.6-fold increase in adipose DNA content between days 12 and 19 of embryonic development (Table 10.15). Hypertrophy (increase in adipocytes volume or lipid filling) is obvious from the 48-fold increase in the triglyceride: DNA ratio between days 12 and 19 of embryonic development (Table 10.15).

Adipose Development/Growth in the Peri-hatching Period

Immediately following hatching, there is decline in adipose tissue weight mainly reflecting mobilization of triglyceride from adipocytes (reflected in a reduction in the triglyceride-to-DNA ratio see Table 10.15).

Table 10.14. Differences in adipocyte characteristics in fat and lean breeds of pigs (at 109 kg live weight) (data from Hood and Allen, 1977)

Parameter	Lean (Hampshire × Yorkshire)	Fat (Minnesota No3 × No 1)
Age (Days)	168	160
Perirenal fat (%)	2.3	3.2[*]
Intramuscular fat (%)	3.1	3.5
Outercutaneous fat (cm)	0.9	1.3[*]
Middle subcutaneous fat (cm)	1.3	2.1[*]
Adipocyte cell volume (pL)		
Perirenal	54	87[*]
Outer subcutaneous	41	73[*]
Middle subcutaneous	50	90[*]
Adipocyte cell number ($\times 10^9$)		
Perirenal	44	3.5
Extramuscular	64	52[*]

[*]Lines differ p<0.05.

Table 10.15. Changes in adipose tissue during embryonic and early posthatch growth in egg-laying lines of chickens[1] (data from Langslow and Lewis, 1974; Pfaff and Austic, 1976)

			Adipose Tissue		
	Age	Depot	Weight	Cellularity DNA— Content mg (Number of Cells × 10⁶)	Triglyceride/mg DNA
Study A[1]	12d Embryonic (E)	Subcutaneous	19	54	0.03
	14dE	Subcutaneous	61	125	0.15
	16dE	Subcutaneous	126	140	0.48
	19dE	Subcutaneous	450	192	1.43
	Hatch				
	1 d	Subcutaneous	525	150	2.15
	8 d	Subcutaneous	137	125	0.84
	15 d	Subcutaneous	150	80	1.03
Study B[2]	2–2.5 W	Abdominal	0.75	180	8.3
	4 W	Abdominal	0.93	251	10.5
	5.5 W	Abdominal	1.2	293	—
	7–7.5 W	Abdominal	5.2	478 (36)	6.7
	9.5 W	Abdominal	6.2	640	—
	12.5–13 W	Abdominal	16	1210 (103)	34
	16 W	Abdominal	36	1515 (117)	57
	20–24 W	Abdominal	54	1669	67
	39 W	Abdominal	90	–(137)	—

[1] Egg laying strains of chickens were employed. Study with subcutaneous fat employed Rhode Island Reds (mixed sex); the data for abdominal fat pad are from female White Leghorns.

Adipose Development/Growth in Chicks Posthatching

Growth of adipose tissue occurs throughout growth and sexual maturation. The growth rate of adipose tissue is initially allometric but later is more rapid than body growth and continues after sexual maturation and the termination of bone growth. Quantitative data on the growth of chicken adipose tissue are summarized in, respectively, Tables 10–15B (a laying hen strain—white Leghorn chickens) together with Table 10.16 and Figure 10.3 (in broiler-type heavy chickens).

In a "light," laying hen strain, growth of adipose tissue is due to increases in both cell number (determined either as DNA or directly) and cell size (determined as triglyceride/DNA ratio) (Pfaff and Austic 1976) (Table 10.15B). Early in posthatch growth (between 2 and 7–7.5 weeks of age), growth is due to hyperplasia; cell number (as reflected by DNA content) increases 2.66-fold. Later, adipose growth is predominantly hypertrophy (a progressively greater triglyceride-to-DNA ratio). There is some continued increase in cell number.

The changes of cellularity and cell volume of adipose tissue have been reported in heavy rapidly growing broiler chickens (Hood 1982; Cherry et al. 1984; March et al. 1984; Cartright et al. 1986), These have been measured in the abdominal fat pad, which is well defined anatomically. Throughout most of posthatch growth, there is both hyperplasia and hypertrophy of the adipose tissue (Tables 10.16 and Figure 10.4).

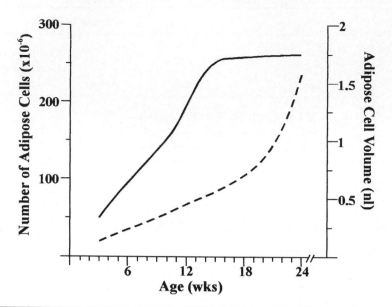

Figure 10.3. Growth of chicken adipose tissue is due to increases in cell number and volume (adapted from Hood, 1982).

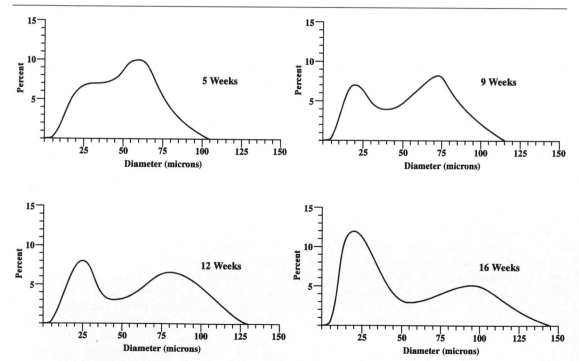

Figure 10.4. Changes in the distribution of large-sized adipocytes during growth of chickens (adapted from March et al., 1984).

Table 10.16. Changes in adipocyte cell number and cell volume in the abdominal fat pad during growth in female broiler chickens

A. *Early growth (data from Cartwright et al., 1986)*

	Age in Weeks (Increase over Previous Age)	
Parameter	4	8
Abdominal fat pad (g)	15	36 (+140%)
Adipocyte number (# × 10^6)	121	233 (+93%)
Adipocyte volume (pL)	117	177 (+51%)

B. *Later growth (data from March et al., 1984)*

	Age in Weeks		
Parameter	7–9	12–16	21–22
Abdominal fat pad (g)	53	172 (+224%)	347 (+102%)
Small Adipocytes			
Number (# × 10^6)	95	394 (+315%)	891 (+116%)
Volume (pL)	10	12 (+15%)	12 (+2%)
Large adipocytes[1]			
Number (# × 10^6)	257	470 (+83%)	558 (+19%)
Volume (pL)	179	367 (+105%)	671 (+83%)

[1]Diameter >50µm.

C. *Changes in adipocyte characteristics during growth of broiler chickens in different depots (data from Merkley and Cartwright, 1989)*

	Age in Weeks			
Depot and Parameter	4	8	12	16
Abdominal fat				
Weight	15.6±1.1	55.2±4.7	130.0±9.9	273.9±17.9
Adipocyte number (# × 10^6)	122±98	213±12	298±20	354±30
Adipocyte volume (pL)	198±11	350±33	501±40	788±43
Back fat				
Weight	2.8±0.2	7.8±0.4	18.0±1.7	37.2±2.1
Adipocyte number (# × 10^5)	25±1	36±2	39±4	55±3
Adipocyte volume (pL)	158±12	285±22	582±35	775±54
Neck fat				
Weight (g)	6.2±0.3	14.9±1.6	29.1±2.5	51.5±5.4
Adipocyte number (# × 10^5)	53±3	69±7	78±6	89±11
Adipocyte volume (pL)	180±5	307±19	475±37	750±38
Thigh fat				
Weight (g)	1.2±0.1	3.2±0.2	5.6±0.4	10.5±1.0
Adipocyte number (# × 10^5)	12±1	16±1	16±1	19±2
Adipocyte volume (pL)	156±9	284±16	447±20	740±36

In early posthatch growth, there are increases in both adipocyte number and cell volume (Table 10.16 and Figures 10.3 and 10.4). Adipose growth between 4 and 8 weeks of age is attributable to an increase in cell number, accounting for about 66% of growth, and an increase in cell volume, accounting for 34%. Later in growth, hypertrophy becomes more important. The average volume of adipocytes is increasing in a logarithmic manner (e.g., Hood 1982; March et al. 1984) (Table 10.16 and Figure 10.3). The number of adipocytes (as determined by Coulter counter) in the abdominal fat pad reaches a plateau at ~14 weeks of age.

Depot

There are very similar patterns of development of adipocyte number and volume in the different adipose depots (Table 10.16C).

Conclusions

As in the pig, there is a bimodal distribution of adipocytes by size (March et al. 1984). Small adipocytes make up <3% of the volume of tissue but >25% of cells (27% at 7–9 weeks of age, 45% at 12–16 weeks of age, and 61% at 21–22 weeks of age) (calculated from Table 10.16). It can be presumed that the small adipocyte population includes the proliferating and differentiating preadipocytes and the large adipose cells that have been recruited, differentiated, and are accumulating triglyceride. Adipose growth predominantly reflects hypertrophy (lipid accumulation) of the large adipose cells (lipid accumulation). This accounts for 63% of growth between 7–9 and 12–16 weeks old and 91% between 12–16 and 21–22 weeks old.

Diet

Nutrient availability affects adipose growth. If chickens receive excess nutrients by overfeeding (via a gavage), there is markedly greater adipose growth (Table 10.17). This is due to hypertrophy. The 91% increase in adipocyte volume accounts for 81% of adipose growth (Table 10.18). Diet obviously can affect the accumulation of adipose tissue with low caloric diets associated with low adipose tissue weights. As is to be expected, diet influences the average volume of individual adipocytes (March et al. 1984) (also see Table 10.18). In addition, the number of adipocytes can be affected with some diets (March et al. 1984). This reflects recruitment and/or proliferation and/or differentiation of adipocyte precursors or lipid filling of very small adipocytes (<5m-diameter missed in counts).

Breeding/Genetics

Compared to unselected random-bred birds, commercial broiler chickens show much greater adiposity. For an example study (Cartwright et al. 1986), see Table 10.19. This increase in adipose tissue is due predominantly to greater hypertrophy, adipocytes being larger, but there is some increase in adipocyte number (Table 10.18). The increase in adipocyte volume (due to triglyceride filling) accounts for about 70% of the increased adiposity in broiler chickens. Changes in adipocyte number account for less than 30%.

Hormones and Adipocyte Characteristics

An inverse relationship exists between either adipocyte volume or number and the circulating concentrations

Table 10.17. Effect of hyperalimentation[1] on growth of adipose tissue and adipocyte characteristics in 44-day-old broiler chickens (data from Cartwright, 1991)

	Control	Overfed	Percentage Increase
Body weight (kg)	1.42	1.65	
Abdominal fat pad (g)	13.9	32.8[*]	136%
Adipocyte volume (pL)	131	250[*]	+81%
Adipocyte number x 10^6	162	200	+19%

[1]Overfed by gavage from 28–40 days of age.
[*]Different to control p<0.05.

Table 10.18. Effect of diet on adipose tissue cellularity in female chickens

Parameters	Strain	Age (w)	Control[1]	High Protein	Low Energy	Reference
Fat Pad Weight (g)	White Leghorn	12.5	32[a]	16[b]	8[c]	Pfaff and Austic, 1976
Number of cells in fat pad (# $\times 10^6$)	White Leghorn	12.5	103[a]	77[b]	54[c]	Pfaff and Austic, 1976
DNA	White Leghorn	9.5	640[a]	460[b]	428[b]	Pfaff and Austic, 1976
Fat Pad Weight (g)	Broiler	4–4.5	17[a]	3.5[b]	—	March et al., 1984[2]
Adipocyte number (# $\times 10^6$)	Broiler	4–4.5	132[a]	77[b]	—	March et al., 1984[2]
Adipocyte volume ($\mu m^3 \times 10^2$)	Broiler	4–4.5	1355[a]	530[b]	—	March et al., 1984[2]

[a,b,c]Different superscript letters indicate different $p < 0.05$.
[1]Control 25% protein; metabolizable energy (ME) 3180 kcal/kg.
  high protein 44% protein; ME 3100 kcal/kg.
  low energy 18% protein; ME 2200 kcal/kg.
[2]Control 20% protein; ME 2370 kcal/kg.
  high protein 30% protein; ME 3270 kcal/kg.

Table 10.19. Differences in adipose tissue characteristics on broiler (selected for growth) and randombred chickens (at 54 days of age) (data from Cartwright et al., 1986)

	Broiler	Randombred/Unselected
Body weight (kg)	1.86	0.8[*]
Abdominal weight (9)	23	6.7[*]
Adipocytes number ($\times 10^6$)	126	90[*]
Adipocyte volume (pL)	120	54[*]

[*]Lines differ $p < 0.01$.

of GH in different lines of chickens (Cartwright 1991). Chronic administration of the β-adrenergic-agonist, cimaterol, did not have a consistent effect on adipocyte characteristics (Merkley and Cartwright 1989).

Monoclonal Antibodies

The growth of adipose tissue is reduced posthatching following the in ovo administration of monoclonal antibodies to adipocyte cell membrane proteins (to the chick embryo) (Wu et al. 2000). The mechanism by which this in ovo treatment affects adipose volume much later in development is unknown. It may involve the antibody-destroying differentiating/differentiated adipocytes, of which there are a limited number.

TRIGLYCERIDE METABOLISM AND ITS CONTROL

Adipose tissue grows predominantly by accretion of triglyceride:

Accretion of triglyceride = Triglyceride synthesis – Triglyceride breakdown (lipolysis)

The synthesis of triglyceride is summarized in Figure 10.5, the rate of triglyceride synthesis depending on both the availability of fatty acids and glycerol-3-phosphate. In turn, fatty acid availability depends on de novo synthesis [in adipose tissue in nonlactating ruminants—cattle and sheep (reviewed Vernon 1980) together with pigs and the liver in chickens] and absorption from the gastrointestinal track. Fatty acids are readily taken up by adipocytes with circulating triglyceride (bound to lipoprotein) hydrolyzed by lipoprotein lipase in close to the adipocytes (reviewed Vernon 1980). Glycerol-3-phosphate is a product of metabolism of glucose (glycolysis).

Control of Lipid Metabolism in Sheep and Cattle

In ruminants, acetate is the major precursor for lipogenesis being incorporated into fatty acids at 10–100 times the rate observed with glucose (reviewed Vernon 1980).

Changes in Lipogenic Capability with Physiological State

There are differences in the lipolytic, lipogenic, and triglyceride synthetic capability of bovine adipocytes with physiological state (reviewed Vernon 1980).

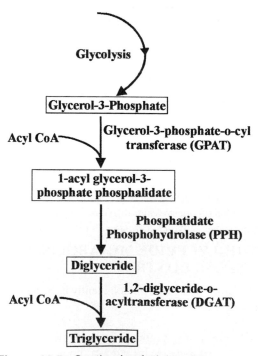

Figure 10.5. Synthesis of triglyceride.

Hormones and Lipid Metabolism

Hormones play a crucial role in controlling the rate of lipogenesis, lipolysis, and triglyceride synthesis by bovine adipocytes. This is summarized in Table 10.20. The major hormones affecting lipolysis are the following: stimulatory—epinephrine and norepinephrine acting via β-adrenergic receptors; and inhibitory—insulin and, acting locally, adenosine. The major hormones affecting lipogenesis are insulin (stimulatory) and epinephrine and norepinephrine (acting via β-adrenergic receptors) (inhibitory) and GH (inhibitory).

Triglyceride Metabolism and Its Control in Pigs

Changes in Lipogenic Capability During Adipocyte Growth

There are marked changes in lipogenic and triglyceride synthetic capability in porcine adipocytes during postnatal growth (see Tables 10.12 and 10.13).

Hormones and Lipolysis/Lipogenesis/Triglyceride Synthesis

Hormones play a crucial role in controlling the rate of lipogenesis, lipolysis, and triglyceride synthesis. The effects of hormones on these in pig adipocytes are summarized in Table 10.21. It is readily apparent that lipolysis is under both stimulatory and inhibitory control. The major lipolytic hormones are epinephrine (E) and norepinephrine (NE). These act via β receptors (probably a mix of β receptor sub-types), G_i, adenylate cyclase, cyclic AMP, and protein kinase A (Mills and Liu 1990). Many but not all β-adrenergic agonists stimulate lipolysis and inhibit lipogenesis (Hu et al. 1987; Peterla and Scanes 1990; Mills 1999).

As might be expected, insulin reduces lipolysis in the presence of β-adrenergic agonists and alone enhances the rate of lipogenesis (e.g., Peterla and Scanes 1990; Mills 1999). Chronic exposure of adipocytes to GH suppresses the lipogenic response to insulin (Walton et al. 1986, 1987).

Lipid Metabolism and Its Control in Poultry

Lipogenesis in Chickens

There is very little lipogenesis (fatty acid synthesis) occurring in chicken adipose tissue (Goodridge 1968a). Hepatocytes are the predominant site of

Table 10.20. Hormonal effects on lipolysis and lipogenesis in cattle and sheep

Hormone	Effect	Reference
Lipolysis		
Glucagon	+/0	Reviewed Vernon, 1980
β-adrenergic agonists including epinephrine	++	Sheep: Thornton et al., 1985;
Cattle: Yang and Baldwin, 1973;		Smith, 1987
GH (acute)	0	Cattle and Sheep: Houseknecht et al., 1996
GH (chronic)	+	Sheep: Watt et al., 1991
IGF-I (acute)	0	Cattle and Sheep: Houseknecht et al., 1996
Insulin	−	Cattle: Yang and Baldwin, 1973
Adenosine	−	Sheep: Doris et al., 1998
Leptin	0	Sheep: Newby et al., 2001
Prostaglandin E$_2$	0	Cattle: Di Marco et al., 1986
ACTH	0	Cattle: Yang and Baldwin, 1973
Lipogenesis		
β-adrenergic agonists	−	Reviewed Vernon, 1980
Insulin	++	e.g., Etherton et al., 1987; Vernon, 1996
GH (chronic effect in the presence of insulin)	−	Etherton et al., 1987; Vernon, 1996
Leptin	0	Newby et al., 2001
Triglyceride synthesis (C^{14}- glucose Æglyceryl in triglyceride)		
Insulin	0	Reviewed Vernon, 1980

Table 10.21. Hormonal effects on lipolysis and lipogenesis in pigs

Hormone	Effect	Reference
Lipolysis		
β-adrenergic agonists	++	Hu et al., 1987; Liu et al., 1989; Peterla and Scanes, 1990; Mills, 1999
Insulin	−	Peterla and Scanes, 1990; Mills, 1999
Adenosine	−	Mills, 1999
Leptin	+	Ramsey, 2001
Lipogenesis		
β-adrenergic agonists	−	Liu et al., 1989; Peterla and Scanes, 1990
Insulin	++	Mills, 1999
Adenosine/adenosine agonists	+	Mills, 1999
GH (chronic effect in the presence of insulin)	-/0	Walton et al., 1986, 1987
Triglyceride synthesis (C^{14}- glucose Æglyceryl in triglyceride)		
β-agonist-isoproterenol	−	Rule et al., 1987
Insulin	0	Rule et al., 1987

lipogenesis in the chicken, with the liver accounting for more than 90% of fatty acid synthesis de novo (O'Hea and Leveille 1969). There is both hormonal and metabolic control of lipogenesis with the role of hormones summarized in Table 10.22. For instance, lipogenesis is greatly reduced following fasting (Yeh and Leveille 1971). This is due presumably to the presence of high circulating concentrations of fatty acids and/or the fasting-related hormones, glucagon together with, perhaps, also E and NE; these are the major anti-lipogenic hormones in the chicken (for hormones, see Table 10.22; fatty acids: Goodridge et al. 1974). Based on studies with specific adrenergic agonists, E and NE effects are mediated predominantly by β receptors (Campbell and Scanes 1985a).

Tremendous changes in the lipogenic capability of chicken hepatocytes occur during growth and development and, in particular, at the time of hatching (Goodridge 1968a) (also see Figure 10.6). There is little lipogenic capacity in embryonic hepatocytes, because there is little need for fatty acid synthesis in the chick embryo that is utilizing yolk, rich in triglyceride, as its nutrient source. Immediately following hatching, hepatocytes become lipogenic rapidly (Figure 10.6). It has been demonstrated using enzymes in hepatocytes from chicken embryos that both insulin and triiodothyronine (T_3) are required to induce lipogenic enzymes (Goodridge et al. 1974; Back et al. 1986b; Wilson et al. 1986) (Table 10.23). A large peak in the circulat-

Table 10.22. Hormonal effects on lipolysis and lipogenesis in chickens

Hormone	Effect	Reference
Lipolysis		
Glucagon	+++	Goodridge, 1968b
Secretin	+/0	Langslow, 1973; Kitadgi et al., 1976
Norepinephrine (β-adrenergic agonists)	+	Langslow and Hales, 1969
Epinephrine (β-adrenergic agonists)	+	Langslow and Hales, 1969
ACTH	+	Langslow and Hales, 1969
GH	+	Campbell and Scanes, 1985b, 1988; Campbell et al., 1993
Insulin	0	Goodridge, 1968b; Langslow and Hales, 1969
Prostaglandin E_1	−	Langslow, 1971
Somatostatin (SRIF)	− −	Strosser et al., 1983; Campbell and Scanes, 1988
Pancreatic Polypeptide (PP)	−/+	McCumbee and Hazelwood, 1977; Oscar, 1993
Adenosine	−	Scanes et al., 1994
Lipogenesis		
Glucagon	− −	Watkins et al., 1977; Back et al., 1986
Norepinephrine (β-adrenergic agonists)	−	Campbell and Scanes, 1985a
Epinephrine (β-adrenergic agonists)	−	Cramb et al., 1982; Campbell and Scanes, 1985a
Insulin	++	Goodridge and Adelman, 1976; Back et al., 1986b
Triiodothyronine (T_3)	+	Goodridge and Adelman, 1976; Back et al., 1986
Insulin +GH	+?	Harvey et al., 1977
Triglyceride synthesis (C^{14}- glucose Æglyceryl)		
Glucagon	−	Goodridge, 1968c
Insulin	+	Goodridge, 1968c; Gomez-Capilla and Langslow, 1977

ing concentrations of T_3 occurs at the right time, in the peri-hatch period (Decuypere et al. 1979), to be responsible for the induction of lipogenic enzymes.

Triglyceride Transportation

Fatty acids are transported from the liver (and also from the gastrointestinal tract and yolk sac in the embryo and newly hatched chick) to the adipocyte via the blood stream. They are transported as triglyceride bound to very low density lipoproteins (VLDL) (Griffin and Whitehead 1982). Accompanying the increase in hepatic fatty acid synthesis in the peri-hatch period (see above) are increases in the circulat-

ing concentration of VLDL (Puvadolpirod et al. 1997). The triglyceride is hydrolyzed by lipoprotein lipase in the capillary bed adjacent to adipocytes to yield fatty acids and glycerol. The fatty acids are taken up by the adipocytes and the glycerol returns to the liver as a gluconeogenic precursor, adipose tissue lacking the critical enzyme, glycerol kinase.

In view of the importance of circulating triglyceride to the availability of fatty acid for adipose triglyceride accretion, it is not surprising that the amount of body fat correlates well with either circulating concentrations of triglyceride or VLDL (Griffin and Whitehead 1982; Griffin et al. 1982).

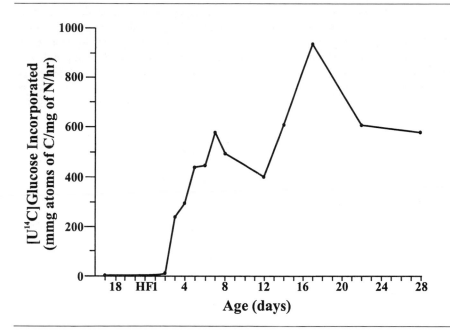

Figure 10.6. Increases in liver fatty acid synthesis during chick development (adapted from Goodridge, 1968a).

Table 10.23. Ability of insulin and triiodothyronine (T_3) to induce lipogenic enzymes in hepatocytes from chicken embryos (data from Back et al., 1986b; Wilson et al., 1986)

Hormone	Malic Enzymic		Fatty Acid Synthase	
	Activity	mRNA	Activity	mRNA
O	2.2	9.3	47	10
Insulin	2.4	9.2	12	11
T_3	33	62	10	50
Insulin + T_3[a]	100	100	100	100
Insulin + T_3 + glucagon	3.2	6.9	27	40

[a]By definition, 100%.

Lipolysis

A number of hormones can influence lipolysis by chicken adipose tissue. Glucagon is the major lipolytic hormone and somatostatin and pancreatic polypeptide are anti-lipolytic (for details see Table 10.21 and Figure 10.7). There is not necessarily good compliance between the hormones that are lipolytic and/or anti-lipolytic in domestic mammals and the same situation in poultry. An example of this is that insulin, which has little effect on lipolysis in chickens, reduces lipolysis in ruminants and pigs.

There are marked changes in the ability of poultry adipose tissue to respond to lipolytic hormones during growth and development. Prior to hatching, the chick embryo is refractory to lipolytic hormones. This is presumably due to the lack of a need for a physiological stimulus for lipolysis because energy needs are met by the absorption of yolk. Embryonic avian adipose tissue either does not respond to lipolytic hormones or responds very poorly (Table 10.23). Immediately following hatch, there is a tremendous increase in responsiveness to either glucagon or NE (Langslow 1972; Langslow and Lewis 1974) (Table 10.23). It is not clear what induces this acquisition of responsiveness, but it may involve one or more of the hormones whose production increases during the peri-hatch period, including triiodothyronine (T_3), corticosterone, or GH (Decuypere et al. 1979; reviewed Scanes et al. 1987).

After 4 weeks of age, the rate of lipolysis in the presence of glucagon or NE declines (Langslow 1972; Langslow and Lewis, 1974) (Table 10.24). As the lipolytic responsiveness to hormones decreases with stage of growth, there are concomitant increases in adipocyte volume (Table 10.15) due to net accretion of triglyceride (triglyceride synthesis/esterification >>lipolysis).

Triglyceride Synthesis

The rate of triglyceride synthesis depends upon fatty acid availability and the rate of glycolysis. There has been relatively little attention placed on triglyceride synthesis in chicken adipose tissue except from the following: The rate is much lower than in the rat (Goodridge 1968c). The rate is enhanced by insulin and reduced by glucagon

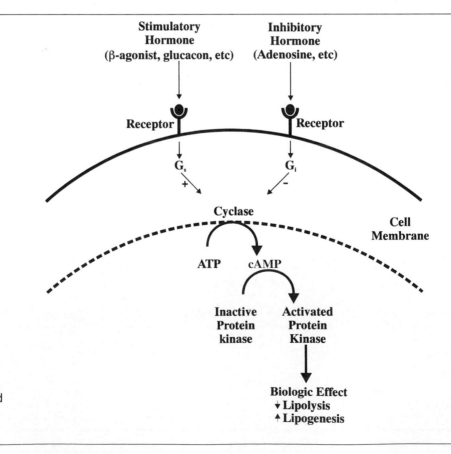

Figure 10.7.
Hormones and lipolysis/ lipogenesis.

(Goodridge 1968c;) (see also Table 10.21). The effect of insulin on glucose oxidation by chicken adipocytes increases during early posthatch growth (Gomez-Capilla and Langslow 1977).

BROWN ADIPOSE TISSUE

Brown adipose tissue plays an important role in maintenance of body temperature, particularly in the newborn mammal. Nonshivering thermogenesis by brown adipose tissue in the neonate is critical to this homeostasis of body temperature. The presence of brown adipose tissue has been definitively identified in newborn lambs (Gemmell et al. 1972) and calves (Alexander et al. 1975). Brown adipose tissue represents approximately 2% of body weight of the newborn calf. The brown adipose tissue is identified by the cellular morphology, including that of the mitachondria (see Figure 10.8), the in vivo increase in temperature/metabolic rate in response to NE, and the presence/gene expression of the uncoupling protein.

The mechanism for nonshivering thermogenesis involves uncoupling tissue respiration from ATP production. There is a specific uncoupling protein. Studies in fetal/neonatal sheep have demonstrated that both thermogenesis and mRNA for the uncoupling protein increases at birth (Casteilla et al. 1989; Clarke et al. 1992). This is probably related to thyroid hormones acting on the brown adipose tissue. Circulating concentrations of T_3 increase around the time of birth (Nathanielsz and Fisher 1979) and thermogenesis is impaired by fetal thyroidectomy (Schermer et al. 1996).

Growth/Development of Brown Adipose Tissue

One of the best-characterized brown adipose tissue depots in ruminants is the perirenal adipose tissue. In the fetal lamb, no detectable perirenal (brown) adipose tissue is detected before 60 days of gestation (Alexander 1978). Subsequently, perirenal adipose tissue grows exponentially. The weight of the perirenal adipose tissue relative to body weight increases in a linear manner to approximately 120 days of gestation with allometric growth thereafter (Alexander 1978) (see Table 10.24). During postnatal life, brown adipose tissue rapidly transforms into white adipose

Table 10.24. Changes in adipose tissue sensitivity to lipolytic hormones during growth of Rhode Island Red chickens (male only, at 12 and 16 weeks old, and in adults) (data from Langslow, 1972; Langslow and Lewis, 1974)

| | | Lipolysis[a] | | |
| | | (Δ) Increase with Glucagon | | (Δ) Increase with Norepinephrine |
Age	Basal	0.25 ng/ml	1.0 ng/ml	10 µg/ml
14ED	1.1	0.1	1.9	—
16ED	0.4	0.1	0.8	<0.1
19ED	0.4	0.1	1.8	0.2
20ED	0.6	0.5	1.4	<0.1
0D	0.8	1.1	9.6	2.9
1D	1.4	11	24	9.0
1W	1.18	19	36	13.0
2W	1.1	16	43	8.8
4W	1.8	37	53	20
8W	1.0	11	34	2
12W	1.8	11	25	2
16W	0.9	3.9	8.8	0.1
Adult	0.6	2.3	12.5	1.4

[a]Glycerol release.
Note: ED—Embryo Day; D—Days or W—Weeks posthatch

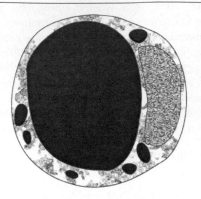

Figure 10.8. Structure of brown adipocyte showing large fat droplet (black), nucleus (grey), and multiple mitochondria (black).

tissue with changes in cell morphology and a loss of the thermogenic response to NE (lambs: Gemmell et al. 1972; calves: Alexander et al. 1975).

Control of Brown Adipose Tissue Growth/Development

Based on studies in sheep, growth/development of brown adipose tissue is under hormonal control. Thyroid hormones affect lipid deposition and probably other aspects of development. Fetal hypophy-sectomy is followed by increases in perirenal adipose tissue (Alexander 1978). Fetal thyroidectomy increases the mass of this adipose depot due to greater lipid deposition (Schermer et al. 1996) (Table 10.25). Growth of the perirenal adipose tissue is affected by nutrient availability. Restriction of nutrients to the dam dramatically reduces growth of the perirenal adipose tissue (Alexander 1978) (Table 10.24). Conversely, elevating glucose availability by continuously infusing glucose into fetal sheep enhanced the weight of both brown and white adipose tissue depots (Stevens et al. 1990) (Table 25).

There is evidence of breed effects on the development of brown adipose tissue. Carstens and colleagues (1997) suggested that the reduced thermogenic activity of calves from Brahman dams compared to Angus dams is due to the former having less brown adipose tissue.

Differences exist between the ability of hormones to influence lipogenesis in developing fetal white and brown adipose tissue. Hormones (insulin and dexamethasone) increase lipogenesis in subcutaneous white adipose tissue from fetal sheep, as is the case with the adult (Vernon 1991) (see Table 10.26); this effect is reduced in the presence of GH (Table 10.26). No such stimulation of lipogenesis is observed with fetal perirenal adipose tissue (developing brown adipose tissue) (Vernon 1991) (see Table 10.27).

Table 10.25. Changes in adipose tissue during development of the fetal lamb (data from or calculated from Alexander, 1978)

| Age | Depot | Adipose Tissue (g/kg Body Weight) | |
		Control	Dam Feed Restricted[1]
125[2]	Perirenal	8.8	7.3
146[3]	Perirenal	7.4[a]	5.7[b]
125	Subcutaneous	3.1[pa]	0.3[b]
146	Subcutaneous	0.3[q]	<0.1

[a,b]Different superscripts in row indicate different p<0.05.
[p,q]Different superscripts in column indicate different p<0.05.
[1]Restricted to ~29% of ad libitum intake.
[2]Fetal weight: controls—2.6 kg, feed restricted 2 kg.
[3]Fetal weight: controls—4.1 kg, feed restricted 3.5 kg.

Table 10.26. Brown adipose tissue development: effects of fetal thyroidectomy or glucose infusion

Treatment	Brown Adipose Tissue Weight[1] (g)	Brown Adipose Tissue Lipid Content[1] (g)	Subcutaneous White Adipose Tissue Weight[1] (g)	Reference
Study A				
Control	19.6±2.1[a]	5.2±1.1	—	Schermer et al., 1996
fetal thyroidectomy[2]	29.3±4.9[b]	12.4±3.7	—	Schermer et al., 1996
Study B				
Control (saline infusion)	22.1±1.2[a]	—	0.9±0.4[a]	Stevens et al., 1990
Continuous glucose infusion[3]	38.2±2.5b	—	4.9±1.7b	Stevens et al., 1990

[a,b]Different superscripts indicate different $p<0.05$.
[1]At birth.
[2]Surgery at day 127 of gestation.
[3]Intravenous beginning day 116 of gestation.

Table 10.27. Effect of hormones on lipogenesis (fatty acid synthesis) in adipose tissue from adult and fetal pigs (data from Vernon, 1991)

Treatment Lipogenesis—μmoles Acetate Incorporated per 2 hr. per g Tissue

	Fetal Subcutaneous	Fetal Perirenal	Adult Subcutaneous Adipose Tissue
Control	8.8[a]	18.4[a]	0.3[a]
Insulin + Dexamethasone	14.2[b]	15.5[b]	1.9[b]
Insulin + Dexamethasone + GH	10.1[a]	14.8[b]	0.2[a]

[a,b]Different superscripts indicate different $p<0.05$.

REFERENCES

Alexander, G. 1978. Quantitative development of adipose tissue in foetal sheep. *Australian Journal of Biological Science* 31:489–503.

Alexander, G., Bennett, J.W., and Gemmell, R.T. 1975. Brown adipose tissue in the new-born calf (Bos Taurus). *Journal of Physiology* 244:223–234.

Anderson, D.B., and Kauffman, R.G. 1973. Cellular and enzymatic changes in porcine adipose tissue during growth. *Journal of Lipid Research* 14:160–168.

Back, D.W., Goldman, M.J., Fisch, J.E., Ochs, R.S., and Goodridge, A.G. 1986a. The fatty acid synthase gene in avian liver. *Journal of Biological Chemistry* 261:4190–4197.

Back, D.W., Wilson, S.B., Morris, S.M., and Goodridge, A.G. 1986b. Hormonal regulation of lipogenic enzymes in chick embryo hepatocytes in culture. *Journal of Biological Chemistry* 261:12555–12561.

Boone,C., Grégoire, F., and Remacle, C. 2000. Culture of stromal–vascular cells in serum-free medium: differential actions of various hormonal agents on adipose conversion. *Journal of Animal Science* 78: 885–895.

Braissant, O., Foufelle, F., Scotto, C., Dauca, M., and Wahli, W. 1996. Differential expression of peroxisome proliferator-activated receptors (PPARs): tissue distribution of PPAR-alpha, -beta and -gamma in the adult rat. *Endocrinology* 137:354–366.

Burt, D.W., Boswell, J.M., Paton, I.R., and Butterwith, S.C. 1992) Multiple growth factor mRNAs are expressed in chicken adipocyte precursor cells. *Biochemical and Biophysical Research Communications* 187:1298–1305.

Butterwith, S.C., and Gilroy, M. (1991) Effects of transforming growth factor β1 and basic fibroblast growth factor on lipoprotein lipase activity in primary cultures of chicken (Gallus domesticus) adipocyte precursors. *Comparative Biochemistry and Physiology* 100A:473–476.

Butterwith, S.C., and Goddard, C. 1991. Regulation of DNA synthesis of chicken adipocyte precursor cells by insulin-like growth factors, platelet-derived growth factor and transforming growth factor-β. *Journal of Endocrinology* 130:203–209.

Butterwith, S.C., Peddie, C.D., and Goddard, C. 1992. Effects of transforming growth factor-β on chicken adipocyte precursor cells in vitro. *Journal of Endocrinology* 134:163–168.

Butterwith, S.C., Peddie, C.D., and Goddard, C. 1993. Regulation of adipocyte precursor DNA synthesis by acid and basic fibroblast growth factors: Interaction with heparin and other growth factors. *Journal of Endocrinology* 137:369–374.

Campbell, R.M., Chen, W.Y., Wiehl, P., Kelder, B., Kopchick, J.J., and Scanes, C.G. 1993. A growth hormone (GH) analog that antagonizes the lipolytic effect but retains full insulin-like (antilipolytic) activity of GH. *Proceedings of the Society for Experimental Biology and Medicine* 203:311–316.

Campbell, R.M., and Scanes, C.G. 1985a. Adrenergic control of lipogenesis and lipolysis in the chicken in vitro. *Comparative Biochemistry and Physiology* 82c:137–142.

Campbell, R.M., and Scanes, C.G. 1985b Lipolytic activity of purified pituitary and bacterially derived growth hormone on chicken adipose tissue in vitro. *Proceedings of the Society for Experimental Biology and Medicine* 180:513–517.

Campbell, R.M., and Scanes, C.G. 1988. Inhibition of growth hormone-stimulated lipolysis by somatostatin, insulin and insulin-like growth factor (somatomedins) in vitro. *Proceedings of the Society for Experimental Biology and Medicine* 189:362–366.

Cao, Z.D., Umek, R.M., and McKnight, S.L. 1991. Regulated expression of three C/EBP isoforms during adipose conversion of 3T3-L1 cells. *Genes and Development* 5:1538–1552.

Carstens, G.E., Mostyn, P.M., Lammoglia, M.A., Vann, R.C., Apter, R.C., and Randel, R.D. 1997. Genotypic effects on norepinephrine-induced changes in thermogenesis, metabolic hormones, and metabolites in newborn calves. *Journal of Animal Science* 75:1746–1755.

Cartwright, A.E. 1991. Adipose cellularity in Gallus domesticus: investigations to control body composition in growing chickens. *Journal of Nutrition* 121:1486–1497.

Cartwright, A.L., Marks, H.L., and Campion, D.R. 1986. Adipose tissue cellularity and growth characteristics of unselected and selected broilers: implications for the development of body fat. *Poultry Science* 65:1021–1027.

Casteilla, L., Champigny, O., Bouilland, F., Robelin, J., and Riquier, D. 1989. Sequential changes in the expression of mitochondrial protein mRNA during the development of brown adipose tissue in bovine and ovine species. *Biochemistry Journal* 257:665–671.

Chen, N.X., Hausman, G.J., and Wright, J.T. 1996. Hormonal regulation of insulin-like growth factor binding proteins and insulin-like growth factor I (IGF-I) secretion in porcine stromal-vascular cultures. *Journal of Animal Science* 74:2369–2375.

Cherry, J.A., Swartworth, W.J., and Siegel, P.B. 1984 Adipose cellularity studies in commercial broiler chicks. *Poultry Science* 63:97–108.

Cianzio, D.S., Topel, D.G., Whitehurst, G.B., Beitz, D.C., and Self, H.L. 1985. Adipose tissue growth and cellularity: changes in bovine adipocyte size and number. *Journal of Animal Science* 60:970–976.

Clarke, L., Van de Waal, S., Lomax, M.A., and Symonds, M.E. 1992. Brown adipose tissue development in the ovine fetus during the final month of gestation. In Neonatal Survival and Growth. *Occasional Publication of the British Society of Animal Production No. 15. M.A. Varley*, P.F.V. Williams, and T.L.J. Lawrence, eds. British Edinburgh: Society of Animal Production.

Cramb, G., Langslow, D.K., and Phillips, J.H. 1982 Hormonal effects on cyclic nucleotides and carbohydrate and lipid metabolism in isolated chicken hepatocytes. *General and Comparative Endocrinology* 46:310–321.

Decuypere, E., Nouwen, E.J., Kuhn, E.R., Geers, R., and Michels, H. 1979. Differences in serum iodohormone concentration between chick embryos with and without the bill in the air chamber at different incubation temperatures. *General and Comparative Endocrinology* 37:364–367.

DiMarco, N.M., Whitehurst, G.B., and Beitz, D.C. 1986. Evaluation of prostaglandin E2, as a regulator of lipolysis in bovine adipose tissue. *Journal of Animal Science* 62:363–369.

Donnelly, L.E., Cryer, A., and Butterwith, S.C. 1993. Comparison of the rates of proliferation of adipocyte precursor cells derived from two lines of chicken which differ in their rates of adipose tissue development. *British Poultry Science* 34:187–193.

Doris, R.A., Kilgour, E., Houslay, M.D., and Vernon, R.G. 1998. Regulation of ATP-binding protein-based antilipolytic system of sheep adipocytes by growth hormone. *Journal of Endocrinology* 158:295-303.

Etherton, T.D., Aberle, E.D., Thompson, E.H., and Allen, C.E. 1981. Effects of cell size and animal age on glucose metabolism in pig adipose tissue. *Journal of Lipid Research* 22:72–80.

Etherton, T.D., Evock, C.M., and Kensinger, R.S. 1987. Native and recombinant bovine growth hormone antagonize insulin action in cultured bovine adipose tissue. *Endocrinology* 121:699–703.

Forman, B. M., Tontonoz, P., Chen, J., Brun, R. P., Spiegelman, B. M., and Evans, R. M. 1995. Deoxy-delta 12, 14-prostaglandin J2 is a ligand for the adiopocyte determination factor PPAR gamma. *Cell* 83:803–812.

Gemmell, R.T., Bell, A.W., and Alexander, G. 1972. Morphology of adipose cells in lambs at birth and during subsequent transition of brown to white adipose tissue in cold and in warm conditions. *American Journal Anatomy* 133:143–163.

Gerfault, V., Louveau, I., and Mourot, J. 1999. The effect of GH and IGF-I on preadipocytes from Large White and Meishan pigs in primary culture. *General and Comparative Endocrinology* 114:396–404.

Glass, C. K., and Rosenfeld, M. G. 2000. The coregulator exchange in transcriptional functions of nuclear receptors. *Genes and Development* 14:121–141.

Gomez-Capilla, J.A., and Langslow, D.R. 1977 Insulin action on glucose utilisation by chicken adipocytes. *International Journal of Biochemistry* 8:417–420.

Goodridge, A.G. 1968a. Conversion of [U-14C]glucose into carbon dioxide, glycogen, cholesterol and fatty acids in liver slices from embryonic and growing chicks. *Biochemical Journal* 108:655–661.

Goodridge, A.G. 1968b. Lipolysis in vitro in adipose tissue from embryonic and growing chicks. *American Journal of Physiology* 214:902–907.

Goodridge, A.G. 1968c. Metabolism of glucose-U-14C in vitro in adipose tissue from embryonic and growing chicks. *American Journal of Physiology* 214:897–901.

Goodridge, A.G., and Adelman, T.G. 1976. Regulation of malic enzyme synthesis by insulin, triiodothyronine, and glucagon in liver cells in culture. *Journal of Biological Chemistry* 251:3027–3032.

Goodridge, A.G., Garay, A., and Silpananta, P. 1974. Regulation of lipogenesis and the total activities of lipogenic enzymes in a primary culture of hepatocytes from prenatal and early postnatal chicks. *Journal of Biological Chemistry* 249:1469–1475.

Griffin, H.D., and Whitehead, C.C. 1982. Plasma lipoprotein concentration as an indicator of fatness in broilers: development and use of a simple assay for plasma very low density lipoproteins. *British Poultry Science* 23:307–313.

Griffin, H.D., Whitehead, C.C., and Broadbent, L.A. 1982. The relationship between plasma triglyceride concentrations and body fat content in male and female broilers—a basis for selection? *British Poultry Science* 23:15–23.

Harvey, S., Scanes, C.G., and Howe, T. 1977. Growth hormone effects on in vitro metabolism of avian adipose and liver tissue. *General and Comparative Endocrinology* 33:322–328.

Hausman, G.J. 2000. The influence of dexamethasone and insulin on expression of CCAAT/enhancer binding protein isoforms during preadipocyte differentiation in porcine stromal-vascular cell cultures: evidence for very early expression of C/EBPb. *Journal of Animal Science* 78:1227–1235.

Hausman, G.J., and Richardson, R.L. 1998. Newly recruited and pre-existing preadipocytes in cultures of porcine stromal-vascular cells: morphology, expression of extracellular matrix components, and lipid accretion. *Journal of Animal Science* 76:48–60.

Hausman, G.J., Wright, J.T., and Richardson, R.L. 1996. The influence of extracellular matrix substrata on preadipocyte development in serum-free cultures of stromal-vascular cells. *Journal of Animal Science* 74:2117–2128.

Hausman, G.J., and Yu, Z.K. 1998. Influence of thyroxine and hydrocortisone in vivo on porcine preadipocyte recruitment, development and expression of C/EBP binding proteins in fetal stromal vascular (S-V) cell cultures. Growth, *Development and Aging* 62:107–118.

Hirsch, J., and Gallian, E. 1968. Methods for the determination of adipose cell size in man and animals. *Journal of Lipid Research* 9:110–119.

Hood, R.L. 1982. The cellular basis for growth of the abdominal fat pad in broiler-type chickens. *Poultry Science* 61:117–121.

Hood, R.L., and Allen, C.E. 1973. Cellularity of bovine adipose tissue. *Journal of Lipid Research* 14:605–610.

Hood, R.L., and Allen, C.E. 1977. Cellularity of porcine adipose tissue: effects of growth and adiposity. *Journal of Lipid Research* 18:275–284.

Houseknecht, K.L., Bauman, D.E., Vernon, R.G., Byatt, J.C., and Collier, R.J. 1996. Insulin-like growth factors-I and II, somatotropin, prolactin, and placental lactogen are not acute effectors of lipolysis in ruminants. *Domestic Animal Endocrinology* 13:239–249.

Hu, C.Y., Novakofski, J., and Mersmann, H.J. 1987. Hormonal control of porcine adipose tissue fatty acid release and cyclic AMP concentration. *Journal of Animal Science* 64:1031–1037.

Kitabgi, P., Rosselin, G., and Bataille, D. 1976. Interactions of glucagon and related peptides with chicken adipose tissue. *Hormones and Metabolic Research* 8:266–270.

Kliewer, S. A., Sundseth, S. S., Jones, S. A., Brown, P. J., Wisely, G. B., Koble, C. S., Devchand, P., Wahli, W., Willson, T. M., Lenhard, J. M., and Lehmann, J. M. 1997. Fatty acids and eicosanoids regulate gene expression through direct interactions with peroxisome proliferator-activated receptors α and β. *Proceedings of the National Academy Sciences of USA* 94:4318–4323.

Langslow, D.R. 1971. The anti-lipolytic action of prostaglandin E1 on isolated chicken fat cells. *Biochimica et Biophysica Acta* 239:33–37.

Langslow, D.R. 1972. The development of lipolytic sensitivity in the isolated fat cells of Gallus domesticus during the foetal and neonatal period. *Comparative Biochemistry and Physiology* 43B: 689–701.

Langslow, D.R. 1973. The action of gut glucagon-like immunoreactivity and other intestinal hormones on lipolysis in chicken adipocytes. *Hormones and Metabolic Research* 5:428–432.

Langslow, D.R., and Hales, C.N. 1969 Lipolysis in chicken adipose tissue in vitro. *Journal of Endocrinology* 43:285–294.

Langslow, D.R., and Lewis, R.J. 1974. Alterations with age in composition and lipolytic activity of adipose tissue from male and female chickens. *British Poultry Science* 15: 267–273.

Liu, C.Y., Boyer, J.L., and Mills, S.E. 1989. Acute effects of beta-adrenergic agonists on porcine adipocyte metabolism in vitro. *Journal of Animal Science* 67:2930-2936.

Lowell, B.B. 1999. PPARγ: an essential regulator of adipogenesis and modulator of fat cell function. *Cell* 99:239–242.

Mangelsdorf, D.J., and Evans, R.M. 1995. The RXR heterodimers and orphan receptors. *Cell* 83:841.

March, B.E., MacMillan, C., and Chu, S. 1984. Characteristics of adipose tissue growth in broiler-type chickens to 22 weeks of age and the effects of dietary protein and lipid. *Poultry Science* 63:2207–2216.

McCumbee, W.D., and Hazelwood, R.L. 1977. Biological evaluation of the third pancreatic hormone (APP): hepatocyte and adipocyte effects. *General and Comparative Endocrinology* 33:518–525.

Merkley, J.W., and Cartwright, A.L. 1989. Adipose tissue deposition and cellularity in cimaterol-treated female broilers. *Poultry Science* 68:762–770.

Mersmann, H.J., Goodman, J.R., and Brown, L.J. 1975. Development of swine adipose tissue: morphology and chemical composition. *Journal of Lipid Research* 16:269–279.

Mills, S.E. 1999. Regulation of porcine adipocyte metabolism by insulin and adenosine. *Journal of Animal Science* 77:3201–3207.

Mills, S.E., and Liu, C.Y. 1990. Sensitivity of lipolysis and lipogenesis to dibutyryl-cAMP and β-adrenergic agonists in swine adipocytes in vitro. *Journal of Animal Science* 68:1017–1023.

Minguell, J.J., Erices, A., and Conget, P. 2001. Mesenchymal stem cells. *Proceedings of the Society of Experimental Biology and Medicine* 226:507–520.

Nathanielsz, P.W., and Fisher, D.A. 1979. Thyroid function in the perinatal period. *Animal Reproduction Science* 257–62.

Newby, D., Gertler, A., and Vernon, R.G. 2001. Effects of recombinant ovine leptin on in vitro lipolysis and lipogenesis in subcutaneous adipose tissue from lactating and nonlactating sheep. *Journal of Animal Science* 79:445–452.

O'Hea, E.K., and Leveille, G.A. 1969. Lipid biosynthesis and transport in the domestic chick (Gallus domesticus). *Comparative Biochemistry and Physiology* 30:149–159.

Oscar, T.P. 1993. Enhanced lipolysis from broiler adipocytes pretreated with pancreatic polypeptide. *Journal of Animal Science* 71:2639–2644.

Peterla, T.A., and Scanes, C.G. 1990. Effect of β-adrenergic agonists on lipolysis and lipogenesis by porcine adipose tissue in vitro. *Journal of Animal Science* 68:1024–1029.

Pfaff, F.E., and Austic, R.E. 1976. Influence of diet on the development of the abdominal fat pad in the pullet. *Poultry Science* 61: 117–121.

Puvadolpirod, S., Thompson, J.R., Green, J., Latour, M.A., and Thaxton, J.P. 1997. Influence of yolk on blood metabolites in perinatal and neonatal chickens. *Growth, Development and Aging* 61:39–45.

Ramsay, T.G. 2001. Porcine leptin alters insulin inhibition of lipolysis in porcine adipocytes in vitro. *Journal of Animal Science* 79:653–657.

Ramsay, T.G., White, M.E., and Wolverton, C.K. 1989a. Insulin-like growth factor 1 induction of differentiation of porcine preadipocytes. *Journal of Animal Science* 67:2452–2459.

Ramsay, T.G., White, M.E., and Wolverton, C.K. 1989b. Glucocorticoids and the differentiation of porcine preadipocytes. *Journal of Animal Science* 67:2222–2229.

Richardson, R.L., Campion, D.R., Hausman, G.J., and Wright, J.T. 1989. Transforming growth factor type β (TGF-β) and adipogenesis in pigs. *Journal of Animal Science* 67:2171–2180.

Richardson, R.L., Hausman, G.J., and Gaskins, H.R. 1992. Effect of transforming growth factor-beta on insulin-like growth factor 1- and dexamethasone-induced proliferation and differentiation in primary cultures of pig preadipocytes. *Acta Anatomica* 145:32–326.

Robelin, J. 1981. Cellularity of bovine adipose tissues: developmental changes from 15 to 65 percent mature weight. *Journal of Lipid Research* 22:452–457.

Rodbell, M. 1964. Localization of lipoprotein lipase in fat cells of rat adipose tissue. *Journal of Biological Chemistry* 239:753–755.

Rule, D.C., Smith, S.B., and Mersmann, H.J. 1987. Effects of adrenergic agonists and insulin on porcine adipose tissue lipid metabolism in vitro. *Journal of Animal Science* 65:136–149.

Scanes, C.G., Hart, L.E., Decuypere, E., and Kuhn, E.R. 1987. Endocrinology of the avian embryo: an overview. *Journal of Experimental Zoology Supplement* 1:253–264.

Scanes, C.G., Peterla, T.A., and Campbell, R.M. 1994. Influence of adenosine or adrenergic agonists on growth hormone stimulating lipolysis by chicken adipose tissue in vitro. *Comparative Biochemistry and Physiology* 107C:243–248.

Schermer, S.J., Bird, J.A., Lomax, M.A., Sheperd, D.A.L., and Symonds, M.E. 1996. Effect of fetal thyroidectomy on brown adipose tissue and thermoregulation in newborn lambs. *Reproduction, Fertility and Development* 8:995–1002.

Steffen, D.G., Phinney, G., Brown, L.J., and Mersmann, H.J. 1979. Ontogeny of glycerolipid biosynthetic enzymes in swine liver and adipose tissue. *Journal of Lipid Research* 20:246–253.

Stevens, D., Alexander, G., and Bell, A.W. 1990. Effect of prolonged glucose infusion into fetal sheep on body growth, fat deposition and gestation length. *Journal of Developmental Physiology* 13:277–281.

Strosser, M.-T., Scala-Guenot, D.D., Koch, B., and Mialhe, P. 1983. Inhibitory effect and mode of action of somatostatin on lipolysis in chicken adipocytes. *Biochimica Biophysica Acta* 763:191–196.

Suryawan, A., and Hu, C.Y. 1997. Effect of retinoic acid on differentiation of cultured pig preadipocytes. *Journal of Animal Science* 75:112–117.

Suryawan, A., Swanson, L.V., and Hu, C.Y. 1997. Insulin and hydrocortisone, but not triiodothyronine, are required for the differentiation of pig preadipocytes in primary culture. *Journal of Animal Science* 75:105–111.

Vernon, R.G. 1980. Lipid metabolism in the adipose tissue of ruminant animals. *Progress in Lipid Research* 19:23–106.

Vernon, R.G. 1991. Depot specific endocrine control of fatty acid synthesis in adipose tissues of foetal lambs. *Domestic Animal Endocrinology* 8:161–164.

Vernon, R.G. 1996. GH inhibition of lipogenesis and stimulation of lipolysis in sheep adipose tissue: involvement of protein serine phosphorylation and dephosphorylation and phospholipase C. *Journal of Endocrinology* 150:129–140.

Walton, P.E., Etherton, T.D., and Chung, C.S. 1987. Exogenous pituitary and recombinant growth hormone induce insulin and insulin-like growth factor-1 resistance in pig adipose tissue. *Domestic Animal Endocrinology* 4:183–189.

Walton, P.E., Etherton, T.D., and Evock, C.M. 1986. Antagonism of insulin action in cultured pig adipose tissue by pituitary and recombinant porcine growth hormone: potentiation by hydrocortisone. *Endocrinology* 118:2577–2581.

Watkins, P.A., Tarlow, D.M., and Lane, M.D. 1977. Mechanism for acute control of fatty acid synthesis by glucagon and 3':5'-cyclic AMP in the liver cell. *Proceedings of the National Academy of Sciences of the USA* 74:1497–1501.

Watt, P.W., Finely, E., Cork, S., Clegg, R.A., and Vernon, R.G. 1991. Chronic control of the α- and β2-adrenergic systems of sheep adipose tissue by growth hormone and insulin. *Biochemistry Journal* 273:39–42.

Wilson, S.B., Back, D.W., Morris, S.M., Jr., Swierczynski, J., and Goodridge, A.G. 1986. Hormonal regulation of lipogenic enzymes in chick embryo hepatocytes in culture. *Journal of Biological Chemistry* 261:15179–15182.

Wright, J.T., and Hausman, G.J. 1995. Insulin like growth factor-1 (IGF-1)-induced stimulation of porcine preadipocyte replication. *In Vitro Cell and Developmental Biology* 31:404–408.

Wu, Y.J., Valdez-Corcoran, M., Wright, J.T., and Cartwright, A.L. 2000. Abdominal fat pad mass reduction by in ovo administration of anti-adipocyte monoclonal antibodies in chickens. Poultry Science 79:1640–1644.

Yang, Y.T., and Baldwin, R.L. 1973. Lipolysis in isolated cow adipose cells. *Journal of Dairy Science* 56:366–374.

Yeh, Y.-Y., and Leveille, G.A. 1971. In vitro and in vivo restoration of hepatic lipogenesis in fasted chicks. *Journal of Nutrition* 101:803–810.

Yu, Z.K., and Hausman, G.J. 1998. Expression of CCAAT/enhancer binding proteins during porcine preadipocyte differentiation. *Experimental Cell Research* 245:343–349.

11
Modeling and Growth

Roberto Sainz and R. Lee Baldwin

Our understanding of the biology of animal growth has increased tremendously over the past 25 years, leading to new opportunities for improving the efficiency and quality of meat animal production. Realization of these opportunities will depend upon our ability to control and predict the outcome of novel technologies in animal feeding and management. Such predictions require the development and use of mathematical models of growth. This chapter presents a few classical, empirical growth functions, then some predictive (nutritional) models, and finally a brief discussion of dynamic, mechanistic nutritional models of growth processes.

France and Thornley (1984) categorized mathematical models as follows:

1. *Static* vs. *Dynamic*; dynamic models incorporate time explicitly and static models do not.
2. *Empirical* vs. *Mechanistic*; empirical models provide a best fit to data obtained at the prediction level (e.g., body weight), whereas mechanistic models incorporate concepts about the underlying biology and data from lower levels of aggregation (e.g., cellular function).
3. *Stochastic* vs. *Deterministic*; deterministic models always give the same solution to a given set of inputs, but stochastic models include some random element(s), giving a distribution of outputs to a given set of inputs.

The mathematical representation and prediction of growth has been a widespread endeavor in biology and a wide range of approaches have been proposed. Objectives in modeling growth may include

1. Description of past observations
2. Prediction of outcomes of different management strategies
3. Explanation of mechanisms

Each of these objectives requires a different approach. Descriptive and predictive models are usually static and empirical, whereas explanatory or mechanistic models require a dynamic appproach. Dynamic models are usually represented as difference equations, which may be solved analytically or (especially for more complex models) numerically.

CLASSICAL EQUATIONS FOR GROWTH

A number of equations have been used to represent growth of an organism and its body conponents. These include the exponential, logistic, Brody, Gompertz, and Richards functions, and many others (Table 11.1).

The exponential growth equation implies that the rate of growth at any point in time is a constant proportion k of weight W at that point. This equation is also used to predict unrestricted growth of populations, and displays a J-curve (Figure 11.1). The monomolecular equation implies that instantaneous growth rate is a constant function k of the difference between current weight W and potential maximum

Table 11.1. Some common growth equations

Equation	Differential	Integral
Exponential	$\dfrac{dW}{dt} = k \cdot W$	$W = W_0 \cdot e^{k \cdot t}$
Monomolecular	$\dfrac{dW}{dt} = k \cdot (A - W)$	$W = A \cdot (1 - e^{-k \cdot t})$
Logistic	$\dfrac{dW}{dt} = k \cdot W \cdot (A - W)$	$W = \dfrac{A}{1 + C \cdot e^{-k \cdot A \cdot t}}$
Gompertz	$\dfrac{dW}{dt} = k \cdot W \cdot \log_e(A/W)$	$W = A \cdot e^{-b \cdot e^{t}}$
Bertalanffy	$\dfrac{dW}{dt} = a \cdot W^c - b \cdot W$	$W = (a/b - e^{-(1-c) \cdot b(t-t)})^{1/(1-c)}$
Richards		$W = A \cdot (1 - b \cdot e^{-k \cdot t})^a$
Janoschek		$W = A - (A - W_0) \cdot e^{-k \cdot r}$
Allometric	$\dfrac{dY}{dt} = b \cdot X^{b-1} + c$	$Y = a \cdot X^b$

weight A. Since this equation contains a maximum weight, it displays hyperbolic or saturation kinetics (Figure 11.1). The logistic equation is a modification of the monomolecular function, such that growth rate is a function k of current weight W and the difference between current and maximum weight A. The logistic equation produces a sigmoid growth curve, with accelerating early growth, a point of inflection, and then decelerating growth as W approaches A (Figure 11.1). Most growth curves are in fact sigmoid, but the point of inflection may vary. In the logistic equation, the point of inflection is always one-half of the adult weight ($W = 1/2\ A$). An alternative approach used widely to describe tissue growth is the Gompertz equation. The Gompertz equation describes body and organ weights within a species from early embryonic life to maturity very well (Laird 1966). Its point of inflection occurs at about 37% of the adult weight. Brody (1945) combined the exponential and monomolecular equations to represent growth before and after, respectively, an empirically defined point of inflection, t^*. Bertalanffy (1957) devised a growth function with anabolic and catabolic elements; its point of inflection is around 30% of mature weight.

Unlike the logistic and Gompertz equations, the point of inflection of the Richards (1959) equation is not a constant fraction of the asymptote, the value being a function of A, b, and M. Therefore, the Richards equation is a generalized form of the others, becoming the monomolecular equation at $M = 1$, the logistic equation at $M = -1$, the Bertalanffy equation at $M = 3$, and the Gompertz equation as M approaches

infinity (positive or negative). Although it is highly flexible, its parameters can exhibit significant colinearity, resulting in difficulties in parameter estimation (Gille and Salomon 1995). Similar to the Richards function, the equation proposed by Janoschek (1957) is very flexible; when $p < 1$, growth is exponential, and when $p > 1$, growth is sigmoidal. The point of inflection is variable, and is dependent upon the values of p and k. Since there is less covariance between the parameters, the Janoschek equation presents fewer problems of convergence (Gille and Salomon 1995).

The allometric equation is derived from a plot of log Y against log X, with b as the slope of the resulting line (Brody 1945). This relationship has also been used to describe a number of physiological and metabolic functions in animals (Adolph 1949; Munro 1969). Values of b that are less than, equal to, or greater than 1 represent body components that grow more slowly, directly proportionately, or more rapidly than the whole body, respectively.

Taylor (1980) emphasized the notion of degree of maturity, which he designated as u. Thus, maturity of protein growth is represented by the following equation:

$$u = P/P_m$$

where P is the current mass of body protein and P_m is the mass of body protein at maturity. This enables scaling of the Gompertz function, which is widely used in nutritional growth modeling, in the following form:

$$dP/dt = B{\cdot}Pm{\cdot}u{\cdot}ln(1/u)$$

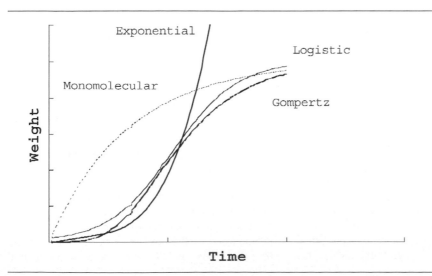

Figure 11.1. Selected growth curves.

which expresses potential growth rate of protein in terms of u, a state variable, and two animal characteristics, a rate parameter, B, and the mature protein parameter Pm. Since $(Pm \cdot B)$ is a constant for a given animal, the potential rate of protein accretion is proportional to $u \cdot log_e(l/u)$. This approach has been applied to modeling growth of poultry (Emmans 1981). The concept of potential growth of pigs in terms of (dP/dt) was applied by Moughan et al. (1987) with the assumption that the values are constant, for a given sex and genotype, over the growth period from 20 to 90 kg. Other workers have used the notion of protein maturity to define rates of body protein synthesis, degradation, and accretion (Whittemore and Fawcett 1976).

All of the equations given above can be and are used to describe the growth of a variety of organisms. However, the parameters are not constant, do not vary systematically across species, and have no useful, underlying biological meaning (Laird 1966). Moreover, the effects of nutritional state are not represented at all, so that they have little predictive value.

PREDICTIVE MODELS OF GROWTH

Nutritional models for growing animals should enable accurate predictions of nutrient requirements, calculation of responses of defined animals to defined feeds, and calculation of optimal nutritional strategies. Feeding systems based upon these models typically handle the utilization of energy, protein, and other nutrients separately. A detailed review of these systems is beyond the scope of this chapter; the interested reader is referred to ARC (1980), Jarrige (1989), and SCA (1990). A brief description of the development of the net energy system for beef cattle (NRC 2000) is given below as an example.

Kleiber (1961) noted that the partial efficiency of energy use for maintenance is greater than that for weight gain. The feeding systems in use at that time (NRC 1963), based on total digestible nutrients (TDN), recognized only one feed energy value and undervalued roughages for maintenance and concentrates for production. To overcome this limitation, which would require a feed's energy value to decrease with level of feeding, Lofgreen and Garrett (1968) introduced a net energy system for growing and finishing beef cattle; with some modifications, it is still the basis for the feeding systems published by the National Research Council (NRC 2000). This system separated the energy requirements for maintenance from those for weight gain; thus feed energy values for both functions were developed. The net energy requirement for maintenance was set equal to the animal's fasting heat production; the net energy requirement for gain was the energy content of the animal's gain. Hence, the net energy for maintenance content of a ration (NE_m) was set as the animal's fasting heat production divided by the amount of feed needed for body energy equilibrium. Similarly, the net energy for gain content of a ration (NE_g) was defined as the energy content of gain divided by the amount of feed fed above that required for body energy equilibrium. Therefore, empty body weight (EBW) gain (EBG) is represented as

$$EBG = 12.341 \cdot EBW^{-0.6837} \cdot RE^{0.9116}$$

where retained energy (RE) in MJ/day is the NE_g available after accounting for the NE_m requirement.

The current net-energy based system for beef cattle (NRC 2000) is quite sophisticated in the sense that significant effort has been directed to development of empirical equations to accommodate sources of variance. For example, adjustment factors have been developed to account for differences in growth due to a wide variety of variables, including diet energy density, breed, sex, current and previous temperature, previous nutrition, hormonal growth promotants, and physical activity, among others. Very large input-output data sets were required to develop these empirical equations. These systems remain static and factorial in nature, since total requirements are the sum of estimated requirements for individual functions and apply to one specific weight and rate of gain. Although adjustment factors are adequate in well-defined conditions, new situations with different sets of input variables than were used to validate the original adjustment factors may make predictions erroneous. This is due to interrelationships among variables and thus a lack of independence among adjustment factors.

MECHANISTIC MODELS OF GROWTH

Early models (Baldwin and Black 1979) of growth of tissues and organ systems were developed based on realization that relative organ weights contribute to differences in fasting heat production and that nutritional, physiological, and environmental interactions determine patterns of nutrient utilization, growth rates, and body composition. Initially, allometric equations were used to estimate tissue and organ weights in growing animals, based on published data. No consistent relationship was found in the values of *a* and *b* among and within species. This lack of interspecific applicability of numerical inputs to the allometric equation was not considered acceptable. For example, the allometric equation under-predicted brain weights in young animals, and over-predicted in older animals. Since nervous tissue has a disproportionate metabolic rate relative to mass, this bias led to concomitant errors in estimating energy expenditure. These deficiencies of allometric equations in describing organ weights during development within a species, together with their lack of a temporal parameter (Brody 1945; Laird 1966), preclude their use in mechanistic models of animal growth.

Robinson (1971) developed the concept first proposed by Enesco and Leblond (1962), that growth of tissues, organ systems, and whole animals occurs in three phases: hyperplasia, hypertrophy, and accretion. Early pre- and postnatal growth is clearly hyperplastic in that it is due to cell proliferation in all tissues. Muscle presents a special case because the number of fiber cells in mammals is fixed near birth. However, the number of nuclei in muscle cells continues to increase for some time as a result of satellite cell proliferation and subsequent fusion with muscle fiber cells (Allen et al. 1979). Thus, a more general definition of hyperplasia might be increases in nuclei or DNA per tissue. Hypertrophic growth was defined by Robinson (1971) as, essentially, increases in protein per unit of DNA to some genetically defined maximum. This is in accord with the DNA unit size hypothesis of Cheek et al. (1971), which holds that each unit of DNA in each tissue of each species expresses the information required for the formation of a specific amount of cell material. These concepts lead to three premises that apparently determine growth in mammals:

1. The primary genetic determinant of organ size is the final amount of deoxyribonucleic acid (DNA). This premise arises from the observations that DNA per diploid nucleus is constant in animals and that a difference in cell number and not cell size is largely responsible for variations in organ weight between mature individuals of different species (Munro and Gray 1969) or strains within a species (Robinson and Bradford 1969).

2. Each unit of DNA specifies, on a genetically defined basis for each tissue and each species, information required for the ultimate formation of a specific amount of cell material. This premise embodies the DNA unit concept discussed by Cheek et al. (1971) and overcomes any complications that may arise from polyploidy. Whether information specified by a unit of DNA leads to the formation of cell material is dependent upon the nutritional and physiological status of the animal. This premise accounts for observed differences in cell size and composition between tissues and across species of mature animals.

3. The specific activities, expressed as units per gram of tissue, of enzymes or groups of enzymes responsible for tissue metabolism and growth vary as an exponential function of organ size (Lin et al. 1959). Also, the kinetic properties of enzymes are reasonably constant across species.

The adequacy of equations based upon these three premises was evaluated by simulating effects of (1) starvation on development of rat liver; (2) nutrient restriction and refeeding on rat liver and brain; (3) normal intake on nine tissues in two strains of mice, rats, sheep, and pigs; and (4) normal intake on brain in several other species, including man (Baldwin and Black 1979). These workers concluded that these premises provide appropriate and adequate bases for mechanistic and dynamic representations of the basic processes that drive the growth process and influence growth rates.

The concepts and equation forms used by Baldwin and Black (1979) served as the starting point for the beef cattle growth model of Oltjen et al. (1986a, 1986b). That model is dynamic; thus differential equations were integrated to estimate gain (or loss) of DNA and body protein. Body fat gain is estimated from the difference between energy intake and energy used in maintenance and protein gain. Empty body weight is the sum of fat and fat-free body masses, where fat-free body mass is body protein ÷ 0.2201 (Garrett and Hinman 1969). Since the model requires initial estimates of whole-body DNA, protein, and fat, empirical relationships between these and animal weight, mature size and condition score are used to set beginning values for model implementation. The Oltjen model has been used widely in feedlot management. For example, this model, coupled with weight and ultrasound measurements of cattle entering the feedlot, was used to sort cattle into more uniform outcome groups (Sainz and Oltjen 1994; Sainz et al. 1995). More recent work based on the Oltjen model includes the introduction of variable maintenance functions (Oltjen and Sainz 2001) and distribution of body fat among different depots (Sainz and Hasting 2000).

Although Oltjen et al. (1986a, 1986b) accounted for variations attributable to initial body composition and mature size, their model does not always yield acceptable estimates of fat gain. This is not unexpected, since fat accretion is computed after energy requirements for maintenance and protein gain are satisfied. Thus, any errors in estimates of maintenance or protein gain result in biased fat-gain predictions. Baldwin and Bywater (1984) showed that factors that affect energy expenditures are normally accounted for within the definition of maintenance. Further, feed energy available for fat accretion is not used at the same net efficiency as for energy gain of protein, as the net energy system assumes. For example, of the major metabolites used for fat synthesis, fatty acids are the most efficient precursor (96%), followed by glucose (80–85%) and, finally, acetate (65–75%). Thus, for diets of similar ME content, the one resulting in absorption of more long-chain fatty acids will support faster energy gains when the composition of gain is relatively greater in fat.

In recent years, attempts have been made to account for variation in nutrient partitioning using dynamic, mechanistic models of digestion, metabolism, and growth (Gill et al. 1984; Black et al. 1986, 1987a, 1987b; France et al. 1987; DiMarco et al. 1989; Sainz and Wolff 1990a,1990b). These models incorporate concepts and data regarding fermentation and digestion of feeds, the metabolism of the products of digestion, and the anabolic and catabolic processes leading to deposition of body protein and fat. Therefore, they are able to account for interactions among previous planes of nutrition, level of feeding, and ration composition. The explicit representation of the products of digestion suggest that feeds must be represented by their chemical constituents in future systems. At present, the complexity and lack of identity (additional experimental data are needed to set parameter values with confidence) of these models impose limits to their practical use. Due to their complexity, these models cannot be solved analytically, and so must be solved numerically.

CONCLUSIONS

Growth models are used for a variety of purposes, including the simple description of observations, prediction of responses to management, and explanation of biological mechanisms. Depending upon the objectives, a number of different approaches may be used, including classical algebraic equations, predictive empirical relationships, and dynamic, mechanistic models. The latter offer the best opportunity to make full use of the growing body of knowledge regarding the biology of animal growth. Continuing development of these types of models and computer technology and software for their implementation holds great promise for improvements in the effectiveness with which fundamental knowledge of animal function can be applied to improve animal agriculture.

REFERENCES

Adolph, E.F. 1949. Quantitative relations in the physiological constitutions of mammals. *Science* 109:579.

Agricultural Research Council. 1980. *The Nutrient Requirements of Ruminant Livestock*. Farnham Royal, Surrey: Commonwealth Agricultural Bureaux.

Allen, R.E., Merkel, R.A., and Young, R.B. 1979. Cellular aspects of muscle growth: myogenic cell proliferation. *Journal of Animal Science* 49:115.

Baldwin, R.L., and Black, J.L. 1979. Simulation of the effects of nutritional and physiological status on the growth of mammalian tissues: description and evaluation of a computer program. *Animal Research Laboratories Technical Paper 6*. Melbourne, Australia: Commonwealth Science and Industrial Research Organization.

Baldwin, R.L., and Bywater, A.C. 1984. Nutritional energetics of animals. *Annual Reviews of Nutrition* 4:101.

Bertalanffy, L. v. 1957. Wachstum. In *Handbuch der Zoologie: Bd.8, 10. Lieferung*. J.G. Helmcke, H.v. Lengerken, and G. Starck, eds. Berlin: W. de Gruyter.

Black, J.L., Campbell, R.G., Williams, I.H., James, K.J., and Davies, G.T. 1986. Simulation of energy and amino acid utilization in the pig. *Research and Development in Agriculture 3:121*.

Black, J.L., Gill, M., Beever, D.E., Thornley, J.H.M., and Oldham, J.D. 1987a. Simulation of the metabolism of absorbed energy-yielding nutrients in young sheep: efficiency of utilization of acetate. *Journal of Nutrition* 117:105.

Black, J.L., Gill, M., Thornley, J.H.M., Beever, D.E., and Oldham, J.D. 1987b. Simulation of the metabolism of absorbed energy-yielding nutrients in young sheep: efficiency of utilization of lipid and amino acid. *Journal of Nutrition* 117:116.

Brody, S. 1945. *Bioenergetics and Growth*. New York: Reinhold.

Cheek, D.B., Holt, A.B., Hill, D.E., and Talbert, J.L. 1971. Skeletal muscle cell mass and growth: the concept of the deoxyribonucleic acid unit. *Pediatric Research* 5:312.

DiMarco, O.N., Baldwin, R.L., and Calvert, C.C. 1989. Simulation of DNA, protein and fat accretion in growing steers. *Agricultural Systems* 29:21.

Emmans, G.C. 1981. A model of the growth and feed intake of ad libitum fed animals, particularly poultry. In *Computers in Animal Production*. G.M. Hillyer, C.T. Whittemore, and R.G. Gunn, eds. Surrey: British Society of Animal Production, Thames Ditton.

Enesco, M., and Leblond, C.P. 1962. Increase in cell number as a factor in the growth of the organs and tissues of the young male rat. *Journal of Embryology* 10:530.

France, J., Gill, M., Thornley, J.H.M., and England, P. 1987. A model of nutrient utilization and body composition in beef cattle. *Animal Production* 44:371.

France, J., and Thornley, J.H.M. 1984. *Mathematical Models in Agriculture*. London: Butterworth.

Garrett, W.N., and Hinman, N. 1969. Reevaluation of the relationship between carcass density and body composition of beef steers. *Journal of Animal Science* 28:1.

Gill, M., Thornley, J.H.M., Black, J.L., Oldham, J.D., and Beever, D.E. 1984. Simulation of the metabolism of absorbed energy-yielding nutrients in young sheep. *British Journal of Nutrition* 52:621.

Gille, U., and Salomon, F.V. 1995. Bone growth in ducks through mathematical models with special reference to the Janoschek growth curve. *Growth, Development and Aging* 59:207.

Gompertz, B. 1825. On the nature of the function expressive of the law of human mortality, and a new mode of determining the value of live contingencies. *Philosophical Transactions of the Royal Society* 182:513.

Janoschek, A. 1957. Das reaktionskinetische Grundgesetz und seine Beziehungen zum Wachs-tums- und Ertragsgesetz. *Statistische Vierteljahresschriften* 10:25.

Jarrige, R. 1989. Ruminant Nutrition. *Recommended Allowances and Feed Tables*. Paris Institut Nationale de Recherche Agronomique.

Kleiber, M. 1961. Metabolic rate and food utilization as a function of body size. *Brody Memorial Lecture I. Missouri Agricultural Experiment Station*, Columbia, Missouri.

Laird, A.K. 1966. Postnatal growth of birds and mammals. *Growth* 30:349.

Lin, E.C.C., Rivlin, R.S., and Knox, W.E. 1959. Effect of body weight and sex on activity of enzymes involved in amino acid metabolism. *American Journal of Physiology* 21:787.

Lofgreen, G.P., and Garrett, W.N. 1968. A system for expressing the net energy requirements and feed values for growing and finishing beef cattle. *Journal of Animal Science* 27:793.

Moughan, P.J., Smith, W.C., and Pearson, G. 1987. Description and validation of a model simulating growth in the pig (28–90 kg liveweight). *New Zealand Journal of Agricultural Research* 30:481.

Munro, H.N. 1969. Evolution of protein metabolism in mammals. In *Mammalian Protein Metabolism*, vol. III. H.N. Munro, ed. New York: Academic Press.

Munro, H.N., and Gray, J.A.M. 1969. The nucleic acid content of skeletal muscle and liver in mammals of different body size. *Comprehensive Biochemistry and Physiology* 28:897.

National Research Council. 1963. *Nutrient Requirements of Beef Cattle*, 4th ed. Washington, D.C.: National Academy Press.

National Research Council. 2000. *Nutrient Requirements of Beef Cattle*, 7th rev. ed. Washington, D.C.: National Academy Press.

Oltjen, J.W., Bywater, A.C., and Baldwin, R.L. 1986a. Evaluation of a model of beef cattle growth and composition. *Journal of Animal Science* 62:98.

Oltjen, J.W., Bywater, A.C., Baldwin, R.L., and Garrett, W.N. 1986b. Development of a dynamic model of beef cattle growth and composition. *Journal of Animal Science* 62:86.

Oltjen, J.W., and Sainz, R.D. 2001. Alternate forms for heat production in ruminant growth and composition models. In *Energy Metabolism in Animals*. A. Chwalibog and K. Jakobsen, eds. *European Association for Animal Production publication* No. 103. Wageningen, The Netherlands: Wageningen Pers.

Richards, F.J. 1959. A flexible growth curve for empirical use. *Journal of Experimental Botany* 10:290.

Robinson, D. W. 1971. Cellular basis for changes in body composition. *Journal of Animal Science* 33:416.

Robinson, D.W., and Bradford, G.E. 1969. Cellular response to selection for rapid growth. *Growth* 33:221.

Sainz, R.D., and Hasting, E. 2000. Simulation of the development of adipose tissue in beef cattle. In *Modelling Nutrient Utilization in Farm Animals*. J.P. McNamara, J. France, and D.E. Beever, eds.. Wallingford, U.K.: CAB International.

Sainz, R.D., and Oltjen, J.W. 1994. Improving uniformity of feeder steers using ultrasound and computer modelling. *Proceedings of the American Society of Animal Science, Western Section* 45:179.

Sainz, R.D. , Smith, J.G., Garnett, I., and Lee Y.B. 1995. Use of ultrasound and computer modeling to predict days on feed and improve beef carcass uniformity. *Proceedings of the American Society of Animal Science, Western Section* 46:148.

Sainz, R.D., and Wolff, J.E. 1990a. Development of a dynamic, mechanistic model of lamb metabolism and growth. *Animal Production* 51:535.

Sainz, R.D., and Wolff, J.E. 1990b. Evaluation of hypotheses regarding mechanisms of action of growth promotants and repartitioning agents using a simulation model of lamb metabolism and growth. *Animal Production* 51:551.

Standing Committee on Agriculture. 1990. Feeding Standards for Australian Livestock. *Ruminants*. Melbourne, Australia: Commonwealth Scientific Industrial Research Organisation.

Taylor, St. C.S. 1980. Live-weight growth from embryo to adult in domesticated mammals. *Animal Production* 31:223.

Whittemore, C.T., and Fawcett, R.H. 1976. Theoretical aspects of a flexible model to simulate protein and lipid growth in pigs. *Animal Production* 22:87.

12
Animal Growth and Meat Quality

Elisabeth Huff-Lonergan, Steven M. Lonergan, and D. H. Beermann

The efficient production of high-quality desirable meat products is a major goal of meat animal production and processing systems. Indeed, as animal agriculture has improved the efficiency of muscle/meat production, some emphasis has shifted toward producing meat products that have quality characteristics that the consumer wants and the processor needs. These characteristics can be classified in two ways: functional (processing) characteristics, and palatability/sensory characteristics. *Functional characteristics* of fresh meat include composition, color, protein extractability, and the ability of the meat to bind and/or retain moisture to name a few. *Sensory characteristics* include those noticeable to the final consumer of the product. Among these characteristics are tenderness, juiciness, flavor, aroma, and overall appearance. Composition of the muscle (amount of lipid, protein, moisture) can affect the functional and sensory qualities of meat. In addition, many characteristics of fresh meat can also be greatly influenced as muscle is converted to meat. For instance, the water-holding capacity of meat and the ability to solubilize and extract myofibrillar protein decrease during the early postmortem period (Lonergan et al. 2001). Because of this, some processors use pork that has been harvested before the muscle has gone into rigor (pre-rigor) to produce sausage products with exceptional bind strength and moisture-retaining capacity. Pre-rigor muscle is superior in these characteristics for ground product. Often times, however, meat that is removed from the carcass prior to the completion of rigor is decidedly less tender, and is therefore not commonly used for whole-muscle products such as steaks and chops. Biochemical changes in the product during the first several hours after exsanguination are responsible for the changes in protein solubility/ extractability, water-holding capacity, tenderness and other quality attributes (see Table 12.1 for a review). Many of these biochemical changes have their roots in the physiology of the muscle in the live animal. In addition to considering how composition of muscle influences functional and sensory qualities, this chapter examines some of the key biochemical changes that occur as muscle is converted to meat. This chapter also discusses how some of these quality characteristics are influenced by factors related to the growth and maturation of domestic meat animals.

CONVERSION OF MUSCLE TO MEAT

Muscle Metabolism

The process of converting muscle to meat is very dynamic and is affected by the metabolism of the animal prior to exsanguination. After harvest, the muscle attempts to maintain homeostasis. For a short period of time, the muscle can still contract and produce heat. The muscle and other tissues and organs also attempt to maintain normal compartmental levels of calcium and other ions and metabolites. Most of these processes require energy in the form of ATP. The biochemical pathways in muscle that produce ATP after exsanguination can greatly affect the final quality of the product.

There are two main ways early postmortem muscle can synthesize ATP. One is by using the compound creatine phosphate and the other is through catabolism of glycogen. Creatine phosphate (CP) can donate a high-energy phosphate to ADP to reform the needed ATP. This reaction is catalyzed by the enzyme creatine phosphokinase.

$$CP + ADP \Rightarrow C + ATP$$

Table 12.1. Common quality defects of fresh meat influenced by postmortem muscle metabolism

Quality Defect	Characteristics	Possible Underlying Cause	Contributing Factors
Pale, soft, and exudative pork	Very light lean color, soft lean texture, excessive loss of moisture as purge (low water-holding capacity)	Accelerated muscle metabolism that carries over into the early postmortem period and results in rapid pH decline	1. Genetic defect in the sarcoplasmic reticulum calcium release channel (ryanodine receptor) compromising the ability of muscle cells to sequester calcium in the sarcoplasmic reticulum 2. Excessive stress in the live animal within a short time before exsanguination—not always due to a genetic defect
Red, soft, and exudative pork	Normal to light lean color, soft lean texture, excessive loss of moisture as	1. Low ultimate pH and/or 2. Moderately accelerated pH decline	1. Abnormally high levels of glycogen stored in the muscle prior purge (low water-holding capacity) to slaughter 2. Unknown
Dark, firm, and dry pork Dark cutting beef	Very dark lean color, "tacky" surface, exceptionally little moisture loss	Very limited pH decline causing a higher-than-normal ultimate pH	Long-term stress resulting in depletion of muscle energy stores prior to slaughter
Two-toned color "heat-ring"	Abnormal dark and light regions within the same muscle, typically manifested as dark outer regions and light inner regions	Differential in pH and temperature decline within the muscle resulting in rapid cooling and slower pH decline in the outer regions of the muscle	1. Inefficient cooling of muscle during the early postmortem period 2. Abnormal muscle metabolism
Lack of tenderness	Meat that is less tender than desired	1. Lack of activity of proteolytic enzymes that degrade structures within muscle cells during postmortem aging 2. Excessive contraction of the muscle after slaughter 3. High levels of connective tissue 4. Connective tissue that is highly crosslinked	1. Inherent differences in the proteolytic capacity of the muscle 2. Excessively rapid chilling leading to overcontraction of the muscle as it enters rigor 3. Muscles that are used frequently for locomotion or endure much mechanical stress 4. Older Animals

In postmortem muscle, this reaction is very short-lived, usually contributing to ATP resynthesis for only several minutes after exsanguination, because this compound can be rapidly depleted (Figure 12.1). In general, the impact of this system on fresh meat quality is thought to be limited.

One of the primary energy reserves (ATP) in muscle is glycogen, the storage form of glucose. This molecule is the starting substrate for glycolysis, which is a prelude to energy production via the TCA cycle and oxidative phosphorylation. Before glucose from glycogen can be used in glycolysis, glycogen must first be degraded by the enzyme glycogen phosphorylase. This enzyme removes glucose units from their β-(1,4) linkages within glycogen. The resulting product is glucose-1-phosphate. This is advantageous for the muscle from a couple of standpoints. First, free glucose itself is biologically inert until it is converted into a labile, phosphorylated form; if the starting material is free glucose, this step would require ATP. However, when the cell produces glucose-1-phosphate from glycogen via glycogen phosphorylase, an ATP is spared. Second, this phosphorylated glucose will not diffuse freely from the muscle cell and will be available for energy production inside the cell. Through a series of successive steps (glycoly-sis), the six-carbon atom molecule, glucose-1-phosphate, is converted to two pyruvate molecules, each containing three carbon atoms. This process of glycolysis generates a net of two (if free glucose is the starting material) or three (if glycogen is the starting material) ATP molecules. In living tissue, the pyruvate undergoes oxidative decarboxylation to form acetyl CoA, carbon dioxide, and hydrogens that are carried on NADH. The final stage of the energy pathway is oxidative phosphorylation in which the NADH is used to produce an additional 36 ATP molecules from each glucose.

Operation of this entire pathway requires the presence of oxygen to fully oxidize glucose. Under anaerobic conditions the only portion of this pathway that can operate is glycolysis. Conditions for anaerobic metabolism are found during periods of very strenuous exercise or after exsanguination. Under anaerobic conditions, the enzyme lactate dehydrogenase catalyzes the reduction of pyruvate to lactic acid (lactate) by NADH. This process also regenerates NAD^+. Since one molecule of glucose produces 2 pyruvates molecules under anaerobic conditions, the final yield of lactate is 2 lactate molecules for every glucose moiety that enters glycolysis. The NAD^+ that is generated from the reduction of pyruvate by NADH is needed

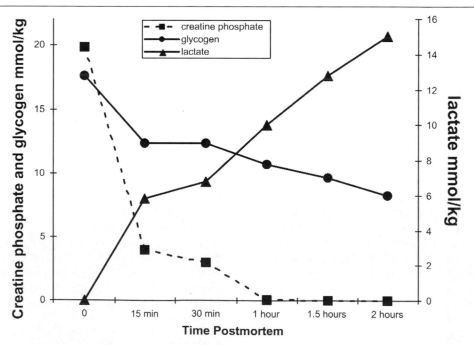

Figure 12.1. Typical postmortem changes in creatine phosphate, glycogen, and lactate in porcine longissimus dorsi muscle over the first two hours after exsanguination.

during an intermediary step in glycolysis. Without NAD+, glycolysis would not continue and no ATP would be generated. This process however, is not self-sustaining for a long period of time. Ultimately, the build-up of lactic acid inactivates the enzymes involved in glycolysis, causing the process to significantly slow, and after death, to cease. In living muscle, the lactic acid is carried away by the circulatory system, but after exsanguination, the lactic acid builds up in the muscle. This buildup of lactic acid is primarily responsible for the gradual fall in pH that is observed during the conversion of muscle to meat.

After an animal is harvested, the major events that are responsible for metabolism to slow and ultimately cease include the following. First, the depletion of oxygen forces the muscle to rely on creatine phosphate (very short term) and glycolysis for the production of ATP. Second, as glycolysis continues, lactic acid accumulates, finally slowing and ultimately inactivating the glycolytic enzymes. Third, since the circulatory system can no longer deliver glucose, the only substrates that are available to the muscle for glycolysis are the glycogen and any glucose that was in the muscle at the time of exsanguination; therefore, when these substrates are consumed, glycolysis can no longer proceed. When all of these processes are considered together, a predictable pattern of high-energy phosphate (ATP and CP) and substrate (glycogen) depletion, lactic acid accumulation, and pH decline can be observed for normal muscles (Figure 12.1). One can also envision that the drop in ATP production almost parallels the decline in pH, and the production of IMP (deaminated single phosphate moiety resulting from degradation of ATP) has an inverse relationship to pH decline (Figure 12.2).

Consequences of ATP Depletion

Two of the major functions of ATP in living muscle include providing energy that is used during a contraction cycle, and providing the energy for maintaining proper calcium levels in the muscle. When signaled by an influx of calcium ($> 10^{-6}$ M), muscle contracts and shortens via the interaction of actin in the thin filament and the myosin heads that protrude from the thick filament. The ATP that is used in contraction is hydrolyzed to ADP and P_i and provides energy to allow the actin/myosin complex (actomyosin) to pull the thin filaments toward the center of the sarcomere, thus shortening the myofibril and ultimately the cell and the muscle. The actomyosin complex will remain associated until a new ATP can replace the ADP. After ATP is depleted, these actomyosin bonds are more or less permanent and the muscle is in rigor.

The other key part of the contraction cycle is the maintenance of calcium levels in the muscle cell. The concentration of free calcium in the cytoplasm of the muscle cell (sarcoplasm) is critical in controlling contraction. For the muscle to be relaxed, the concentration of calcium in the sarcoplasm needs to be maintained below 10^{-6} M. This is accomplished by ionic pumps located in the membranes of the sarcoplasmic reticulum and the mitochondria—two major stores of calcium in the muscle cell. These pumps work against a concentration gradient; thus they require energy in the form of ATP to transport calcium from a region of relatively low concentration, the sarcoplasm, to a region of relatively high concentration (sarcoplasmic reticulum or mitochondria). Therefore, as the level of ATP falls in postmortem muscle, the amount of calcium in the sarcoplasm begins to rise because the pumps begin to fail. After ATP is sufficiently depleted, calcium levels remain high enough to signal contraction. This, combined with the fact that there is also insufficient ATP to allow dissociation of actin and myosin, causes rigor to begin.

Impact of Postmortem Muscle Metabolism on Meat Quality

From the preceding discussion, it can be noted that the metabolic state of muscle at the time of exsanguination is critical in controlling the processes of pH decline and rigor development in postmortem tissue. For example, a muscle that has very little substrate for glycolysis (glycogen and/or glucose) at the time of exsanguination will undergo very limited pH decline because there are fewer glucose moieties in the muscle to be converted to lactic acid. Limited substrate at slaughter will also translate to limited ATP production. Therefore, muscles with less glycogen will probably also enter rigor more quickly than a muscle that had normal amounts of substrate for glycolysis at harvest. This condition is most often caused by long-term stress encountered by the animal prior to harvest. Injury, loss of appetite due to stress and long periods of being "off-feed" will contribute to this condition by depleting the energy stores (primarily glycogen) in muscle. The resulting product has a very high pH, has high water-binding capacity, will be dark in color and has a greater tendency for off-flavor development. In addition, because of the higher pH, the product has reduced shelf-life.

Product (meat) from muscles that have a very high rate of metabolism at the time of slaughter and have adequate supplies of available glucose and glycogen for glycolysis to continue will have very different

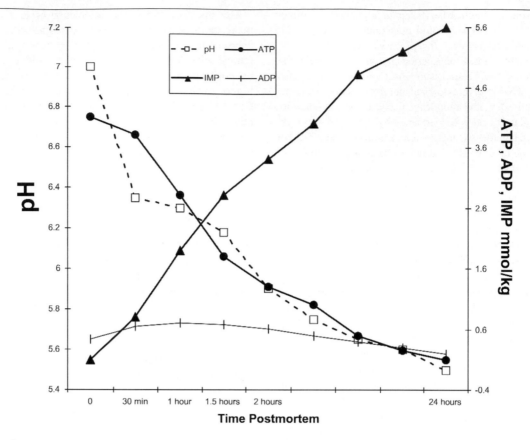

Figure 12.2. Typical postmortem changes in pH, adenosine triphosphate (ATP), adenosine diphosphate (ADP), and inosine monophosphate (IMP, inosinate) in porcine longissimus dorsi over the first 24 hours after exsanguination.

quality traits. In this case, the metabolism rate "carries over" into the postmortem phase resulting in rapid glycolysis in the muscle after exsanguination. Rapid glycolysis leads to rapid depletion of glycogen reserves and, consequently, rapid production of lactic acid. This can allow the muscle to reach its ultimate pH before the muscle is properly chilled. The resulting acidic pH and relatively high muscle temperature can cause dramatic denaturation of muscle proteins involved in water-holding capacity, color, and texture. In some pigs this can be caused by a genetic mutation. This particular genetic defect results in an abnormality in the calcium release channel in the sarcoplasmic reticulum (ryanodine receptor) that causes the channel to be inefficient in retaining calcium. The resulting inappropriate "leakage" of calcium into the sarcoplasm causes intolerance to stress, muscle tremors, and accelerated metabolism in the live animal. These pigs are often very lean and very muscu-

lar, but in the early postmortem muscle, the exaggerated rate of metabolism causes an excessively rapid drop in pH such that ultimate pH can be attained within 45 minutes to an hour after exsanguination. The resulting product is often very pale in color, soft in texture, and loses much moisture in the form of exudate. This product is often referred to as PSE (pale, soft, and exudative). A genetic test is available to swine producers that allows them to select against this defect in their breeding herd. The phenomenon of PSE meat can also be observed in product from pigs that are free of the genetic defect of the ryanodine receptor but have been excessively agitated immediately prior to harvest. This short-term stress carries over as the rapid metabolism that is seen in postmortem muscle and also can result in milder forms of PSE meat.

Poor quality product can also be obtained from muscles that have a normal rate of pH decline, but ends up with lower pH than normal. This is most often seen in pork. A normal ultimate (24 hours postmortem) pH for pork would be between approximately 5.5–5.9. Pork that has an ultimate pH below that has a tendency to be more exudative. This product may be difficult to detect visually because it is typically not as light in color as PSE pork. This product can occur when very high levels of glycogen (starting material for glycolysis) are present in the muscle at harvest. High levels of glycogen provide the potential for the muscle to produce greater amounts of lactic acid. One potential solution to this problem in normal pigs is to withdraw feed a few hours before loading them on a truck for transport to the processing facility. This can limit the amount of available glycogen in the muscle during the early postmortem period.

Low ultimate pH of pork can also be associated with a genetic condition known as the RN⁻ gene. Because it was first observed in the Hampshire breed, it has also been referred to as the Hampshire effect. This genetic defect occurs in the signaling pathway associated with glycogen use/sparing and results in high levels of glycogen in muscle of the animal. As is the case for the defect in the ryanodine receptor, a genetic test now exists that can allow breeders to identify this gene in the breeding population.

LIPID CONTENT

Intramuscular lipid (marbling) was once thought to accumulate late in the finishing phase of growth. Recent results suggest that marbling increases linearly over time and may not be as closely related to subcutaneous adipose tissue growth as once thought (Figure 12.3, compliments of Gene Rouse, Iowa State University). Marbling is the visible fat present in the intrafasicular spaces of a muscle. This lipid consists primarily of triglycerides and is associated with the perimysium. Although there is considerable variation in lipid content (Figure 12.3), intramuscular fat increases with increasing age, decreasing levels of activity, and increasing energy consumption. Intramuscular lipid contributes to the *flavor* and *juiciness* and, to some extent, *tenderness* of meat products (Tables 12.2, 12.3). Because USDA beef grading standards use degree of marbling as a major parameter for U.S. Quality grades, intramuscular lipid content is an important value-defining parameter for beef carcasses.

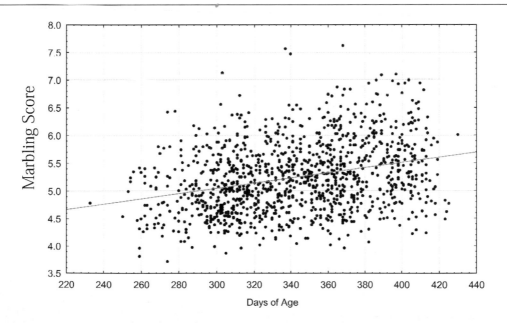

Figure 12.3. Increase in marbling score over time. Marbling score was predicted using real-time ultrasound. Steers (n = 407) were scanned over the feeding period. Marbling score of 4.0 = Slight, 5.0 = Small, 6.0 = Modest, 7.0 = Moderate. Predicted marbling score increased linearly over time (marbling score = 3.6414 + (0.0047 x days of age). (Data compliments of Dr. Gene Rouse, Iowa State University.)

Table 12.2. Influence of marbling on Warner-Bratzler shear force and sensory traits of beef top loin steaks (Shackelford et al. 1994b)

Marbling Score	Warner-Bratzler Shear Force (kg)	Sensory Tenderness[a]	Sensory Juiciness[b]	Beef Flavor Intensity[c]
Traces (or lower)	6.06[d]	4.64[g]	4.95[g]	4.83[e]
Slight	5.45[e]	4.90[f]	5.09[f]	4.86[e]
Small	4.82[f]	5.21[e]	5.25[e]	4.96[d]
Modest (or higher)	4.28[g]	5.41[d]	5.46[d]	4.92[d,e]

[a]8 = Extremely tender; 1 = extremely tough.
[b]8 = Extremely juicy; 1 = extremely dry[c].
[c]8 = Extremely intense; 1 = extremely bland.
[d,e,f,g]Different letters indicate different p<0.05.

Table 12.3. Summary of reported phenotypic correlations between tenderness traits and calpastatin activity, intramuscular lipid content, or marbling in longissimus steaks

Tenderness Trait	24-hour Calpastatin Activity (μ/g)	Intramuscular Lipid Content	Marbling	Number of Animals	Reference
WBS (d7 and d9)	.27	−.27	—	555	Shackelford et al., 1994a
WBS (d7)	.14	—	.00	89	Miller et al., 1996
WBS	—	—	−.12	2,453	Koch et al., 1982
WBS (d 7)	.27	—	−.17	392	Wulf et al., 1996
WBS (d 9)	—	−.16	−.24	1,594	Gregory et al., 1995
WBS (d 7)	—	−.15	−.11	888	Wheeler et al., 1996
WBS (d 7)	.40	—	−.15	575	O'Connor et al., 1997
Sensory panel tenderness	—	.17	.20	1,594	Gregory et al., 1995
Sensory panel tenderness	—	.16	.12	888	Wheeler et al., 1996
Sensory panel tenderness	−.14	—	.19	392	Wulf et al., 1996

The importance of marbling in predicting cooked beef palatability has been the focus of numerous research investigations over the years. The inclusion of marbling in quality grading criteria has received criticism, because it appears to account for only a small amount of variation in tenderness (Koohmaraie 1992; Parrish 1981). Smith et al. (1987) demonstrated that, across the entire range of marbling and maturity, quality grade accounted for 40% of the variation in overall palatability and 25% of the variation Warner-Bratzler shear force values in cooked beef loin steaks. A tenderness advantage exists for "Modest" and other degrees of marbling greater than "Small" (Table 12.2). Premium beef merchandising programs, such as Certified Angus Beef, rely on this relationship (along with specified aging periods) to market beef that will be palatable and tender.

The association between marbling and tenderness loses some of its "predictive power" when the focus is on differences in tenderness within quality grades. Many studies (reviewed by Parrish 1981) have shown very little difference in WBS in steaks with Slight and Small marbling. This is a crucial comparison, because the 2002 National Beef Quality Audit reported that 33% and 42% of graded carcasses had Slight and Small degrees of marbling, respectively (McKenna et al. 2002). It can be concluded that quality grade does little to predict tenderness in a majority of the graded beef.

Increasing marbling through genetic selection for visible marbling scores or intramuscular lipid (determined chemically) is achievable as heritability for this trait is moderately high. However, selection for increased marbling can also decrease retail product yield (Shackelford et al. 1994a; Wheeler et al. 1996; Gregory et al. 1995, Koch et al. 1982). Thus, genetic selection for increased marbling has the potential to result in less efficient production of lean meat.

Pork flavor, juiciness, and tenderness are influenced by intramuscular lipid content (Jones et al. 1994). The influence of intramuscular lipid on objective measures of tenderness in pork is not consistent. Some researchers (Candek-Potokar et al. 1998; Blanchard et al. 2000; Huff-Lonergan et al. 2002) demonstrated significant, negative relationships between intramuscular lipid and objective measures of textural integrity. These relationships are typically not strong. Other reports have reported no relationship between intramuscular lipid and instrumental measures of textural integrity

(Hovenier et al. 1993; Jones et al. 1994). Clearly the potential of intramuscular lipid to affect WBS also depends on other factors that impact textural properties. These other properties include amount of postmortem proteolysis of myofibrillar and cytoskeletal proteins. Lipid content is positively correlated with fresh pork flavor and pork firmness. A minimum of 2.5% lipid has been suggested to improve the possibility of a positive eating experience (DeVol et al. 1988). This is of importance because it has been well documented that selection for lean growth has the potential to decrease intramuscular lipid content in pork loin muscle (Cameron et al. 1999; Lonergan et al. 2001).

MODELS OF LEAN GROWTH: MEAT QUALITY CASE STUDIES

Several examples of novel conditions among genetic strains of livestock provide evidence that changes in muscle metabolism during growth may affect meat quality. Muscle metabolism in the early postmortem period has a profound impact on meat quality. The composition of muscle, specifically lipid content, also influences meat quality. With this in mind, it should be apparent that changes in muscle metabolism during growth affect meat quality.

CALLIPYGE

Callipyge, a novel form of muscle hypertrophy associated with extensive muscling in the loin and hindquarters of sheep, has been identified and characterized (Cockett et al., 1994; see also Chapter 2). In callipyge lambs, the muscular phenotype develops gradually after 3 weeks of age. Callipyge lambs produce leaner, more muscular carcasses. Muscle hypertrophy in the callipyge model is associated with an increase in the proportion of Type IIB (fast glycolytic) muscle fibers compared to Type IIA and Type I fibers (Figure 12.4). Further evidence of hypertrophy is presented when fiber diameter within each fiber type is examined (Figure 12.5). The increase in protein accretion in muscle has been suggested to be due to a reduction in protein degradation rather than an increase in protein synthesis (Koohmaraie et al. 1995).

A change in living muscle metabolism has the potential to influence the early postmortem events in muscle that impact meat quality. Little postmortem proteolysis of myofibrillar proteins and myofibrillar fragmentation is observed in callipyge sheep muscles that exhibit hypertrophy. This decrease in postmortem proteolysis is hypothesized

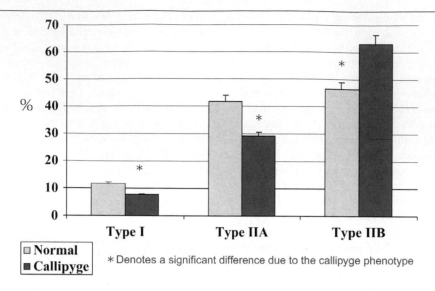

Figure 12.4. Effect of callipyge phenotype on muscle fiber type distribution in longissimus muscle (Carpenter et al. 1996).

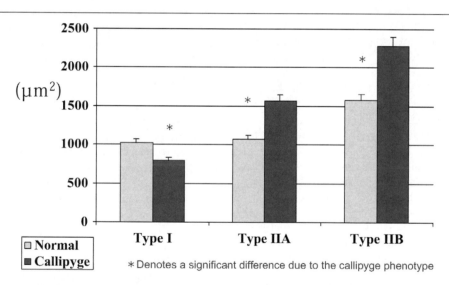

Figure 12.5. Effect of callipyge phenotype on muscle fiber area (μm²) in longissimus muscle (Koohmaraie et al. 1995).

to be caused by higher calpastatin activities at slaughter and throughout the aging period (Table 4; Koohmaraie et al. 1995).

Double Muscling

Double muscling is an inherited condition in cattle. The condition is classified as a syndrome, which implies that it is associated with many physiological characteristics in addition to muscle hypertrophy (see review by Arthur 1995). Expression of the double muscled phenotype is normally observed in the regions of the proximal fore and hind quarter. Cattle expressing the phenotype typically demonstrate higher carcass dressing percentages, greater percentage of carcass lean, and less carcass fat than normal cattle. Other names such as "doppellender,"

Table 12.4. Effect of callipyge phenotype on calpastatin activity, Myofibrillar Fragmentation Index, and Warner-Bratzler shear force values (Koohmaraie et al. 1995)

	Normal	Callipyge
Calpastatin activity (units/g tissue)		
0 hour	3.2	5.8
7 days postmortem	1.2	2.2
21 days postmortem	0.9	1.9
Myofibrillar Fragmentation Index		
1 day postmortem	59.5	43.1
7 days postmortem	79.1	51.1
21 days postmortem	82.4	52.2
Warner-Bratzler shear force (kg)		
1 day postmortem	7.5	10.9
7 days postmortem	4.7	10.1
21 days postmortem	3.3	8.2

"double rumped," and "bottle thighed" have been used to describe this condition.

The double muscling condition in cattle is due to a mutation in myostatin (Grobet et al. 1997, 1998; Kambadur et al. 1997). Different mutations in myostatin are observed in different breeds. Myostatin mutations have been identified in Belgian Blue, Piedmontese, Charolais, Maine-Anjou, and Asturiana cattle (Smith et al. 1998). The double muscling phenotype has often been mistakenly referred to as a muscle hypertrophy phenotype. Observed increases in muscle growth are due to hyperplastic and, to a lesser extent, hypertrophic growth. In contrast to the callipyge model, the double muscling condition in cattle results in a greater number of muscle cells rather than an increase in cell size. Gerrard et al. (1991) observed that double muscled cattle possess roughly twice as many muscle cells as normal cattle, even at birth.

Because the mechanism of growth is different, we should expect to see differences in the textural integrity of the product. Meat from double muscled cattle is at least comparable and is often more tender than beef from normal cattle—despite a much lower intramuscular lipid concentration (Bouton et al. 1978). Muscles from double muscled cattle have less total collagen than muscles from normal cattle (up to 40% less on a dry matter basis) (Lawrie et al. 1964; Uytterhaegen et al. 1994, Ngapo et al. 2002a). The majority of this difference in collagen content appears to be in perimysial connective tissue. A lower collagen concentration has the potential to decrease the *background toughness* in cooked meat. Alterations in the collagen maturation may also influence background toughness. The concentration (mol/mol collagen) of a collagen crosslink, histidinohydroxymerodesmosine, is lower in the semitendinosus muscle of double muscled cattle compared to normal or hetertozygous animals (Ngapo et al. 2002b). This same report demonstrated a significant positive correlation between histidinohydroxymerodesmosine content and the structural integrity of uncooked semitendinosus muscle.

The double muscling condition offers additional evidence that muscle metabolism and growth has the potential to impact meat quality and composition. Studies focused on meat quality of double muscled beef have shed new light on how muscle composition, structure, and histochemical properties can impact the characteristics of fresh beef.

Genetic Selection for Lean Growth

One of the prime considerations in the meat industry is to produce—at the least cost—the highest quantity of muscle tissue for conversion to meat. Since growth and carcass characteristics are moderately highly heritable, it is possible to achieve improvement in carcass composition using genetic selection. Selection for lean growth efficiency in a closed herd of Duroc pigs demonstrated this effect (Table 12.5). This change in composition and growth would be expected to result in a change in the response to the early postmortem environment. In this study, a more rapid pH decline was observed in the longissimus muscle in pigs in the selected line. No difference was noted in the ultimate pH. The change in the response to the early postmortem environment did however result in a greater amount of product weight lost as drip (Figure 12.6), higher Warner-Bratzler shear force values, and less proteolysis of the myofibrillar protein troponin-T.

In another study, Brocks et al. (2000) compared the histochemical traits of muscle from pigs selected for either a fast rate of growth or lean growth.

They demonstrated that the biceps femoris muscle from pigs in the lean growth line had a lower percentage of type I fibers and a higher percentage of type IIB fibers. Decreased leanness appeared to be more closely related to a higher percentage of oxidative fibers and a lower percentage of glycolytic fibers. In general, one would expect this change in morphology to result in differences in the response to handling and processing during the early postmortem period.

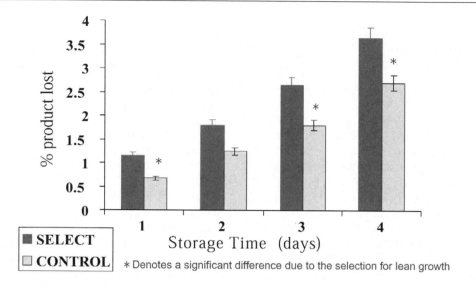

Figure 12.6. Influence of selection for lean growth on drip loss from longissimus dorsi chops (Lonergan et al. 2001).

Table 12.5. Effect of selection for lean growth efficiency on lean gain and carcass composition in Duroc pigs (Lonergan et al. 2001)

Trait	Select Line	Control Line	P-Value
Lean gain/day (kg)	0.292	0.218	<0.01
Loin eye area (cm^2)	30.5	26.4	<0.05
10th rib fat (cm)	2.3	3.6	<0.01
Average backfat (cm)	2.8	3.7	<0.01
Percent lean	49.4	41.5	<0.01
WBS (kg force)	3.12	2.62	<0.01
Longissimus pH			
15 minutes	6.41	6.61	<0.01
30 minutes	6.25	6.46	<0.01
45 minutes	6.09	6.35	<0.01
24 hours	5.45	5.51	0.26

Selection for improved growth rate and carcass composition will typically result in improvement in these traits. Animal scientists must be aware of changes in metabolism of muscle that are associated with improvement in growth and monitor how those changes will impact the quality of the product.

Case Study Summary

A fundamental principle in meat science is that any alteration of muscle metabolism, physical structure, or composition has the potential to alter the response of that muscle to the postmortem environment during the conversion of muscle to meat. This response is the critical factor in understanding how our industry can be better prepared to consistently and efficiently produce a high-quality meat product.

REFERENCES

Arthur, P.F. 1995. Double muscling in cattle: a review. *Australian Journal of Agricultural Research* 46:1493–1515.

Blanchard, P.J., Willis, M.B., Warkup, C.C., and Ellis, M. 2000. The influence of carcass backfat and intramuscular fat level on pork eating quality. *Journal of the Science of Food and Agriculture* 80:145–151.

Bouton, P.E., Harris, P.V., Shorthose, W.R., and Ellis, R.W. 1978. Comparison of some properties of meat from normal steers and steers heterozygous for muscular hypertrophy. *Meat Science* 2:1392–1396.

Brocks, L., Klont, R.E., Buist, W., de Greef, K., Tiemenan, M., and Engle, B. 2000. The effect of selection of pigs on growth rate vs leanness on histochemical characteristics of different muscles. *Journal of Animal Science* 78:1247–1254.

Cameron, N.D., Nute, G.R., Brown, S.N., Enser, M., and Wood, J.D. 1999. Meat quality of Large White pig genotypes selected for components of efficient lean growth rate. *Animal Science* 68:115–127.

Candek-Potokar, M., Zlender, B., Lefoucheur, L., and Bonneau, M. 1998. Effects of age and/or weight at slaughter on longissimus muscle: Biochemical traits and sensory quality in pigs. *Meat Science* 48:287–300.

Carpenter, C.E., Rice, O.D., Cockett, N.E., and Snowder, G.D. 1996. Histology and composition of muscles from normal and callipyge lambs. *Journal of Animal Science* 74:388–393.

Cockett, N.E., Jackson, S.P., Shay, T.L., Nielsen, D., Moor, S.S., Steele, M.R., Barendse, W., Green, R.D., and Georges, M. 1994. Chromosomal localization of the callipyge gene in Sheep (Ovis aries) using bovine DNA markers. *Proceedings of the National Academy of Sciences of the United States of America* 91:3019–3023.

DeVol, D.L., McKeith, F.K., Bechtel, P.J., Novakofski, J., Shanks, R.D., and Carr, T.R. 1988. Variation in composition and palatability traits and relationships between muscle characteristics in a random sample of pork carcasses. *Journal of Animal Science* 66:385–395.

Gerrard, D.E., Thrasher, K.H., Grant, A.L., Lemenager, R.P., and Judge, M.D. 1991. Serum-induced myoblast proliferation and gene expression during development of double muscled and normal cattle. *Journal of Animal Science* 69 (Supplement 1):317.

Gregory, K.E., Cundiff, L.V., and Koch, R.M. 1995. Genetic and phenotypic (Co)-variances for growth and carcass traits of purebred and composite populations of beef cattle. *Journal of Animal Science* 73:1920–1926.

Grobet, L., Martin, L.J., Poncelet, D., Pirottin, D., Brouwers, B., Riquet, J., Schoeberlein, A., Dunner, S., Menissier, F., Massabanda, J., Fries, R., Hanset, R., and Georges, M. 1997. A deletion in the bovine myostatin gene causes the double-muscled phenotype in cattle. *Nature: Genetics* 17:71–74.

Grobet, L., Poncelet, D., Royo, L.J., Brouwers, B., Pirottin, D., Michaux, C., Menissier, F., Zanotti, M., Dunner, S., and Georges, M. 1998. Molecular definition of an allelic series of mutations disrupting the myostatin function and causing double-muscling in cattle. *Mammalian Genome* 9:210–213.

Hovenier, R., Kanis, E., and Verhoeven, J.A.M. 1993. Repeatability of taste panel tenderness scores and their relationship to objective pig meat quality traits. *Journal of Animal Science* 71:2018–2025.

Huff-Lonergan, E., Baas, T.J., Malek, M., Dekkers, J.C.M., Prusa, K., and Rothschild, M.F. 2002. Correlations among selected pork quality traits. *Journal of Animal Science* 80:617–627.

Jones, S.D.M., Tong, A.K.W., Campbell, C., and Dyck, R. 1994. The effects of fat thickness and degree of marbling on pork color and structure. *Canadian Journal of Animal Science* 74:155–157.

Kambadur, R., Sharma, M., Smith, T.P., and Bass, J.J. 1997. Mutations in myostatin (GDF8) in double-muscled Belgian Blue and Piedmontese cattle. *Genome Research* 9:910–916.

Koch, R.M., Cundiff, L.V., and Gregory, K.E. 1982. Heritabilities and genetic, environmental and phenotypic correlations of carcass traits in a population of diverse biological types and their implications in selection programs. *Journal of Animal Science* 55:1319–1329.

Koohmaraie, M. 1992. Role of neutral proteinases in postmortem muscle degradation and meat tenderness. *Proceedings of the Reciprocal Meat Conference* 45:63–71.

Koohmaraie, M., Shackelford, S.D., Wheeler, T.L., Lonergan, S.M., and Doumit, M.E. 1995. A muscle hypertrophy condition in lamb (callipyge): Effects and possible modes of action. *Journal of Animal Science* 73:3596–3607.

Lawrie, R.A., Pomeroy, R.W., and Williams, D.R. 1964. Studies in the muscles of meat animals IV. Comparative composition from 'doppelender' and normal sibling heifers. *Journal of Agricultural Sciences* 62:89–92.

Lonergan, S.M., Huff-Lonergan, E., Rowe, L.J., Kuhlers, D.L., and Jungst, S.B. 2001. Selection for lean growth efficiency in Duroc pigs: Influence on pork quality. *Journal of Animal Science* 79:2075–2085.

McKenna, D.R., Roeber, D.L., Bates, P.K., Schmidt, T.B., Hale, D.S., Griffin, D.B., Savell, J.W., Brooks, J.C.,

Morgan, J.B., Montgomery, T.H., Belk, K.E., and Smith, G.C. 2002. National Quality Beef Audit-2000: Survey of targeted cattle and carcass characteristics related to quality, quantity, and value of fed steers and heifers. *Journal of Animal Science* 80:1212–1222.

Miller, R.K., Taylor, J.F., Sanders, J.O., Lunt, D.K., Davis, S.K., Turner, J.W., Savell, J.W., Kallel, F., Ophir, J., and Lacey, R.E. 1996. Methods for improving meat tenderness. *Proceedings of the Reciprocal Meat Conference* 49:106–113.

Ngapo, T.M., Berge, P., Culioli, J., and De Smet, S. 2002a. Perimysial collagen crosslinking in Belgian Blue double-muscled cattle. *Food Chemistry* 77:15–26.

Ngapo, T.M., Berge, P., Culioli, J., Dransfield, E., De Smet, S., and Claeys, E. 2002b. Perimysial collagen crosslinking and meat tenderness in Belgian Blue double-muscled cattle. *Meat Science* 61:91–102.

O'Connor, S.F., Tatum, J.D., Wulf, D.M., Green, R.D., and Smith, G.C. 1997. Genetic effects on beef tenderness in Bos indicus composite and Bos taurus Cattle. *Journal of Animal Science* 75:1822–1830.

Parrish, F.C. 1981. Relationships between beef carcass quality indicators and palatability. *Proceedings of the National Beef Grading Conference*. Iowa State University Cooperative Extension Service. CE-1633:46–67.

Shackelford, S.D., Koohmaraie, M., Cundiff, L.V., Gregory, K.E., Rohrer, G.A., and Savell, J.W. 1994a. Heritabilities and phenotypic and genetic correlations for bovine postrigor calpastatin activity, intramuscular fat content, Warner-Bratzler shear force, retail product yield and growth rate. *Journal of Animal Science* 72:857–863.

Shackelford, S.D., Koohmaraie, M., and Wheeler, T.L. 1994b. The efficacy of adding a minimum adjusted fat thickness requirement to the USDA beef quality grading standards for select grade beef. *Journal of Animal Science* 72:1502–1507.

Shackelford, S.D., Koohmaraie, M., Whipple, G., Wheeler, T.L., Miller, M.F., Crouse, J.D., and Reagan, J.O. 1991.

Predictors of tenderness: Development and verification. Journal of Food Science 56:1130.

Smith, G.C., Savell, J.W., Cross, H.R., Carpenter, Z.L., Murphey, C.E., Davis, G.W., Abraham, C.C., Parrish, F.C., and Berry, B.W. 1987. Relationship of USDA quality grades to palatability of cooked beef. *Journal of Food Quality* 10:269–286.

Smith, T.P., Casas, E., Fahrenkrug, S.C., Stone, R.T., Kappes, S.M., and Keele, J.W. 1998. Myostatin mutations cause double muscling in cattle. *Proceedings of the Reciprocal Meat Conference* 51:112–117.

Uytterhaegen, L., Claeys, E., Demeyer, D., Lippens, M., Fiems, L.O., Boucque, C.Y., Van de Voorde, G., and Bastiaens, A. 1994. Effects of double-muscling on carcass quality, beef tenderness and myofibrillar protein degradation in Belgian Blue white bulls. *Meat Science* 38:255–267.

Wheeler, T.L., Cundiff, L.V., Koch, R.M., and Crouse, J.D. 1996. Characterization of biological types of cattle (Cycle IV): Carcass traits and longissimus palatability. *Journal of Animal Science* 74:1023–1035.

Wheeler, T.L., Koohmaraie, M., Cundiff, L.V., and Dikeman, M.E. 1994. Effects of cooking and shearing methodology on variation in Warner-Bratzler shear force values in beef. *Journal of Animal Science* 72:2325–2330.

Whipple, G., Koohmaraie, M., Dikeman, M.E., and Crouse, J.D. 1990b. Predicting beef longissimus tenderness from various biochemical and and histological traits. *Journal of Animal Science* 68:4193–4199.

Whipple, G., Koohmaraie, M., Dikeman, M.E., Crouse, J.D., Hunt, M.C., and Klemm, R.D. 1990a. Evaluation of attributes that affect longissimus muscle tenderness in Bos taurus and Bos indicus cattle. *Journal of Animal Science* 68:2716–2728.

Wulf, D.M., Tatum, J.D., Green, R.D., Morgan, J.B., Golden, B.L., and Smith. G.C. 1996. Genetic influences on beef longissimus palatability in Charolais- and Limousin-sired steers and heifers. *Journal of Animal Science* 74:2394–2405.

13
Growth of the Mammary Gland

Colin G. Scanes

The characteristic of mammals is the presence of mammary glands. These produce milk and are suckled by the young (neonates). The mammary glands are of critical importance to agriculture; they are the basis for the dairy industry and critical to beef, pork, and lamb production due to the postpartum nutrition of calves, piglets, and lambs.

The mammary glands are located on the ventral surface and usually lateral to the midline (on either side). The number of mammary glands varies from species to species and in some cases within a species: cow 4, sheep 2, horses 2, and pigs 12 (ranging from 2–18 in pairs). The location of mammary glands also varies from species to species: inguinal (groin)—cow, sheep, horse; abdominal—pig; and thoracic to inguinal—rabbit.

The growth, differentiation (development), and functioning of the mammary gland is under intricate hormonal control:

- *Prepubertal stage.* Estrogens (e.g., estradiol), growth hormone/somatotropin (GH), adrenal steroids
- *Postpubertal ("virgin") stage.* Estrogen, GH, adrenal steroids (the ductal system becomes *very branched*)
- *Pregnancy stage.* Estrogen, progesterone, prolactin, placental lactogen, GH acting via insulin-like growth factor-I (IGF-I), adrenal steroids (in livestock—both the glucocorticoid, cortisol, and the mineralocorticoid, aldosterone) (further development of the ducts and the formation of the alveoli)

This is covered in more detail in the following sections.

ANATOMICAL CHANGES (MAMMOGENESIS) AND ITS HORMONAL CONTROL

The mammary gland consists of the following tissues: alveoli, ducts, connective tissue (stroma) including loose connective areolar tissue, and the teat (or nipple). The glandular tissue (alveoli and ducts) is referred to as parenchymal tissues/cells. There are several stages in the development of the mammary gland (mammogenesis): prepubertal stage, postpubertal ("virgin") stage and pregnancy stage. The anatomical changes for each developmental stage are discussed in the following sections.

Mammary Growth Prior to Puberty

The anatomy of the prepubertal mammary gland consists of relatively simple ducts extending from the teat. Mammary growth has been extensively studied in cattle, because of the importance of milk production—and in sheep, as cheaper surrogates for cattle.

Cattle

Following birth, the growth of the mammary gland is first *isometric*, growing at the same rate as the body. Subsequently but prior to puberty, mammary growth becomes *allometric* (faster than body growth). Mammary growth prior to puberty is first independent of the ovary and then becomes dependent on the ovary. Growth of the mammary gland includes increases in parenchymal tissue (initially ducts plus endothelial cells).

Ovarian Hormones and Mammary Growth Prior to Puberty

During the stages of prepubertal growth, the mammary gland becomes able to respond to ovarian hormones, such as the estrogen, estradiol (E_2). Growth of the mammary gland goes from being independent of the ovary to dependent on the ovary (Ellis et al. 1998). Mammary growth is reduced in heifer calves whose ovaries have been surgically removed (ovariectomy) (Purup et al. 1993). Ovariectomy decreases mammary growth in terms of the total weight of the gland and weight of parenchymal tissue (Purup et al. 1993) There is a change with age in the ability of the mammary gland to respond to injections of ovarian hormones (E_2 and progesterone, P_4). Heifer calves received injections of a mixture or cocktail of E_2 and P_4. The effects varied with the age of the calves receiving the injections: No effects are found at 4 and 7 months (i.e., the mammary gland cannot respond) but for 10-month heifers, there is increased mammary weight (i.e., the mammary gland can now respond).

The effect of E_2 is to increase the number of ductal cells. In vitro, it stimulates proliferation (cell division) of these ductal cells. E_2 also enhances the proliferation of endothelial cells. These latter cells form new blood vessels and hence bring oxygen, nutrients, and hormones to the growing mammary gland (Woodward et al. 1993)

Pituitary Hormones and Mammary Growth Prior to Puberty

Prepubertal mammary growth appears to be also dependent on the pituitary hormone, growth hormone (GH) (or somatotropin) (ST). In studies with heifers on different levels of feed, prepubertal mammary growth (parenchymal weight and DNA) was correlated with the circulating concentrations of GH. On the other hand, mammary adipose tissue was inversely correlated with circulating concentrations of GH (Sejrsen et al. 1983). Moreover in another study by the same group, administration of GH was found to result in increased growth of the mammary parenchymal tissue (Radcliff et al. 1997). This effect of GH on mammary growth in cattle is observed consistently (Purup et al. 1993; reviewed Sejrsen et al. 1999).

Sheep

Mammary growth in very young prepubertal sheep is thought to be independent of ovarian hormones. As in very young cattle, mammary growth in lambs was found to be unaffected by ovariectomy at 10 days of age or by E_2 administration. The indices of mammary growth measured included mammary weight, parenchymal weight, stromal weight, and parenchymal DNA at 6 and 13 weeks of age (Ellis et al. 1998). Early growth of the mammary glands in cattle is independent of ovarian hormones.

Teat Growth

Teat growth appears to be affected by the ovary in the prepubertal ruminant based on studies in the sheep. Teat length is reduced following ovariectomy in lambs and increased by E_2 in intact or ovariectomized lambs (Ellis et al. 1998).

Postpubertal ("Virgin") Mammary Growth

At this stage, the ductal system becomes very branched. Postpubertal mammary growth is hormone-dependent. There is a strong role for sex steroids and mammary growth.

The development of the ductal system (becoming very branched) occurs under the influence of estrogen. (There may be cyclical changes in the ducts during the estrous cycle.) The evidence for this comes from the ability of E_2 to stimulate mammary growth even prior to puberty and the increases in E_2 released into the blood stream by the now fully functional ovary (postpuberty).

There is also a role for GH. In studies with heifers on different levels of feed, post pubertal mammary growth (percentage parenchymal tissue) was correlated with circulating concentrations of GH. Mammary adipose tissue was inversely correlated with circulating concentrations of GH. (Sejrsen et al. 1983). Moreover, GH administration is thought to increase mammary growth following puberty, but this does not necessarily increase subsequent milk yield (reviewed Sejrsen et al. 1999). Some studies involving hormone administration extend from the prepubertal stage to postpuberty. Increases in mammary parenchyma and mammary DNA were observed in heifers receiving bGH with this effect more marked when on a high energy/protein diet formulated for high growth (Radcliff et al. 1997).

Mammary Growth During Pregnancy

The growth and differentiation (development) of the mammary gland is completed during pregnancy. This includes the further development of the ducts and the formation of the alveoli. This is under the control of multiple hormones together with growth factors released from and acting within the mammary gland. The role of each of these hormones is considered in the following sections.

Estrogen/Progesterone

During pregnancy, E_2 and P_4 continue to play a critical role in mammogenesis and lactogenesis. Indeed, a complete mammogenesis and lactogenesis can be induced in cows simply by E_2 and P_4 treatment (injected twice daily for 7 days) (Smith and Schanbacher 1973). The lactation is only at a slightly lower level that the normal lactation, and is decreased by 18% compared to the previous lactation (Smith and Schanbacher 1973).

Progesterone and Ductal Development

During pregnancy, P_4 binding to P_4 receptors stimulates side branching of ducts and development of the ductal epithelium (Brisken et al. 2000). Studies with Wnt-4-/- mice demonstrate that P_4/P_4- receptor activation of the protooncogene Wnt-4 is essential to the action of P_4 in activating ductal branching (Brisken et al. 2000).

Prolactin

Prolactin plays a critical role in mammary development at the end of pregnancy. A large peak in circulating concentrations of prolactin occurs at the time of parturition. Is this prolactin surge required for mammary development and subsequent milk yield? To examine this, a study was conducted by Akers and colleagues (1981). There were four treatment groups:

- "Positive" controls—untreated cattle
- A low prolactin group in which prolactin secretion had been suppressed by injections of the dopamine agonist CB154 (2-bromo-α-cryptine), starting before anticipated parturition
- Prolactin injected to cattle also receiving CB154
- "Negative" control—mammary tissue from cows sacrificed 10 days before anticipated parturition

Milk yield was reduced with CB154 treatment (by 80% on day 1 of lactation, by ~30% on day 10). This effect was overcome by prolactin injections.

Mammary DNA and fatty acid synthesis were increased following parturition, but there was no effect of treatment with either CB154 or the combination of CB154 and prolactin. Mammary RNA and both lactose and milk protein (α-lactalbumin) synthesis increased following parturition. These responses were attenuated by CB154 treatment but not with CB154 and prolactin (Akers et al. 1981). Fully differentiated mammary epithelium was observed following parturition. Differentiation was reduced by CB154 treatment, with prolactin overcoming the effect of CB154. Similarly, prolactin increased mammary growth (weight, DNA, and differentiation) in heifers primed with E_2 and P_4 but receiving CB154 to suppress prolactin secretion (Byatt et al. 1994). CB154 treatment during lactogenesis (late pregnancy) in cows markedly reduces milk production in the following lactation (e.g. Johke and Hodate 1978).

There is additional strong evidence for a role of prolactin in both mammogenesis and lactogenesis from studies in goats and rodent models. Reduction of circulating prolactin concentrations was achieved in pregnant goats by hypophysectomy or CB154 treatment. Either approach decreased both mammary lobulo-alveolar tissue and milk production (Buttle et al. 1979). In E_2 primed rodents, prolactin increases the expression of osteoprotegerin-ligand (OPGL), which in turn induces the differentiation of the alveoli (Fata et al. 2000) (for more details of the role of OPGL, see the section "Osteoprotegerin—Ligand (OPGL) and Alveolar Development," below).

Placental Lactogen (PL)

Placental lactogen (PL) rises in pregnancy. It is reasonable to question whether PL may play a role in stimulating mammogenesis and lactogenesis. In fact, PL is both mammogenic and lactogenic. The mammogenic effect of PL was demonstrated by increases in mammary weight, DNA, and differentiation in heifers that were primed with E_2 and P_4 but receiving CB154 (prolactin secretion suppressed) (Byatt et al. 1994).

Growth Hormone/Somatotropin

Administration of GH during pregnancy consistently increases mammary parenchymal growth in ruminants, and there appears to be a carryover effect in milk yield. It is probable that the GH effect is mediated by insulin-like growth factor I (IGF-I) (reviewed Sejrsen et al. 1999).

Role of Growth Factors in Mammary Development

There is evidence that locally produced/acting (paracrine) growth factors are involved in the control of mammary development. For a more extensive discussion of insulin-like growth factor I (IGF-I), see Chapter 5; for information about other growth factors, See chapter 6.

Insulin-Like Growth Factor I (IGF-I)

Studies with rodents have demonstrated that IGF-I plays a critical role in mammary development. Mammary development at puberty is greatly reduced (gland area decreased by 93% and number of terminal end buds by 83%) in mice in which IGF-I production is genetically "knocked-out." These mice do not respond to GH. Administration of IGF-I (irrespective of with or without E_2) to the knock-out mice increased gland area, number of terminal end buds, and number of ducts (Ruan and Kleinberg 1995).

Evidence for the mechanism by which GH/IGF-I influences mammary development comes from studies with hypophysectomized and gonadectomized sexually immature rats (that is, lacking both pituitary and gonadal hormones). Treatment with either GH or IGF-I stimulates mammary development (terminal end buds and number of alveolar structures) in these rats, but only if E_2 is injected. Similarly, GH increases IGF-I expression in mammary tissue in vivo—but again only with E_2 replacement therapy (Ruan et al. 1995).

In vitro studies with mouse mammary tissue also indicate that GH and IGF-I stimulate ductal/alveolar development. Mice were pretreated with E_2 and P_4. Ductal and alveolar development were observed with GH or IGF-I (Plaut et al. 1993). This effect was intensified in the presence of epidermal growth factor (EGF) (Plaut et al. 1993).

A source of the IGF-I influencing mammary development is the adipose tissue closely associated with mammary tissue. Increased IGF-I expression is observed following GH treatment of hypophysectomized/gonadectomized rats, and the effect is augmented in the presence of E_2 (which has no effect alone) (Walden et al. 1998). A model for GH, IGF-I, and E_2 is shown in Figure 13.1.

The role of IGF-I in mammogenesis of livestock is not well established but is probably similar to the model in Figure 13.1. IGF-I and insulin stimulate proliferation/DNA synthesis in bovine mammary cells in vitro (Baumrucker and Stemberger 1989; McGrath et al. 1991) (see Figure 13.2). The IGF-I effect is augmented by EGF (McGrath et al. 1991). The concentrations of insulin that stimulate proliferation were very high and, thus, the insulin could be acting via the IGF type I receptor (see Chapter 5). Maximal "insulin" stimulation of cell division (H^3-thymidine incorporation into DNA) was observed in cells from lactating cows compared to pregnant cows. Similarly, insulin increases cell proliferation (^{3}H-thymidine incorporation) in porcine mammary tissue (Buttle and Lin 1991). There is little basal- or insulin-stimulated DNA synthesis in bovine mammary cells in which lactation was induced by the presence of prolactin, GH, glucocorticoid, thyroid hormone, and insulin (Baumrucker and Stemberger 1989). This suggests that mammary cells can either divide or differentiate.

Both insulin and IGF-I increase the synthesis of IGFBP3 by a bovine mammary cell line (MAC-T) in culture (Cohick and Turner 1998). The addition to IGFBP3 cell cultures would be expected to reduce the effectiveness of IGF-I to stimulate proliferation of bovine mammary cells. However, if the mammary cells are transfected and express high levels of IGFBP3, this acts either in an autocrine manner acting at the cell surface or in an intracrine manner to augment the effectiveness of IGF-I (Cohick 1998).

Figure 13.1. A possible model of action of GH and IGF-I on mammary development.

Model

$$E_2 \text{ pre-exposure}$$
$$\Downarrow \qquad\qquad\qquad \Downarrow$$

GH $\Rightarrow$ IGF-I $\Rightarrow$ mammary ductal development
                Mammary
            adipose tissue

Osteoprotegerin-Ligand (OPGL) and Alveolar Development

Osteoprotegerin-ligand (OPGL) is required for the proliferation of alveolar progenitor cells and survival (prevention of apoptosis) of both these cells and alveolar cells (Fata et al. 2000). Mice which are ogpl-/- or rank-/- do not show alveolar differentiation (Fata et al. 2000). OPGL is expressed in the mammary epithelial cells that are the progenitors for the alveolus, and only during late pregnancy under the influence of prolactin, P_4, or parathyroid hormone-related peptide after E_2 priming (Fata et al. 2000).

Epidermal Growth Factor (EGF)/Transforming Growth Factor α (TGFα)

It is hypothesized that transforming growth factor α (TGFα) influences mammogenesis (reviewed Plaut 1993). A possible model of action is shown in Figure 13.3. It might be noted that the same receptor binds EGF and TGFα (also see Chapter 6). EGF evokes a small stimulation of proliferation of bovine mammary cells and augments proliferation in response to IGF-I (McGrath et al. 1991). TGFα is expressed in bovine mammary tissue during preg-

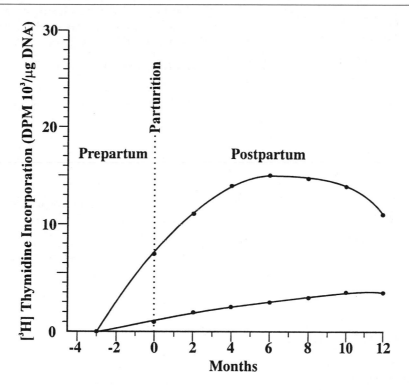

Figure 13.2. Effect of insulin (surrogate for IGF-I) on proliferation of bovine mammary cells. (Data adapted from Baumrucker and Stemberger, 1989.)

Figure 13.3. A possible model of action of EGF and TGFα on mammary development.

$$E_2/P_4 \text{ exposure}$$
$$\Downarrow \qquad\qquad \Downarrow$$
$$TGF\alpha\Uparrow \Rightarrow EGF \text{ receptor}\Uparrow \Rightarrow \text{ mammary ductal development}$$

nancy and lactation. One transcript (observed at high stringency) is observed only late in pregnancy (Koff and Plaut 1995).

Fibroblast Growth Factors (FGF)

There is evidence that members of the FGF family of growth factors (FGF1, 2 and 7 along with FGF receptor) are expressed in the bovine mammary gland. Tissue levels of both FGF1 and 2 are high in late pregnancy when mammogenesis is occurring, but fall during lactation (Plath et al. 1998). Expression of FGF-1, 2, and 7 has been detected in the bovine mammary gland, particularly due to involution (Plath et al. 1998). During lactogenesis and galactopoiesis, expression of FGF-2 is largely limited to the myoepithelial cells (Plath et al. 1998). An FGF2-like growth factor has been purified from bovine colostrum (Hironaka et al. 1997).

Transforming Growth Factor-β1 (TGF-β1)

There is evidence that Transforming Growth Factor-β1 (TGF-β1) is involved in mammary growth and/or development. There is considerable specific binding of TGF-β1 in mammary tissue at times when mammary growth is occurring rapidly. For instance, bovine mammary tissue exhibits marked specific TGF-β1 binding that is maximal during postpubertal mammary development and minimal in early lactation (Plaut and Maple 1995). This is consistent with a role for TGF-β1 in mammary development.

Tumor Necrosis Factor (TNFα)

TNFα stimulates the proliferation of ductal epithelial cells leading to the branching of the lobulo-alveolar ducts (Ip et al. 1992; Lee et al. 2000.).

LACTOGENESIS AND ITS HORMONAL CONTROL

In mammals including ruminants, lactogenesis (the initiation of lactation) requires several hormones including prolactin. The hormonal control of lactogenesis in ruminants is less well understood than in rodent models. The lactogenic hormone complex includes prolactin, insulin, cortisol, and GH together, probably, with P_4 and E_2 plus PL.

Lactogenesis In Vivo (Estrogen/Progesterone)

During pregnancy, E_2 and P_4 play a critical role in lactogenesis. Indeed, a complete lactation can be induced

in cows by E_2 and P_4 treatment (Smith and Schanbacher 1973). The E_2/P_4 treatment probably acts both to prime the mammary tissue to respond to lactogenic hormones and to increase the release of prolactin (a major lactogenic hormone). Some of the priming effect of E_2/P_4 treatment is to induce an increase in the expression of prolactin receptors. This has been observed in the mammary gland of postpubertal ewes (Cassy et al. 2000). It should be remembered that the steroid-treated cows still have the normal repertoire of pituitary and metabolic hormones (Keller et al. 1977). To examine which hormones are actually needed, in vitro studies have been performed.

Smith and Schanbacher (1973) induced cows to lactate with E_2/P_4 treatment. Similarly, lactation in prepubertal heifers can be induced by administration of E_2/P_4 plus dexamethasone (Ball et al. 2000). This may be a useful approach for determining whether mammary-linked gene constructs can be expressed in transgenic cattle.

Lactogenesis In Vitro

Lactogenesis can be induced by the lactogenic complex of the following hormones in vitro in mammary tissue from pregnant cows:

- Prolactin
- Placental lactogen
- GH via IGF-I
- Insulin
- Adrenal steroids—cortisol and aldosterone
- Thyroid hormones
- Estrogen

Mammary fatty acid synthesis requires prolactin and insulin. In studies with mammary tissue from pregnant cows, neither insulin alone nor with cortisol-induced lipogenesis (Collier et al. 1977). Fatty acid synthesis was increased with prolactin together with insulin (Collier et al. 1977). Another index of lactogenesis is lactose synthesis, and this requires prolactin, insulin, and cortisol (Collier et al. 1977). It should be noted that the mammary tissue was from pregnant cows and, hence, had been exposed to the hormones of pregnancy prior to the in vitro studies. It may be questioned whether the hormones of pregnancy prime the mammary tissue so that they can respond to the lactogenic hormones. This appears to be the case. The ability of prolactin (along with insulin and cortisol) to induce lactogenesis in vitro is augmented by co-incubation in the presence of P_4 and E_2 (Nickerson et al. 1978).

Lactogenesis also involves the initiation of the synthesis of milk proteins. The expression of β casein, by mammary cells, can be induced by lactogenic hormones (insulin, cortisol, aldosterone, and prolactin) in vitro. This requires E_2/P_4 priming (Maple et al. 1998).

Other Factors and Lactogenesis

Placental Lactogen (PL)

The lactogenic effect of PL has been demonstrated. PL markedly increases the concentration of the milk protein α-lactalbumin in the circulation in heifers primed with E_2 and P_4 (with prolactin secretion suppressed) (Byatt et al. (1994). Ovine PL can induce lactogenesis by sheep mammary tissue in vitro; it is much less potent than prolactin (Houdebine et al. 1985).

Growth Factors

Growth factors play a modulatory role in the control of lactogenesis. For instance, TNFα modulates (depresses) the expression of genes related to lactogenesis (Shea-Eaton et al. 2001).

MILK PRODUCTION (GALACTOPOIESIS)

This section discusses the hormonal control of milk production (galactopoiesis) in nonruminants and ruminants. In particular, the relative roles of GH and prolactin are considered.

Mammals Excluding Ruminants (Galactopoiesis Reguires Prolactin and GH)

Prolactin is the major galactopoietic hormone in nonruminants. Milk production requires prolactin. Suckling increases prolactin release, and this increases milk production. Not only is prolactin required for milk production, but there is a strong correlation between indicators of milk synthesis and mammary prolactin binding but not circulating prolactin concentrations. An inverse relationship exists due to prolactin down-regulating its receptor (Plaut et al. 1989).

Both prolactin and GH (and probably other metabolic hormones) appear to be required for the maintenance of lactation in nonruminants (that is: both prolactin and GH are galactopoietic). Evidence for this comes from an elegant study by David Flint and Dick Vernon in 1998. In rats, milk production (and mammary DNA) is greatly decreased following the administration of CB154 (suppressed prolactin release). These effects are overcome by injecting the rats daily with prolactin. Similarly, when rats were injected with both bromocryptine and antisera against rat GH (which makes the rat's GH unavailable), there were also marked reductions in both milk production and mammary DNA. As might be expected, injections of prolactin to rats (receiving both bromocryptine and antisera against rat GH) increased milk production and mammary DNA. The prolactin injections did not, however, fully restore either milk production or mammary DNA to the level in the control rats. Injections of bovine GH (not cross-reacting with the antisera to rat GH) to rats receiving both bromocryptine and antisera against rat GH resulted in increases in milk production and mammary DNA. This provides definitive evidence that GH is required for milk production and the maintenance of the functioning mammary gland in the rat.

A similar situation exists is the pig. Not only can injected GH increase milk yield in pigs (Table 13.1) (Harkins et al. 1989), but it also is likely to be one of the endogenous galactopoetic hormones.

Galactopoiesis in Ruminants

This section discusses the hormonal control of milk production in ruminants, particularly cows.

Table 13.1. Effect of porcine GH (pGH) on milk yield (kg/d) in sows (data from Harkins et al., 1989)

Treatment	Milk Yield (kg/day) on Day of Lactation	
	Day 22	Day 28
Control	8.9	9.0
pGH	9.9[*]	11.0[*]

[*]$p < 0.05$.

GH and Galactopoiesis

Milk production in ruminants requires GH. Exogenous bovine GH (bGH) increases milk production (reviewed Bauman 1992, 1999). Table 13.2 summarizes some of the studies by Dale Bauman's group at Cornell University demonstrating the effectiveness of bGH. Administration of bGH increases milk production in high-yielding dairy cows irrespective of whether they are early in, in the middle of, or late in a lactation (Peel et al. 1983).

In November 1993, the U.S. Food and Drug Administration FDA) approved the commercial use of bGH for dairy cattle. This (marketed by Monsanto under the brand name Posilac) is now used extensively in the United States to improve the economic efficiency of milk production. The advantages of bGH include the following: Increased profitability for farmers is likely (the cost of the Posilac, and the increased feed consumed was more than offset by the receipts from the sale of the increased milk produced). A referred paper examined on-farm profitability (Tauer and Knoblauch 1997), and did not provide conclusive support for this. Commercial use of bGH by New York dairy farms increased milk receipts over operating costs ($120/cow). The increased net farm income ($27/cow) was statistically insignificant (Tauer and Knoblauch 1997). There is increased efficiency of production (reductions in feed per unit milk produced and in capital costs (facilities, equipment, etc.) and, hence, providing a benefit to the consumer with reduced cost of milk. Improvements to the environment are likely because there is less animal waste produced per unit of milk. The hormone favors good management because the effectiveness of bGH is related to cow health and good nutrition. The technology is supposedly size-neutral technology; however, adoption/usage has been greater with large producers.

Safety

The FDA review concluded that there are no problems with food safety and animal health with bGH. Human safety was demonstrated by the following:

- The absence of any changes of milk quality with no increase in concentration of bGH in the milk
- Degradation of bGH (and other hormones/growth factors) during digestion
- The inability of bGH to act in humans (reviewed Juskevich and Guyer 1990)

It is been demonstrated that bGH does not bind to the human GH receptor or improve growth rate in hypopituitary dwarfs.

The animal safety conclusion by FDA was based on trials with several hundred thousand cows. There was no discernible effect of bGH treatment on the incidence of mastitis per cow and a slightly lower incidence per unit of milk. More recently, an extensive study examined health effects of bGH treatment in ~100,000 primiparous and ~170,000 multiparous cows. No effects were observed on clinical mastitis or reproductive indices. There were some increases in therapeutic medication (Collier et al. 2001). Similarly, no effect of bGH treatment on the incidence of mastitis was observed in a Michigan study (Judge et al. 1997).

Terminology

Discussion of bGH and its stimulatory effect on milk production is fraught with an issue of terminology. Dairy scientists in universities and industry tend to refer to the hormone as bovine somatotropin or bST. Opponents of its commercial application use the term bovine GH or BGH (sic) or BGROWTH HORMONE. Endocrinologists use the term growth hormone for the hormone in all species including livestock, rodents, and humans. This book uses the term GH.

Table 13.2. Effect of bGH on milk production in dairy cattle

	Milk Yield kg/d	Fat Yield kg/d	Protein Yield kg/d	Reference
Vehicle	34.4	1.23	—	Peel et al., 1981
bGH	37.7[*]	1.51[*]	—	Peel et al., 1981
Vehicle	13.4	0.53	0.50	Fronk et al., 1983
bGH	17.4[*]	0.71[*]	0.59[*]	Fronk et al., 1983
Vehicle	27.9	1.00	0.95	Bauman et al., 1985
bGH	34.4[*]	1.31[*]	1.17[*]	Bauman et al., 1985

[*]$p<0.05$

Historical Background

The first study to suggest that bGH could increase milk production in dairy cattle occurred in the 1930s in what was then the Soviet Union (Asimov and Krouze 1937). A single injection of a "crude" bGH-containing preparation increased milk production. Research in the United Kingdom prior to and during World War II, showed that bGH, purified from the anterior pituitary glands, increases the amount of milk produced per cow. This could have had practical importance given the shortage of food in Britain. There was insufficient food production and, hence, a history of importing food. Insufficient food could be imported due to the torpedoing of ships, particularly in the North Atlantic Ocean. Moreover, it was viewed as economically feasible to inject bGH (derived from pituitary glands) given the unusual wartime situation (Young 1947).

The use of bGH, from cattle pituitary glands, to increase milk production was not economically feasible thereafter. Research in the late 1960s/early 1970s definitively established that bGH and not another pituitary hormone stimulated milk production (Machlin 1973).

Bacteria were first bioengineered to produce recombinant bGH in the 1970s and extensive research demonstrated that bGH increased milk yield even in very high-producing cows (reviewed Bauman 1992, 1999) (also see Table 13.2). It was critically important to demonstrate that bGH could stimulate milk production in today's dairy cows, which are high-producing due to genetic improvement. The ability of bacteria to produce large quantities of bGH relatively cheaply was critical to bGH's successful commercialization.

This was one of the first uses of biotechnology in animal agriculture. It should be noted that others had developed and used biosynthetic enzymes (renin) for cheese making and recombinant vaccines had been adopted.

Mechanism of Action

The mechanism by which bGH increases production/synthesis of milk involves the following:

- Increases in both circulating and local production of IGF-I
- Increases in hepatic gluconeogenesis
- Increases in lipolysis in response to epinephrine
- Decreases in fat synthesis

The bovine liver expresses GH receptor 1A, and other tissues—including adipose tissue and the mammary gland—express GH receptor 1B (Lucy et al. 1998). The GH receptor is expressed in alveolar and duct cells of cows during mammogenesis and lactation (Sinowatz et al. 2000).

In cattle during mammogenesis and lactation, there is expression of IGF-I by mammary adipocytes but not by alveolar or ductal cells (Plath-Gabler et al. 2001). It is likely that the IGF-I affecting galactopoiesis is of peripheral (hepatic) origin with some coming from mammary adipose tissue.

bGH on the Web

Web sites on the issue of bGH include www.nalusda.gov/bic/BST/BST.html (the United States Department of Agriculture) together with www.monsanto.com/dairy/documents/FDA-rbST.html. Several sites exist strongly opposed to bGH with links to others. These include www.benjerry.com/bgh/index.html and www.enviroweb.org/issues/biotech/bgh/index.html.

Social Issues

There has been strong opposition to bGH from a variety of groups. These include the following: consumer, animal welfare and environmental groups, vegetarians, activists against "factory-farming," "corporate farming," agricultural chemical companies, and biotechnology. The concerns perhaps stemmed from bGH being the first extensive use of biotechnology in animal agriculture. Opponents of biotechnology targeted bGH in the same way that they have more recently targeted genetically modified crops (GMOs). Arguments against bGH include the issue of food safety together with lack of trust of the federal regulatory processes and of science. The food safety issues raised include the presence of increased IGF-I in milk and possible increases in mastitis, thereby increasing both somatic cells in milk and use of antibiotics to treat mastitis. There are very stringent federal regulations on use of antibiotics and testing of milk. Particularly in Europe, the similarity in the name bST and BSE ("mad cow disease") is a source of confusion.

Under U.S. law, the FDA can permit labeling only if there is a substantial difference between products. The U.S. works on the basis that we look at "products" not the "process" to get there. There is not a substantial difference between the milk of bST-treated cows and nontreated cows (indeed not a discernible difference). However, there is the strong argument that opposition to labeling is "hiding something from the public."

Other Hormones and Milk Production

Insulin

There is evidence that insulin increases the synthesis of milk protein. In a study at Cornell University, dairy cows were assigned to four treatments (2x2): casein (protein supplement) or water infused into the abomasum and insulin intravenous infusion (with euglycemia being maintained by glucose "clamping"), with pretreatment as control. Milk protein yield was increased with insulin treatment in animals receiving casein into the abomasum (see Table 13.3 for details). This nutritional supplementation partially overcame the pronounced reduction in circulating concentrations of branched chain amino acids that occurs with insulin infusion (Griinari et al. 1997a) (see Table 13.3). The milk protein response to insulin appears to be constrained by amino-acid availability.

The effect of insulin infusion has also been examined in cattle in the presence or absence of abomosal infusions of casein together with branched chain amino acids. Again, insulin infusion with a glucose clamp (euglycemia) increased mammary protein production (casein or whey) (Mackle et al. 2000) (see Table 13.3). The addition of branched chain amino acids to the abomosal infusion in study B (Mackle et al. 2000) did not appear to be any more effective that casein alone (Table 13.3).

It is not clear whether insulin increases milk protein production directly or indirectly via IGF-I. There is evidence for both. Insulin administration increases circulating concentrations of IGF-I (Mackle et al. 2000) (Table 13.3). Direct effects of insulin are favored by both in vivo and in vitro studies. Intramammary infusion of insulin affects milk yield or production of either protein or fat (Mackle et al. 2000) (Table 13.3). The mammary gland synthesizes triglyceride de novo. Insulin influences mammary triglyceride synthesis in vitro. In a transformed bovine mammary cell line (MAC-T cells), insulin increased *sn*-glycerol-3-phosphate acyltransferase and lysophosphatidate acyl transferase activities (Morand et al. 1998). However in vivo, infusion of insulin reduces milk fat percentage (Griinari et al. 1997b).

Glucocorticoids/Cortisol

There does not appear to be an absolute requirement for adrenal glucocorticoids to *maintain* milk production. If lactating sheep are adrenalectomized and subsequently receive injections of deoxycorticosterone (a mineralocorticoid to maintain mineral balance), milk production is maintained (Ely and Balwin 1975).

Prolactin

Prolactin is not a major galactopoetic hormone in cattle, but it may have minor effects. Suppression of

Table 13.3. Effect of insulin[1] on milk protein production in dairy cows

Parameter	Treatment			
	Control	Casein[2]	Insulin	Casein + Insulin
Study A (Griinari et al. 1997a)				
Milk protein yield kg/d (% of control)	0.81 (100)	0.84[+] (104)	0.89[+] (110)	1.04[+] (128)
Circulating branched amino acids[3] ng/ml	95	105[++]	26[++]	38[++]
Study B (Mackle et al. 2000)				
Milk protein production				
Casein kg/d (% of control)	0.67[a] (100)	0.68[a] (101)	0.76[b] (113)	0.79[b] (117)
Whey kg/d (% of control)	0.18[a] (100)	0.17[a] (98)	0.20[b] (115)	0.22[b] (122)
Plasma IGF-I ng/ml	102[a]	103[a]	132[b]	131[b]

[+]Casein effect $p<0.001$; insulin effect $p<0.01$, interaction $p<0.05$.
[++]Insulin effect $p<0.001$.
[a,b]Different superscript letters indicate different $p<0.05$.
[1]Insulin administration as an intravenous infusion with euglycemia maintained by a glucose clamp.
[2]Abomosal infusion of (500 g/d) casein (study A) and (400 g/d) casein supplemented with 88 g/d branched chain amino-acids.
[3]Leucine, isoleucine, and valine.

prolactin release by CB154 does not prevent milk production after a lactation is established (see the earlier section, "Galactopoiesis Reguires Prolactin and GH"). In vitro studies support a role for prolactin in maintaining the activities of critical enzymes for milk production. The activities of both *sn*-glycerol-3-phosphate acyltransferase and lysophosphatidate acyl transferase are increased by prolactin with a bovine mammary cell line (Morand et al. 1998).

Parathyroid Hormone-Related Protein

The mammary gland produces a hormone or hormone-like protein, parathyroid hormone-related protein (PTHrP). This was first characterized as a tumor protein; some tumors have the ability to induce hypercalcemia due to their production of PTHrP. The cells in the mammary gland that synthesize PTHrP are nests of epithelial cells during mammogenesis and the alveolar epithelial cells during lactogenesis and lactation (Rakopoulos et al. 1992).

Based on studies in the goat, it would appear that mammary output of PTHrP peaks at about the time of parturition (Ratcliffe et al. 1992) due to stimulation of the mammary gland by prolactin. Evidence for the latter comes from the ability of bromocryp-

tine to suppress prolactin secretion and reduce secretion of PTHRP (Ratcliffe et al. 1992), and in vitro studies. Production of PTHrP from bovine mammary cells in vitro is increased by the presence of prolactin through a mechanism possibly involving EGF (Okada et al. 1996) (Figures 13.3 and 13.4).

MILK LET DOWN AND ITS HORMONAL CONTROL

Milk is stored in the teat and mammary cisterns (~20%) together with the lobulo-alveolar system (~80%). Milk in the cisterns is immediately available for removal. The rest requires the milk let down response. This is the oxytocin inducting the contraction of the myoepithelial cells. These cells surround the alveoli and small milk ducts (reviewed Bruckmaier and Blum 1998).

Oxytocin and Milk Let Down

The release of oxytocin is a neuroendocrine reflex involving the following: tactile stimulation of the teat and nervous connections to the brain (anterior and posterior inguinal nerves to the lumbar nerves and then via the nerves in the spinal column to the hypothalamus). Oxytocin is synthesized in neurosecretory cell bodies in the supraoptic nucleus and

Figure 13.4. A model of action of hormones during lactogenesis on mammary development (assumes mammary development complete).

Possible model
(assumes mammary development complete)

$$\begin{array}{ccc} E_2 & E_2 & \text{Insulin, cortisol, aldosterone, GH?} \\ \Downarrow & \Downarrow & \Downarrow \\ \text{Prolactin secretion} \Uparrow & \Rightarrow \text{Prolactin receptor} \Uparrow \Rightarrow \text{lactogenesis} \\ & \Uparrow \\ & \text{PL} \end{array}$$

Figure 13.5. Interactions of prolactin and PTHRP.

Parturition $\Rightarrow$ Pituitary
    Gland $\Rightarrow$ Prolactin $\Uparrow$

$$\Downarrow$$

Mammary gland $\Rightarrow$ PTHRP $\Uparrow$

$$\Downarrow$$

Local/peripheral effects +
    $\Rightarrow$ bone/kidney

paraventricular nuclei and released from neurosecretory terminals in the posterior pituitary gland. Oxytocin is transported in the circulation to the mammary gland where it stimulates contraction of the myoepithelial cells.

Oxytocin is released rapidly from the posterior pituitary gland during milking of cows (e.g., Gorewit et al. 1983; Wachs et al. 1984) (see Figure 13.6). Circulating concentrations of oxytocin increase to a peak rapidly (within 1–2 minutes) of teat stimulation (e.g., after machine milking is initiated) and decline precipitously at the end of milking (Wachs et al. 1984). The maximum increment in circulating concentrations of oxytocin (Δ oxytocin) is higher in early than in late lactation (Wachs et al. 1984) (Table 13.4). There are also changes in the magnitude of the oxytocin response during pregnancy. Oxytocin release in response to teat stimulation in early pregnancy (~100 days) is less than that occurring later in pregnancy (150–250 days) (Lefcourt and Akers 1991). Teat stimulation does not appear to effect circulating concentrations of epinephrine (E) or norepinephrine (NE).

Stress and Milk Let Down

Stress adversely affects milk let down. For instance, there is a negative effect of the presence of a rough versus a gentle handler on milk let down with more residual milk in the mammary gland (Rushen et al.

1999). The inhibitory effects of stress on milk let down are probably mediated by the catecholamines, E and/or NE. These may be either adrenal medulla or sympathetic nervous origin. There is some relationship between milk let down and E/NE. Large oxytocin responses to teat stimulation have been predominantly observed when circulating concentrations of NE were low (Lefcourt and Akers 1991). This is consistent with the negative effect of E and/or NE on milk letdown. Injections of E reduce milk let down/yield (Gorewit and Aromando 1985). E has no effect on the rapid (within 2 minutes) oxytocin response to the milking machine (Gorewit and Aromando 1985). Injections of E evoked a marked (~95%) reduction in mammary blood flow and hence delivery of oxytocin to the mammary gland (Gorewit and Aromando 1985).

Table 13.4. Variation in maximal increase in circulating concentration of oxytocin between early and late lactation (data from Wachs et al., 1984)

	Maximal Oxytocin Increment (Δ oxytocin-$\Delta\mu$U/ml)
Early Lactation	22.1±4.5
Late Lactation	12.3±2.3[*]

[*]Different $p<0.05$.

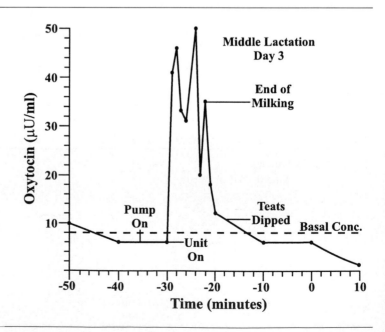

Figure 13.6. Oxytocin release during milking of cows. (Data adapted from Wachs et al., 1984.)

MAMMARY BLOOD FLOW

It would seem self-evident that, for there to be greater milk production by the mammary gland, there should be more blood flow providing essential nutrients together with oxygen. There are both acute (rapid) and chronic (longer-term) changes in mammary blood flow (e.g., Dhondt et al. 1973; also reviewed Prosser et al. 1996).

Acute Changes in Mammary Blood Flow

There is evidence from a number of approaches that mammary blood flow can be changed rapidly. For instance, angiotensins cause vasoconstriction in the bovine mammary artery (Gorewit et al. 1993). This would be anticipated to reduce mammary blood flow. In lactating sheep, mammary blood flow is reduced by suckling, hand milking, or oxytocin administration (McBride et al. 1986). This may be due to myo-epithelial cell contraction, and hence both an increase in resistance in the capillary bed and possibly constriction of blood vessels. Mammary blood flow has been found to be stimulated by prostacyclin (prostaglandin I_2), by low concentrations of prostaglandin E_2 (Nielsen et al. 1995), adenosine (Prosser et al. 1996), and nitric oxide donors (Lacasse et al. 1996). The stress hormones, epinephrine and norepinephrine, have been observed to reduce mammary blood flow in some studies (e.g., Dhondt et al. 1973; Gorewit and Aromando 1985) but not others (McBride et al. 1986).

Chronic Changes in Mammary Blood Flow

There are chronic changes in mammary blood flow. An example is the major increase in mammary blood flow on the day of parturition and the day following (Ratcliffe et al. 1992). Some of the chronic changes in mammary blood flow are hormone-mediated. The effect of GH on milk production is well documented (see above) and is mediated at least partially by locally produced IGF-I. It is, therefore, not surprising that mammary blood flow is elevated by IGF-I (Prosser et al. 1990; Fleet et al. 1992; Prosser and Davis 1992). Bromocryptine does not affect mammary blood flow (Ratcliffe et al. 1992). It is unlikely that either dopamine or prolactin influences mammary blood flow.

DAYLENGTH AND LACTATION

Milk production in dairy cattle can be increased by supplementary light (imposing a long daily photoperiod) compared to natural daylength (Stanisiewski et al. 1985; Bilodeau et al. 1989; Miller et al. 1999). Cows on the long photoperiod have slightly higher circulating concentrates of IGF-I (Dahl et al. 1997). In contrast, exposing cows to short daylength during the dry period is followed by increased milk production in the subsequent lactation (Miller et al. 2000).

REFERENCES

Akers, R.M., Bauman, D.E., Capuco, A.V., Goodman, G.T., and Tucker, H.A. 1981. Prolactin regulation of milk secretion and biochemical differentiation of mammary epithelial cells in periparturient cows. *Endocrinology* 109:23–30.

Asimov, G.J., and Krouze, N.K. 1937. The lactogenic preparations from the anterior pituitary and the increase of milk yield in cows. *Journal of Dairy Science* 20:289–306.

Ball, S., Polson, K., Emeny, J., Eyestone, W., and Akers, R.M. 2000. Induced lactation in prepubertal Holstein heifers. *Journal of Dairy Science* 83:2459–2463.

Bauman, D.E. 1992. Bovine somatotropin: a review of an emerging animal technology. *Journal of Dairy Science* 75:3432–3451.

Bauman, D.E. 1999. Bovine somatotropin and lactation: from basic science to commercial practice. *Domestic Animal Endocrinology* 17:101–116.

Bauman, D.E., Eppard, P.J., de Geeter, M.J., and Lanza, G.M. 1985. Responses of high-producing dairy cows to long-term treatment with pituitary somatotropin and recombinant somatotropin. *Journal of Dairy Science* 68:1352–1362.

Baumrucker, C.R., and Stemberger, B.H. 1989. Insulin and insulin-growth factor-I stimulate DNA synthesis in bovine mammary tissue in vitro. *Journal of Animal Science* 67:3503–3514.

Bilodeau, P.P., Petitclerc, D., St. Pierre, N., Pelletier, G., and St. Laurent, G.J. 1989. Effects of photoperiod and pair-feeding on lactation of cows fed corn or barley grain in total mixed rations. *Journal of Dairy Science* 72:2999–3005.

Brisken, C., Heineman, A., Chavarria, T., Elenbaas, B., Tan, J., Dey, S.K., McMahon, J.A., McMahon, A.P., and Weinberg, R.A. 2000. Essential function of Wnt-4 in mammary gland development downstream of P4 signaling. *Genes and Development* 14:650–654.

Bruckmaier, R.M., and Blum, J.W. 1998. Oxytocin release and milk removal in ruminants. *Journal of Dairy Science* 81:939–949.

Buttle, H.L., Cowie, A.T., Jones, E.A., and Turvey, A. 1979. Mammary growth during pregnancy in hypophsectomized or bromocriptine-treated goats. *Journal of Endocrinology* 80:343–351.

Buttle, H.L., and Lin, C.L. 1991. The effect of insulin and relaxin upon mitosis (in vitro) in mammary tissue from pregnant and lactating pigs. *Domestic Animal Endocrinology* 8:565–571.

Byatt, J.C., Eppard, P.J., Veenhuizen, J.J., Curran, T.L., Curran, D.F., McGrath, M.F., and Collier, R.J. 1994.

Stimulation of mammogenesis and lactogenesis by bovine placental lactogen in steroid-primed dairy heifers. *Journal of Endocrinology* 140:33–43.

Cassy, S., Charlier, M., Bélair, L., Guillomot, M., Land, K., and Djiane, J. 2000. Increase in prolactin receptor (PRL-R) mRNA level in the mammary gland after hormonal induction of lactation in virgin ewes. *Domestic Animal Endocrinology* 18:41–55.

Cohick, W.S. 1998. Role of the insulin-like growth factors and their binding proteins in lactation. *Journal of Dairy Science* 81:1769–1777.

Cohick, W.S., and Turner, J.D. 1998. Regulation of IGF binding protein synthesis by a bovine mammary epithelial cell line. *Journal of Endocrinology* 157:327–336.

Collier, R.J., Bauman, D.E., and Hays, R.L. 1977. Lactogenesis in explant cultures of mammary tissue from pregnant cows. *Endocrinology* 100:192–1200.

Collier, R.J., Byatt, J.C., Denham, S.C., Eppard, P.J., Fabellar, A.C., Hintz, R.L., McGrath, M.F., McLaughlin, C.L., Shearer, J.K., Veenhuizen, J.J., and Vicini, J.L. 2001. Effects of sustained release bovine somatotropin (Sometribove) of animal health in commercial dairy herds. *Journal of Dairy Science* 84:1098–1108.

Dahl, G.E., Elsasser, T.H., Capuco, A.V., Erdman, R.A., and Peters, R.R. 1997. Effects of a long daily photoperiod on milk yield and circulating concentrations of insulin-like growth factor-I. *Journal of Dairy Science* 80:2784–2789.

Dhondt, G., Houvenaghel, A., Peeters, G., and Verschooten, F. 1973. Influence of vasoactive hormones on blood flow through the mammary artery in lactating cows. *Archives of Internal Pharmacodynamics* 204:89–104.

Ellis, S., McFadden, T.B., and Akers, R.M. 1998. Prepubertal ovine mammary development is unaffected by ovariectomy. *Domestic Animal Endocrinolgy* 15:217–225.

Ely, L.O., and Balwin, R.L. 1975. Effects of adrenalectomy upon liver and mammary function during lactation. *Journal of Dairy Science* 59:491–502.

Fata, J.E., Kong, Y.-Y., Li, J., Sasaki, T., Irie-Sasaki, J., Moorehead, R.A., Elliott, R., Scully, S., Voura, E.B., Lacey, D.L., Boyle, W.J., Khokha, R., and Penninger, J.M. 2000. The osteoclast differentiation factor osteoprotegerin-ligand is essential for mammary gland development. *Cell* 103:41–50.

Fleet, I.R., Davis, A., Richardson, M., and Heap, R.B. 1992. The effects of recombinantly-derived insulin-like growth factor-I and insulin-like growth factor-II on mammary vasodilatation in the goat. *Journal of Physiology* 446:69P.

Flint, D.J., and Vernon, R.G. 1998. Effects of food restriction on the responses of the mammary gland and adipose tissue to prolactin and growth hormone in the lactating rat. *Journal of Endocrinology* 156:299–305.

Fronk, T.J., Peel, C.J., Bauman, D.E., and Gorewit, R.C. 1983. Comparison of different patterns of exogenous growth hormone administration on milk production in Holstein cows. *Journal of Animal Science* 57:699–705.

Gorewit, R.C., and Aromando, M.C. 1985. Mechanisms involved in the adrenaline-induced blockade of milk ejec-

tion in dairy cattle. *Proceedings of the Society for Experimental Biology and Medicine* 180:340–347.

Gorewit, R.C., Jiang, J., and Aneshansley, D.J. 1993. Responses of the bovine mammary artery to angiotensins. *Journal of Dairy Science* 76:1278–1284.

Gorewit, R.C., Wachs, E.A., Sagi, R., and Merrill, W.G. 1983. Current concepts on the role of oxytocin in milk ejection. *Journal of Dairy Science* 66:2236–2250.

Griinari, J.M., McGuire, M.A., Dwyer, D.A., Bauman, D.E., Barbano, D.M., and House, W.A. 1997a. The role of insulin in the regulation of milk protein synthesis in dairy cows. *Journal of Dairy Science* 80:2361–2371.

Griinari, J.M., McGuire, M.A., Dwyer, D.A., Bauman, D.E., and Palmquist, D.L. 1997b. Role of insulin in the regulation of milk fat synthesis in dairy cows. *Journal of Dairy Science* 80:1076–1084.

Harkins, M., Boyd, R.D., and Bauman, D.E. 1989. Effect of recombinant porcine somatotropin on lactational performance and metabolite patterns in sows and growth of nursing pigs. *Journal of Animal Science* 67:1997–2008.

Hironaka, T., Ohishi, H., and Masaki, T. 1997. Identification and partial purification of a basic fibroblast growth factor–like growth factor derived from bovine colostrum. *Journal of Dairy Science* 80:488–495.

Houdebine, L.-M., Djiane, J., Dusanter-Fourte, I., Martel, P., Kelly, P.A., Devinoy, E., and Servely, J.-L. 1985. Hormonal action controlling mammary action. *Journal of Dairy Science* 68:489–500.

Ip, M.M., Shoemaker, S.F., and Darcy, K.M. 1992. Regulation of rat mammary epithelial cell proliferation and differentiation by tumor necrosis factor a. *Endocrinology* 130:2833–2844.

Johke, T., and Hodate, K. 1978. Effects of CB154 on serum hormone level and lactogenesis in dairy cows. *Endocrinologia Japonica* 25:67–74.

Judge, L.J., Erskine, R.J., and Bartlett, P.C. 1997. Recombinant bovine somatotropin and clinical mastitis: Incidence, discarded milk following therapy, and culling. *Journal of Dairy Science* 80:3212–3218.

Juskevich, J.C., and Guyer, C.G. 1990. Bovine growth hormone: human food safety evaluation. *Science* 249:875–884.

Keller, H.F., Chew, B.P., Erb, R.E., and Malven, P.V. 1977. Estrogen dynamics and hormonal differences associated with lactational performance of cows induced to lactate. *Journal of Dairy Science* 60:1617–1623.

Koff, M.D., and Plaut, K. 1995. Expression of transforming growth factor-α-like messenger ribonucleic acid transcripts in the bovine mammary gland. *Journal of Dairy Science* 78:1903–1908.

Lacasse, P., Farr, V.C., Davis, S.R., and Prosser, C.G. 1996. Local secretion of nitric oxide and the control of mammary blood flow. *Journal of Dairy Science* 79:1369–1374.

Lee, P.-P.H., Hwang, J-J., Murphy, G., and Ip, M.M. 2000. Functional significance of MMP-9 in tumor necrosis factor-induced proliferation and branching morphogenesis of mammary epithelial cells. *Endocrinology* 141:3764–3773.

Lefcourt, A.M., and Akers, R.M. 1991. Teat stimulation-induced oxytocin and catecholamine release in pregnant and lactating Holstein heifers. *Domestic Animal Endocrinology* 8:235–243.

Lucy, M.C., Boyd, C.K., Koenigsfeld, A.T., and Okamura, C.S. 1998. Expression of somatotropin receptor messenger ribonucleic acid in bovine tissues. *Journal of Dairy Science* 81:1889–1895.

Machlin, L.J. 1973. Effect of growth hormone on milk production and feed utilization in dairy cows. *Journal of Dairy Science* 56:575–580.

Mackle, T.R., Dwyer, D.A., and Bauman, D.E. 2000. Intramammary infusion of insulin or Long R3 insulin-like growth factor-I did not increase milk protein yield in dairy cows. *Journal of Dairy Science* 83:1740–1749.

Maple, R.L., Akers, R.M., and Plaut, K. 1998. Effects of steroid hormone treatment on mammary development in prepubertal heifers. *Domestic Animal Endocrinology* 15:489–498.

McBride, G.E., and Christopherson, R.J. 1986. Effects of adrenaline, oxytocin and 2-Br-α-ergocryptine on mammary blood flow in the lactating ewe. *Canadian Journal of Animal Science* 66:983–993.

McGrath, M.F., Collier, R.J., Clemmons, D.R., Busby, W.H., Sweeney, C.A., and Krivi, G.G. 1991. The direct in vitro effect of insulin-like growth factors IGFs on normal bovine mammary cell proliferation and production of IGF binding proteins. *Endocrinology* 129:671–678.

Miller, A.R.E., Erdman, R.A., Douglass, L.W., and Dahl, G.E. 2000. Effects of photoperiodic manipulation during the dry period of dairy cows. *Journal of Dairy Science* 83:962–967.

Miller, A.R.E., Stanisiewski, E.P., Erdman, R.A., Douglass, L.W., and Dahl, G.E. 1999. Effects of long daily photoperiod and bovine somatotropin (Trobest) on milk yield in cows. *Journal of Dairy Science* 82:1716–1722.

Morand, L.Z., Morand, J.N., Matson, R., and German, J.B. 1998. Effect of insulin and prolactin on acyltransferase activities in MAC-T bovine mammary cells. *Journal of Dairy Science* 81:100–106.

Nickerson, S.C., Heald, C.W., Bibb, T.L., and McGilliard, M.L. 1978. Cytological effects of hormones and plasma on bovine mammary tissue in vitro. *Journal of Endocrinology* 79:63–383.

Nielsen, M.O., Fleet, I.R., Jakobsen, K., and Heap, R.B. 1995. The local differential effect of prostacyclin, prostaglandin E2 and prostaglandin F2α on mammary blood flow of lactating goats. *Journal of Endocrinology* 145:585–591.

Okada, H., Schanbacher, F.L., McCauley, L.K., Weckmann, M.T., Capen, C.C., and Rosol, T.J. 1996. In vitro model of parathyroid hormone-related protein secretion from mammary cells isolated from lactating cows. *Domestic Animal Endocrinology* 13:399–410.

Peel, C.J., Bauman, D.E., Gorewit, R.C., and Sniffen, C.J. 1981. Effect of exogenous growth hormone on lactation performance in high yielding dairy cows. *Journal of Nutrition* 111:1662–1671.

Peel, C.J., Fronk, T.J., Bauman, D.E., and Gorewit, R.C. 1983. Effect of exogenous growth hormones in early and late lactation on lactational performance of dairy cows. *Journal of Dairy Science* 66:76–782.

Plath, A., Einspanier, R., Gabler, C., Peters, F., Sinowwatz, F., Gospodarowicz, D., and Schams,D. 1998. Expression and localization of members of the fibroblast growth factor family in the bovine mammary gland. *Journal of Dairy Science* 81:2604–2613.

Plath-Gabler, A., Gabler, C., Sinowwatz, F., Berisha, B., and Schams, D. 2001. The expression of the IGF family and GH receptor in the bovine mammary gland. *Journal of Endocrinology* 168:39–48.

Plaut, K. 1993. Role of epidermal growth factor and transforming growth factors in mammary development and lactation. *Journal of Dairy Science* 76:1526–1538.

Plaut, K., Ikeda, M., and Vonderhaar, B.K. 1993. Role of growth hormone and insulin-like growth factor I in mammary development. *Endocrinology* 133:1843–1848.

Plaut, K., and Maple, R.L. 1995. Characterization of binding of Transforming Growth Factor-β to bovine mammary tissue. *Journal of Dairy Science* 78:1463–1469.

Plaut, K.I., Kensinger, R.S., Griel, L.C., and Kavanaugh, J.F. 1989. Relationships among prolactin binding, prolactin concentrations and metabolic activity of the porcine mammary gland. *Journal of Animal Science* 67:1509–1519.

Prosser, C.G., and Davis, S.R. 1992. Milking frequency alters the milk yield and mammary blood flow response to intra-mammary infusion of insulin-like growth factor-I in the goat. *Journal of Endocrinology* 135:311–316.

Prosser, C.G., Davis, S.R., Farr, V.C., and Lacasse, P. 1996. Regulation of blood flow in the mammary microvasculature. *Journal of Dairy Science* 79:1184–1197.

Prosser, C.G., Fleet, I.R., Corps, A.N., Froesch, E.R., and Heap, R.B. 1990. Increase in milk secretion and mammary blood flow by intra-arterial infusion of insulin-like growth factor-I into the mammary gland of the goat. *Journal of Endocrinology* 126:437–443.

Purup, S., Sejrsen, K., Foldager, J., and Akers, R.M. 1993. Effect of exogenous bovine growth hormone and ovariectomy on prepubertal mammary growth, serum hormones and acute in-vitro proliferative response of mammary explants from Holstein heifers. *Journal of Endocrinology* 139:19–26.

Radcliff, R.P., Vandehaar, M.J., Skidmore, A.L., Chapin, L.T., Radke, B.R., Lloyd, J.W., Stanisiewski, E.P., and Tucker, H.A. 1997. Effect of diet and bovine somatotropin on heifer growth and mammary development. *Journal of Dairy Science* 80:1996–2003.

Rakopoulos, M., Vargas, S.J., Gillespie, M.T., Ho, P.W.M., Diefenbach-Jagger, H., Leaver, D.D., Grill, V., Moseley, J.M., Danks, J.A., and Martin, T.J. 1992. Production of parathyroid hormone-related protein by the rat mammary gland in pregnancy and lactation. *American Journal of Physiology* 263:E1077–E1087.

Ratcliffe, W.A., Thompson, G.E., Care, A.D., and Peaker, M. 1992. Production of parathyroid hormone-related protein by the mammary gland of the goat. *Journal of Endocrinology* 133:87–93.

Ruan, W., Catanese, V., Wieczorek, R., Feldman, M., and Kleinberg, D.L. 1995. E2 enhances the stimulatory effect of insulin-like growth factor I (IGF-I) on mammary development and growth hormone induced-IGF-I messenger ribonucleic acid. *Endocrinology* 136:1296–1302.

Ruan, W., and Kleinberg, D.L. 1999. Insulin-like growth factor I is essential for terminal end bud formation and ductal morphogenesis during mammary development. *Endocrinology* 140:5075–5081.

Rushen, J., De Passille, A.M.B., and Munksgaard, L. 1999. Fear of people by cows and effects on milk yield, behavior, and heart rate at milking. *Journal of Dairy Science* 82:720–727.

Sejrsen, K., Huber, J.T., and Tucker, H.A. 1983. Influence of amount fed on hormone concentrations and their relationship to mammary growth in heifers. *Journal of Dairy Science* 66:845–855.

Sejrsen, K., Purup, S., Vestergaard, M., Weber, M.S., and Knight, C.H. 1999. Growth hormone and mammary development. *Domestic Animal Endocrinology* 17:117–129.

Shea-Eaton, W.K., Lee, P.-P.H., and Ip, M.M. 2001. Regulation of Milk Protein Gene Expression in Normal Mammary Epithelial Cells by Tumor Necrosis Factor. *Endocrinology* 142:2558–2568.

Sinowatz, F., Schams, D., Kölle, S., Plath, A., Lincoln, D., and Waters, M.J. 2000. Cellular localisation of GH receptor in the bovine mammary gland during mammogenesis, lactation and involution. *Journal of Endocrinology* 166:503–510.

Smith, K.L., and Schanbacher, F.L. 1973. Hormone induced lactation in the bovine. I. Lactation performance following injections of 17β-E2 and P4. *Journal of Dairy Science* 56:738–743.

Stanisiewski, E.P., Mellenberger, R.W., Anderson, C.R., and Tucker, H.A. 1985. Effect of photoperiod on milk yield and milk fat in commercial dairy herds. *Journal of Dairy Science* 68:1134–1140.

Tauer, L.W., and Knoblauch, W.A. 1997. The empirical impact of bovine somatotropin on New York dairy farms. *Journal of Dairy Science* 80:1092–1097.

Wachs, E.A., Gorewell, R.C., and Currie, W.B. 1984. Oxytocin concentrations of cattle in response to milking stimuli through lactation and mammary involution II. *Domestic Animal Endocrinology* 1:141–154.

Walden, P.D., Ruan, W., Feldman, M., and Kleinberg, D.L. 1998. Evidence that the mammary pad mediates the action of growth hormone in mammary gland development. *Endocrinology* 139:659–662.

Woodward, T.L., Beal, W.E., and Akers, R.M. 1993. Cell interactions in the initiation of epithelial proliferation by E2 and P4 in prepubertal heifers. *Journal of Endocrinology* 136:149–157.

Young, F.G. 1947. Experimental stimulation (galactopoiesis) of lactation. *British Medical Bulletin* 5:155–160.

14
Nutrition and Growth

Douglas C. McFarland

Animal growth is influenced by many factors, including environment, genetics, sex, disease status, and nutrition. The effect of nutrition on growth and development is quite profound because nutrients contribute to and become incorporated into not only the structural components of animals, but they are also key players in the physiological and biochemical events leading to the formation of tissues and organs.

Even before birth or hatching, adequate nutrition is important to the development of the embryo and fetus before it can successfully commence an independent existence. As reviewed by Palsson (1955), severe maternal malnutrition has no noticeable effects on very early fetal development. However, during later fetal development, malnutrition has the greatest impact on those tissues that normally grow at faster rates during the period of nutritional insult.

In mammals the placenta serves a key role in regulating the nutrient supply from the dam to the fetus and removal of waste products (for review, see Garnica and Chan 1996). Levels of maternal circulating nutrients are a major factor influencing fetal nutrition. Additionally, the size of the placenta correlates well with fetal blood flow rates, and with ultimate birth weight. Lowered blood flow results in decreased nutrient transport and oxygen supply to the fetus. In fact, small placental size is a major determinant of intrauterine growth retardation in humans. The placenta is also responsible for the production of hormones to maintain pregnancy and support the growth of the embryo and fetus. Free fatty acids are the major forms of lipid that transverse the placenta to the fetus. Triglycerides are apparently not transported in either direction across the placenta. Maternal glucose and amino acids utilize specific transport systems to enter fetal circula-

tion through the placenta. It is interesting that substantial amounts of fetal glucose are, in turn, utilized to support placental metabolism. Among the important hormones produced by the placenta and secreted into maternal circulation is placental lactogen. Placental lactogen acts as an antagonist of insulin action and alters maternal carbohydrate and lipid metabolism to "favor" fetal supply of these nutrients. Placental lactogen is similar in structure and function to growth hormone. By stimulating lipolysis, elevated free fatty acids become available for eventual transport to the fetus. Additionally, glucose uptake and gluconeogenesis in maternal tissues are inhibited, shunting more glucose and amino acids to fetal circulation. Although maternal placental lactogen levels are much higher than found in fetal circulation, it is thought that this hormone plays an anabolic role in the development of the fetus. Several fetal tissues have been demonstrated to increase DNA synthesis, mitogenesis, amino acid transport, and IGF-I release when exposed to placental lactogen.

Most animals undergo differential growth of the various tissues giving rise to variable body proportions during development. But in the case of fish, which experience indeterminate growth (i.e., attain no set maximum size), the young are miniatures of the adult form. Hammond (1932; and reviewed by Palsson 1955) examined the growth of the various tissues and structures of sheep and determined that there are "growth waves" of structures at different time points during development. Early development was characterized by rapid development of the nervous system. This was followed by a wave of bone growth, then muscle deposition, and finally, fat. Within tissues, there is also variation in deposition rates. For instance, mesenteric fat is laid down early, followed by kidney fat, intermuscular fat, subcutaneous fat, and finally, marbling fat. These growth waves are illustrated in Figure 14.1. Similar growth waves occur with other species. Differential growth of structures during development accounts for variation in the body form of young and mature animals. The characteristic "leggy" appearance of foals is due to advanced prenatal development of legs in this species. In fact, postnatally, very little growth of the leg occurs below the hock joint in the horse. Nutritional deficiency during the growth period can result in variation in anatomical proportions compared to well-fed individuals of the same age.

Differential growth rates of tissues also impact the feed efficiency of animals fed different planes of nutrition during the growth period. McMeekan (1940a, 1940b, 1940c), in his classic study, fed four groups of growing pigs the following feeding programs until they reached 200 lbs live weight:

1. High plane of nutrition throughout
2. High plane of nutrition to 16 weeks of age followed by low plane
3. Low plane of nutrition to 16 weeks of age followed by high plane
4. Low plane of nutrition throughout

Figure 14.2 illustrates the growth curves for the 4 groups. Pigs fed the high plane throughout the study had a feed/gain ratio of 5.05, and pigs fed the high plane during the first 16 weeks followed by a low plane of nutrition had a feed/gain ratio of 4.28. The improved feed efficiency of this latter group is believed to be due to the fact that the period of decreased nutrition coincided with the growth wave of adipose tissue. As the economy of feed conversion to fat is low compared to other tissues, the results are an improvement in overall feed efficiency. As expected, those pigs started with a low plane of nutrition and then switched to a high plane of nutrition (during the fat tissue growth wave) had the highest feed/gain efficiency (5.61)—i.e., they were the least efficient. Pigs fed the low plane throughout the growth period also demonstrated low efficiency, with a feed/gain ratio of 5.17. As can be seen in Figure 14.2, it took much longer for these animals to reach 200 lbs., so that a higher proportion of their intake was used to satisfy the maintenance requirement, resulting in lower feed efficiency. Similar results have been seen with cattle.

Following birth or hatching, nutritional deprivation continues to most influence those tissues that would have normally experienced highest rates of growth. When nutritional intake dips below maintenance requirements, tissues are catabolized in the reverse order of their development to provide for the animal's needs. In other words, fat is first utilized, then muscle, and then bone. Nervous tissue, which is laid down very early in development, is not utilized to maintain the nutritionally deprived animal, because the animal would die before this point was ever reached. Nutritional deprivation results in attenuation and lengthening of the growth waves (Figure 14.1B). The order of tissue growth waves is not changed, but the time required for tissue and

---

Figure 14.1. Rate of increase in weight, illustrating the order of development of various tissues and parts of the body. Curve B illustrates the effect of a lowered level of nutrition on the growth waves. (Data adapted from Palsson, 1955, page 437.)

A= Early maturity with high plane of nutrition
B= Late maturity with low plane of nutrition
Curves:

1	2	3	4
head	neck	thorax	loin
brain	bone	muscle	fat
cannon	tibia-fibula	femur	pelvis
kidney fat	intermuscular fat	subcutaneous fat	marbling fat

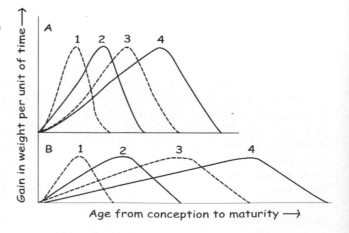

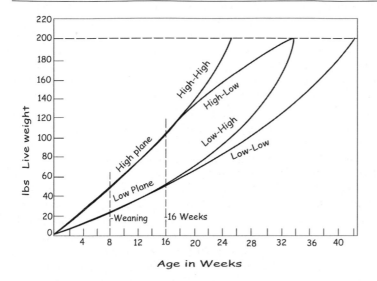

Figure 14.2. Effect of plane of nutrition on the shape of growth curves. (Data adapted from Palsson, 1955, page 402.)

structural maturation to occur is extended. If nutritional deprivation has not been severe, the affected organs may grow and attain their normal weights when adequate nutrients are supplied. Early maturing breeds of cattle are much more susceptible to permanent growth stunting following feed restriction than later maturing breeds.

The recovery that occurs following the reintroduction of adequate nutrition is called "compensatory gain." Compensatory gain is marked by a faster and more efficient accretion of body mass. Much of this is due to lowered net energy for gain (NE_g) and lowered maintenance requirement during the compensatory period (Ferrell et al. 1986; Carstens et al. 1991).

In the following sections, the various nutrient groups and their importance in growth and development are covered. For the required dietary levels of these nutrients for growth, one should consult the most current National Research Council (NRC) nutrient requirement books for the species of interest. For further details of nutritional biochemistry one should consult one of the excellent texts available (for example, Brody 1994).

PROTEIN

The protein fraction of the diet may have several different functions. A major proportion of protein undergoes digestion in the stomach and small intestine, yielding single amino acids and short peptides for absorption. The resulting amino acids serve as the substrates for new protein synthesis within the various tissues of the body. Other proteins appear to remain intact and exert various biological effects at the gut level or in the body proper.

In the acid environment of the stomach or abomasum of mammals and the proventriculus of birds, dietary protein is denatured, exposing protease-labile sites in its structure to digestion by the enzyme pepsin. As digesta enters the duodenum, gastric acid is buffered by an influx of bicarbonate from glands in the region. In the near-neutral pH environment of the duodenum, proteases from the pancreas mix with the digesta and continue to cleave the peptide bonds in the dietary protein, reducing the peptide chain lengths further. These enzymes include trypsin, chymotrypsin, carboxypeptidases, and elastase, each having their own specificity as to cleavage sites. Individual amino acids resulting from the digestion of protein are transported into the enterocytes lining the GI tract. Amino acids are absorbed from the small intestine and even as distal as the colon (Silk et al. 1985). There are several types of transport systems, having different affinities for the individual amino acids. These transport systems are as follows:

- Imino acid system for secondary amines (such as proline)
- Alpha amino-monocarboxylic acid system for neutral amino acids
- Cationic system for basic amino acids
- Anionic system for acidic amino acids

Much of protein degradation results in oligopeptides that are further reduced to di- and tripeptides by the action of several types of peptidases on the intestinal brush border. The resulting di- and tripeptides are transported into the enterocytes by an active mechanism and there reduced to single amino acids by the action of dipeptidase, aminotripeptidase, or proline dipeptidase. There is good evidence that the absorption of these short peptides represents the major route of amino acid assimilation from the GI tract (Adibi and Kim 1981). The resulting free amino acids are then transported out of the enterocytes, enter the portal circulation and are routed to the liver. In the liver, amino acids may be utilized for protein synthesis, catabolized, or returned to circulation for use by other tissues and organs.

The quality of ingested protein refers to the ability of a protein to provide amino acids to support growth, maintenance, and/or production of animals. Although 22 different amino acids are required for the synthesis of protein, only some of these are required to be present in the diet. These are referred to as essential (or indispensable) amino acids. They are either not synthesized in the body or are synthesized at levels insufficient to meet the nutritional needs of the animal. Nonessential or dispensable amino acids may be synthesized from other amino acids or other carbon compounds or may be obtained from the diet. In the mature ruminant, essential amino acids are provided by the action of rumen microbes; in the very young ruminant, these amino acids need to be provided in the diet until the rumen has developed.

Proteins whose amino acid profile closely meets animal nutritional needs are often of higher quality than those proteins with profiles considerably different than requirements. Another major factor impacting protein quality is digestibility. Proteins that are resistant to proteolytic degradation are of low value. This may be due to the configuration of the protein, amino acid sequence, or the presence of other compounds, such as plant protease inhibitors, in the diet. Proteins may also be of poor quality if they produce amino acid imbalances, antagonisms, or toxicities (for review, see Scott et al. 1982). Amino acid imbalances result when the amino acid profile of a protein is considerably different than requirements. In this situation, feed intake becomes depressed, negatively impacting growth rates. Imbalances may be overcome by supplying additional levels of the amino acid(s) most limiting. Amino acid antagonisms result when there are improper ratios of amino acids with similar structures. For instance, the growth depressing effects of excess dietary leucine may be overcome by additional isoleucine and valine in the diet. Lysine–arginine antagonism is particularly a potential problem in poultry. Excess levels of dietary lysine results in elevated arginase enzyme levels in kidney mitochondria. This enzyme, which is responsible for degrading arginine to ornithine and urea may decrease arginine levels such that growth depression occurs. Finally, some amino acids may actually be toxic at high levels, but this is not expected to occur in practical diets.

Consumption of a poor quality protein is not likely to have an immediate impact on the protein nutrition of the animal ingesting it. Endogenous protein from gut secretions and sloughed off mucosal cells represent from between one-third and one-half of the protein present in the intestinal lumen (Nasset 1957; Nixon and Mawer 1970a, 1970b). This large influx of endogenous protein, with a less-variable amino acid profile, serves to buffer the effects of short-term ingestion of poor quality protein. Thus, large fluctuations in gut luminal amino acid profiles and levels are prevented.

Intact peptides and proteins in the diet may also have direct physiological functions apart from supplying amino acids (for review, see Donovan and Odle 1994). Colostrum and milk provide a number of growth factors that may impact the growth of the GI tract and other organs as well (Donovan and Odle 1994; Itoh et al. 2002):

- Epidermal Growth Factor (EGF)
- Insulin
- Insulin-like Growth Factor-I (IGF-I)
- Insulin-like Growth Factor-II (IGF-II)
- Nerve Growth Factor (NGF)
- Relaxin
- Transforming Growth Factor-alpha (TGF-alpha)
- Transforming Growth Factor-beta$_1$ & -beta$_2$ (TGF-ß$_1$ & TGF-ß$_2$)
- Hepatocyte Growth Factor (HGF)

This is likely of more importance in the newborn whose digestive system is less mature and not as efficient in the digestion of protein. Milk and colostrum stimulates the GI tract growth of the neonatal piglet. Colostrum-fed piglets also experience greater fractional protein synthesis rates of visceral organs and skeletal muscle, compared to milk-fed controls, suggesting that growth factors may enter circulation of the newborn and impact tissue growth directly.

Early cell culture studies demonstrated the presence of factors in milk capable of stimulating cell division of hepatocytes and intestinal enterocyte cells. One such mitogen, epidermal growth factor (EGF), influences visceral growth as well as tooth eruption and eyelid opening in the neonate. Suckling rats, pigs, and calves administered oral insulin respond with hypoglycemia, indicating that insulin is absorbed from the GI tract and enters the circulatory system intact. In fact, insulin levels of colostrum-fed piglets and calves were several-fold higher than control animals fed mature milk, which contains lower levels of insulin. Ingested insulin also accelerates GI tract development and maturation in the neonate. Milk transforming growth factor-alpha (TGF-alpha) also interacts through the EGF receptor and may affect developmental events.

Insulin-like growth factors -I and -II (IGF-I and -II) are also present in both colostrum and mature milk. These factors bind to receptors on the crypt cells of the intestinal lining and are believed to stimulate proliferation of enterocytes. Studies with radiolabeled IGF-I have also demonstrated that a small amount of IGF-I may be absorbed intact, enter circulation, and influence tissue growth peripherally. Milk nerve growth factor (NGF) is also absorbed intact from the neonatal gut and is found in circulation. NGF serves as a survival or trophic factor for peripheral neurons, and when fed to neonatal mice, was shown to induce nerve cell hypertrophy. Transforming growth factor-beta, which has various effects, depending on the tissue, inhibits proliferation of intestinal enterocytes and stimulates differentiation.

A major proportion of the protein fraction of colostrum consists of the immunoglobulins. IgG, IgM, and IgG classes of immunoglobulins are found in colostrum and are critical in imparting passive immunity to the neonate for a short period following birth. By several days following parturition, the ability of the small intestine to absorb the immunoglobulins is greatly reduced, a process called "closure." The ability to acquire passive immunity in this manner is extremely important to the health of the neonate.

CARBOHYDRATES

The carbohydrate faction of the diet consists of simple sugars, short chain carbohydrates (oligosaccharides), and longer chain carbohydrates (polysaccharides). Simple sugars resulting from the hydrolysis of carbohydrates are of major importance in meeting the energy requirements of animals. The resulting ATP generated through glycolysis and the TCA cycle is necessary for operating the many biochemical pathways required for growth. Additionally, carbohydrates are required for synthesis of glycoproteins, nucleic acids, the storage carbohydrate glycogen, and many other essential compounds. Carbohydrates may also provide the carbon backbone for the synthesis of nonessential amino acids and lipids.

Most dietary carbohydrates consist of polysaccharides and oligosaccharides. In practical diets, starch comprises the greater proportion of dietary carbohydrates. Starch is made up of amylose, which consists of long alpha-1,4 chains of glucose, and amylopectin, which is similar to amylose, but it has alpha-1,6 linkages of alpha-1,4 chains giving it a branching or tree-like structure.

Starch digestion begins in the mouth of most animals by the secretion of amylase in the serous secretions of the salivary glands. However, the pig and the chicken lack salivary amylase. The products of starch digestion are maltose (glu-glu), maltotriose (glu-glu-glu), and mixtures of short chain carbohydrates (dextrins) containing the alpha-1,6 branch points. Any dietary glycogen is digested similarly. More extensive digestion of starch occurs in the duodenum by the action of pancreatic amylase. The resulting short chain oligosaccharides are reduced to glucose by the action of enzymes bound to the intestinal enterocyte cells. One of these enzymes, maltase, cleaves maltose to 2 glucose molecules and maltotriose to 3 glucose molecules. The other enzyme, isomaltase, cleaves the dextrins to maltose and glucose. These enzymes are located throughout the intestine, but are highest in the mid-jejunum and upper ileum. Other hydrolases found associated with enterocytes include

- Sucrase, which cleaves sucrose to glucose and fructose
- Lactase, which cleaves lactose to glucose and galactose
- Trehalase, which cleaves trehalose to glucose

The lactase enzyme is very important to the neonatal mammal consuming milk, because milk contains high levels of lactose. The neonate is very efficient in digesting lactose, but this ability generally decreases with age. Trehalase is only important to those animals consuming single cell organisms, such as yeasts, bacteria, and algae, which contain trehalose. Other carbohydrates, such as raffinose and stachyose found in beans, are not digested by the hydrolases of the GI tract, and are thus, unavailable. Enzymes required for the breakdown of cellulose and hemicellulose are also not produced in the GI tract. Nevertheless, these carbohydrates are important substrates for ruminant animals whose rumen microbial populations convert it to acetate, propionate, and butyrate. These volatile fatty acids are converted in the ruminant tissues to glucose, amino acids, and lipids. Polysaccharides and lignin not digested by endogenous hydrolases are termed fiber. Up to approximately 30% of dietary fiber may be degraded in adult monogastric animals to short-chain fatty acids by the gut microflora of the large intestine and cecum, contributing to the energy requirement of the host animal. Dietary fiber is also important in maintenance of normal gut peristalsis and functioning.

Glucose and galactose are the major sugars resulting from carbohydrate digestion in practical diets of monogastric animals. They are actively transported from the gut through the same transport system. It is estimated that approximately 10% of the absorbed glucose is metabolized locally, with the rest entering portal circulation. Fructose, which results primarily from the feeding of sucrose, is absorbed by passive diffusion into the enterocyte. There it is largely converted to glucose or lactate before passing into intestinal portal drainage. Xylose is a major pentose actively absorbed from the GI tract.

LIPIDS

Dietary lipids consist of triglycerides, phospholipids, cholesterol, cholesteryl esters, and the fat soluble vitamins (A, D, E, and K). Cholesterol is used as a substrate for the synthesis of steroid hormones and bile salts and may be supplied in the diet or synthesized by the liver. Triglycerides are important sources of energy, having approximately 2.25-fold greater energy content than an equal weight of the carbohydrate starch. These compounds are also important as sources of the essential fatty acids, linoleic acid and linolenic acid. Linoleic acid and linolenic acid are incorporated into membrane phospholipids and are also the substrates for synthesis of several important classes of hormones: prostaglandins, leukotrienes, and thromboxanes. A deficiency of linoleic acid results in integumentary system problems, such as scaly skin, hair loss, and impaired wound healing. A deficiency of linolenic acid, at least in primates, has been demonstrated to lead to neurological and vision

problems. Unlike most species, cats are unable to convert linoleic acid to arachidonic acid, so arachidonic acid must be provided in the diet of this species.

Fatty acids may also be synthesized from carbohydrates and the products resulting from amino acid catabolism. The site of fatty acid synthesis is species-dependent. In birds, most fatty acid synthesis, elongation, and desaturation occurs in the liver. In mammals, this occurs in both the liver and adipose tissue to different extents, depending on the species. For example, in swine, most occurs in the adipose tissue; in rats, about two-thirds occurs in the adipose tissue; and in humans, it is mostly in the liver.

Lipid digestion begins in the mouth, at least in humans and rodents. A lingual lipase is present, which is active in the acid environment of the stomach and does not require bile salts for activation. A gastric lipase, resistant to degradation in the stomach and secreted by the fundus of the stomach, is particularly important in the neonate. This enzyme serves to cleave a large proportion of triglycerides during the early period when pancreatic lipase levels are low. This enzyme continues to be active in the duodenum, further breaking down the fat droplet structure. As fat passes into the duodenum, it is further acted upon by pancreatic lipase. Together with bile salts, the fat droplets are further broken down and emulsified to yield increasingly smaller mixed micelles containing fatty acids, 2-acylglycerides, cholesterol, and fat soluble vitamins (A, D, E, and K). These mixed micelles migrate to the microvilli structure of the intestinal villi and are absorbed by the enterocytes. Within the enterocytes, the monoglycerides are re-esterified to triglycerides and combined with apolipoproteins, fat soluble vitamins, and cholesteryl esters to form chylomicron particles. In mammals, chylomicrons enter the lymphatic drainage of the intestine, flowing to increasingly larger lymphatic vessels until they are secreted into the bloodstream at the thoracic duct on the subclavian vein. In birds, which do not have the same type of lymphatic system as mammals, chylomicrons exit the enterocytes and are transported to the liver by the portal blood drainage system.

After they are in the blood stream, chylomicrons are degraded by lipoprotein lipase bound to the capillary walls of tissues such as muscle and adipose. The resulting free fatty acids cross the cell membrane and are absorbed. There the fatty acids may be utilized as an energy source, or in the case of adipocytes, re-esterified and stored as triglycerides. Triglycerides may be mobilized from the adipose tissue by action of hormone-sensitive lipase, which causes the release of fatty acids and the glycerol backbone into circulation. Circulating free fatty acids, largely associated with serum albumin, may be released and absorbed by various tissues and utilized as an energy source.

VITAMINS

Vitamins are small organic compounds that are required for growth, production, reproduction, and maintenance of animals. Although some of them may be synthesized in the body proper, they are generally not produced at levels adequate to meet nutritional requirements. An exception to this is vitamin D, which may be synthesized from precursors in the skin exposed to sunlight. Ascorbic acid (vitamin C) is synthesized by most vertebrates at adequate levels for growth. However, primates, including humans, guinea pigs, and several species of birds, lack the ability to synthesize ascorbic acid, so it must be provided in their diet. Vitamins are effective at very low levels, and although some are essential in energy transformation, they are not, themselves, consumed as energy sources. Others are required for regulation of the activities of structures, such as membranes, but are not structural units. A number of the vitamins serve as important cofactors in the many metabolic pathways that operate in the body.

Historically, vitamins have been classified as either fat-soluble or water-soluble. The fat-soluble vitamins are absorbed along with lipids within micelles from the small intestine. They may be found as pro-vitamins in plant feedstuffs and converted to active vitamins in animal tissues. For example, plant beta-carotene is converted to vitamin A in the intestinal wall and plant ergosterol may be converted to vitamin D by sunlight. Cats are unusual in that they lack the enzyme required to convert beta-carotene to vitamin A. Water-soluble vitamins do not have pro-vitamin forms, yet most undergo metabolic conversion within animal tissues to their active form. Water-soluble vitamins are largely involved in energy regulation as cofactors. In fact, more than 50% of enzymes require organic cofactors.

While ruminant animals require the same vitamins as nonruminant animals, rumen microbe and tissue synthesis of vitamins is generally adequate to meet requirements. Rumen synthesis of B-vitamins

and vitamin K is inadequate in young cattle prior to development of the rumen microflora population. Therefore, it is necessary to supplement these vitamins in their rations. Dairy cattle of all ages require supplemental vitamins A and E (Miller 1979).

Table 14.1 lists the vitamins, their active chemical forms and many of their major functions. For additional details of the functions of vitamins as well as their requirements and deficiency symptoms, see one of the excellent texts available (for example, McDowell 2000; Combs 1992).

In addition to the vitamins listed here, there are a number of other nutrients that may be called "conditional" or "quasi-" vitamins, because they are required by certain species under particular conditions. For instance, choline is required for growth of young poultry and prevention of the joint disorder perosis. Choline is a component of phosphatidylcholine, an important structural compound in membranes, and is needed in the formation of the neurotransmitter, acetylcholine. Through its conversion to betaine, it functions as a source of methyl groups for transmethylation reactions. Another such compound, carnitine, is required for the transport of fatty acids into mitochondria for fatty acid oxidation. As carnitine is synthesized from the essential amino acid lysine, conditions of protein malnutrition may impact its synthesis, resulting in impaired energy metabolism. The pathway of carnitine biosynthesis in neonatal humans and other species is not well developed. Therefore, feeding of soy-based formulas and rations that contain little or no carnitine may put these individuals at risk. Taurine, while synthesized in adequate amounts by most species, must be supplied in the diets of cats. The absence of taurine in the diet causes central retinal degeneration and blindness in this species. Inositol is incorporated into phosphatidylinositol and is required in the diet of certain species of fish, and the gerbil. In most species, inositol is synthesized in adequate amounts from glucose in a number of tissues. Phosphorylated inositol compounds function in cellular responses involving Ca^{+2} fluxes, as well as in the formation of eicosanoids.

MINERALS

Minerals may be divided into three categories depending on the levels required for adequate nutrition: major or macronutrients, trace or micronutrients, and ultra-trace minerals. The major minerals consist of calcium (Ca), phosphorus (P), potassium (K), sodium (Na), chlorine (Cl), magnesium (Mg),

Table 14.1. Active forms and functions of vitamins

Vitamin	Active Forms	Functions
Fat-Soluble Vitamins		
Vitamin A	Retinol, retinal, retinoic acid	Vision; cell differentiation; skeletal development; immune responses
Vitamin D	1,25-dihydroxyvitamin D	Calcium and phosphorus homeostasis: Ca and P uptake from GI tract, bone mineralization and demineralization, kidney reabsorption of Ca and P; cell growth and differentiation
Vitamin E	Isomers of tocopherols and tocotrienols	Biological antioxidant; membrane formation and protection; prostaglandin synthesis; immune function
Vitamin K	Menaquinone (K_2), phylloquinone (K_1)	Carboxylation of glutamic acids of proteins leading to formation of blood clotting factors; bone formation and remodeling
Water-Soluble Vitamins		
Thiamin (B_1)	Thiamine pyrophosphate	Decarboxylation reactions: TCA cycle, pentose pathway, amino acid catabolism; nerve function
Riboflavin (B_2)	Flavin mononucleotide (FMN), Flavin adenine dinucleotide (FAD)	Electron transfer in oxidation-reduction reactions involving carbohydrate, fat, and amino acid metabolism
Niacin (B_3)	Nicotinamide adenine dinucleotide (NAD) Nicotinamide adenine dinucleotide phosphate (NADP)	H+ transfer reactions in carbohydrate, fatty acid, and amino acid metabolism
Vitamin B_6	Pyridoxal phosphate, pyridoxamine phosphate	Many reactions in amino acid metabolism; porphyrin synthesis; glycogen phosphorylase activity; neurotransmitter synthesis; amino acid transport; immune function
Pantothenic Acid	Component of acyl carrier protein and coenzyme A	CoA serves as a carrier of carboxylic acids in amino acid, carbohydrate, and fat metabolism; synthesis of neurotransmitters, steroid hormones, porphyrins, and hemoglobin. ACP serves as an acyl carrier in fatty acid synthetase
Biotin	Lysine-bound biotin in enzymes	Serves as a carboxyl carrier in enzymes of amino acid metabolism, purine synthesis, fatty acid synthesis, and carbohydrate metabolism
Folate	Polyglutamate tetrahydrofolic acid	One carbon transfers (formyl, formimino, methylene, methyl) in synthesis of purines, pyrimidines, methionine, and choline; serine glycine interconversion; histidine degradation
Vitamin B_{12}	Adenosylcobalamin, methylcobalamin	Required by methylmalonyl CoA mutase, leucine mutase, and methionine synthetase
Vitamin C	Ascorbic acid	Oxidation of lysine and proline residues in collagen formation; biological antioxidant, immune function; hydroxylation reactions; carnitine biosynthesis; absorption and mobilization of minerals; catecholamine biosynthesis

and sulfur (S). Trace elements consist of iron (Fe), iodine (I), zinc (Zn), manganese (Mn), copper (Cu), molybdenum (Mo), selenium (Se), and chromium (Cr). Ultra-trace elements consist of vanadium (V), fluorine (F), silicon (Si), boron (B), lithium (Li), nickel (Ni), arsenic (As), and probably others. Cobalt (Co) is required in the diet of ruminant animals for the synthesis of vitamin B_{12} by rumen microbes. There are many additional minerals found in animal tissues, some of which may or may not have a biochemical function. As with other nutrients, minerals may vary in terms of their biological availability depending on the chemical form they are in, as well as the presence and levels of other minerals and nutrients in the diet. It is very unlikely that a deficiency of any of the ultra-trace elements will occur in animals fed practical rations.

Table 14.2 lists the known mineral nutrients and major functions. The functions may be divided into 3 broad categories. They may serve a structural role such as Ca, P, Mg, F, and Si in bones and teeth. Minerals are important constituents in body fluids and other tissues where they serve to maintain osmotic pressure, acid-base balance, and membrane responsiveness. Some minerals also serve as catalysts or activators of enzymes and others as a component of hormone systems. Unlike organic nutrients, minerals are not metabolized to inactive forms. Excess minerals are eliminated through the urine, intestinal mucosa, and digestive glands, and through the skin.

There are a number of remarkable species differences in terms of mineral requirements. For instance, growing chicks have nearly twice the dietary Ca requirement and about a twenty-fold higher requirement for Mn as do growing pigs. Animals in production may also have considerably higher mineral requirements. Because milk contains relatively high levels of Ca and P, the mineral requirement for dairy cows is higher than for non-lactating animals. A similar situation is seen with layer hens in production, which also require higher levels of Ca and P in the diet. Mineral requirements for growth may be lower than for production or other processes. Lowering the Cu levels in growing sheep rations may not affect growth rates, but could have a big impact on wool growth and quality. This is because Cu is involved in the process of pigmentation and keratinization of wool. Likewise, in sheep the Zn requirement for growth is considerably lower than the requirement for testicular development and spermatogenesis. Therefore, animals selected for

breeding purposes will have a different requirement for this nutrient.

Minerals are mostly obtained from the feed, but in some situations significant amounts may be obtained from the water supply. Grazing animals may be supplemented with minerals through the use of sodium chloride–based mineral blocks that may contain other essential minerals, such as Co, P, Mg, Cu, or Se.

HORMONAL RESPONSE TO NUTRITION

Following absorption of nutrients, a number of physiological changes occur to direct these compounds to be utilized in the most appropriate manner. For instance, if energy intake is low, some amino acids may not be utilized in protein synthesis, but rather may be degraded and the carbon skeletons used in energy-yielding pathways. The disposition of absorbed glucose, amino acids and fat is largely regulated by the action of the pancreatic hormones insulin and glucagon.

As circulating levels of glucose increase following absorption from the small intestine, the pancreas responds by releasing insulin. Insulin stimulates the uptake of glucose by cells and the storage of energy by stimulating the enzymes involved in glycogen formation and fatty acid synthesis. Glycogen synthesis occurs mainly in the liver and skeletal muscle, but the sites of fatty acid synthesis are species-dependent. When circulating glucose levels decrease, glucagon is released from the pancreas. Glucagon increases the release of energy stores by stimulating key enzymes in glycogenolysis, glycolysis and the TCA cycle, lipolysis, and protein degradation. The ratio of glucagon/insulin is, therefore, a key factor regulating the overall energy metabolism of animals.

Elevation of insulin following meal consumption results in the synthesis and release of the hormone leptin by adipocytes (for review, see Ahima and Flier 2000; Woods et al. 1998). Conversely, feed restriction and low levels of circulating insulin result in decreased leptin levels. This 16 KDa protein is the product of the *ob* gene, which is defective in the obese mouse model. Circulating levels of leptin correlate with body fat stores and act to depress feed intake and regulate energy balance. Leptin is also produced by skeletal muscle, placenta, gastric mucosa, and mammary epithelium. Leptin stimulates skeletal muscle cell proliferation (Lamosova and Zeman 2001) and increases glucose uptake into

Table 14.2. Functions of the essential minerals

Mineral	Functions
Macrominerals	
Calcium (Ca)	Major structural component of bones and teeth; blood clotting; muscle contraction; neural activity; cofactor for enzymes; cellular signaling
Phosphorus (P)	Major structural component of bones and teeth; phosphorylated compounds involved in most metabolic pathways; phospholipids; nucleic acids
Potassium (K)	Acid-base and osmotic balance; nerve transmission; muscle contraction; enzyme cofactor; amino acid transport
Sodium (Na)	Acid-base and osmotic balance; sugar and amino acid transport; muscle contraction; nerve transmission
Chloride (Cl)	Acid-base and osmotic balance; nutrient transport; nerve transmission; gastric HCl; activator of amylase
Magnesium (Mg)	Structural component of bones and teeth; activates enzymes; ATP metabolism and oxidative phosphorylation; muscle contraction; protein synthesis; immune function
Sulfur (S)	Component of the amino acids cysteine and methionine, sulfate in extracellular matrix compounds; component of coenzyme A, acyl carrier protein, hemoglobin, cytochromes, glutathione, and many other compounds
Trace Elements	
Iron (Fe)	Component of cytochromes, hemoglobin, myoglobin; component or activator of numerous enzymes and other proteins including oxidases and oxygenases, transferrin, ferritin, succinate dehydrogenase
Iodine (I)	Component of the thyroid hormones triiodothyronine and thyroxine which play major roles in metabolism, growth, differentiation, and development
Zinc (Zn)	Component and activator of enzymes; involved in nucleic acid, protein, and carbohydrate metabolism; hormone action; spermatogenesis and male reproductive tissue development; integumentary system; immune function
Manganese (Mn)	Component and activator of enzymes; mucopolysaccharide and glycoprotein synthesis; reproduction; choline biosynthesis; blood clotting; membrane integrity; immune function
Copper (Cu)	Hemoglobin synthesis; Fe absorption and mobilization; collagen crosslinking; hair and wool pigmentation and keratinization; phospholipid synthesis; reproductive function; immune response; lipid metabolism
Molybdenum (Mo)	Component of enzymes; purine, pyrimidine, pteridine, aldehyde, and sulfite metabolism; electron transport; niacin metabolism
Selenium (Se)	Component of glutathione peroxidase, which serves to protect membranes from oxidative damage; immune function; component of types 1 and 3 iodothyronine deiodinases; protective effect against some heavy metals; mitochondrial structural protein
Chromium (Cr)	Component of the glucose tolerance factor, which potentiates the effect of insulin
Ultra-Trace Elements	
Vanadium (V)	Unidentified role in the metabolism of hormones, glucose, lipids, bones and teeth; reproduction
Fluorine (F)	Decreases incidence of dental caries in humans; other beneficial effects are unclear
Silicon (Si)	Glycosaminoglycan and collagen synthesis; skeletal development
Boron (B)	Parathyroid regulation; bone metabolism
Lithium (Li)	Reproduction; central nervous system function
Nickel (Ni)	Possible role as a cofactor or structural component of metalloenzymes; component of rumen bacterial urease enzyme
Arsenic (As)	Unidentified role in skin and skeletal formation and reproduction
Cobalt (Co)	Required by ruminants for the formation of vitamin B_{12} by ruminant microbes

cultured skeletal muscle myotubes, at least in part by recruiting GLUT4 glucose transporters to the cell surface (Berti and Gammeltoft 1999). The hormone is secreted into colostrum and absorbed by the neonate. It appears that a major site of action of leptin is the hypothalamus. Specific regions of the hypothalamus known to function in feeding behavior and energy balance possess leptin receptors. Leptin action is thought to be mediated through a number of neuropeptides and neurotransmitters arising from this area of the hypothalamus. The presence of leptin and its expression in the placenta and in many fetal tissues suggests that it also has a role in early growth and development.

The signals regulating appetite and energy homeostasis are complex and not completely understood. In addition to leptin, insulin itself will reduce food intake. Cholecystokinin (CCK), which is released during meal consumption and serves to stimulate release of pancreatic proteases and bile (important in protein and fat digestion), is also believed to act as a satiety signal in the brain. Other potential peptides affecting satiety include bombesin, gastrin-releasing peptide, neuromedin B, and glucagon.

Fasting in humans results in a rapid drop in serum T3 levels as well as in the ratio of T3 to T4. Although sufficient thyroid precursor (iodinated thyroglobulin) may be stored within the thyroid gland for up to 100 days of an iodine-deficient diet, long-term I deficiency results in enlarged thyroid gland (goiter) and characteristic developmental abnormalities called cretinism (Brody 1994).

During early development, mammals and birds differ in terms of their energy metabolism. Lipid from the yolk sac is the primary source of energy for the avian embryo, and maternal glucose is more important in the developing mammalian fetus. Avian species largely rely on gluconeogenesis from protein stores for glucose during this time. Following hatching, and consumption of a carbohydrate-containing diet, the young bird makes a major transition in its energy metabolism. Because relatively little glucose is absorbed by the ruminant animal, these animals also rely heavily on gluconeogenesis to maintain blood glucose levels.

Nutritional status has a major effect on the growth hormone (GH)–insulin-like growth factor (IGF) axis (for review, see Breir 1999). Most studies have demonstrated that undernutrition results in elevated serum growth hormone (GH) and depressed IGF-I levels. Furthermore, GH receptor levels are decreased, resulting in lowered synthesis of IGF-I in

tissues including the liver, the latter being the primary source of circulating IGF-I (Sjogren et al. 1999). In fact, nutritional status and response to nutritional support in human patients is often assessed by measuring circulating IGF-I levels (Underwood 1999). Patients with either protein-calorie malnutrition or protein malnutrition alone exhibit depressed IGF-I levels. However, when fed diets containing adequate protein and inadequate caloric content, IGF-I levels were normal. Circulating IGF-I levels appear to be particularly sensitive to the status of essential amino acids in the diet. Glucocorticoids, which are elevated during malnutrition, also inhibit GH stimulation of IGF-I transcription in the liver and other tissues (Butler and Le Roith 2001). Elevated GH levels are likely caused by the hypoglycemia, stress, and lowered serum free fatty acids resulting from undernutrition, as well as decreased feedback regulation of its release by lowered circulating levels of IGF-I. GH serves to decrease protein catabolism to maintain nitrogen balance and stimulates lipolysis to provide free fatty acids for tissue needs. The IGF binding proteins also respond to nutritional changes and may impact the activity of the IGFs during undernutrition. IGF binding protein-1 (IGFBP-1) and IGFBP-2 levels in the serum increase with reduced nutritional intake, the latter specifically responding to decreased dietary protein. At the same time, IGFBP-3 and –4 levels decrease under these conditions. It is thought that because IGFBP-3 is the major circulating BP, these changes would shift the distribution of IGFs from the circulating pool toward tissue usage. Furthermore, IGFBP-3 specific protease, which reduces the affinity of IGFs for this BP, is induced, leading to further decease in circulating IGFs.

Studies to determine the effects of the timing of maternal protein restriction on rat fetal plasma and hepatic IGF-I levels revealed that early and brief malnutrition had no impact on IGF-I levels or birth weights (Muaku et al. 1995). However, protein malnutrition of the dam during the final week of pregnancy or throughout pregnancy resulted in depressed birth weights and lowered liver and circulating IGF-I levels. Long or short-term malnutrition of the dam had no measurable effect on circulating or hepatic IGF-II levels. These results demonstrate that fetal growth and IGF-I synthesis are closely tied with maternal amino acid supply during periods of rapid growth and likely explain, at least partially, the observations of Palsson (1955) discussed earlier.

NUTRIENT-GENE INTERACTIONS

Aside from their direct incorporation into biological compounds, certain nutrients have an additional role in that they may influence the expression of certain genes. The following illustrate a few examples of this relationship. (For additional details and reviews, see Hesketh et al. 1998; Clarke and Abraham 1992).

It has long been known that dietary Zn increases the levels of metallothionein, a major storage protein for Zn, by affecting transcription of this protein (Durnam and Palmiter 1981). This is mediated by binding Zn to the appropriate transcription factor (Magis et al. 1996). Furthermore, zinc finger structures of transcription factors control genes involved in growth factor signaling, and Zn may also serve directly in cell signaling (Beyersmann and Haase 2001). Another mineral, iodine, has a profound effect on growth and development due to its incorporation into thyroid hormone. A deficiency of iodine results in major developmental defects, including mental retardation (for review, see Dauncey et al. 2001). Thyroid hormone (especially T-3) binds to a receptor protein, which in turn binds to thyroid-responsive elements of DNA, and this influences the rates of transcription of a number of mRNAs to elicit biological responses. Thyroid hormone stimulates basal metabolic rate and influences protein synthesis and degradation rates. Thyroid status is a key factor in inducing skeletal muscle fiber transition (type I slow fibers to type II fast fibers) and the conversion of cardiac myosin isoforms during development. Lowered dietary energy intake results in depressed thyroid hormone status contributing to reduced growth, development, and metabolism.

Vitamin A, in addition to its role in vision, is a major player in early limb pattern development and the differentiation of many cell types (for review, see Petkovich 1992). All-*trans* retinoic acid and 9-*cis* retinoic acid enter cells and bind to a number of different nuclear receptors, which in turn, interact with DNA to affect the transcription of genes important in development. Metabolism of vitamin D in the liver and kidney results in the formation of 1, 25- dihydroxyvitamin D the active hormone form of the vitamin. This steroid hormone interacts with nuclear receptors and affects the transcription of various genes involved in Ca and P metabolism.

Glucose stimulates the transcription of genes involved in lipogenesis and glycolysis in adipose tissue, liver, and pancreatic beta cells (Girard et al. 1997). By stimulating the expression of hepatic glucokinase, glucose serves to increase its uptake and metabolism. Several genes, including the gene for acetyl-coenzyme A carboxylase, have been shown to possess glucose response elements in their structures. Furthermore, specific fatty acid-regulated transcription factors have been identified that are involved in regulation of cell metabolism, cell growth, and differentiation (Jump and Clarke 1999). The feeding of low fat diets to previously fasted animals results in a marked induction of fatty acid synthase and glycerol-3-phosphate acyltransferase, key enzymes involved in fatty acid and triglyceride synthesis (Sul and Wang 1998).

Nutrition not only has a central role in the early structural development of animals, it also has long-term effects that may not be obvious until later in life (for review, see Koletzko et al. 1998; Dauncey and Bicknell 1999). This includes life-long effects on health, disease, and mortality risks. For example, peak bone mass, which occurs during adolescence and is influenced by nutrition, is a major indicator of the occurrence of osteoporosis in later years. In addition to its importance in the development of the brain structure, nutrition is known to play an important part in brain function. Malnutrition negatively impacts development of structures important in memory and learning and is a factor in the development of schizophrenia and other mental illnesses.

In recent years there has been increasing interest in the physiological functions of specific compounds in foods, some of which are not presently known to be directly involved in growth and developmental processes. This has given rise to the concept of "functional foods." Functional foods demonstrate beneficial function(s) in the body that lead to "improved state of health and well-being and/or reduction of risk of disease" (Contor 2001). This includes foods that contain compounds that are anti-mutagenic and may help prevent cancer (Kinae, et al. 2000; Go et al. 2001), control cholesterol levels (Bouic 2001), improve gut function (Li and Zhang 2001), and promote growth of beneficial gut microflora (Floch and Hong-Curtiss 2001). As more knowledge is gained in the function of these and other compounds, it is anticipated that significant changes may be made in the design of diets to incorporate their beneficial effects.

REFERENCES

Adibi, S.A., and Kim, Y.S. 1981. Peptide absorption and hydrolysis. In Physiology of the Gastrointestinal Tract. L.R. Johnson, ed. New York: *Raven Press.*

Ahima, R.S., and Flier, J.S. 2000. Leptin. *Annual Reviews of Physiology* 62:413–437.

Berti, L., and Gammeltoft, S. 1999. Leptin stimulates glucose uptake in C2C12 muscle cells by activation of ERK2. *Molecular and Cellular Endocrinology* 157:121–130.

Beyersmann, D., and Haase, H. 2001. Functions of zinc in signaling, proliferation and differentiation of mammalian cells. *BioMetals* 14:331–341.

Bouic, P.J. 2001. The role of phytosterols and phytosterolins in immune modulation: a review of the past 10 years. *Current Opinion in Clinical Nutrition and Metabolic Care* 4:471–475.

Breier, B.H. 1999. Regulation and energy metabolism by the somatotropic axis. *Domestic Animal Endocrinology* 17:209–218.

Brody, T. 1994. Nutritional Biochemistry. San Diego: *Academic Press.*

Butler, A.A and Le Roith, D. 2001. Control of growth by the somatotropic axis: growth hormone and the insulin-like growth factors have related and independent roles. *Annual Reviews of Physiology* 63:141–164.

Carstens, G.E., Johnson, D.E., Ellenberger, M.A., and Tatum, J.D. 1991. Physical and chemical components of the empty body during compensatory growth in beef steers. *Journal of Animal Science* 69:3251 3264.

Clarke, S.D., and Abraham, S. 1992. Gene expression: nutrient control of pre- and posttranscriptional events. *The FASEB Journal* 6:3146–3152.

Combs, Jr., G.F. 1992. The Vitamins: Fundamental Aspects in Nutrition and Health. San Diego: Academic Press.

Contor, L. 2001. Functional food science in Europe. *Nutrition, Metabolism, and Cardiovascular Diseases* 11:suppl:20–23.

Dauncey, M.J., and Bicknell, R.J. 1999. Nutrition and neurodevelopment: mechanisms of developmental dysfunction and disease in later life. *Nutrition Research Reviews* 12:231–253.

Dauncey, M.J., White, P., Burton, K.A., and Katsumata, M. 2001. Nutrition-hormone receptor-gene interactions: implications for development and disease. *Proceedings of the Nutrition Society.* 60:63–72.

Donovan, S.M., and Odle, J. 1994. Growth factors in milk as mediators of infant development. *Annual Reviews of Nutrition* 14:147–167.

Durnam, D.M., and Palmiter, R.D. 1981. Transcriptional regulation of the mouse metallothionein-I gene by heavy metals. *Journal of Biological Chemistry* 256:5712–5716.

Ferrell, C.L., Koong, L.J., and Nienaber, J.A. 1986. Effect of previous nutrition on body composition and maintenance energy costs of growing lambs. *British Journal of Nutrition* 56:595–605.

Floch, M.H., and Hong-Curtiss, J. 2001. Probiotics and functional foods in gastrointestinal disorders. *Current Gastroenterology Reports* 3:343–350.

Garnica, A.D., and Chan W.-Y. 1996. The role of the placenta in fetal nutrition and growth. *Journal of the American College of Nutrition* 15:206–222.

Girard, J., Ferre, P., and Foufelle, F. 1997. Mechanisms by which carbohydrates regulate expression of genes for glycolytic and lipogenic enzymes. *Annual Reviews of Nutrition* 17:325–352.

Go, V.L., Wong, D.A., and Butrum, R. 2001. Diet, nutrition and cancer prevention: where are we going from here? *The Journal of Nutrition* 131:suppl:3121S–3126S.

Hammond, J. 1932. Growth and Development of Mutton Qualities in the Sheep. London: *Oliver and Boyd.*

Hesketh, J.E., Vasconcelos, M.H., and Bermano, G. 1998. Regulatory signals in messenger RNA: determinants of nutrient-gene interaction and metabolic compartmentation. *British Journal of Nutrition* 80:307–321.

Itoh, H., Itakura, A., Kurauchi, O., Okamura, M., Nakamura, H., and Mizutani, S. 2002. Hepatocyte growth factor in human breast milk acts as a trophic factor. *Hormone and Metabolic Research* 34:16–20.

Jump, D.B., and Clarke, S.D. 1999. Regulation of gene expression by dietary fat. *Annual Reviews of Nutrition* 19:63–90.

Kinae, N., Masuda, H., Shin, I.S., Furugori, M., and Shimoi, K. 2000. Functional properties of wasabi and horseradish. *BioFactors* 13:265–269.

Koletzko, B., Aggett, P.J., Bindels, J.G., Bung, P., Ferre, P., Gil, A., Lentze, M.J., Roberfroid, M., Strobel, S. 1998. Growth, development and differentiation: a functional food science approach. *British Journal of Nutrition* 80:Suppl. 1:S5–S45.

Lamosova, D., and Zeman, M. 2001. Effect of leptin and insulin on chick embryonic muscle cells and hepatocytes. *Physiological Research* 50:183–189.

Li, S.Q., and Zhang, Q.H. 2001. Advances in the development of functional foods from buckwheat. *Critical Reviews in Food Science and Nutrition* 41:451–464.

Magis, W., Fiering, S., Groudine, M., and Martin, D.I.K. 1996. An upstream activator of transcription coordinately increases the level and epigenetic stability of gene expression. *Proceedings of the National Academy of Sciences USA* 93:13914–13918.

McDowell, L.R. 2000. Vitamins in Animal and Human Nutrition. Ames: *Iowa State University Press.*

McMeekan, C.P. 1940a. Growth and development in the pig, with special reference to carcass quality characters. I. *Journal of Agricultural Science* 30:276–343.

McMeekan, C.P. 1940b. Growth and development in the pig, with special reference to carcass quality characters. Part II. The influence of the plane of nutrition on growth and development. *Journal of Agricultural Science* 30:387–435.

McMeekan, C.P. 1940c. Growth and development in the pig, with special reference to carcass quality characters. Part III. Effect of the plane of nutrition on the form and composition of the bacon pig. *Journal of Agricultural Science* 30:511–569.

Miller, W.J. 1979. Vitamin requirements of dairy cattle. In Dairy Cattle Feeding and Nutrition. Tony J. Cunha, ed. Orlando, Florida: *Academic Press.*

Muaku, S.M., Underwood, L.E., Selvais, P.L., Ketelslegers, J.M., and Maiter, D. 1995. Maternal protein restriction early or late in rat pregnancy has differential effects on fetal growth, plasma insulin-like growth factor-I (IGF-I) and liver IGF-I gene expression. *Growth Regulation* 5:125–132.

Nasset, E.S. 1957. Role of the digestive tract in the utilization of protein and amino acids. *Journal of the American Medical Association* 164:172–177.

Nixon, S.E., and Mawer, G.E. 1970a. The digestion and absorption of protein in man. 1. The site of absorption. *British Journal of Nutrition* 24:227–240.

Nixon, S.E., and Mawer, G.E. 1970b. The digestion and absorption of protein in man 2. The form in which disgested protein is absorbed. *British Journal of Nutrition* 24:241–258.

Palsson, H. 1955. Chapter 10. "Conformation and Body Composition." In Progress in the Physiology of Farm Animals vol. 2. John Hammond, ed. London: *Butterworths Scientific Publications.*

Petkovich, M. 1992. Regulation of gene expression by vitamin A: The role of nuclear retinoic acid receptors. *Annual Reviews of Nutrition* 12:443–471.

Scott, M.L., Nesheim, M.C., and Young, R.J. 1982. Proteins and Amino Acids. In *Nutrition of the Chicken.* Geneva, N.Y.: W.F. Humphrey Press, Inc.

Silk, D.B.A., Grimble, G.K., and Rees, R.G. 1985. Protein digestion and amino acid and peptide absorption. *Proceedings of the Nutrition Society* 44:63–72.

Sjogren, K., Liu, J.-L, Blad, K., Skrtic, S., Vidal, O., Wallenius, V., LeRoith, D., Tornell, J., Isaksson, O.G.P., Jansson, J.-O., and Ohlsson, C. 1999. Liver-derived insulin-like growth factor I (IGF-I) is the principal source of IGF-I in blood but is not required for postnatal body growth in mice. *Proceedings of the National Academy of Science USA* 96:7088–7092.

Sul, H.S., and Wang, D. 1998. Nutritional and hormonal regulation of enzymes of fat synthesis: studies of fatty acid synthase and mitochondrial glycerol-3-phosphate acyltransferase gene transcription. *Annual Reviews of Nutrition* 18:331–351.

Underwood, L.E. 1999. Clinical uses of IGF-I and IGF binding protein assays. 617–628. In: The IGF System—molecular biology, physiology, and clinical applications. R.G. Rosenfeld and C.T. Roberts, Jr. Totowa, N..J.: *Humana Press.*

Woods, S.C., Seeley, R.J., Porte Jr., D., and Schwartz, M.W. 1998. Signals that regulate food intake and energy homeostasis. *Science* 280:1378–1383.

15
Genetics and Growth

Archie C. Clutter

A comprehensive picture of the relationship of genetics to growth would include all genes encoding proteins in pathways underlying growth processes. However, a distinction can be drawn between genes critical to growth and development but fixed in species or subpopulations, and those that contribute to variation in growth and development between species, between breeds within species, and within breeds or lines. Knowledge of the genes important to mammalian biological and physiological pathways is expanding at a rapid pace (see, for example, Chapter 5), often without accompanying knowledge of whether the genes are fixed or segregating in relevant populations. It is the genetic variation in components of growth and development that is the raw material of genetic change within and divergence between populations and, consequently, the primary focus of this chapter. Although the species focus of the chapter is mammalian livestock (cattle, sheep, and pigs), there are cases in which more basic knowledge exists—for example, in model species—and examples are provided from those species for context.

The earliest development of a mammal occurs in utero, and knowledge of the genetic control of embryonic and fetal development in livestock is rapidly expanding. Although this chapter covers only postnatal development, readers can find recent reviews of early development in cattle (Thatcher et al. 2001) and pigs (Maddox-Hyttel et al. 2001). In contrast to this early development in which single genes have been identified with functions hypothesized to determine the success or failure of the developing embryo, most of the genetic variation in postnatal growth is quantitative. In other words, variation in traits of postnatal growth is mostly expressed as a continuous distribution and thought to be the result of more subtle differences in the effects of many genes in combination with the environment. Results from genetic analyses of body size, tissue growth, and animal maturity, and from controlled selection on growth traits, is used to describe this quantitative genetic variation.

In addition to physical measurements and linear descriptions of growth (e.g., body weight, fat thickness, average daily gain), much progress has been achieved in the mathematical modeling of the biology of tissue growth, and in some cases genetic variation in the parameters of such models has been estimated. The linking of biological models to quantitative variation will be discussed, and an example of an associated strategy for genetic improvement will be described.

Diverse breeds or selection lines have been used in some cases to identify physiological mechanisms through which genetic differences are expressed, and the tools now exist for the discovery of specific genes that cause genetic variation in growth processes. Progress in this new frontier of gene discovery, as a way to gain greater understanding of existing genetic variation and to enhance genetic improvement in growth characteristics of livestock species, is also reviewed.

EFFECTS OF MAJOR GENES

There are several graphic examples of sequence variation in single genes (i.e., gene alleles) that greatly affect aspects of tissue growth and development in livestock species. In some, such as ovine hereditary chondrodysplasia or spider lamb syndrome (Cockett et al. 1999), a single allele causes severely abnormal or lethal changes, but in others a viable animal results with characteristics drastically different than its contemporaries. For example, inheritance of alleles of a single gene were reported many years ago to cause dwarfism in Hereford cattle, the heterozygote expressing a compressed body size intermediate to that of normal Herefords and the usually lethal homozygous mutant (Chambers et al. 1954). More recently, mutations in single genes have been studied in cattle and sheep that have major effects on tissue development, but that results in animals with viable production potential.

The condition in cattle known as double muscling, named for extreme skeletal muscle development, was first reported in the 1800s and is characteristic of the Belgium Blue and Piedmontese breeds. The pattern of inheritance supports the hypothesis of a single gene for which a nonrecessive allele causes extreme muscle hypertrophy (Arthur 1995). Casas et al. (1998) evaluated progeny of F1 Piedmontese x Angus and Belgian Blue x MARC III sires heterozygous for the muscle hypertrophy (mh) allele mated to homozygous (+/+) dams. Hence, progeny were either mh/+ or +/+. For most of the carcass traits measured, genotype differences either approached or exceeded one standard deviation. In residual standard deviation units, differences between the genotype groups (mh/+ minus +/+) for birth weight, rib eye area, retail product yield, birth weight, marbling score, USDA yield grade, carcass fat thickness, and kidney, pelvic, and heart fat were 0.41, 1.35, 1.6, −1.01, −1.42, −.84, and −.86. The genotype groups did not differ for calving ease or shear force measurements of meat tenderness. Allelic effects were similar in Belgian Blue and Piedmontese progeny.

Short et al. (2002) used F2 calves from Piedmontese (mh/mh) grandsires to quantify differences among all three genotypes (0, 1, or 2 copies of the mh allele). F2 grandprogeny of Hereford and Limousin sires were also produced in the study so that Piedmontese-cross calves with varying double muscling genotypes could be compared with crossbred calves from these two other breeds of similar mature size but with normal and moderately greater degrees of muscling, respectively. Birth weight and adjusted efficiency (adjusted for primal cut weights) of Piedmontese F2 progeny increased in a linear fashion with increasing number of copies of the mh allele, but increases in longissimus and semitendinosus area and decreases in fat thickness were nonlinear with greater differences between mh/mh and mh/+ than between mh/+ and +/+, suggesting dominant gene action for the body composition traits. Postweaning gain was less in Piedmontese than in either Limousin or Hereford, and did not differ between doubling muscling genotypes. Longissimus area of Limousin was greater than that of Hereford, and Piedmontese progeny without a copy of the double muscling allele (i.e., +/+) did not differ from Hereford.

Extreme muscle hypertrophy in some of the progeny of a Dorset ram was first reported in the early 1990s (Jackson and Green 1993). Jackson et al. (1997) reported subsequent progeny ratios from designed matings that supported the hypothesis of a single, autosomal locus with nonrecessive gene action. The condition was termed *callipyge* for the distinct postnatal development of the hindquarter that occurs in heterozygous lambs (Figure 15.1).

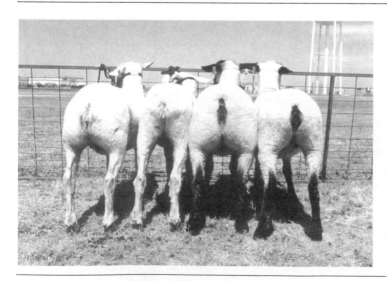

Figure 15.1. Expression of the major callipyge gene for muscle hypertrophy in two different breed backgrounds. From left, callipyge lambs are first and third in line.

Freking et al. (1998) reported growth and carcass traits in callipyge heterozygotes versus non-callipyge contemporaries in a Dorset x Romanov F2. Callipyge lambs did not differ from their contemporaries in body weight at any of the measured ages from birth to 140 days. Lambs were serially slaughtered at 3-week intervals beginning at 23 weeks of age. Rates of protein and fat accretion at the mean age were 22.5% greater and 16.4% less, respectively, in callipyge than in non-callipyge lambs. The distribution of carcass protein was shifted slightly to the posterior in callipyge lambs. Duckett et al. (2000) reported that muscle hypertrophy in callipyge lambs does not occur until between 7 and 20 kg body weight (19 and 100 days of age), and results in 40% heavier longissimus and semimembranosus muscles between 20 and 69 kg liveweight. The greater lean yield in callipyge lambs is accompanied by a greater calpastatin activity and Warner-Bratzler shear force values, suggesting reduced meat tenderness (Koohmaraie et al. 1995; Duckett et al. 2000).

Recent developments in technology have allowed the chromosomal location of the genes causing double muscling in cattle and callipyge in sheep to be determined. In a later section of this chapter, "Molecular Genetic Factors—Segregating Genes," the novel gene action associated with callipyge and specific mutations causing double muscling will be described.

QUANTITATIVE GENETIC VARIATION

The genes with major effects on growth and development of livestock described in the previous section are the exception rather than the rule. If one considers typical differences among individuals for traits such as body size, rate of growth, muscling, or body composition at maturity that can be observed in a given population, it becomes clear that individuals cannot easily be categorized into discrete classes but rather express a continuous distribution of values (phenotypes). This continuous or quantitative variation results from the presence of many genes, each with a relatively small effect on the trait. The co-segregation of alleles for these genes means that at any given time there is an array of individuals in the population with different combined genotypes. The slightly different genetic value for the trait associated with each of these different combined genotypes, along with variation due to nongenetic or environmental sources, creates

the continuous, quantitative variation. See Falconer and Mackay (1996) for a more detailed description of the concepts of quantitative genetics. This theory, of quantitative variation due to many genes—each with small effect—has not only stood the test of time as the foundation of modern animal breeding (Hill 1999), but is supported by results from recent efforts to discover genes affecting quantitative traits, as will be discussed in a later section of this chapter.

Between- and Within-Breed or Line Variation

Although ranges of between-breed differences are not as great in livestock species as within the widely referenced canine species, there is substantial between-breed variation for traits of growth and development in cattle, swine, and sheep. Although in rare cases a significant part of a breed difference in a characteristic of growth and development can be attributed to an allele of a major gene (e.g., the contribution of the myostatin gene to muscling characteristics of Piedmontese and Belgian Blue relative to other cattle breeds), most between-breed variation is due to polygenic effects.

A long-term comprehensive evaluation of cattle breeds has been conducted by the USDA Meat Animal Research Center (Gregory et al. 1979; Laster et al. 1979; Cundiff et al. 1998; Thallman et al. 1999; see also http://www.marc.usda.gov/). Bulls from diverse sire breeds have been mated to Hereford and Angus dams, and growth, carcass, and female reproduction traits measured in the F1 progeny. The project has occurred in several cycles in which different sire breeds were used, and Cundiff et al. (1993) presented an overview of Cycles I through IV that included 26 *Bos indicus* and *Bos taurus* breeds. There were significant differences between all of the sire breeds for body weights at different ages, body composition of steers at slaughter, and age of puberty and mature size of female progeny.

Mean birth weight ranged from 89 lb in Brahman progeny to 66 lbs in Jersey progeny. Ranges for weaning weight, postweaning ADG of steers, and 400-day weight, 550-day weight, and age of puberty of heifers were 73 lb (479 for Charolais versus 406 for Longhorn), .70 lb/day (2.89 in Charolais versus 2.19 in Longhorn), 148 lb (781 in Charolais versus 633 in Longhorn), 168 lb (903 in Charolais versus 735 in Jersey), and 122 days (439 in Brahman versus 317 in Jersey), respectively. Because these are mean differences between progeny of sires of the breeds, they reflect transmitting ability and thus only half of the genetic difference that exists between the breeds.

The range of means for backfat thickness was .25 inch (.57 for Santa Gertrudis versus .31 for Piedmontese); mean backfat thickness for the Hereford x Angus reciprocals was .63 inch. The range for rib-eye area was 2.87 square inches (13.19 for Piedmontese versus 10.32 for Jersey). Although Piedmontese sires were assumed to be homozygous for the myostatin double muscling mutation and their progeny heterozygous, while all other progeny were homozygous for the wild-type allele, the ranges in body composition traits were nearly as great when excluding Piedmontese (e.g., mean backfat thickness was .32 inch for Chianina and mean rib-eye area was 12.56 square inches for Charolais).

There was a tendency for sire breeds to rank similarly for body weights taken at birth, at weaning, and at 400 and 550 days of age. Those breeds with greater birth weights and weaning weights also experienced more calving difficulty and greater preweaning mortality. Breeds with greater mature size (e.g., Charolais, Chianina, Maine Anjou) tended to have a greater percentage of retail product and a lesser percentage of fat trim when adjusted to a standard slaughter age than those with lesser mature size (e.g., Jersey, Longhorn, Red Poll). Although there was also a tendency for breeds with greater mature size to produce heifers that reached puberty at an older age than those with lesser mature size, there were exceptions. *Bos indicus* breeds (Brahman, Nellore, and Sahiwal) reached puberty at older ages than any of the *Bos taurus* breeds, regardless of mature size, and breeds with a history of selection for milk production (e.g., Holstein, Simmental) reached puberty sooner than breeds with similar mature size that do not have a history of selection for milk production (e.g., Charolais, Chianina).

Similar breed differences for characteristics of growth and development, and relationships between rates of whole-body growth and maturation, and tissue deposition also exist in swine and sheep. In pigs, there are not only significant differences in characteristics of growth among western breeds, but great diversity between western and Chinese breeds. Jones (1998) reviewed the origin and characteristics of common domesticated swine breeds, including results from a 1995 U.S. national evaluation of ter-

minal sire lines. Extremes between commercial pigs from U.S. sire pure breeds (reflecting differences in transmitting ability or 1/2 the additive genetic difference between the breeds) were between 5 and 10% of the mean for daily feed intake, postweaning gain, and carcass lean percentage. Chinese breeds tend to be slower growing and earlier maturing than western breeds, with much greater fat deposition at a market weight. Females in some Chinese breeds reach sexual maturity as early as 60 days of age at body weights less than 50 kg, and females in western breeds reach puberty at ages greater than 150 days and weights greater than 100 kg.

In addition to the between-breed differences that exist for traits of growth and development, there is also significant genetic variation in these same traits within breeds and lines. Estimates of direct heritability reflect the proportion of observed phenotypic variation in a trait that is due to additive genetic effects of individuals. The genetic potential of the individual is clearly an important determinant of variation in growth and body size beginning at the earliest ages. Koots et al. (1994a) reported that weighted average estimates of direct heritability from numerous studies of cattle were .31, .29, and .24 for birth weight, preweaning gain, and weaning weight, respectively. Fogarty (1995) reviewed literature estimates in sheep and reported average heritabilities for weaning weight of .33, .21, and .20 in wool, meat, and dual-purpose breeds, respectively; average heritability for birth weight was approximately .20. In addition to the genetic potential of the individual, maternal environment can contribute significantly to variation in growth traits of livestock early in life and in some cases beyond the time in which the young animal is dependent on its mother for nourishment. For example, reported average estimates of maternal heritabilities, reflecting variation in a trait due to genetic differences among dams, were .14, .24, and .13 for birth weight, preweaning gain, and weaning weight in cattle (Koots et al. 1994a), but also ranged from .09 to .21 for mature weight in cattle (Rumph et al. 2002).

Clutter and Brascamp (1998) summarized literature estimates of heritabilities for traits of postweaning growth, efficiency and body composition in pigs. Feed intake, postweaning ADG, feed conversion ratio, backfat thickness, and lean tissue growth rate were all moderately to highly heritable (average heritabilities of .29, .31, .30, .49, and .34, respectively). A similar proportion of direct genetic variation exists for postweaning production and carcass traits in other livestock species as well. For example, average estimates of heritabilities for feed intake, postweaning gain, feed conversion ratio, yearling weight, yearling height, fat thickness, and rib-eye area in cattle were .34, .31, .32, .33, .61, .44, and .42, respectively. Mature weight is also moderately to highly heritable. Examples of estimates of direct heritability in cattle and sheep are .49 to .86 (mature cow weight: Koots et al. 1994; Rumph et al. 2002) and .23 (31-month weight: Mousa et al. 1999), respectively.

Genetic correlations reflect the degree to which the same genes, or linked genes, contribute to variation in the same traits. Estimates of genetic correlations between growth, body composition, and mature size reveal some of the same tendencies described for breed differences. The average genetic correlations between birth weight in cattle with weaning weight, postweaning gain, yearling weight, and mature cow weight were .50, .32, .55, and .67 (Koots et al. 1994b), indicating that those animals within breeds that had greater genetic potential for weight at birth also tended to have greater potential for growth rate and body size through maturity. Average genetic correlations between postweaning gain and feed conversion ratio (−.67), rib-eye area (.31), and lean percentage (.31), mean that cattle with greater potential for gain tended to have more potential for efficiency and depositing a greater amount of lean than fat through slaughter age. Mousa et al. (1999) reported that birth weight in sheep was not genetically correlated with 31-month weight (r = −.01), but genetic correlations of weaning weight and postweaning ADG with 31-month weight were .32 and .69, respectively.

An alternative to single or multitrait analyses of body weights or size measurements taken on an animal at different stages in its life is the characterization of changes in those discrete measurements with a continuous function. Parameters from functions describing sigmoidal growth curves have been used to quantify rate and degree of maturation and estimate associated genetic variances and covariances in cattle (e.g., Fitzhugh and Taylor 1971; Kaps et al. 2000) and sheep (Stobart et al. 1986). Reported estimates of heritabilities for degree of maturity in immature animals have been similar in magnitude to corresponding heritabilities for body weight at the same ages. Genetic correlations between body weight and degree of maturity at the same age were positive, indicating that animals selected to be heavier at a given age will tend to be more mature at that

and adjacent ages (Fitzhugh and Taylor 1971; Stobart et al. 1986). Animals genetically heavier than average at maturity tended to be less mature than average at each of the younger ages measured. Maternal effects were also reported to affect temporal patterns of maturity (Kaps et al. 2000), with a tendency for an advantageous maternal environment to result in earlier maturation.

Recently, statistical methods for random regression previously applied for analysis of longitudinal data in human growth studies have been used to model livestock growth and extended to quantify genetic variation and covariation in growth measurements over time (Meyer and Hill 1997). In contrast to the more traditional methods described above in which measurements at different ages have been treated as different distinct traits, or growth functions have been fitted to the data and the resulting parameters subjected to genetic analysis, random regression can generate covariance functions that describe the genetic variance and covariance for all ages represented in the data, even those ages for which there are no data. For example in pigs, Huisman et al. (2002) applied random regression to body weight and reported daily heritabilities from 50 to 220 days of age. Daily heritabilities fluctuated around .17, the mid-range of estimated heritabilities from the multitrait analysis of body weights at approximately 70, 135, and 190 days (.14, .17, and .19, respectively), but were greatest at earliest ages, dropped, and then increased again over time. Meyer (1999) fitted a random regression model to body weights of Hereford cows and cows from a synthetic breed (Wokalup) and presented daily heritabilities as well as 3-dimensional plots of genetic correlations across the entire age range. It was obvious from the results that longitudinal weights of cows through their adult life cannot be considered repeated measurements of the same trait with constant variances and heritabilities, and that much more genetic information can be generated with random regression relative to multitrait analyses. The continued development of random regression methods for genetic analysis of livestock growth data will enhance understanding of the genetic control of growth processes and could suggest refinements to selection methods to capitalize on periods of greatest genetic variation or optimum genetic covariation (e.g., between easily obtainable early measurements and economically important end points).

From the breed evaluations described here, it is clear that large differences can exist within a species for characteristics of growth and development, not because of one gene with very large effect, but rather due to the summed smaller effects of the alleles of many genes that differ between the breeds. The differences in allele frequencies between breeds that underlie these distinct phenotypic differences have come about in large part by the breeder's actions to close breed populations and practice selection not only for specific superficial characteristics such as coat color, but also body size, growth performance, and body composition. Estimates of genetic variation and covariation suggest that similar changes in these characteristics can still occur within breeds or lines.

Selection for Quantitative Traits

The potential for making dramatic changes in quantitative traits of a breed or line through selection is well documented in plants and laboratory animal species. (Dudley 1977; Bunger et al. 1994) Great amounts of cumulative response and associated divergence in growth and tissue deposition have also been produced by selection within livestock populations. For example, divergent, single-trait selection for postweaning ADG in a composite population of swine produced large differences in feed intake, growth rate, and body composition (Woltmann et al. 1992; Clutter et al. 1998). The results summarized in Table 15.1 reflect 10 generations of selection and the resulting divergence between the fast and slow growth rate lines. Pigs from the fast line consumed 36% (~4 SD) more feed per day, grew at a rate 47% faster (~5SD), and deposited 13% (~1 SD) more backfat than pigs from the slow line. Thus, selection characteristics for growth and development can create divergence

within a line at least as great as many of the existing between-breed differences.

Largely due to the short generation interval and high reproductive rate in pigs, and the magnitude of the pork industry, a great deal of experimental selection for traits of growth and development has been carried out in the pig (see Clutter and Brascamp 1998, for a review). Experiments involving single-trait selection similar to that reported by Clutter et al. (1998; Table 15.1) provide a realized picture of genetic correlations between components of growth and development. In general, single-trait selection for growth rate with ad libitum access to feed has resulted in correlated increases in daily feed intake and lean tissue growth rate. The increase in daily gain generally offsets the increase in feed intake, resulting in an improved feed conversion ratio, and the increase in lean tissue gain is usually but not always accompanied by increased fat deposition. Correlated responses to selection for daily feed intake varied by population in a comprehensive study of selection for components of efficiency of lean tissue growth at the Roslin Institute (Cameron and Curran 1994). Single-trait selection for increased daily feed intake resulted in fewer days on test and greater backfat thickness in a Large White population, but did not change days on test or fatness in a Landrace population. Differences in correlated responses to selection for either body weight gain or daily feed intake may be due to the relative capacities of the population for feed intake and protein deposition, as discussed in the next section ("Biological Models of Growth and Genetic Variation").

In the search for methods to improve the economic efficiency of pork production, classical index

Table 15.1. Direct and correlated responses[a] to divergent selection for growth rate within a closed population of pigs[b]

Trait[c]	Line F[d]	Line S
DFI, kg/d	2.83 ± 0.04	1.77 ± 0.05
ADG, kg/d	0.95 ± 0.01	0.65 ± 0.01
FE	0.328 ± 0.003	0.301 ± 0.003
BF, mm	31.01 ± 0.41	27.50 ± 0.60

[a]Least squares means ± SE averaged across barrows and gilts.
[b]Adapted from Clutter et al., 1998.
[c]DFI = average daily feed intake from 9 weeks of age to 100 kg; ADG = average daily gain from 9 weeks of age to 100 kg; FCR = gain/feed; BF = ultrasound backfat thickness at the last rib adjusted to 105 kg.
[d]Line F = selection for fast postweaning ADG; Line S = selection for slow postweaning ADG.

selection has been extensively studied and applied in pigs. A typical index is derived to estimate an aggregate breeding value that includes components of lean tissue feed conversion (e.g., rate of gain, carcass lean and feed intake) based on measured performance phenotypes (e.g., weight per day of age or postweaning ADG, and ultrasound measurements of backfat thickness and loin-eye area at off-test). Individual feed intake is not typically one of the measured phenotypes, but rather is changed through genetic correlations with gain and ultrasound measurements. Index selection has been successfully used to improve lean tissue growth rate and feed conversion (Clutter and Brascamp 1998), but the correlated response in daily feed intake to these indexes depended on the relative emphasis (value) given to gain versus leanness traits. Indexes with greater emphasis on leanness versus gain tended to improve lean tissue feed conversion largely through a decline in feed intake. In the Roslin study, the following selection criteria in addition to daily feed intake were compared: selection for lean growth rate (predicted lean content from ultrasound) or lean feed conversion (predicted lean content and individual feed intake) with ad libitum access to feed (LGA and LFC, respectively), and selection for lean growth rate in a testing environment with restricted feeding in which animals are allowed access to an amount of feed scaled to their predicted requirements for lean tissue growth (LGS). Improved lean feed conversion in LFC was primarily through decreased appetite accompanied by a reduced rate of fat growth, with little change in lean growth rate. Both lean growth rate and lean feed conversion were improved in LGA without a decrease in appetite, but rate of fat growth was not reduced (Cameron and Curran 1995). Selection in LGS seemed to achieve the best of both LGA and LFC: increased lean gain and decreased fat gain without reduced appetite. These results clearly show the importance of a biological approach to achieve optimum genetic selection for growth and tissue deposition in the pig.

Experimental selection for production traits in sheep and cattle has focused primarily on body weights at a standard age (e.g., weaning weight in sheep: Lasslo et al. 1985; Jurado et al. 1994; weaning, yearling, or 18-month weight in cattle: Koch et al. 1974; Buchanan et al. 1982; Frahm et al. 1985; Irgang et al. 1985; Aaron et al. 1986; Baker et al. 1991; Parnell et al. 1997) or postweaning growth rate (e.g., in cattle: Bailey and Lawson 1986; Irgang et al. 1985). Consistent with estimates of heritabilities for these traits, significant

responses have been achieved. In cattle, examples of reported realized heritabilities based on selection response are .24 and .30 for weaning weight (Hereford and Angus, respectively: Frahm et al. 1985; Aaron et al. 1986), .31 to .38 for yearling weight (Baker et al. 1991; Parnell et al. 1997) and .18 to .57 for postweaning gain (Bailey and Lawson 1986; Irgang et al. 1985). Correlated responses to selection for growth have also generally been consistent with estimates of genetic correlations. Morris et al. (1992) reported that realized genetic correlations from selection for either yearling weight or 18-month weight were on average .93 with feed intake, .51 with carcass fat depth, .18 with age at puberty, and .37 with weight at puberty.

Archer et al. (1998) studied the effects of divergent selection for yearling gain in cattle on parameters of a Gompertz growth function. Selection lines were significantly different in height and weight at birth and maturity. Although upward selection increased both the weight and height of cows at maturity relative to downward selection, the lines did not differ in rate of maturation in either weight or height. In other words, even though cows from the two lines reached maturity at different weights, the age at which they reached their mature weights were similar, and the same held true for their mature heights. Steers from the lines slaughtered at a constant age differed in body weight, but not body composition, demonstrating that it was the degree of maturity at slaughter rather than the gain to slaughter weight that determined relative deposition of fat and lean. After scaling to remove differences in mature weight, rate of maturation was higher in the line selected for greater yearling gain than in the line selected for lesser yearling gain. These results indicated that selection had indeed not only changed the scale, but also the shape, of the growth curve.

Genetic variation in traits of growth and development has been successfully exploited through selection in all of the livestock species, and selection can result in within-breed or line differences at least as large as some differences between breeds. Correlated responses to selection can reveal the genetic interrelationships among phases of growth and maturation.

Biological Models of Growth and Genetic Variation

Although the traits traditionally used by animal breeders to describe growth and development of livestock have been rather broadly defined to reflect important economic aspects of production (e.g., yearling weight, weight per day of age, lb of feed/lb of gain, subcutaneous fat thickness), much progress has been made in the modeling of the more basic biology of growth and development in mathematical terms (see Chapter 11). Estimation of genetic variation in parameters of these biological models has been relatively rare, probably due to the large number of parameters in most models, the large number of observations on family members needed to make such estimates with much precision, and the difficulty and cost associated with measuring the basic biological traits. There have been examples, however, of genetic analysis of biological models.

Whittemore (1986) proposed a model for growth in pigs based on a linear plateau relationship between energy intake and protein deposition. The model assumes that the pig's genetic potential for maximum protein deposition is relatively constant beginning at an early age and over most or all of the finishing period (Figure 15.2). The maximum rate of protein deposition (PD_{max}) is expressed only if sufficient energy is made available, and early in the pig's life energy is partitioned almost entirely to protein deposition, with only a marginal amount of fat deposition. If feed intake capacity (FIC) exceeds the minimum amount required for expression of PD_{max} (FI_0), the animal begins to deposit fat more rapidly. The fact that the model has relatively few parameters (FIC, PD_{max}, and the marginal rate of lipid deposition) makes it attractive for investigations of genetic variation.

Eissen (2000) used restrictive feeding and serial slaughter to estimate the relative FIC and PD_{max} in boars, barrows, and gilts from different commercial lines. In several cases, FIC was below optimum (FI_0), most often for gilts (rather than barrows) and for sire lines used to produce terminal cross pigs. These results confirm that in some lines selection for increased feed intake may be necessary to realize PD_{max}; thus feed intake has a positive economic value in the selection objective. But as pointed out by de Vries and Kanis (1992), the cost of feed sets the weighting for feed intake in the objective of a conventional economic index and will always be negative. They used the linear plateau model to calculate the impact on net revenue of changes in FIC under different levels of PD_{max}, thereby deriving optimum economic weightings for FIC and providing the framework for selection indicies based on the parameters of a biological growth model.

FACTORS UNDERLYING GENETIC VARIATION

The idea that greater understanding will result from studying biological components of broadly defined

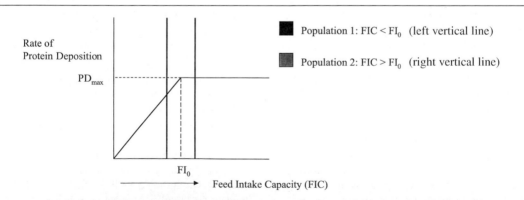

Figure 15.2. The linear plateau relationship between feed intake capacity and protein deposition in pigs, taken conceptually from Whittemore (1986). The model assumes that the pig's genetic potential for maximum protein deposition is relatively constant, beginning at an early age and over most or all of the finishing period. The maximum rate of protein deposition (PD_{max}) is expressed only if sufficient energy is made available. Early in the pig's life, energy is partitioned almost entirely to protein deposition with only a marginal amount of fat deposition. If feed intake capacity (FIC) exceeds the minimum amount required for expression of Pd_{max} (FI_0), the animal begins to deposit fat more rapidly (e.g., Population 2). Eissen (2000) reported that in some commercial populations of pigs, FIC does not reach FI_0 and PD_{max} is not expressed (e.g., Population 1).

traits through mathematical models can be extended to the search for those basic physiological or molecular genetic factors that contribute to variation in growth and development. In theory, genetic variation in each quantitative trait can be described by a series of pathways anchored by a complex of genes. Although far from a trivial task, the combination of novel populations and increasingly powerful technical tools has allowed this search to begin.

Physiological Factors

At least until the rather recent technological advancements in the development of molecular genetics tools, there has been great incentive to identify underlying physiological indicators of growth processes that could be used to enhance genetic selection, especially selection for the efficiency of lean tissue growth, which may be difficult with conventional methods (Blair et al. 1990). Choice of a candidate factor or pathway is burdened not only by the complexity of growth and development, but also the fact that there may not be genetic variation associated with some important components of growth processes. Despite those challenges and given a growing body of information on the physiology of growth and development, a relatively small number of studies have been conducted to understand genetic variation at the level of the somatotropic axis and for putative regulators of appetite.

One widely cited approach to discerning physiological factors responsible for growth is the comparison of closely related breeds of dogs with greatly divergent size. Eigenmann et al. (1984) described a stepwise decline in concentrations of circulating IGF-I measured in standard, toy, and miniature poodles, respectively. There are some reports of physiological differences between breeds in livestock species as well. For example, Buonomo et al. (1987) reported that pigs from a cross of larger, faster growing breeds (1/4 Large White $\times$ 1/4 Landrace $\times$ 1/2 Duroc) had 24 and 105% greater levels of IGF-I than smaller, slower growing Yucatan micro and Hanford miniature pigs. Physiological comparisons between breeds, however, are often confounded with factors other than the traits of interest due to the complex selection histories involved. Evaluations of experimental lines selected for traits of growth or efficiency can provide a picture of the physiological factors underlying selection response that is relatively free of confounding factors.

Circulating concentrations of growth hormone and IGF-I, as well as pulsatility of growth hormone, were compared in ram lambs from lines selected either for or against backfat thickness (Suttie et al. 1993). The lines differed in backfat thickness by 3.24 mm (5.1 in the fat line versus 1.86 in the lean line) at the time of the study. Mean GH and pulse amplitude did not differ between the lines, but pulse frequency was greater in the fat than in the lean line. Concentration of circulating IGF-I was also greater in the fat line than in the lean line, but IGF binding proteins were not characterized, so it is difficult to speculate as to how differences between the lines relate to available IGF-I.

Secretion of GH, thyrotropin, and prolactin were studied in Targhee rams selected for 1.5 generations for rate and efficiency of gain relative to Targhee rams from a line unselected for 20 years (Dodson et al. 1983). Selected rams had greater overall mean GH and overall mean thyrotropin, and greater baseline thyrotropin than rams from the unselected line. There were no differences between the lines in characteristics of prolactin secretion. Together, these results from sheep indicate that response to selection for either fatness or rate and efficiency of gain may be in part through changes in the somatotrophic axis.

Clutter et al. (1995b) studied characteristics of GH and IGF-I in lines of pigs derived from divergent selection for postweaning ADG and expressing greatly different growth performance and body composition (see Table 15.1). Serial blood samples from gilts of the fast and slow lines revealed no differences in mean GH concentration nor pulsatility of GH secretion, but there was greater mean concentration of IGF-I in the fast line than in the slow line. In addition to the greater amount of circulating IGF-I, there was also less activity of IGF binding proteins (IGFBP-2 and IGFBP-3) in fast line pigs relative to slow line pigs, suggesting a greater availability of active IGF-I.

Because much of the growth response observed in these divergent lines could be attributed to changes in daily feed intake (Woltmann et al. 1992), the putative satiety hormone cholecystokinin-8 (CCK) was also studied. Clutter et al. (1998) reported that when serial blood samples were collected from fast and slow line pigs after overnight deprivation of feed and during a subsequent 2-hour period with free access to feed, CCK per unit of feed intake was significantly greater in slow line pigs than in fast line pigs. A subsequent experiment in which pigs were infused with synthetic CCK during free access to feed revealed that feed intake was reduced more in slow line pigs than in fast line pigs, suggesting a greater sensitivity in the slow line to the CCK satiety signal (Clutter et al. 1995a).

The experimental lines of pigs produced from divergent selection for components of efficient lean tissue growth at the Roslin Institute have also been compared for candidate determinants of feed intake and growth. Based on their respective putative roles in appetite stimulation and inhibition, serum concentrations of neuropeptide Y (NPY) and leptin were studied in lines divergently selected with ad libitum access to feed for either daily feed intake (DFI), lean feed conversion (LFC), or lean growth rate (LGA) (Cameron et al. 2000; Cameron et al. 2002). The line selected for upward DFI had a greater level of serum leptin and was fatter than either a control or the line selected for downward DFI, but the divergent DFI lines did not differ in NPY concentration. Upward versus downward selection in LGA resulted in greater feed intake, growth rate, protein relative to lipid weight, and NPY concentration, but no change in serum leptin. Similar to DFI, downward selection in LFC (poorer LFC) also resulted in increased fatness and greater leptin concentration. NPY concentration was also increased by downward selection in LFC even though feed intake was not changed. Correlations of leptin with fat deposition and feed intake indicated that the response in leptin was primarily due to greater fat deposition rather than greater energy intake per se. The results suggest that response to selection for greater feed intake is more likely due in part to decreased sensitivity to leptin rather than insufficient leptin production. In general, NPY concentration was not highly correlated with energy intake. The DFI and LGA lines were also studied, along with lines divergently selected for lean growth rate with restricted access to feed (LGS), to determine serum IGF-I concentrations (Cameron et al. 2001). There were significant differences in IGF-I at 6 weeks of age between the DFI lines (158 versus 104 ug/l in the high and low lines; SED = 22), and IGF-I at 90 kg was different between divergent lines LGA (198 versus 153 ug/l; SED = 13) and LGS (214 versus 178 ug/l).

Taken in total, these results shed some light on the physiological factors that may underlie divergent selection for postweaning performance in pigs. It appears that selection for postweaning ADG has acted in part to alter the secretion of IGF-I and asso-

ciated binding proteins so that more active IGF-I may be available in pigs selected for fast gain than in those selected for slow gain (Clutter et al. 1995b). Further, selection may have both increased the amount of CCK circulating in response to feed intake and the sensitivity to the CCK satiety signal in pigs selected for slow gain relative to those selected for fast gain, the latter suggesting a change in CCK receptor characteristics (Clutter et al. 1995a; Clutter et al. 1998). Results from the Roslin populations for IGF-I (Cameron et al. 2001) also indicate an alteration in IGF-I secretion due to selection for postweaning performance, either for daily feed intake or for lean tissue gain, but suggest that the timing of the IGF-I response may depend on the trait selected. Clearly the response to selection for daily feed intake and correlated response in fat deposition has not been through insufficient leptin, leaving the possibility that a decrease in sensitivity to leptin may have occurred (Cameron et al. 2000). Divergence in energy intake has apparently not been driven by changes in NPY concentration (Cameron et al. 2002). Given that each set of divergent lines originated from a single base population and that only a single selection criterion (postweaning ADG, daily feed intake, lean tissue gain, or lean efficiency) was applied since closing of the lines, physiological differences between the lines can be attributed to founder effects that may have occurred by chance in the derivation of the lines from the base population, random drift in gene frequency due to non-infinite line size and chance, or the selection applied. Although the effects of these factors are confounded, it is clear that there was intense single-trait selection achieved in these studies, and it is likely that the physiological differences observed are associated with the divergent genetic merit of the lines for feed intake, growth, and tissue deposition.

As mentioned previously, a potential benefit of an advanced understanding of physiological factors underlying within-breed or line genetic variation is the identification of an indicator trait or index of indicator traits that could be used to enhance selection. From the evaluations of the Roslin lines, IGF-I at 6 weeks of age as an indicator of daily feed intake and leptin concentration as an indicator of carcass lean content have been presented as selection candidates (Cameron et al. 2000; Cameron et al. 2001). Blair et al. (1990) reported that seven generations of divergent, family selection for plasma IGF-I in the mouse resulted in a realized heritability for IGF-I of .15 and a significant correlated response in body weight (the high IGF-I line exceeded the low IGF-I line in body weight by up to 25%), results consistent with the aforementioned results in pigs. A study was subsequently begun in Angus cattle to practice divergent selection for serum IGF-I (Davis et al. 1995). Data from that selected cattle population was used to estimate genetic parameters associated with IGF-I and growth (Davis and Simmen 1997). The estimated heritability for mean IGF-I concentration was .48, confirming that IGF-I should respond to selection in cattle, but estimates of the genetic correlations of IGF-I with body weights at different ages ranged from –.21 to –.54 and averaged –.38, indicating that selection should be for less postweaning IGF-I in order to increase growth rate. Practical implementation of physiological indicators will require not only confirmation of the specific genetic relationships between indicators and breeding objectives within target populations, but also opportunity costs of using physiological markers versus emerging molecular genetic markers in selection.

Molecular Genetic Factors— Segregating Genes

Although comparisons of divergent lines produced by single-trait selection can successfully identify contributing physiological factors that likely reflect changes in gene frequency due to the selection applied, it is impossible from these comparisons to determine whether the physiological difference is due to selected sequence variation at the locus encoding the candidate protein or at some other locus or combination of loci elsewhere in the pathway. In the early 1990s, the use of restriction enzymes and the newly available methods for polymerase chain reaction (PCR) allowed the extension of the candidate approach from the protein to the gene level.

Genetic markers, many based on comparative sequence from the human and mouse, have been developed in livestock species for several peptides with established or putative effects on feed intake, growth, and development (e.g., GH: Jiang et al. 1996; IGF-I: Kirkpatrick 1992; Leptin: Sasaki et al. 1996; Pomp et al. 1997). These markers become potential tools for studies to detect associations between the candidate gene and traits of interest. In cattle, Moody et al. (1996) tested informative markers for the GH, IGF-I, and PIT1 genes for associations with birth weight and preweaning gain

expected progeny differences (EPD) in an inbred line of Herefords and reported several significant associations, the largest of which was an association between the IGF-I locus and birth weight, which accounted for 16% of the variation in EPD. Ge et al. (2001) reported an association between a marker for IGF-I and weight gain in the first 20 days after weaning lines of Angus cattle that were being divergently selected for serum IGF-I concentration. The association was significant in one of the divergent lines, but not in the other.

Yu et al. (1995) studied birth and weaning weights, postweaning gain and market weight fat thickness in Meishan-based reference families of pigs and reported an association of the PIT1 locus with birthweight and fatness, a result later supported by a study of additional animals and markers in the PIT1 region (Yu et al. 1999). Kim et al. (2000) tested a marker for the melanocortin-4 receptor (MC4R) locus in several lines of commercial pigs and a Meishan composite line. Although the associations were not consistent across all lines, there were significant overall associations with feed intake, growth (days to 110 kg), and fatness. The most extensive association study of the porcine leptin locus was conducted by Jiang and Gibson (1999), who evaluated four different PCR-based polymorphisms in Duroc, Hampshire, Landrace, and Large White pigs selected from a large carcass dissection project for their extreme (high and low) backfat thickness. Only one of the polymorphisms (at position 3469) was significantly associated with backfat, and only in the sample of Large White pigs. However, in a second replicate of Large White pigs, sampled from the same population, there was no association of the 3469 polymorphism with backfat. Inconsistencies in results between populations for candidate gene markers can be caused by epistatic effects in different genetic backgrounds, or because the causal gene is in fact linked to the candidate gene (i.e., in linkage disequilibrium), and linkage phase between the causal gene and candidate marker varies between or within populations.

Although several associations between candidate gene markers and production traits in livestock have been reported, the approach in which candidate genes are chosen solely on knowledge of the biology or physiology underlying the trait has inherent limitations. First, it is difficult to effectively choose candidates from the large pool of known genes with biological functions that may be related to a given trait. This challenge is exemplified by the relative lack of significant associations between the growth hormone gene and growth traits, not only in livestock (e.g., Casas et al. 1997b), but also in the mouse (Pomp 1997), a species in which there have already been extensive searches for genes causing variation in growth. Second, although information on new genes is being generated at a rapid pace in the mouse and human, there are still many undiscovered genes that are not available in the candidate pool. Finally, the quantitative nature of traits of growth and development suggests that many genes, each with relatively small effect, contribute to variation in each component trait. Thus it is likely that many of the segregating genes of interest do not encode proteins at the end of physiological pathways, but have deeper regulatory functions. The theory of such a complex genetic architecture underlying quantitative traits is supported by recent results from model species (e.g., Mackay 2001).

A more comprehensive approach to gene searches makes use of anonymous markers at regularly spaced intervals along each of the chromosomes. This approach became available to researchers of livestock species in the 1990s with the development of markers based on simple sequence repeats (SSRs) scattered throughout the genomes of cattle, sheep, and pigs that can be easily amplified with PCR. Anonymous markers were quickly used to map major genes, such as the spider syndrome (Cockett et al. 1999) and callipyge (Cockett et al. 1994) genes in sheep, and the double muscling gene in cattle (Charlier et al. 1995). Subsequent finemapping in the identified chromosomal regions has revealed much about the molecular basis for these major gene effects. In the case of spider lamb syndrome and double muscling in cattle, comparative chromosomal regions in the mouse and human provided candidate genes (i.e., "comparative positional candidate genes") that led to the discovery of the causal mutations (Cockett 1999; Grobet et al. 1998). Fine-mapping of the callipyge locus has revealed a novel type of genetic imprinting in which only heterozygotes that inherit the mutation from their sire express the phenotype (Cockett et al. 1996), and has also enhanced selection of positional candidate genes (Bidwell et al. 2001).

Anonymous markers have been used in a similar way to scan the genomes of cattle and pigs for the locations of genes contributing to variation in quantitative traits (Quantitative Trait Loci: QTL). The first reported genome-wide QTL scan in livestock was for growth and fatness QTL in a Wild Boar x

Large White F2 by Andersson et al. (1994). There have subsequently been reports of several scans for growth and carcass trait QTL in pigs using this same Wild Boar x Large White population (Andersson-Eklund et al. 1998), F2s from Meishan x commercial breed crosses (Paszek et al. 1999; Harlizius et al. 2000; Rohrer 2000; Bidanel et al. 2001; de Koning et al. 2001), half-sib families from divergent selection lines (Casas et al. 1997b), and F2s from crosses of two commercial breeds (Nezer et al. 1999; Malek et al. 2001). Some consensus regions that have emerged through these numerous scans are now the target of fine-mapping and comparative mapping efforts. For example, a region on chromosome 4 first reported by Andersson et al. (1994) to account for 20% of phenotypic variation in average backfat and abdominal fat in a Wild Boar x Large White F2 has been detected in several other scans and is presently being fine-mapped in a repeated backcross design (Knott et al. 2002). Paternally imprinted alleles at a locus on the distal tip of chromosome 2p account for up to 30% or more of phenotypic F2 variance in muscle mass and leanness. The region was detected in two independent F2 populations (Jeon et al. 1999; Nezer et al. 1999) and, through a combination of comparative and physical fine-mapping, IGF2 has been identified as a likely positional candidate for the causal gene. In total, several putative QTL regions representing many of the 18 autosomes and the X chromosome have been detected for body weights at standard ages throughout the finishing period, for early and postweaning gain and for fatness and lean content. Although the QTL effects on chromosomes 4 and 2 are relatively large, the majority of putative QTL effects detected are consistent with a quantitative model in which many genes contribute to variation. Indeed in an analysis of published QTL results from the pig, Hayes and Goddard (2001) concluded that the likely distribution of QTL for a typical production trait is one in which there are few of large effect and many of small to moderate effect (.25 PSD or less).

Scans for QTL affecting growth and carcass traits are also progressing in cattle. Davis et al. (1998) reported putative QTL for birth weight on five different chromosomes (5, 6, 14, 18, and 21) segregating in half-sib families of three *Bos taurus* x *Bos indicus* sires, but only one of the regions was significant in multiple sire families. Grosz and MacNeil (2001) detected a QTL for birth weight on chromosome 2 using a backcross design originating from the Line 1 Hereford. The QTL was estimated to account for .64

residual standard deviations in birthweight, without significantly affecting preweaning gain, suggesting the region as a candidate for marker-assisted selection to decrease birthweight. Stone et al. (1999) used selective genotyping in a *Bos indicus* x *Bos taurus* backcross design and detected several putative QTL for growth and body composition; the strongest evidence was for a region on chromosome 5 of Brahman origin that increased fat thickness and decreased dressing percentage. Casas et al. (2001) extended the use of the resource families in which the double muscling locus had been mapped to conduct a comprehensive genome scan for QTL affecting growth and carcass, as well as meat quality traits. Because the sires (Belgian Blue x MARC III and Piedmontese x Angus) were heterozygous, QTL effects could be estimated in backgrounds segregating alternative forms of the myostatin allele. There was significant evidence of QTL for postweaning ADG and hot carcass weight on chromosome 4, for birth weight and yearling weight on chromosome 6, and for fat thickness, yield grade, and retail product yield on chromome 5. Based on these published results for chromosome 5, Li et al. (2002) used identity-by-descent mapping of haplotypes in the region to verify and fine-map the putative QTL in commercial lines of *Bos taurus*.

The availability of PCR-based polymorphic markers throughout the genomes of cattle, pigs, and sheep has allowed comprehensive searches for genes underlying variation in growth and development traits. Although much progress has been made in the coarse mapping of major genes and QTL affecting important traits in livestock, this is a relatively new research frontier that is sure to accelerate along with development of marker technologies and comparative genome sequences.

CONCLUSION

A tremendous amount of genetic variation exists in traits of growth and development in livestock species, not only between breeds but also within breeds and lines. Only in relatively rare cases is this variation explained by segregation of genes with very large effect, large enough to allow the categorization of animals into discrete classes. Rather, most variation is continuous and the result of the co-segregation of many genes in combination with environmental effects. Breed differences reveal tendencies for relationships among rates of growth and maturation and tissue composition of market animals that are also observed through genetic correlations for these traits

within breeds. These relationships are the foundation for genetic selection strategies and the improved efficiency of livestock production. Selection efforts can be enhanced by linking biological models to genetic variation, and by expanded knowledge of the physiological and molecular genetic factors that underlie genetic differences. The new frontier of livestock genomics continues to grow, fueled by the developing genome maps of the human and various model species. The result will be an increasingly clearer picture of genetic variation in growth and development of livestock.

ACKNOWLEDGMENTS

The author is grateful to Professor Neil Cameron for providing unpublished results from physiological evaluations of the Roslin selection lines, and to Dr. Sam Jackson for permission to use the photograph of callipyge lambs.

REFERENCES

Aaron, D.K., Frahm, R.R., and Buchanan, D.S. 1986. Direct and correlated responses to selection for increased weaning or yearling weight in Angus cattle. 2. Evaluation of response. *Journal of Animal Science* 62:66–76.

Andersson, L., Haley, C.S., Ellegren, H., Knott, S.A., Johansson, M., Andersson, K., Andersson-Eklund, L., Edfors-Lilja, I., Fredholm, M., Hansson, I., Hakansson, J., and Lundstrom, K. 1994. Genetic mapping of quantitative trait loci for growth and fatness in pigs. *Science* 263:1771–1774.

Andersson-Eklund, L., Marklund, L., Lundstrom, K., Haley, C.S., Andersson, K., Hansson, I., Moller, M., and Andersson, L. 1998. Mapping quantitative trait loci for carcass and meat quality traits in a Wild Boar x Large White intercross. *Journal of Animal Science* 76:694–700.

Archer, J.A., Herd, R.M., Arthur, P.F., and Parnell, P.F. 1998. Correlated responses in rate of maturation and mature size of cows and steers to divergent selection for yearling growth rate in Angus cattle. *Livestock Production Science* 54:183–192.

Arthur, P.F. 1995. Double muscling in cattle: A review. *Australian Journal of Agricultural Research* 46:1493–1515.

Bailey, D.R.C., and Lawson, J.E. 1986. Genetic progress through selection for postweaning gain in Angus and Hereford cattle. *Third World Congress on Genetics applied to Livestock Production*, Lincoln, NE XII:210–214.

Baker, R.L., Morris, C.A., Johnson, D.L., Hunter, J.C., and Hickey, S.M. 1991. Results of selection for yearling or 18-month weight in Angus and Hereford cattle. *Livestock Production Science* 29:277–296.

Bidanel, J.P., Milan, D., Iannuccelli, N., Amigues, Y., Boscher, M.Y., Bourgeois, F., Caritez, J.C., Gruand, J., LeRoy, P., Lagant, H., Quintanilla, R., Renard, C., Gellin,

J., Ollivier, L., and Chevalet, C. 2001. Detection of quantitative trait loci for growth and fatness in pigs. *Genetics, Selection and Evolution* 33:289–309.

Bidwell, C.A., Shay, T.L., Georges, M., Beever, J.E., Berghmans, S., and Cockett, N.E. 2001. Differential expression of the GTL2 gene within the callipyge region of ovine chromosome 18. *Animal Genetics* 32:248–256.

Blair, H.T., McCutcheon, S.N., and Mackenzie, D.D.S. 1990. Components of the somatotropic axis as predictors of genetic merit for growth. *Proceedings of the 4th World Congress on Genetics Applied to Livestock Production.* Edinburgh.

Buchanan, D.S., Nielsen, M.K., Koch, R.M., and Cundiff, L.V. 1982. Selection for growth and muscling score in beef cattle. 2. *Genetic parameters and predicted response. Journal of Animal Science* 55:526–532.

Bunger, L., Renne, U., and Dietl, G. 1994. Sixty generations of selection for an index combining high body weight and high stress resistance in laboratory mice. *Proceedings of the 5th World Congress on Genetics Applied to Livestock Production.* Guelph, Ontario, Canada, 19:16–19.

Buonomo, F.C., Lauterio, T.L., Baile, C.A., and Campion, D.R. 1987. Determination of IGF-I and IGF binding protein levels in swine. *Domestic Animal Endocrinology* 4:23–27.

Cameron, N.D., and Curran, M.K. 1994. Selection for components of efficient lean growth rate in pigs 4. Genetic and phenotypic parameter estimates and correlated responses in performance test traits with ad libitum feeding. *Animal Production* 59:281–291.

Cameron, N.D., and Curran, M.K. 1995. Genotype with feeding regime interaction in pigs divergently selected for components of efficient lean growth rate. *Animal Science.* 61:123–132.

Cameron, N.D., McCullough, E., Troup, K., and Penman, J.C. 2002. Serum neuropeptide Y (NPY) and leptin concentrations in pigs selected for components of efficient lean growth. *Domestic Animal Endocrinology* (in press).

Cameron, N.D., McCullough, E., Troup, K., Penman, J.C., and Pong-Wong, R. 2001. Serum IGF-1 concentration in pigs divergently selected for daily food intake or lean growth rate. *Proceedings of Annual EAAP Meeting.* Budapest. Paper no. 5.3.

Cameron, N.D., Penman, J.C., and McCullough, E. 2000. Serum leptin concentration in pigs selected for high or low daily food intake. *Genetical Research Cambridge* 75:209–213.

Casas, E., Keele, J.W., Shackelford, S.D., Koohmaraie, M., Sonstegard, T.S., Smith, T.P.L., Kappes, S.M., and Stone, R.T. 1998. Association of the muscle hypertrophy locus with carcass traits in beef cattle. *Journal of Animal Science* 76:468–473.

Casas, E., Prill-Adams, A., Price, S.G., Clutter, A.C., and Kirkpatrick, B.W. 1997a. Relationship of growth hormone and insulin-like growth factor-1 genotypes with growth and carcass traits in swine. *Animal Genetics* 28:88–93.

Casas, E., Prill-Adams, A., Price, S.G., Clutter, A.C., and Kirkpatrick, B.W. 1997b. Mapping genomic regions associated with growth rate in pigs. *Journal of Animal Science* 75:2047–2053.

Casas, E., Stone, R.T., Keele, J.W., Shackelford, S.D., Kappes, S.M., and Koohmaraie, M. 2001. A comprehensive search for quantitative trait loci affecting growth and carcass composition of cattle segregating alternative forms of the myostatin gene. *Journal of Animal Science* 79:854–860.

Chambers, D., Whatley, J.A., and Stephens, D.F. 1954. The inheritance of dwarfism in a comprest Hereford herd. Abstract. *Journal of Animal Science* 13:956.

Charlier, C., Coppieters, W., Farnir, F., Grobert, L., Leroy, P.L., Michaux, C., Mni, M., Schwers, A., Vanmanshoven, P., Hanset, R., and Georges, M. 1995. The mh gene causing double muscling in cattle maps to bovine chromosome 2. *Mammalian Genome* 6:788–792.

Clutter, A.C., and Brascamp, E.W. 1998. Genetics of Performance Traits. In *The Genetics of the Pig.* M.V. Rothschild and A. Ruvinsky, eds. New York: CAB International.

Clutter, A.C., Jiang, R., McCann, J.P., and Buchanan, D.S. 1995a. Evaluation of a satiety hormone in pigs with divergent genetic potential for feed intake and growth. *Oklahoma Agricultural Experiment Station Research Report* P943:5–10.

Clutter, A.C., Jiang, R., McCann, J.P., and Buchanan, D.S. 1998. Plasma cholecystokinin-8 in pigs with divergent genetic potential for feed intake and growth. *Domestic Animal Endocrinology* 15:9–21.

Clutter, A.C., Spicer, L.J., Woltermann, M.D., Grimes, R.W., Hammond, J.M., and Buchanan, D.S. 1995b. Plasma growth hormone, IGF-I, and IGF binding proteins in pigs with divergent merit for postweaning average daily gain. *Journal of Animal Science* 73:1776–1783.

Cockett, N.E., Jackson, S.P., Shay, T.L., Farnir, F., Berghmans, S., Snowder, G.D., Nielsen, D.M., and Georges, M. 1996. Polar overdominance at the ovine callipyge locus. *Science* 273:236–238.

Cockett, N.E., Jackson, S.P., Shay, T.L., Nielsen, D., Moore, S.S., Steele, M.R., Barendse, W., Green, R.D., and Georges, M. 1994. Chromosomal location of the callipyge gene in sheep (Ovis aries) using bovine DNA markers. *Proceedings of the National Academy of Science USA* 91:3019–3023.

Cockett, N.E., Shay, T.L., Beever, J.E., Nielsen, D., Albretsen, J., Georges, M., Peterson, K., Stephens, A., Vernon, W., Timofeevskaia, O., South, S., Mork, J., Maciulis, A., and Bunch, T.D. 1999. Localization of the locus causing Spider Lamb Syndrome to the distal end of ovine Chromosome 6. *Mammalian Genome* 10:35–38.

Cundiff, L.V., Gregory, K.E., and Koch, R.M. 1998. Germplasm evaluation of beef cattle—Cycle IV: Birth and weaning traits. *Journal of Animal Science* 76:2528–2535.

Cundiff, L.V., Szabo, F., Gregory, K.E., Koch, R.M., Dikeman, M.E., and Crouse, J.D. 1993. Breed comparisons in the germplasm evaluation program at MARC. *Proceedings of the Beef Improvement Federation 25th Anniversary Conference*, Asheville, NC.

Davis, G.P., Hetzel, D.J.S., Corbet, N.J., Scacheri, S., Lowden, S., Renaud, J., Mayne, C., Stevenson, R., Moore, S.S., and Byrne, K. 1998. The mapping of quantitative trait loci for birth weight in a tropical beef herd.

Proceedings of the 6th World Congress on Genetics Applied to Livestock Production. Armidale, NSW, Australia 26:441–444.

Davis, M.E., Bishop, M.D., Park, N.H., and Simmen, R.C.M. 1995. Divergent selection for blood serum IGF-I concentration in beef cattle: I. Nongenetic factors. *Journal of Animal Science* 73:1927–1932.

Davis, M.E., and Simmen, R.C.M. 1997. Genetic parameter estimates for serum IGF-I concentration and performance traits in Angus beef cattle. *Journal of Animal Science* 75:317–324.

de Koning, D.J., Rattink, A.P., Harlizius, B., Groenen, M.A.M., Brascamp, E.W., and van Arendonk, J.A.M. 2001. Detection and characterization of quantitative trait loci for growth and reproduction traits in pigs. *Livestock Production Science* 72:185–198.

de Vries, A.G., and Kanis, E. 1992. A growth model to estimate economic values for food intake capacity in pigs. *Animal Production* 55:241–246.

Dodson, M.V., Davis, S.L., Ohlson, D.L., and Ercanbrack, S.K. 1983. Temporal patterns of growth hormone, prolactin and thyrotropin secretion in Targhee rams selected for rate and efficiency of gain. *Journal of Animal Science* 57:338–342.

Duckett, S.K., Snowder, G.D., and Cockett, N.E. 2000. Effect of the callipyge gene on muscle growth, calpastatin activity, and tenderness of three muscles across the growth curve. *Journal of Animal Science* 78:2836–2841.

Dudley, J.W. 1977. Seventy-six generations of selection for oil and protein percentage in maize. *Proceedings of the International Conference on Quantitative Genetics*, Ames, IA, USA.

Eigenmann, J.E., Patterson, D.F., and Froesch, E.R. 1984. Body size parallels IGF-I levels but not growth hormone secretory capacity. *Acta Endocrinologia* 106:448–453.

Eissen, J.J. 2000. Breeding for feed intake capacity in pigs. Doctoral thesis. *Animal Breeding and Genetics Group*. Wageningen University.

Falconer, D.S., and Mackay, T.G.C. 1996. *Quantitative Genetics, 4th ed.* Boston: Addison-Wesley.

Fitzhugh, H.A., and Taylor, St. C.S. 1971. Genetic analysis of degree of maturity. *Journal of Animal Science* 33:717–725.

Fogarty, N.M. 1995. Genetic parameters for live weight, fat and muscle measurements, wool production and reproduction in sheep: a review. *Anim. Breed. Abstr.* 63:101.

Frahm, R.R., Nichols, C.G., and Buchanan, D.S. 1985. Selection for increased weaning or yearling weight in Hereford cattle. *Journal of Animal Science* 60:1385–1395.

Freking, B.A., Keele, J.W., Nielsen, M.K., and Leymaster, K.A. 1998. Evaluation of the ovine callipyge locus: II. Genotypic effects on growth, slaughter and carcass traits. *Journal of Animal Science* 76:2549–2559.

Ge, W., Davis, M.E., Hines, H.C., Irvin, K.M., and Simmen, R.C.M. 2001. Association of a genetic marker with blood serum insulin-like growth factor-I concentration and growth traits in Angus cattle. *Journal of Animal Science* 79:1757–1762.

Gregory, K.E., Laster, D.B., Cundiff, L.V., Smith, G.M., and Koch, R.M. 1979. Characterization of biological types of cattle—Cycle III: II. Growth rate and puberty in females. *Journal of Animal Science* 49:461–471.

Grobet, L., Martin, L.J., Poncelet, D., Pirottin, D., Brouwers, B., Riquet, J., Schoeberlein, A., Dunner, S., Menissier, F., Massabanda, J., Fries, R., Hanset, R., and Georges, M. 1998. Molecular definition of an allelic series of mutations disrupting the myostatin function and causing double muscling in cattle. *Mammalian Genome* 9:210–213.

Grosz, M.D., and MacNeil, M.D. 2001. Putative quantitative trait locus affecting birth weight on bovine chromosome 2. *Journal of Animal Science* 79:68–72.

Harlizius, B., Rattink, A.P., de Koning, D.J., Faivre, M., Joosten, R.G., van Arendonk, J.A.M., Groenen, M.A.M. 2000. The X chromosome harbors quantitative trait loci for backfat thickness and intramuscular fat content in pigs. *Mammalian Genome* 11:800–802.

Hayes, B., and Goddard, M.E. 2001. The distribution of the effects of genes affecting quantitative traits in livestock. Genetics, *Selection and Evolution* 33: 209–229.

Hill, W.G. 1999. Advances in quantitative genetics theory. In From Jay L. *Lush to Genomics: Visions for Animal Breeding and Genetics* (http://agbio.cabweb.org).

Huisman, A.E., Veerkamp, R.F., and van Arendonk, J.A.M. 2002. Genetic parameters for various random regression models to describe the weight data of pigs. *Journal of Animal Science* 80:575–582.

Irgang, R., Dillard, E.U., Tess, M.W., and Robison, O.W. 1985. Selection for weaning and postweaning gain in Hereford cattle. 2. Response to selection. *Journal of Animal Science* 60:1142–1155.

Jackson, S.P., and Green, R.D. 1993. Muscle trait inheritance, growth performance and feed efficiency of sheep exhibiting a muscle hypertrophy phenotype. *Journal of Animal Science* 71Suppl.1:241.

Jackson, S.P., Green, R.D. and Miller, M.F. 1997. Phenotypic characterization of Rambouillet sheep expressing the callipyge gene: I. Inheritance of the condition and production characteristics. *Journal of Animal Science* 75:14–18.

Jeon, J.T., Carlborg, O., Tornsten, A., Giuffra, E., Amarger, V., Chardon, P., Andersson-Eklund, L., Andersson, K., Hansson, I., Lundstrom, K., and Andersson, L. 1999. A paternally expressed QTL affecting skeletal and cardiac muscle mass in pigs maps to the IGF2 locus. *Nature: Genetics* 21:157–158.

Jiang, Z., and Gibson, J. 1999. Genetic polymorphisms in the leptin gene and their association with fatness in four pig breeds. *Mammalian Genome* 10:191–193.

Jiang, Z., Rottmann, O.J., and Pirchner, F. 1996. HhaI enzyme reveals genetic polymorphisms at the second exon of the porcine growth hormone gene. *Journal of Animal Breeding and Genetics* 133:553–558.

Jones, G.F. 1998. Genetic Aspects of Domestication, Common Breeds and Their Origin. In *The Genetics of the Pig*, CAB International, M.V. Rothschild and A. Ruvinsky, eds. New York: CAB International.

Jurado, J.J., Alonso, A.A., and Alenda, R. 1994. Selection response for growth in a Spanish Merino flock. *Journal of Animal Science* 72:1433–1440.

Kaps, M., Herring, W.O., and Lamberson, W.R. 2000. Genetic and environmental parameters for traits derived from the Brody growth curve and their relationships with weaning weight in Angus cattle. *Journal of Animal Science* 78:1436–1442.

Kim, S.K., Larsen, N., Short, T., Plastow, G., and Rothschild, M.F. 2000. A missense variant of the porcine melanocortin-4 receptor (MC4R) gene is associated with fatness, growth and feed intake traits. *Mammalian Genome* 11:131–135.

Kirkpatrick, B.W. 1992. Identification of a conserved microsatellite site in the porcine and bovine IGF-I gene 5' flank. *Animal Genetics* 23:543–548.

Knott, S.A., Nystrom, P.E., Andersson-Eklund, L., Stern, S., Marklund, L., Andersson, L., and Haley, C.S. 2002. Approaches to interval mapping of QTL in a multigeneration pedigree. *Animal Genetics* 33:26–32.

Koch, R.M., Cundiff, L.V., and Gregory, K.E. 1974. Selection in beef cattle. I. Selection applied and generation interval. *Journal of Animal Science* 39:449–458.

Koohmaraie, M., Shackelford, S.D., Wheeler, T.L., Lonergan, S.M., and Doumit, M.E. 1995. A muscle hypertrophy condition in lamb (callipyge): Characterization of effects on muscle growth and meat quality traits. *Journal of Animal Science* 73:3596–3607.

Koots, K.R., Gibson, J.P., Smith, C., and Wilton, J.W. 1994a. Analyses of published genetic parameter estimates for beef production traits. 1. Heritability. *Animal Breeding Abstracts* 62:309–338.

Koots, K.R., Gibson, J.P., and Wilton, J.W. 1994b. Analyses of published genetic parameter estimates for beef production traits. 2. Phenotypic and genetic correlations. *Animal Breeding Abstracts* 62:825–853.

Lasslo, L.L., Bradford, G.E., Torell, D.T., and Kennedy, B.W. 1985. Selection for weaning weight in Targhee sheep in two environments. I. Direct response. *Journal of Animal Science* 61:376–386.

Laster, D.B., Smith, G.M., Cundiff, L.V., and Gregory, K.E. 1979. Characterization of biological types of cattle (Cycle II) II. Post-weaning growth and puberty of heifers. *Journal of Animal Science* 48:500–508.

Li, C., Basarab, J., Snelling, W.M., Benkel, B., Murdoch, B., and Moore, S.S. 2002. The identification of common haplotypes on bovine chromosome 5 within commercial lines of Bos Taurus and their associations with growth traits. *Journal of Animal Science* 80:1187–1194.

Mackay, T.F.C. 2001. The genetic architecture of quantitative traits. *Annual Review of Genetics* 35:303–339.

Maddox-Hyttel, P., Dinnyes, A., Laurincik, J., Rath, D., Niemann, H., Rosenkranz, C., and Wilmut, I. 2001. Gene expression during pre- and peri-implantation embryonic development in pigs. *Reproduction Supplement* 58:175–189.

Malek, M., Dekkers, J.C.M., Hakkyo, K.L., Baas, T.J., and Rothschild, M.F. 2001. A molecular genome scan analysis to identify chromosomal regions influencing economic traits in the pig. I. *Growth and body composition.* *Mammalian Genome* 12:630–636.

Meyer, K. 1999. Estimates of genetic and phenotypic covariance functions for postweaning growth and mature weight of beef cows. *Journal of Animal Breeding and Genetics* 116:181–205.

Meyer, K., and Hill, W.G. 1997. Estimation of genetic and phenotypic covariance functions for longitudinal or "repeated" records by restricted maximum likelihood. *Livestock Production Science* 47:185–200.

Moody, D.E., Pomp, D., Newman, S., and MacNeil, M.D. 1996. Characterization of DNA polymorphisms in three populations of Hereford cattle and their associations with growth and maternal EPD in Line 1 Herefords. *Journal of Animal Science* 74:1784–1793.

Morris, C.A., Baker, R.L., and Hunter, J.C. 1992. Correlated responses to selection for yearling or 18-month weight in Angus and Hereford cattle. *Livestock Production Science* 30:33–52.

Mousa, E., Van Vleck, L.D., and Leymaster, K.A. 1999. Genetic parameters for growth traits for a composite terminal sire breed of sheep. *Journal of Animal Science* 77:1659–1665.

Nezer, C., Moreau, L., Brouwers, B., Coppieters, W., Detilleux, J., Hanset, R., Karim, L., Kvasz, A., LeRoy, P., and Georges, M. 1999. An imprinted QTL with major effect on muscle mass and fat deposition maps to the IGF2 locus in pigs. *Nature: Genetics* 21:155–156.

Parnell, P.F., Arthur, P.F., and Barlow, R. 1997. Direct response to divergent selection for yearling growth rate in Angus cattle. *Livestock Production Science* 49: 297–304.

Paszek, A.A., Wilkie, P.J., Flickinger, G.H., Rohrer, G.A., Alexander, L.J., Beattie, C.W., and Schook, L.B. 1999. Interval mapping of growth in divergent swine cross. *Mammalian Genome* 10:117–122.

Pomp, D. 1997. Genetic dissection of obesity in polygenic animal models. *Behavior Genetics* 27: 285–306.

Pomp, D., Zou, T., Clutter, A.C., and Barendse, W. 1997. Rapid communication: Mapping of leptin to bovine chromosome 4 by linkage analysis of a PCR-based polymorphism. *Journal of Animal Science* 75:1427.

Rumph, J.M., Koch, R.M., Gregory, K.E., Cundiff, L.V., and Van Vleck, L.D. 2002. Comparison of models for estimation of genetic parameters for mature weight of Hereford cattle. *Journal of Animal Science* 80:583–590.

Sasaki, S., Clutter, A.C., and Pomp, D. 1996. Assignment of the porcine obese (leptin) gene to chromosome 18 by linkage analysis of a new PCR-based polymorphism. *Mammalian Genome* 7:471.

Short, R.E., MacNeil, M.D., Grosz, M.D., Gerrard, D.E., and Grings, E.E. 2002. Pleiotropic effects in Hereford, Limousin, and Piedmontese F2 crossbred calves of genes controlling muscularity including the Piedmontese myostatin allele. *Journal of Animal Science* 80:1–11.

Stobart, R.H., Bassett, J.W., Cartwright, T.C., and Blackwell, R.L. 1986. An analysis of body weights and maturing patterns in western range ewes. *Journal of Animal Science* 63:729–740.

Stone, R.T., Keele, J.W., Shackelford, S.D., Kappes, S.M., and Koohmaraie, M. 1999. A primary screen of the bovine genome for quantitative trait loci affecting carcass and growth traits. *Journal of Animal Science* 77:1379–1384.

Suttie, J.M., Veenvliet, B.A., Littlejohn, R.P., Gluckman, P.D., Corson, I.D., and Fennessy, P.F. 1993. Growth hormone pulsatility in ram lambs of genotypes selected for fatness or leanness. *Animal Production* 57:119–125.

Thallman, R.M., Cundiff, L.V., Gregory, K.E., and Koch, R.M. 1999. Germplasm evaluation in beef cattle—Cycle IV: Postweaning growth and puberty of heifers. *Journal of Animal Science* 77:2651–2659.

Thatcher, W.W., Guzeloglu, A., Mattos, R., Binelli, M., Hansen, T.R., and Pru, J.K. 2001. Uterine-conceptus interactions and reproductive failure in cattle. *Theriogenology* 56:1435–1450.

Whittemore, C.T. 1986. An approach to pig growth modeling. *Journal of Animal Science* 63:615–621.

Woltmann, M.D., Clutter, A.C., Buchanan, D.S., and Dolezal, H.G. 1992. Growth and carcass characteristics of pigs selected for fast or slow gain in relation to feed intake and efficiency. *Journal of Animal Science* 70:1049–1059.

Yu, T.P., Tuggle, C.K., Schmitz, C.B., and Rothschild, M.F. 1995. Associations of PIT1 polymorphisms with growth and carcass traits in pigs. *Journal of Animal Science* 73:1282–1288.

Yu, T.P., Wang, L., Tuggle, C.K., and Rothschild, M.F. 1999. Mapping genes for fatness and growth on pig chromosome 13: a search in the region close to the pig PIT1 gene. *J. Anim. Breed. Genet.* 116:269–280.

16
Environment and Growth

Colin G. Scanes

Factors in the environment influence the growth of domestic animals. These include stress, microorganisms, parasites, facilities/housing/transportation, daylength, and toxicants. The mechanisms involve changes in feed intake (usually reductions), effects via the endocrine system, and with toxicants/microorganisms, direct tissue effects.

STRESS (PHYSICAL, PSYCHOLOGICAL, AND SOCIAL) AND GROWTH

Exposure of animals to environmental, social, and management stresses have a number of systematic effects on an animal. These responses to stresses include the following:

- Activation of the hypothalamic-pituitary-adrenal axis, increasing the release of
  - Corticotropin releasing hormone (CRH)
  - Adrenocorticotropin (ACTH)
  - Glucocorticoids (in domestic mammals: cortisol; in poultry: corticosterone)
- Release of epinephrine and norepinephrine from the adrenal medulla/sympathetic nervous system terminals
- Suppression of immune functioning and behavioral changes

Based on the growth suppressive effects of adrenal glucocorticoids (see Chapter 5) and the importance of the immune system in combating disease, severe stress will be associated with poor performance/reduced growth. In addition, in domestic and other animals, stress affects the circulating concentrations of hormones other than those of the hypothalamo-pituitary-adrenal-cortical axis. For instance in pigs, acute stress increases the circulating concentrations of GH, prolactin and T_3, in addition to those of cortisol (Farmer et al. 1991).

Some of the physiological responses are associated with only some stresses or are manifest only under some circumstances. This can depend on the novelty of the situation to the animal and psychological factors, including fear, discomfort, and pleasure. For instance, Grandin (1997) noted that "cattle trained and habituated to a squeeze chute may have baseline cortisol levels and be behaviorally calm, whereas extensively reared animals may have elevated cortisol levels in the same chute." The extent to which an animal has been subject to chronic stress influences the magnitude of response to an acute stress. Pigs that had been subjected to tethering for ~10 weeks showed reduced ACTH responses to acute stress (Janssens et al. 1994). This reduction in the acute stress response is mediated via a central nervous endogenous opioid mechanism (Janssens et al. 1995). Studies employing a different chronic/repeated stress did not evoke this attenuating effect, reducing the adrenal cortical response. Repeated intermittent stress (restraint) of pigs had little effect on the adrenal cortical response to ACTH challenge (Klemcke 1994).

It is not possible at this time to provide a definitive series of physiological responses as a corollary to the magnitude of the stress or distress that an animal is experiencing. Moreover, stimuli may be have a positive effect and these can be referred to as "eustressors."

Stresses can suppress immune functioning. This is due in part to glucocorticoid hormones, and is partially independent of the adrenal axis. For instance, in lambs, restraint and isolation stress increase plasma concentrations of cortisol and suppress immune function as assessed by lymphocyte proliferation induced by mitogens. However, elevating circulating concentrations of cortisol to the same magnitude achieved by cortisol administration has no discernable effect on the immune parameters measured (Minton et al. 1995).

STRESSORS AND THE HYPOTHALAMO-PITUITARY-ADRENAL AXIS

Physical and social stresses markedly affect the hypothalamo-pituitary-adrenal axis. An example is given in Table 16.1. Another example of an acute stress is transportation. This is accompanied by activation of the hypothalo-pituitary-adrenocortical axis with increases in circulating concentrations of cortisol (e.g., in pigs: Becker et al. 1985a). The stress of transportation also reduces the number of unoccupied glucocorticoid receptors in muscle (Nyberg et al. 1988). Transportation stress involves several components: temperature/wind, a novel social group, absence of feed and water, and motion (including vibrations) (Lambooij and van Putten 1993). These can have independent effects. For instance, vibrations alone increase the release of both ACTH and cortisol in piglets (Perremans et al. 2001).

Stressed Animals with Reduced Growth Rates

There are examples of animals that are chronically stressed and show the expected effects of elevated circulating concentrations of glucocorticoids and (concomitant) reduction in growth rate. For example, tethering growing pigs decreases growth, because there is a modest increase in circulating concentrations of cortisol (von Borell and Ladewig 1989) (see Table 16.1 for details). In studies with older gilts (10 months old), tethering initially elevated circulating concentrations of cortisol, but these returned to normal within eight hours (Becker et al. 1985b).

Stressed Animals with Increased Growth Rates

There are some examples where stressed animals show increased growth rates. Transportation stress markedly increases circulating concentrations of cortisol (see above). Exposure of pregnant cows to repeated transportation stress is accompanied by increased growth of the fetal calves (Lay et al. 1997) (see Table 16.2). There are also cases where an effect of growth is observed without a major change in the hypothalamo-pituitary-adrenal-cortical axis.

Table 16.1. Effect of chronic stress (rearing tethered) on growth and adrenocortical functioning in young pigs (based on von Borell and Ladewig, 1989)

	Control		Stressed (as % Change Compared to Control)
Average daily gain (g)	460±32	**	307±30 (−33%)
Increase in cortisol in response to ACTH challenge (area under curve)	383±42	*	505±38 (+32%)

*p<0.05; **p<01 compared to control.

Table 16.2. Effect of repeated transportation stress of pregnant cows on the growth of the fetal calves (based on Lay et al., 1997)

Treatment	Body Weight (kg)
Control	23.1±1.1
Stressed dam	28.7±2.5*

*Different from control p<0.05.

There is an improvement in growth rate in early-weaned compared to late-weaned pigs, but little difference in the glucocorticoid stress response (Hohenshell et al. 2000).

FACILITIES/HOUSING/TRANSPORTATION (INCLUDING PHYSICAL AND SOCIAL STRESSES)

Housing markedly affects the growth rate of livestock species. This can reflect sanitary conditions (exposure to microorganisms/clinical and subclinical disease) and/or the presence/absence of specific stressors. Examples of the influence of house/environment are numerous, and only a few examples are considered in the following sections.

Facilities/Housing for Pigs

Off-Site Nursery

Weanling pigs show superior growth (increased by 40%) when reared in an experimental nursery located at a distance away from other swine facilities and with carefully controlled environmental temperatures compared to a conventional on-farm nursery (Table 16.3) (Coffey and Cromwell 1995). The improved growth seems to be due to the reduced adverse effects of disease organisms because spray-dried porcine plasma (containing antibodies) overcame the "growth-drag" in the conventional facilities (Table 16.3) (Coffey and Cromwell 1995).

Specific-Stress-Free Housing

Both transportation and mixing of livestock (that is, introducing new animals into an existing social order or mixing all new animals so that a new social hierarchy needs to be established) are thought to stress the animal. For instance, salivary cortisol concentrations are elevated following mixing pigs (Ekkel et al. 1995).

A system for rearing pigs with the elimination of the specific stresses of transportation has been developed so that pigs are reared with the same group of contemporaries in the same pen throughout growth. This is accompanied by a marked reduction in injuries (associated with aggressive social interaction) and improved growth (see Table 16.4; Ekkel et al. 1995). However, it should be noted that other studies do not support the rationale, although they don't affect the veracity of the data (in Table 16.4). Examples include the following: Social mixing alone has been reported not to influence growth rate (Heetkamp et al. 1995). Moving pigs from individual pens to group housing led to acute responses, including fighting and increased circulating concentrations of cortisol. However, after the social order was established (in less than a day), glucocorticoid levels returned to basal (Barnett et al. 1981). These acute effects are unlikely to influence growth rate.

Space Requirement for Animals

It is not easy to determine the space requirements for animals. There is a very strong case to having sufficient space to provide for animal welfare. Indeed, insufficient space is likely to impair growth. It is not easy to definitively establish this contention. For instance, group size did not affect growth rate of pigs in a wean-to-finish production system (Wolter et al. 2001). On the other hand, some effects of farrow crate design on piglet growth have been reported (Curtis et al. 1989).

Facilities/Housing for Veal Calves

Production of special-fed veal calves involves tethering in individual stalls. Comparison of this production system with tethering in larger stalls or rearing in pens of various sizes but without tethering revealed no difference in growth rate (Terosky et al. 1997). There were some differences in circulating concentrations of

Table 16.3. Comparison of growth of weanling pigs (17 days old) in an experimental nursery (off-site) with that in a conventional nursery (on-site) in the presence and absence of dried porcine plasma (SDPP) on the diet (data from Coffey and Cromwell, 1995)

Treatments	Growth Rate	ADG over 14 Days
Diet	0	+SDPP
Conventional nursery (on-site)	203[a]	269[b]
Experimental nursery (off-site)	284[b]	300[b]

[a,b]Different superscript letters indicate different p<0.001.

Table 16.4. Effect of a system for housing pigs with the specific stresses of social mixing pigs and transportation eliminated (specific-stress-free, SSF) (data from Ekkel et al., 1995)

Growth Rate (g/d)	Control Conventional		SSF
26–60 days	479	*	528
60–143 days	721	**	814
Number of clinical injuries			
26–60 days	72	**	13
60–143 days	130	**	13

*Different from control/conventional p<0.05.
**Different from control/conventional p<0.001.

cortisol (elevated transiently in calves in pens) and behavior (Wilson et al. 1999).

Facilities/Housing for Chickens

There are considerable effects of environment on the growth of broiler chickens. There is a substantial higher growth rate in birds on floor pens between 4 and 6 weeks of age compared to in cages. Average rate of daily gain was 71.3 g/d (floor pen) and 58.4 g/d (cages) (calculated from Suk and Washburn 1995).

There are five environmental factors that affect the growth/development of avian embryos: temperature, humidity, oxygen partial pressure, carbon dioxide partial pressure, and turning (reviewed Christensen 1995). These environmental factors are thought to exert the effects directly, either stimulating or inhibiting chemical reactions. In addition, there is evidence that light may affect hatching time and/or embryonic groups/chickens: Lauber and Shutze 1964; Shutze et al. 1962; turkeys: Fairchild and Christensen 2000).

SEASON AND GROWTH

There are marked seasonal differences in growth rate in livestock species. This is due principally to

environmental effects, including temperature and photoperiod but probably not light intensity. Obviously an additional factor for pasture animals is availability/quality of feed. Feedlot cattle in Northern latitudes show seasonal changes in growth rate (see Table 16.5). Growth rates in the winter are considerably reduced compared to the rest of the year (Young 1981) (see below and Table 16.5).

Temperature and Growth

Temperature and Growth in Pigs

Pigs show some susceptibility to the adverse effects of high temperatures. For instance, elevated temperatures decrease growth rate in growing pigs. Rearing temperatures of about 30°C reduce growth rate of neonatal pigs (Matteri and Becker 1994) (see Table 16.6). Similarly, elevated temperature (32°C) reduced growth rate of piglets between 3 days old and either 4 or 6 weeks of age (Carroll et al. 1999). Rearing at 32°C had little effect on the hypothalamo-pituitary-GH-IGF-I axis, with the exception of an increase in liver GH receptor expression at 6 weeks of age (Carroll et al. 1999).

Table 16.5. Effect of season/temperature on growth in cattle in feedlots (based on Young, 1981)

Location	Growth Average		Daily Gain[+]		Average Temperature (°C)	
	Winter		Rest of Year		Winter	Rest of Year
Colorado	1.08		1.49		1.6	11.7
Saskatchewan	1.20		1.54		–9.8	12.5
Alberta	1.15		1.46		–13.6	14.6

[+]Statistical analysis not reported.

Biology of Growth of Domestic Animals

Table 16.6. Effect of elevated temperature (~30°C) on growth in piglets (data from Matteri and Becker, 1994)

Age	Body Weight (kg)		
Treatment Time (Weeks)	Control-Moderate Temperature (20°C)		Elevated Temperature (27–32°C)
2	4.9	*	4.0
3	5.9	*	5.4

*Different from control p<0.05.

Temperature and Growth in Poultry

Poultry are particularly susceptible to the adverse effects of either low or high temperatures.

Elevated Temperatures

There is considerable industry and anecdotal evidence that high ambient temperatures reduce growth in poultry. Moreover, in controlled environment studies, elevated temperatures have been demonstrated to markedly depress growth rate in poultry. Hurwitz and colleagues (1980) reported lower growth rate of broiler chickens raised under elevated temperatures compared to lower temperatures. For instance, the growth rate of either male or female chickens between 5 and 8 weeks of age was lower at 28°C than 19°C and even lower at 34°C than 28°C (Hurwitz et al. 1980). Elevated environmental temperature adversely affects growth rate carcass composition in broiler chickens. For instance, Temim and colleagues (2000) observed detrimental effects on growth rate, carcass fat (abdominal fat), and carcass protein (breast muscle) in birds reared at 32°C compared to 22°C in male broiler chickens (see Table 16.7).

In chickens, the adverse effect of elevated temperatures is progressively greater with increased age (toward market age) or weight (toward market weight). May and colleagues (1998) reported much reduced gains in 4-, 5-, and 6-week-old broilers raised at elevated temperatures. Moreover, the adverse effect of elevated temperature became progressively worse. For instance, rearing broiler chickens at 31.1°C compared to 21.1°C resulted in no change in growth rate between 3 and 4 weeks of age, but thereafter an attenuation in growth rate was evident. This is exemplified by the following: 3–4 weeks old, ~0% change in growth; 4–5 weeks old, 22% decrease in growth; 5–6 weeks old, 34% reduction in growth; and 6–7 weeks old, 40% reduction in growth rate (May et al. 1998).

An ingenious approach to temperature stress in poultry has been developed by Yahav and Hurwitz (1996). If young broiler chickens are exposed to high temperature (36°C for 24 hours at 5 days old), they are more resistant to a temperature stress

Table 16.7. Comparison of rearing (until 6 weeks old) at 22°–32°C on performance of broiler chickens[1] (data from Temim et al., 2000)

Parameter	Temperature Control		
	22°C		32°C
Live weight (kg)	2.27	*	1.87
Abdominal fat as % of body weight	1.6	*	2.2
Breast muscle as % of body weight	15.9	*	13.8

*Different from control p<0.05.
[1]Receiving 28% protein in diet.

challenge at 42 days. Mortality is reduced from 36% in control thermally challenged chickens to 23% in conditioned chickens. The temperature stress conditioning does not appear to affect overall growth (Yahav and Hurwitz 1996).

In contrast to the detrimental effects of elevated temperatures during the rearing period, in the first week of life high environmental temperatures are advantageous. Elevated temperatures between hatching and 7 days old, do not appear to affect growth, but do markedly reduce mortality in broiler chicks. The mortalities in males reported by May and Lott (2000) were 7.0% at 26–28°C, 0.9% at 27–30°C, and 1.5% at 28–30°C. In females, mortalities were 5.9% at 26–28°C, 2.0% at 27–30°C, and 1.9% at 28–30°C. In turkeys, growth is reduced by high temperature. For instance, growth rate was reduced when turkeys were exposed to an elevated rearing temperature of 32°C compared to temperatures in the low 20s (Hurwitz et al. 1980). Similarly, a recent study examined the relationship between temperature and growth in turkeys (Veldkamp et al. 2000). The reported growth rates were gain between 1–134 days: 18.8 kg at low temperatures and 17.7 kg at elevated temperatures (Veldkamp et al. 2000).

Low Temperature

Reduced brooding temperatures in the first 3 weeks of life has been associated with increased mortality and mortality due to ascites at 6 weeks old but no change in body weight (growth) (Deaton et al. 1996).

Temperature and Growth in Cattle and Sheep

Although cattle are relatively cold-hardy (Young 1981), low temperatures of winter are associated with reduced growth (Young 1981) (also see Table 16.5) and decreased feed:gain efficiency. Circulating concentration of IGF-I are also reduced with low environmental temperatures (Sarko et al. 1994). Cattle show adverse effects on growth rate, with elevated temperatures in part due to reduced feed intake (e.g., Morrison 1983). Sheep are cold-hardy, but growth rate is reduced with moderate increases in temperature (see Table 16.8) (Schanbacher et al. 1982). An inverse relationship between temperature and growth rate in sheep was described by the following equation (Schanbacher et al. 1982):

$$ADG = 327 - 4.46 \text{ (temperature in degrees Celsius)}$$

Photoperiod and Growth

There are distinct effects of daylength on growth in at least some domestic animals (reviewed Forbes 1982; Tucker et al. 1984) (also see Table 16.9). In sheep, long daylength improves growth rate (e.g., Forbes et al. 1975; 1979a) (also see Table 16.9). These effects are observed irrespective of sex (Table 16.8), environmental temperature (5° or 18° or 31°C) (Schanbacher et al. 1982), or feed intake (Forbes et al. 1975, 1979a, 1979b). Long daylength is also associated with improved feed efficiency (some studies only), carcass weight, and elevated circulating concentrations of prolactin (e.g., Pelletier 1973; Forbes et al. 1975, 1979b; Schanbacher and Crouse 1980; reviewed Tucker et al. 1984). In contrast, photoperiod does not appear to influence growth or circulating concentrations of prolactin in pigs (e.g., Minton and Wettemann 1988).

In cattle supplementary lighting above natural winter daylength can improve rate (Peters et al. 1978, 1980) (also see Table 16.10). Continuous lighting does not enhance growth in the way observed with supplementary lighting (Peters et al. 1980). This would be supportive of long daylength, but not continuous light, being capable of entraining

Table 16.8. Effect of temperature on growth of ewe lambs (on short daylength) (data from Schanbacher et al., 1982)

Temperature (°C)	Average Daily Gain (kg/d)
5	0.29[a]
18	0.24[b]
31	0.15[c]

[a,b,c]Different letters indicate difference.

Table 16.9. Effect of photoperiod on growth

| Species | Age/Sex | Growth (Average Daily Gain kg/d) | | Reference |
		Short Day 8L:16D	Long Day 16L:8D	
Cattle	Prepubertal heifers	1.03	1.06	Zinn et al., 1986
Cattle	Postpubertal heifers	1.24	1.08*	Zinn et al., 1986
White Tail Deer	Fawns	0.16	0.12*	Abbott et al., 1984
Sheep	Castrate males	0.20	0.23*	Forbes et al., 1975
	Ewe lambs	0.23	0.27**	Schanbacher et al., 1982
	Ram lambs	0.34	0.41*	Schanbacher and Crouse, 1980

*Different from short daylength p<0.05.
**Different from short daylength p<0.01.

a circannual rhythm underlying the growth rate. There were no differences in basal circulating concentrates of GH, prolactin, or glucocorticoids with different lighting regimens in the second study (Peters et al. 1980). Studies in beef breeds found no effect from supplementary light on growth, but it did hasten puberty (Hansen et al. 1983). There were no differences in the rates of growth (ADG), protein accretion, or lipid accretion in prepubertal heifers reared under long (16L:8D) or short (8L:16D) photoperiods (Zinn et al. 1986) (also see Table 16.9). In contrast, in postpubertal heifers, rates of growth and lipid accretion were greater with short daylengths than with long daylengths (Zinn et al. 1986).

In poultry, there appears to be some small effect of photoperiod on growth. For instance Sorensen and colleagues (1999) reported a 5.3% increase in growth rate in broiler chickens raised on long than on short daily photoperiods. Body weights at 35 days were 1.70 kg (for 8L:16D) and 1.79 kg (for 16L:8D). There was, however, an increase in tibial dyschondroplasia (Sorensen et al. 1999).

In a single study of white tail deer fawns, growth was greater from short than from long daylength (Abbott et al. 1984) (also see Table 16.9). The increased growth was due to increases in skeletal muscle, with concomitant reductions in lipogenesis (Abbott et al. 1984).

Photoperiod and Growth: Mechanism

The mechanism by which daylength influences growth is not clear, but it is possibly hormonal. Jean Pelletier (1973) first identified the link between daylength and circulating concentrations of prolactin in sheep. Changes in the circulating concentration of hormones other than prolactin are less consistently observed. However, a role for prolactin in the stimulation of growth is not definitively established. Chronic suppression of prolactin secretion in sheep on long daylength reduced growth (Eisemann et al. 1984). In contrast, elevating prolactin levels in sheep on short daylengths has no effect on growth rate (Eisemann et al. 1984). Although photoperiod may be responsible or partially responsible for sev-

Table 16.10. Effect of supplementary lighting to impose a 16L:8D photoperiod on growth in Holstein heifers

| | Natural Photoperiod (Winter) | Growth (ADG kg/d) | | Reference |
		Supplementary Lighting	Constant Lighting	
Study 1	0.78	0.86	—	Peters et al., 1978
Study 2	0.84[a]	0.98[b]	0.88[a]	Peters et al., 1980

[a,b]Different superscript letters indicate different p<0.05.

eral differences in growth rate, it is also possible that changes in daylength act either directly on the central nervous system/growing tissue or act to entertain an endogenous circannual rhythm.

A definitive study examined growth rate and circulating concentrations of prolactin and GH in lambs with artificial daylength, either adjusted to reflect actual changes in a year or the annual changes compressed into six months. In both groups, plasma concentrations of prolactin were parallel to daylength. Plasma concentrations of GH were maximal with increasing daylength (from ~10L to ~14D). Growth rate increased with increasing daylength (Barenton et al. 1988). These data are consistent with a role for either hormone in mediating the photoperiodic response and for either model for photoperiodic effects (either direct central nervous effect or entraining the circannual rhythm).

Light Intensity

There is little evidence that light intensity influences either growth or the hormonal control system(s). For instance, increasing the intensity of light from 22 to 540 lux did not affect circulating concentrations of GH, T_4 or cortisol in young cattle (Leining et al. 1980).

Light Spectra and Poultry Growth

There are reports that the spectra of the environmental lighting may affect the growth rate of broiler chickens (reviewed Rozenboim et al. 1999). There has been some lack of consistency in the responses, however. Recently, broiler chickens exposed to monochromatic green light (560 nm) from light emitting diodes had improved growth, compared to either blue or white light (Rozenboim et al. 1999).

MICROORGANISMS AND GROWTH

Microorganisms in the environment affect the growth of domestic animals. Evidence for this comes from the increased growth rate of animals reared in an environment depleted of microorganisms ("germ-free"). For instance, chicks in a germ-free environment grow more rapidly than in a conventional environment (Coates et al. 1963). Similarly, improved sanitation improves growth rate and feed efficiency in domestic animals—e.g., chicks (Hill et al. 1952; Lillie et al. 1952; Libby and Schaible 1955); pigs (see Table 16.3); etc. Bacterial diseases have been directly found to adversely affect growth in control studies. For instance, turkeys challenged with *Pasteurella multocida* exhibited very marked reductions in growth rate and in the circulating concentration of IGF-I (Anthony et al. 1999).

Administration of antibiotics (by definition reducing microorganisms) also improves growth rate and feed efficiency in chicks (Coates et al. 1963), pigs, and cattle (e.g., Rogers et al. 1995). Environmental microorganisms (both pathogenic and nonpathogenic) reduce growth due to one or more of the following: overt and subclinical disease, immune responses, and hormonal and cytokines released in response to the microorganisms.

Immune Challenge and Growth

Exposure to disease results in an immune response and reduced performance. In a controlled study with postweaning piglets (Dritz et al. 1996), disease was simulated by the administration of *E.coli* endotoxin lipopolysaccharide. This regimen resulted in reduced performance/growth (see Tables 16.11 and 16.12).

Table 16.11. Effect of immune challenge on growth in early weaned pigs (14 days old) with diets not containing antibiotics (data from Dritz et al., 1996)

	Control	LPS-Challenged
Pig weight (kg) day 18 postweaning (% decrease over control)	9.3	8.2* (−12%)
Pig weight (kg) day 32 postweaning (% decrease over control)	17.2	15.8* (−8%)
Average daily gain kg/d (% decrease over control)	0.45	0.40* (−12%)

LPS is *E.coli* endotoxin lipopolysaccharide.
*Different from control.

Table 16.12. Effects of immunogens on growth in birds (data from Klasing et al., 1987)

Treatment	Gain g/d (% Vehicle)	Feed Efficiency	Feeding Regimen	Strain
Vehicle	14[a] (100)	2.63[a]	Ad libitum	Leghorn
Sheep Red Blood Cells (SRBC)	11.7[b] (84)	3.12[a,b]	Ad libitum	Leghorn
Sephadex	11.7[b] (84)	2.78[a]	Ad libitum	Leghorn
SSBC+Sephadex	8.4[c] (60)	3.44[b]	Ad libitum	Leghorn
Vehicle	17.0[a] (100)	1.64	Ad libitum	Broiler
E. coli (lipopolysaccharide)	14.9[b] (88)	1.75	Ad libitum	Broiler
Vehicle	31.5[a] (100)	1.89[a]	Restricted[1]	Broiler
SSBC	28.5[a,b] (90)	2.08[a,b]	Restricted[1]	Broiler
Sephadex	28.7[a,b] (91)	2.08[a,b]	Restricted[1]	Broiler
SSBC+Sephadex	27.5[b] (87)	2.17[b]	Restricted[1]	Broiler
E. coli lipopolysacchide	25.8[b] (82)	2.33[b]	Restricted[1]	Broiler
S. typhimurium lipopolysacchide	26.8[b] (85)	2.22[b]	Restricted[1]	Broiler
S. aureum lipopolysacchide	25.7[b] (82)	2.33[b]	Restricted[1]	Broiler

[a,b]Different superscripts indicate difference from respective control.
[1]Pair-fed to chicks injected with *S. typhimurium* lipopolysaccharide.

When animals are challenged with immunogens (e.g., sheep red blood cells, Sephadex, *E.coli* endotoxin lipopolysaccharide), growth rate is attenuated (see Table 16.12). This effect has two components: decreased growth due to a reduction in voluntary food intake (anorexia) and reduced growth that is independent of food intake. This is supported by a series of elegant studies by Kirk Klasing and his colleagues (1987). Chicks receiving immunogen injections exhibited reduced growth rates compared to both *ad libitum* and pair-fed control groups (see Table 12.2). Thus, the immunogens evoked a reduction in growth rate induced both by anorexia and an effect independent of food intake. This latter effect is related at least partially to changes in circulating concentrations of glucocorticoids and cytokines. Administration of *E.coli* endotoxin lipopolysaccharide to growing chicks has been found to increase the circulating concentrations of both corticosterone and interleukin-1 (IL-1) (Klasing et al. 1987; also see Table 16.12). Moreover both IL-1 and glucocorticoids have been demonstrated to inhibit growth. Klasing and colleagues (1987) demonstrated that IL-1 reduced growth rate of chicks, with most of the effect being attributable to the reduced food intake (~69%) but with a component independent of the induction of anorexia (Table 16.12). The same group demonstrated that a preparation containing IL-1 stimulated protein degradation while not affecting synthesis in muscle in vitro. Assuming that these effects reflect the in vivo situation, IL-1 will depress muscle protein accretion. In an analogous but different manner, corticosterone reduces growth and muscle protein accretion by depressing protein synthesis (Tables 16.13 and 16.14).

Table 16.13. Acute effect of bacteria endotoxins on circulating interleukin-1 (IL-1) activity and concentrations of corticosterone (B) in broiler chicks (data from Klasing et al., 1987)

	Serum IL-1	B
Vehicle	1.4[a]	1.0[a]
E. coli lipopolysaccharide	2.2[b]	3.3[b,c]
Salmonella typhimurium	—	4.2[c]
S. aureus	—	4.4[c]

[a,b,c]Different superscript letters indicate different p<0.05.

Table 16.14. Effect of IL-1 or corticosterone on growth (average daily gain, ADG) and muscle protein metabolism (data from Klasing et al., 1987)

	ADG in Vivo	Muscle Protein Degradation in Vitro	Muscle Protein Synthesis in Vitro
Control	17.0[a]	0.34[a]	0.40[a]
IL-1	14.4[c]	0.42[b]	0.38[a,b]
Corticosterone	15.3[b]	0.33[a]	0.33[b]
Pair-fed to IL-1	15.2[b]	Not applicable	Not applicable

[a,b,c]Different superscript letters indicate different $p<0.05$.

Bacterial Infection and Growth

Bacterial infection adversely affects growth. This is partially due to the acute effects of bacterial endotoxins. For instance, *Escherichia coli* endotoxin induces fever (elevated temperature) together with hypoglycemia and hypocalcemia in cattle (Elsasser et al. 1996). The effects on blood glucose and calcium concentrations are partially ameliorated by GH administration (Elsasser et al. 1996).

Protozoan Infections and Growth

Infection with protozoa can result in attenuation of the growth rate. For instance, infection of growing cattle with *Sarcocystin cruzi* reduces their growth (see Table 16.15) (Elsasser et al. 1996, 1998). This can be attributed to both decreased food intake and an impairment of the hypothalamic-pituitary GH-IGF-I axis. Although plasma concentrations of GH are relatively unaffected by infection, plasma IGF-I concentrations are decreased. Thus, the GH-IGF-I axis appears to be uncoupled with reduced IGF-I synthesis and expression (Table 16.15). This may be explicable in terms of reduced numbers of hepatic GH receptors and decreased circulating concentrations of

T_3 (due to GH-dependent hepatic monodeiodinase activity). A similar situation exists with stunting/spiking mortality in chickens (see below).

Coccidiosis is caused by an intracellular infection, particularly of the gastrointestinal mucosa, by *Eimeria* protozoa. Growth is profoundly depressed with broiler chickens with coccidiosis. Table 16.16 provides an example study of the effect of innoculation of broiler chicks with *Eimeria*. Both the infection and its growth restarting effects are overcome by coccidiostats, ionophores such as salinomycin, etc. (see Table 16.16). Similarly in turkeys, the coccidiostat monensin improved performance (feed:gain ratio) while tending to reduce mortality (see Table 16.17) (Chapman and Saleh 1999). There was, however, no effect on growth rate per se.

Stunting/Spiking Mortality in Poultry

Chicks can exhibit spiking mortality/stunting. While the organism is not well established, this can be reproduced experimentally. Accompanying the dramatic reduction in growth, there are concomitant decreases in plasma concentrations of IGF-I and some increase in those of GH (Davis et al. 1995). This is explicable by uncoupling of the

Table 16.15. Effect of protozoan parasite (*Sarcocystis cruzi*) on growth and the hypothalamic-pituitary-GH axis in calves (data from Elsasser et al., 1986, 1998)

	Control	Infected	Pair Fed to Infected
Growth			
Protein Gain	123[b]	52[a]	109[b]
Fat Gain	85[c]	11[a]	43[b]
Plasma GH (ng/ml)	6.1	6.5	7.2
Plasma IGF-I (ng/ml)	142[b]	94[a]	138[b]
Plasma T_3 (ng/ml)	1.6[b]	0.2[a]	1.2[b]
Plasma T_4 (ng/ml)	99	37	51

[a,b,c]Different superscript letters indicate different $p<0.05$.

Table 16.16. Effect of coccidial infection (*Eimeria inoculated*) in the presence or absence of the ionophore, Narosin, on the growth in broiler chickens (data from Waldenstedt et al., 1999)

	Mortality (%)	Body Weight at 36 Days (kg)	Feed:Gain
Control	1.4[a]	1.61[a]	1.77[a]
Inoculated with *Eimeria*	11.4[b]	1.21[b]	1.93[c]
Inoculated with *Eimeria* and receiving narosin[1]	2.9[a]	1.64[a]	1.85[b]

[a,b,c]Different superscript letters indicate different p<0.05.
[1]With 5-day withdrawal period.

Table 16.17. Effect of monensin on growth (at 10 weeks) of male Large White turkeys reared on floor pens (data from Chapman and Saleh, 1999)

	Mortality (%)	Growth ADG (g)	Feed:Gain
Control	10.4	108	1.94
Monensin	4.7	111	1.83*

*Different from control p<0.05.

GH-IGF-I axis, perhaps due to loss of GH receptors. The disease in turkeys, poult enteritis and mortality syndrome (PEMS), is analogous or possibly identical to spiking mortality/stunting in chickens. In this case, the causal agents may include entero-like viruses, bacteria (e.g., *Salmonella, E. coli, Campylobacter, Clostridia*), and protozoa (*Cryptosporidia* and *Cochlosoma*). In poults that survive infection with an inoculum, growth is markedly reduced, as is nutrient absorption/retention, and there is an absence of compensatory growth (Odetallah et al. 2001).

Parasites and Growth

In geographical areas where there is a significant nematode prevalence—for instance, in pastures—parasitic infections have a marked inhibitory effect on growth. This contention is supported by the ability of anthelmintics to enhance the rate of growth (e.g., Purvis and Whittier 1996; Ryan et al. 1997; Mejía et al. 1999) (see Table 16.18).

TOXICANTS AND GROWTH

It would appear to be intuitively obvious that toxicants reduce the overall health of an animal and prevent the realization of the maximum potential growth rate. In many but not all cases, toxicants do reduce growth rate of domestic animals. The decline in the growth rate may be attributable to

- Direct effect on the growing tissues
- Interference with the endocrine axes controlling growth (the hypothalamo-pituitary-growth

Table 16.18. Effect of nematodes infestation/the anthelmintic, ivermectin on growth (average daily gain) in Holstein cattle raised on pasture with bovine nematodes (data from Mejía et al., 1999)

Age	Growth Rate Control (Parasitized)	Ivermectin (Anthelmintic)
0–20 weeks old	0.55	0.65* (+18%)
20–34 weeks old	0.31	0.40 (+29%)
34–48 weeks old	0.28	0.45* (+80%)

*Different from control p<0.05

hormone (GH) growth, or the hypothalamo-pituitary-adrenal and hypothalamo-pituitary-thyroid axes)

- Reduced feed intake due to
  - Reduction of food palatability
  - Induction of a general malaise/inactivity with reduced appetite
  - Specific decreases in appetite
  - Shifts in metabolism that in turn reduces appetite

Environmental Estrogens

Environmental estrogens exert a marked stimulatory effect on growth in domestic animals particularly ruminants (see Chapter 17 for details).

Minerals

Aluminum/Acidity

Acid precipitation has been associated with decreases in growth in wild birds; accompanying decreases in pH, the availability/solubility of aluminum is greatly increased (Driscoll and Schecher 1989). Both acidity and aluminum are associated with decreased growth rate in domesticated birds. Acidified diets reduce growth rate in broiler chickens (Pritzil and Kienholz 1973; Capdevielle and Scanes 1995a). Similarly, aluminum decreases growth in broiler chicks (Storer and Nelson 1968; Wisser et al. 1990; Capdevielle and Scanes 1995a) and mallard duck (Capdevielle and Scanes 1995b). Growth is greatly depressed by acidity and/or aluminum, due, presumably, to decreased feed intake and/or local tissue effects. However, the effects on the hormones of the hypothalamic-pituitary GH-IGF-I axis are relatively mild, if present. In view of the role of glucocorticoid hormones as stress hormones, it is surprising that secretion of corticosterone was not influenced directly by either aluminum sulfate or sulfuric acid. Young chicks receiving aluminum sulfate in the diet have increased plasma concentrations of corticosterone, as do chicks receiving sulfuric acid in their diet. However, this seems to be due to the reduction of food intake, because the plasma concentrations of corticosterone did not differ between chicks receiving aluminum sulfate or sulfuric acid and the respective pair-fed controls (Capdevielle et al. 1996).

Copper

High concentrations of copper increase growth in pigs; see Chapter 17 for details.

Selenium

Selenium is required for growth (being critical for thyroid hormone synthesis). However, selenium, at high concentrations, does exert a toxic effect, including decreasing growth rate (e.g., Kim and Mahan 2001).

Zinc

High concentrations of zinc increase growth in pigs; see Chapter 17 for details.

Mycotoxins

Myotocin contaminates a significant proportion of feedstuffs, with estimates of approximately 25% of the world's crops contaminated (CAST 1989). More than 300 mycotoxins have been identified. van Heugten (2001) concluded that the most problematic of these, based on prevalence and toxicity, are aflatoxin (from *Asperigillus* species), deoxyniralenol (vomitoxin) (from *Fusarium* species), zearalenone (from *Fusarium* species), fumonisin (from *Fusarium* species), and T-2 toxin (from *Fusarium* species). Mycotoxins can markedly depress growth rate (see below for examples). There is, however, little information available on the specific effects of mycotoxins on the hypothalamo-pituitary-GH-IGF-I axis.

Aflatoxin

Addition of aflatoxin to feed greatly reduces growth in chickens (e.g., Clarke et al. 1987) and turkeys (Weibking et al. 1994).

Fumonisins

Poultry growth can be affected by fumonisin contamination of corn. Fumonisins B_1 together with A_1, A_2, B_2, B_3, and B_4, are produced by *Fusarium monoliforme*. In chickens, growth is reduced in diets containing fumonisin B_1 but there is no effect on the feed-to-gain ratio (Weibking et al. 1993). Other mycotoxins [Deoxynivalenol (vomitoxin) and T-2] produced by *Fusarium* also inhibit growth in birds (Huff et al. 1986; Kubena et al. 1988, 1989). Similarly, monoliformin (produced by *Fusarium* species) inhibits broiler growth. Average daily gains were 47 g/day (control) and 36 g/day (moniliformin 100 mg/kg feed) (Li et al. 2000).

Ochratoxins

Ochratoxins are secondary fungal metabolites of *Aspergillus* and *Penicillium* that can infect corn/ maize.

An example is ochrotoxin A. These mycotoxins can have adverse effect on nonruminants and at very high concentrations on ruminants (Marquardt and Frohlich 1992; Höhler et al. 1999). Both ochratoxin A and cyclopriazonic acid are produced by *Aspergillus* species. These mycotocins reduce growth in poultry (e.g., Gentles et al. 1999); ADG for the first 3 weeks was 30g/d in controls, 23g/d with ochratoxcin A, 24 g/d with cyclopriagonic acid, and 19 g/d with ochratoxin A and cyclopriazonic acid.

Ergot Mycotoxins

Unlike many mycotoxins, sorgum ergot (produced by *Claviceps* species) does not appear to exert deleterious effects in broiler chickens (Bailey et al. 1999).

REFERENCES

Abbott, M.J., Ullrey, D.E., Ku, P.K., Schmitt, S.M., Romsos, D.R., and Tucker, H.A. 1984. Effect of photoperiod on growth and fat secretion in white-tailed doe fawns. *Journal of Wildlife Management* 48:776–784.

Anthony, N.B., Nestor, K.E., Emmerson, D.A., Saif, Y.M., Vasilatos-Younken, R., and Bacon, W.L. 1999. Effect of feed withdrawal or challenge with Pasteurella multocida on growth, blood metabolites, circulating growth hormone, and insulin-like growth factor-I concentrations in eight-week–old turkeys. *Poultry Science* 78:1268–1274.

Bailey, C.A., Fazzino, J.J., Ziehr, M.S., Sattar, M., Haq, A.U., Odvody, G., and Porter, J.K. 1999. Evaluation of sorghum ergot toxicity in broilers. *Poultry Science* 78:1391–1397.

Barenton, B., Ravault, J.-P., Chabanet, C., Daveau, A., Pelletier, J., and Ortavant, R. 1988. Photoperiodic control of growth hormone secretion and body weight in rams. *Domestic Animal Endocrinology* 5:247–255.

Barnett, J.L., Cronin, G.M., and Winfield, C.G. 1981. The effects of individual and group penning of pigs on total and free plasma corticosteroids and the maximum corticosteroid binding capacity. *General and Comparative Endocrinology* 44:219–225.

Becker, B.A., Ford, J.J., Christenson, R.K., Manak, R.C., Hahn, G.L., and DeShazer, J.A. 1985a. peropheral concentrations of cortisol as an indicator of stress in the pig. *American Journal of veterinary Research* 46:1034–1038.

Becker, B.A., Ford, J.J., Christenson, R.K., Manak, R.C., Hahn, G.L., and DeShazer, J.A. 1985b. Cortisol response of gilts in tether stalls. *Journal of Animal Science* 60:264–270.

Capdevielle, M.C., Carsia, R.V., and Scanes, C.G. 1996. Effect of acid or aluminum on growth and adrenal function in young chickens. *General and Comparative Endocrinology* 103:54–59.

Capdevielle, M.C., and Scanes, C.G. 1995a. Effect of dietary acid or aluminum on growth and growth related hormones in young chickens. *Toxicology and Applied Pharmacology* 133:164–171.

Capdevielle, M.C., and Scanes, C.G. 1995b. Effect of dietary acid or aluminum on growth and growth related hormones in mallard ducklings (Anas platyrhynchos). *Archives of Environmental Contamination and Toxicology* 29,462–468.

Carroll, J.A., Buonomo, F.C., Becker, B.A., and Matteri, R.L. 1999. Interactions between environmental temperature and porcine growth hormone (pGH) treatment in neonatal pigs. *Domestic Animal Endocrinology* 16:103–113.

CAST. 1989. Mycotoxins: economic and health risks. In: *Task Force Report* 116. Ames, Iowa:CAST.

Chapman, H.D., and Saleh, E. 1999. Effects of different concentrations of monensin and monensin withdrawal upon the control of coccidiosis in the turkey. *Poultry Science* 78:50–56.

Christensen, V.L. 1995. Factors affecting hatchability of turkey embryos. *Poultry Avian Biology Review* 6:71–82.

Clarke, R. N., J. A. Doerr, and M. A. Ottinger. 1987. Age-related changes in testicular development and reproductive endocrinology associated with aflatoxicosis in the male chicken. *Biology of Reproduction* 36:117–124.

Coates, M.E., Fuller, R., Harrison, G.F., Lev, M., and Suffolk, S.F. 1963. A comparison of the growth of chicks in the Gustafsson germ-free apparatus and in conventional environment, with and without dietary supplements of penicillin. *British Journal of Nutrition* 17:141–150.

Coffey, R.D., and Cromwell, G.L. 1995. The impact of environment and antimicrobial agents on the growth response of early-weaned pigs to spray-dried porcine plasma. *Journal of Animal Science* 73:2532–2539.

Curtis, S.E., Hurst, R.J., Widowski, T.M., Shanks, R.D., Jensen, A.H., Gonyou, H.W., Bane, D.P., Muehling, A.J., and Kesler, R.P. 1989. Effects of sow-crate design on health and performance of sows and piglets. *Journal of Animal Science* 67:80–93.

Davis, J.F., Castro, A.E., delaTorre, J.C., Scanes, C.G., Radecki, S.V., Vasilatos-Younken, R., Doman, J.T., and Teng, M. 1995. Hypoglycemia, enteritis, and spiking mortality in Georgia broiler chickens: experimental reproduction in broiler breeder chicks. *Avian Diseases* 39:162–174.

Deaton, J.W., Branton, S.L., Simmons, J.D., and Lott, B.D. 1996. The effect of brooding temperature on broiler performance. *Poultry Science* 75:1217–1220.

Driscoll, C.T., and Schecher, W.D. 1989. Aqueous chemistry of aluminum. In *Aluminum and Health*. H.J. Gitelman, ed. New York: Marcel Dekker.

Dritz, S.S., Owen, K.Q., Goodband, R.D., Nelssen, J.L., Tokach, M.D., Chengappa, M.M., and Blecha, F. 1996. Influence of lipopolysaccharide-induced immune challenge and diet complexity on growth performance and acute-phase protein production in segregated early-weaned pigs. *Journal of Animal Science* 74:1620–8.

Eisemann, J.H., Bauman, D.E., Hogue, D.E., and Travis, H.F. 1984. Evaluation of a role for prolactin in growth and the photoperiod-induced growth response in sheep. *Journal of Animal Science* 59:86–94.

Ekkel, E.D., vanDoorn, C.E.A., Hessing, M.J.C., and Tielen, M.J.M. 1995. The specific-stress-free housing system has positive effects on productivity, health, and welfare of pigs. *Journal of Animal Science* 73:1544–1551.

Elsasser, T.H., Hammond, A.C., Rumsey, T.S., and Fayer, R. 1986. Perturbed metabolism and hormonal profiles in calves infected with Sarcocystis cruzi. *Domestic Animal Endocrinology* 3:277–287.

Elsasser, T.H., Richards, M., Collier, R., and Hartnell, G.F. 1996. Physiological responses to repeated endotoxin challenge are selectively affected by recombinant bovine somatotropin administration to calves. *Domestic Animal Endocrinology* 13:91–103.

Elsasser, T.H., Sartin, J.L., McMahon, C., Romo, G., Fayer, R., Kahl, S., and Blagburn, B. 1998. Changes in somatotropic axis response and body composition during growth hormone administration in progressive cachectic parasitism. *Domestic Animal Endocrinology* 15:239–255.

Fairchild, B.D., and Christensen, V.L. 2000. Photostimulation of turkey eggs accelerates hatching times without affecting hatchability, liver or heart growth, or glycogen content. *Poultry Science* 79:1627–1631.

Farmer, C., Dubreuil, P., Couture, Y., Brazeau, P., and Petitclerc, D. 1991. Hormonal changes following an acute stress in control and somatostatin-immunized pigs. *Domestic Animal Endocrinology* 8:527–536.

Fensterheim, R.J. 1993. Documenting temporal trends of polychlorinated biphenyls in the environment. *Regulatory Toxicology and Pharmacology* 18:181–201.

Forbes, J.M. 1982. Effects of lighting pattern on growth, lactation and food intake of sheep, cattle and deer. *Livestock Production Science* 9:361–374.

Forbes, J.M., Driver, P.M., Brown, W.B., Scanes, C.G., and Hart, I.C. 1979b. The effect of daylength on the growth of lambs. 2. Blood concentrations of growth hormone, prolactin, insulin and thyroxine, and the effect of feeding. *Animal Production* 29:43–51.

Forbes, J.M., Driver, P.M., El Shahat, A.A., Boaz, T.G., and Scanes, C.G. 1975. The effect of daylength and level of feeding on serum prolactin in growing lambs. *Journal of Endocrinology* 64:549–554.

Forbes, J.M., El Shahat, A.A., Jones, R., Duncan, J.G.S., and Boaz, T.G. 1979a. The effect of daylength on the growth of lambs. 1. Comparisons of sex, level of feeding and shearing and breed of sire. *Animal Production* 29:33–42.

Gentles, A., Smith, E.E., Kubena, L.F., Duffus, E., Johnson, P., Thompson, J., Harvey, R.B., and Edrington, T.S. 1999. Toxicological evaluations of cyclopiazonic acid and ochratoxin A in broilers. *Poultry Science* 78:1380–1384.

Gorsline, J., and Holmes, W.N. 1982. Suppression of adrenocortical activity in mallard ducks exposed to petroleum-contaminated food. *Archives of Environmental Contamination and Toxicology* 11:497–502.

Grandin, T. 1997. Assessment of stress during handling and transport. *Journal of Animal Science* 75:249–257.

Hansen, P.J., Kamwanja, L.A., and Hauser, E.R. 1983. Photoperiod influences age at puberty of heifers. *Journal of Animal Science* 57:985–992.

Heetkamp, M.J.W., Schrama, J.W., de Jong, L., Swinkels, J.W.G.M., Schouten, W.G.P., and Bosch, M.W. 1995.

Energy metabolism in young pigs as affected by mixing. *Journal of Animal Science* 73:3562–3569.

Hill, D.C., Branion, H.D., Slinger, S.J., and Anderson, G.W. 1952. Influence of environment on the growth response of chicks to penicillin. *Poultry Science* 32:464–466.

Hohenshell, L.M., Cunnick, J.E., Ford, S.P., Kattesh, H.G., Zimmerman, D.R., Wilson, M.E., Matteri, R.L., Carroll, J.A., and Lay, D.C. 2000. Few differences found between early- and late-weaned pigs raised in the same environment. *Journal of Animal Science* 78:38–49.

Höhler, D., Südekum, K.-H., Wolffram, S., Frohlich, A.A., and Marquardt, R.R. 1999. Metabolism and excretion of ochratoxin A fed to sheep. *Journal of Animal Science* 77:1217–1223.

Huff, W.E., Kubena, L.F., Harvey, R.B., Hagler, W.M., Swanson, S.P., Phillips, T.D., and Creger, C.R. 1986. Individual and combined effects of aflatoxin and deoxynivalenol (DON, Vomitoxin) in broiler chickens. *Poultry Science* 65:1291–1298.

Hurwitz, S., Weiselberg, M., Eisner, U., Bartov, I., Riesenfeld, G., Sharvit, M., Niv, A., and Bornstein, S. 1980. The energy requirements and performance of growing chickens and turkeys as affected by environmental temperature. *Poultry Science* 59:2290–2299.

Janssens, C.J.J.G., Helmond, F.A., Loyens, L.W.S., Schouten, W.G.P., and Wiegant, V.M. 1995. Chronic stress increases the opioid-mediated inhibition of the pituitary-adrenocortical response to acute stress in pigs. *Endocrinology* 136:1468–1473.

Janssens, C.J.J.G., Helmond, F.A., and Wiegant, V.M. 1994. Increased cortisol response to exogenous adrenocorticotropic hormone in chronically stressed pigs: influence of housing conditions. *Journal of Animal Science* 72:1771–1777.

Kim, Y.Y., and Mahan, D.C. 2001. Comparative effects of high dietary levels of organic and inorganic selenium on selenium toxicity of growing-finishing pigs. *Journal of Animal Science* 79:942–948.

Klasing, K.C., Laurin, D.E., Peng, R.K., and Fry, D.M. 1987. Immunologically mediated growth depression in chicks: influence of feed intake, corticosterone and interleukin-1. *Journal of Nutrition* 117:1629–1637.

Klemcke, H.G. 1994. Responses of the porcine pituitary-adrenal axis to chronic intermittent stressor. *Domestic Animal Endocrinology* 11:133–149.

Kubena, L.F., Harvey, R.B., Huff, W.E., and Corrier, D.E. 1989. Influence of ochratoxin A and T-2 toxin singly and in combination on broiler chickens. *Poultry Science* 68:867–872.

Kubena, L.F., Huff, W.E., Harvey, R.B., and Corrier, D.E. 1988. Influence of ochratoxin A and deoxynivalenol on growing broiler chicks. *Poultry Science* 67:253–260.

Lambooj, E., and Van Putten, G. 1993. Transport of pigs. In *Livestock Handling and Transport*. T. Grandin, ed. Wallingford, U.K.: CAB International.

Lauber, J.K., and Shutze, J.V. 1964. Accelerated growth of embryo chicks under the influence of light. *Growth* 28:179–190.

Lay, D.C., Randel, R.D., Friend, T.H., Carroll, J.A., Welsh, T.H., Jenkins, O.C., Neuendorff, D.A., Bushong, D.M., and Kapp, G.M. 1997. Effects of prenatal stress on the fetal calf. *Domestic Animal Endocrinology* 13:73–80.

Leining, K.B., Tucker, H.A., and Kesner, J.S. 1980. Growth hormone, glucocorticoid and thyroxine response to duration, intensity and wavelength of light in prepubertal bulls. *Journal of Animal Science* 51:932–942.

Li, Y.C., Ledoux, D.R., Bermudez, A.J., Fritsche, K.L., and Rottinghaus, G.E. 2000. Effects of moniliformin on performance and immune function of broiler chicks. *Poultry Science* 79:26–32.

Libby, D.A., and Schaible, P.J. 1955. Observations on growth response to antibiotics and arsenic acids in poultry feeds. *Science* 121:733–734.

Lillie, R.J., Sizemore, J.R., and Bird, H.R. 1952. Environment and stimulation of growth of chicks by antibiotics. *Poultry Science* 32:466–475.

Marquardt, R.R., and Frohlich, A.A. 1992. A review of recent advances in understanding ochratoxicosis. *Journal of Animal Science* 70:3968–3988.

Matteri, R.L., and Becker, B.A. 1994. Somatotroph, lactotroph and thyrotroph function in three-week-old gilts reared in a hot or cool environment. *Domestic Animal Endocrinology* 11: 217–226.

May, J.D., and Lott, B.D. 2000. The effect of environmental temperature on growth and feed conversion of broilers to 21 days of age. *Poultry Science* 79:669–671.

May, J.D., Lott, B.D., and Simmons, J.D. 1998. The effect of environmental temperature and body weight on growth rate and feed:gain of male broilers. *Poultry Science* 77:499–501.

Mejía, M., Gonzalez-Iglesias, A., Díaz-Torga, G.S., Villafane, P., Formía, N., Libertun, C., Becú-Villalobos, D., and Lacau-Mengido, I.M. 1999. Effects of continuous ivermectin treatment from birth to puberty on growth and reproduction in dairy heifers. *Journal of Animal Science* 77:1329–1334.

Minton, J.E., Apple, J.K., Parson, K.M., and Blecha, F. 1995. Stress-associated concentrations of plasma cortisol cannot account for reduced lymphocyte function and changes in serum enzymes in lambs exposed to restraint and isolation stress. *Journal of Animal Science* 73:812–817.

Minton, J.E., and Wettemann, R.P. 1988. The influence of duration of photoperiod and hemicastration on growth and testicular and endocrine functions of boars. *Domestic Animal Endocrinology* 5:71–80.

Morrison, S.R. 1983. Ruminant heat stress: Effect on production and means of alleviation. *Journal of Animal Science* 57:1594–1600.

Nyberg, L., Lundström, K., Edfors-Lilja, I., and Rundgren, M. 1988. Effects of transport stress on concentrations of cortisol, corticosteroid-binding globulin and glucocorticoid receptors in pigs with different halothane genotypes. *Journal of Animal Science* 66:1201–1211.

Odetallah, N.H., Ferket, P.R., Garlich, J.D., Elhadri, L., and Kruger, K.K. 2001. Growth and digestive function of turkeys surviving the poult enteritis and mortality syndrome. *Poultry Science* 80:1223–1230.

Pelletier, J. 1973. Evidence for photoperiodic control of prolactin release in rams. *Journal of Reproductive Fertility* 35:143–147.

Perremans, S., Randall, J.M., Rombouts, G., Decuypere, E., and Geers, R. 2001. Effect of whole-body vibration in the vertical axis on cortisol and adrenocorticotropic hormone levels in piglets. *Journal of Animal Science* 79:975–981.

Peters, R.R., Chapin, L.T., Emery, R.S., and Tucker, H.A. 1980. Growth and hormonal response of heifers to various photoperiods. *Journal of Animal Science* 51:1148–1153.

Peters, R.R., Chapin, L.T., Leining, K.B., and Tucker, H.A. 1978. Supplemental lighting stimulates growth and lactation in cattle. *Science* 199:911–912.

Pritzil, M.C., and Kienholz, E.W. 1973. The effect of hydrochloric, sulfuric, phosphoric, and nitric acids in diets for broiler chicks. *Poultry Science* 52:1979–1981.

Purvis, H.T., II, and Whittier, J.C. 1996. Effects of ionophore feeding and anthelmintic administration on age and weight at puberty in spring-born beef heifers. *Journal of Animal Science* 74:736–744.

Rogers, J.A., Branine, M.E., Miller, C.R., Wray, M.I., Bartle, S.J., Preston, R.L., Gill, D.R., Pritchard, R.H., Stilborn, R.P., and Beechtol, D.T. 1995. Effects of dietary virginiamycin on performance and liver abscess incidence in feedlot cattle. *Journal of Animal Science* 73:9–20.

Rohrer, G.A. 2000. Identification of quantitative trait loci affecting birth characters and accumulation of backfat and weight in a Meishan-White Composite resource population. *Journal of Animal Science* 78:2547–2553.

Rozenboim, I., Biran, I., Uni, Z., Robinzon, B., and Halevy, O. 1999. The effect of monochromatic light on broiler growth and development. *Poultry Science* 78:135–138.

Ryan, W.G., Crawford, R.J., Jr., Gross, S.J., and Wallace, D.H. 1997. Assessment of parasite control and weight gain after use of an ivermectin sustained-release bolus in calves. *Journal of American Veterinary Medicine Association* 211:754–756.

Sarko, T.A., Bishop, M.D., and Davis, M.E. 1994. Relationship of air temperature, relative humidity, precipitation, photoperiod, wind speed and solar radiation with serum insulin-like growth factor I (IGF-I) concentration in Angus beef cattle. *Domestic Animal Endocrinology* 11:281–290.

Schanbacher, B.D., and Crouse, J.D. 1980. Growth and performance of growing-finishing lambs exposed to long or short photoperiods. *Journal of Animal Science* 51:943–948.

Schanbacher, B.D., Hahn, G.L., and Nienaber, J.A. 1982. Effects of contrasting photoperiods and temperatures on performance traits of confinement-reared ewe lambs. *Journal of Animal Science* 55:620–626.

Shutze, J.V., Lauber, J.K., Kato, M., and Wilson, W.O. 1962. Influence of incandescent and colored light on chicken embryos during incubation. *Nature* 196:594–595.

Sorensen, P., Su, G., and Kestin, S.C. 1999. The effect of photoperiod:scotoperiod on leg weakness in broiler chickens. *Poultry Science* 78:336–342.

Storer, N.L., and Nelson, T.S. 1968. The effects of various aluminum compounds on chick performance. *Poultry Science* 47: 244–247.

Suk, Y.O., and Washburn, K.W. 1995. Effects of environment on growth, efficiency of feed utilization, carcass fatness, and their association. *Poultry Science* 74:285–296.

Temim, S., Chagneau, A.M., Guillaumin, S., Michel, J., Peresson, R., and Tesseraud, S. 2000. Does excess dietary protein improve growth performance and carcass characteristics in heat-exposed chickens? *Poultry Science* 79:312–317.

Terosky, T.L., Wilson, L.L., Stull, C.L., and Stricklin, W.R. 1997. Effects of individual housing design and size on special-fed holstein veal calf growth performance, hematology, and carcass characteristics. *Journal of Animal Science* 75:1697–1703.

Tucker, H.A., Petitclerc, D., and Zinn, S.A. 1984. The influence of photoperiod on body weight gain, body composition, nutrient intake and hormone secretion. *Journal of Animal Science* 59:1610–1620.

van Heugten, E. 2001. Mycotoxins and other antinutritional factors in swine feeds. In *Swine Nutrition (eds. A.J. Lewis and L.L. Southern)*: CRC Press, Boca Raton, Florida. pp.563–583.

Veldkamp, T., Ferket, P.R., Kwakkel, R.P., Nixey, C., and Noordhuizen, J.P.T.M. 2000. Interaction between ambient temperature and supplementation of synthetic amino acids on performance and carcass parameters in commercial male turkeys. *Poultry Science* 79:1462-1477.

von Borell, E., and Ladewig, J. 1989. Altered adrenocortical response to acute stressors or ACTH(1-24) in intensively housed pigs. *Domestic Animal Endocrinology* 6:299–309.

Waldenstedt, L., Elwinger, K., Thebo, P., and Uggla, A. 1999. Effect of betaine supplement on broiler performance during an experimental coccidial infection. *Poultry Science* 78:182–189.

Weibking, T. S., Ledoux, D. R., Bermudez, A. J., and Rottinghaus, G. E. 1994. Individual and combined effects of feeding Fusarium moniliforme culture material containing known levels of Fumonisin B1, and aflatoxin in the young turkey poult. *Poultry Science* 73:1517–1525.

Weibking, T. S., Ledoux, D. R., Bermudez, A. J., Turk, G. E., Rottinghaus, G. E., Wang, E., and Merrill, A. H. 1993. Effects of feeding Fusarium moniliforme culture material, containing known levels of Fumonisin B1 in the young broiler chick. *Poultry Science* 72:456–466.

Wilson, L.L., Terosky, T.L., Stull, C.L., and Stricklin, W.R. 1999. Effects of individual housing design and size on behavior and stress indicators of special-fed Holstein veal calves. *Journal of Animal Science* 77:1341–1347.

Wisser, L.A., Heinrichs, B.S., and Leach, R.M. 1990. Effect of aluminum on performance and mineral metabolism in young chickens and laying hens. *Journal of Nutrition* 120:493–498.

Wolter, B.F., Ellis, M., Curtis, S.E., Augspurger, N.R., Hamilton, D.N., Parr, E.N., and Webel, D.M. 2001. Effect of group size on pig performance in a wean-to-finish production system. *Journal of Animal Science* 79:1067–1073.

Yahav, S., and Hurwitz, S. 1996. Induction of thermotolerance in male broiler chickens by temperature conditioning at an early age. *Poultry Science* 75:402–406.

Young, B.A. 1981. Cold stress as it affects animal production. *Journal of Animal Science* 52:154–163.

Zinn, S.A., Purchas, R.W., Chapin, L.T., Petitclerc, D., Merkel, R.A., Bergen, W.G., and Tucker, H.A. 1986. Effects of photoperiod on growth, carcass composition, prolactin, growth hormone and cortisol in prepubertal and postpubertal Holstein heifers. *Journal of Animal Science* 63:1804–1815.

17

Performance Enhancement

Colin G. Scanes

The efficiency of production of meat is enhanced using a variety of growth promoters. This chapter considers products that are currently used in commercial production of livestock and poultry in the U.S. and elsewhere. They include sex steroids (estrogens/ androgens) (growth promotants/performance enhancers, particularly in beef cattle), β-adrenergic agonists (growth promotants/performance enhancers, particularly in pigs), antibiotics (including ionophores, copper, and zinc), and probiotics, growth hormone (GH) (somatotropin) The advantages of sex steroids are that they are slow release implants. β-adrenergic agonists and antibiotics are given mixed in the feed. Somatotropin/growth hormone, itself, would have to be administered as relatively short-lived (~2 weeks) implants, but at least one agent that stimulated GH release is orally active.

In addition, it is possible that other uses and/or different agents will gain approval and be used more extensively. These include β-adrenergic agonists as growth promotants/performance enhancers in beef cattle and turkeys, and GH (and/or agents that increase GH release) in growing pigs and beef cattle (see Chapter 5 for detailed discussion) and to improve nitrogen balance in aged horses. Possible transgenic approaches are considered in this chapter and immune approaches are discussed in Chapter 18.

SEX STEROIDS (ESTROGENS/ANDROGENS) AS GROWTH PROMOTANTS

In many mammals, males grow faster than females. This is in part due to the male sex hormones—the androgens, testosterone being the major androgen in most mammals. Androgens increase musculature in rodent models and in people. In fact, they are used illegally by athletes (e.g., weight lifters, etc.). It is reasonable to expect androgens to exert a similar role in livestock and they do. Androgens have been classified as being androgenic and/or anabolic. This is because of their ability to stimulate growth of respectively secondary sexual organs and muscle in the rat. It was unexpected that estrogens would prove able to improve growth and carcass composition in ruminants, particularly beef cattle.

Beef Cattle

History

The synthetic estrogen, diethylstilbestrol (DES), was used as a growth promotant in beef cattle between 1954 and 1979. This follows the pioneering work of Wise Burrows of Iowa State University. It was observed that feeding DES to cattle, at critical concentrations, stimulated growth. There was very widespread use of DES in the beef industry with the DES delivered either as a feed additive or as an implant. Approval of DES required action by the FDA after demonstration that DES worked (efficacy) and was safe (nondetectable DES residues in meat).

The use of DES was subject to considerable controversy. There was concern that DES residue in meat may have negative health effects on consumers, particularly cancer, and perhaps also estrogenic effects, such as feminization of boys. Initial concerns were based on rodent studies and the effects of DES on carcinogenesis/tumor development. The issue came particularly to the fore following reports of genital cancer in the daughters of mothers who had received administration of very high concentrations of DES during their pregnancy to prevent miscarriages. In 1979, DES was withdrawn from the market by the FDA. It might be concluded that this was due to a mix of political pressure and strict interpretation of the regulations. It should be noted that meat from untreated cattle still contains estrogens (of ovarian and adrenal origin) and that plants also contain phytoestrogens.

The history of DES is covered in the book *Cancer from Beef: DES, Federal Food Regulation, and Consumer Confidence* by Alan I. Marcus (1994). This book focuses on the role of advocacy groups, industry, Land Grant Universities' colleges of agriculture/agricultural experiment stations, and federal regulators in the decision by the FDA to ban DES and the political tribulations that led to that decision.

The Present

Sex steroids or synthetic/natural analogues (predominantly estrogens and androgens) are used as growth promotants in cattle. Some progesterone/synthetic progestagens are also used. A number of formulations of these are used (see Table 17.1). They may be synthesized to meet the following criteria. They are identical to natural hormones, such as estradiol (estrogen) or testosterone (androgen). They are very similar to natural hormones but modified to change the absorption and/or half-life in the animal, such as estradiol benzoate or testosterone propionate. They are synthetic androgen (trenbolone acetate) or a progestagen with androgenic activity (melengestrol acetate or MGA). Another example is zeranol. This is a mycotoxin (a toxin produced by the fungus, *Gibberella zeae*) with estrogenic activity. In virtually all cases, the sex steroid or its analogue is given as a slow release implant. Most frequently, implants are placed subcutaneously (under the skin) in the ear. Implanting occurs at different stages of growth (see Table 17.1), with different implants for steers and heifers of different stages of growth.

Mechanism

Estrogens exert their effects through estrogen receptors (ER). It is not clear, however, whether ERα and/or ERβ is involved. Not only does 17β estradiol bind to either receptor but so does zearalenone, albeit at a slightly lower potency. Using in vitro assays (radioreceptor assays using recombinant human ERα or ERβ), zearalenone had potencies of, respectively, 10.3% and 18.3% that of estradiol (Based on Kuiper et al. 1998).

Revalor-S is an implant for steers that contains both estradiol and trenbolone acetate (see Table 17.1). This markedly increases the rate of both gain (e.g., Holgerholt et al. 1992) and of protein accretion (rate of accumulation or "laying down" of protein) in the carcass (e.g., Holgerholt et al. 1992; Johnson et al. 1996a; also see Table 17.2). Accompanying the increased protein accretion is a decline in plasma urea nitrogen, indicating a decline in breakdown/degradation of protein/amino-acids in the whole body (e.g., Holgerholt et al. 1992). However, muscle protein synthesis, degradation, and accretion have been estimated in steers (Table 17.3). Rate of protein accretion is equal to the rate of synthesis minus the rate of degradation.

In practice, the rate of synthesis and accretion are determined with degradation estimated by difference (rate of degradation = rate of synthesis − rate of protein accretion). Thus, it would seem that the small increase in the fractional rate of protein synthesis with no change in protein degradation is responsible for the marked increase in protein accretion.

Implants and Their Effects on Other Hormones

One of the mechanisms by which implants act is by stimulation of the hypothalamo-pituitary GH–IGF-I axis (e.g., see Table 17.4; also see Figure 17.1). Revalor-S–implanted steers show marked improvement in performance (Johnson et al. 1996a) and have elevated concentration of GH-dependent growth factors and GH-dependent growth factor binding protein. There are relatively short-term increases in the circulating concentration of both IGF-I and IGFBP-3 at 21 and 40 days of implantation but not thereafter (Johnson et al. 1996b). Significant increases in basal GH release have not been consistently observed in Revalor-implanted steers (Holgerholt et al. 1992). However, implanted steers did show increased responsiveness to GHRH (Holgerholt et al. 1992).

Implants and Meat Quality

Implants are extensively used in beef cattle due to the improvement in both rate of gain and gain efficiency. There is some evidence that marbling and quality grades might be adversely affected by implants. Duckett and colleagues (1996) performed a meta-analysis of 37 trials and reported a decrease (14.5%) in the number of carcasses grading as choice and a reduction in marbling. More recently the same group reported reduction in marbling and rib-eye steak fatty acids (Duckett et al. 1999; also see Table 17.5).

Table 17.1. Growth promotants used in beef cattle

Brand Name	Composition in Pellet	Dosage in Pellet	Recipient	Source
Ralgro	Zeranol (estrogenic)	36 mg	Beef calves, growing cattle, feedlot steers, and heifers	Schering-Plough Animal Health
Ralgro Magnum	Zeranol (estrogenic)	72 mg	Steers	Schering-Plough Animal Health
Synovex C	Estradiol and progesterone	10 mg+	Beef calves under 400 lb.	Fort Dodge Animal Health
Synovex H	Estradiol and testosterone	20 mg+	Beef heifers over 400 lb.	Fort Dodge Animal Health
Synovex S	Estradiol benzoate and progesterone	20 mg+	Steers over 400 lb.	Fort Dodge Animal Health
Synovex Plus high-performance				Fort Dodge Animal Health
Compudose	Estradiol	24 mg	Heifers and steers	Ivey Animal Health
Component E-S	Progesterone and estradiol benzoate	200 mg+20 mg	Steers over 400 lb.	Ivey Animal Health
Component E-H	Testosterone propionate and estradiol benzoate	200 mg+	Heifers over 400 lb.	Ivey Animal Health
Component T-H	Trenbolone acetate	200 mg	Feedlot heifers	Ivey Animal Health
Component TE-S	Trenbolone acetate and estradiol	120 mg+24 mg	Feedlot steers	Ivey Animal Health
Encore	Estradiol		Confined beef heifers and steers	Ivey Animal Health
Revalor-H	Trenbolone acetate and estradiol	200 mg +20 mg	Heifers	Intervet
Revalor-S	Trenbolone acetate and estradiol	140 mg+28 mg	Steers	Intervet
Finaplex-H	Trenbolone acetate	200 mg	Feedlot heifers	Intervet
Finaplex-S	Trenbolone acetate	140 mg	Feedlot steers	Intervet
MGA200,500	Melengestrol (feed)		Growing cattle	Pharmacia Animal Health

Table 17.2. Effect of trenbolone acetate and/or 17β-estradiol on muscle protein synthesis and degradation in yearling steers (data from Hayden et al., 1992)

	Control	Trenbolone Acetate	17β-Estradiol	Trenbolone Acetate + 17β-Estradiol
ADG (kg) (% change from control)	1.13[a]	1.21[a,b] (+7%)	1.36[b] (+20%)	1.55[c] (+37%)
Skeletal muscle protein accretion g/d (% change from control)	71.6	74.6 (+4%)	95.4 (+33%)	119.5 (+67%)
Whole body muscle protein degradation-N-methyl[τ] histidine excretion as mmoles/d (% change from control)	1.68	1.69 (+1%)	1.70 (+1%)	1.85 (+10%)

[a,b,c]Different superscripts indicate different $p<0.05$.

Table 17.3. Effect of trenbolone acetate and/or 17β-estradiol on growth and protein metabolism in yearling steers (data from Hayden et al., 1992)

	Control	Trenbolone Acetate	17β-Estradiol	Trenbolone Acetate + 17β-Estradiol
Fractional protein synthesis rate %/d (% change from control)	1.65	1.63 (–1%)	1.70 (+3%)	1.77 (+7%)
Fractional protein degradation rate %/d (% change from control)	1.40	1.38 (–1%)	1.39 (–1%)	1.40 (0%)
Fractional protein accretion rate %/d (% change from control)	0.24[x]	0.25[x] (+4%)	0.31[y] (+29%)	0.37[y] (+54%)

[x,y]Significant estradiol effect $p<0.01$.

Table 17.4. Effect of trenbolone acetate and/or 17β-estradiol implants on circulating hormone concentration (mean of 31 and 72 days of implantation) in yearling steers (data from Hayden et al., 1992)

	Control	Trenbolone Acetate	17β-Estradiol	Trenbolone Acetate + 17β-Estradiol
Estradiol pg/ml	7.7	8.6	11.0	12.1
Trenbolone ng/ml	<0.01	0.68	<0.01	1.39
GH ng/ml	3.8	3.4	5.0	3.3
Cortisol (F) ng/ml	2.8	1.9	3.7	1.5

Restrictions on Sale of Beef from Implanted Cattle

The use of hormonal growth promotants is widely used in the United States and Canada. Some beef is produced *without* hormone implants or antibi-

otics (including ionophores). This is sold to specialty markets as natural beef. In addition, beef that is certified as organic does not receive either growth promotants or antibiotics. There is an ongoing trade dispute between the European Union and the U.S. together with Canada on the

Figure 17.1. Mechanisms of action of implants.

i. All androgens ➔ Androgen receptor ➔ Gene Expression ➔ Effects within cell
via released hormones

ii. Aromatizable androgens ➔ Estrogens ➔ Estrogen receptor ➔ Gene Expression

⬇

Effects within cell
and via released hormones
e.g. GH,
GH receptors ⇑
and IGF-I ⇑

iii. Estrogens ➔ Estrogen receptor ➔ Gene Expression ➔ Effects within cell
and via released hormones e.g. GH⇑?;
GH receptors ⇑
and via GH dependant factors:-
IGF-I (⇑) and IGFBP-3 (⇑)

Table 17.5. Effect of implanting on beef meat quality (data from Duckett et al., 1999)

Parameter	Treatment Control	Implant-Single Estradiol (28 mg) + Trenbolone (200 mg)	Implanted Twice
Marbling score	5.48[a]	5.12[b]	4.86[b]
Ribeye area (cm²)	78.9[a]	81.6[b]	88.1[c]
Fatty acids (g)	4.3[a]	3.6[b]	3.4[b]
Cholesterol (% of fatty acids)	0.43	0.49	0.48
Saturated fatty acids (% of fatty acids)	41.6[a]	43.2[b]	43.3[b]
Monounsaturated fatty acids (% of fatty acids)	49.3[a]	47.1[b]	46.9[b]

[a,b,c]Different superscripts indicate different $p<0.05$.

use of hormonal-growth promotants. The European Union does not allow these and has banned the import of North American meat. This has been argued by Canada and the U.S. as being a trade restriction and by the EU to be based on health considerations. The World Trade Organization (WTO) found in favor of the U.S. and Canada.

Sex Steroids and Performance in Pigs

Administration of a mixture of estrogens (DES) and androgens (methyltestostosterone) can influence growth/performance in pigs (Baker et al. 1967; Lucas et al. 1971). The effects on performance include reduced growth rate in barrows but not gilts;

improved feed:gain efficiency in both barrows and gilts, in some but not all trials; more muscling/lean with increased loin-eye area in both barrows and gilts; reduced fat—e.g., backfat thickness in both barrows and gilts but lower palatability of meat; and increased adverse aroma and flavor of pork. Growth promoting implants for pigs have not been developed because the treatment adversely influences meat quality.

Sex Steroids and Poultry Growth

The administration of androgens and/or estrogens to chickens *reduces* their rate of growth. Not surprisingly, these hormones are not used commercially in production of broiler or roaster chickens. In contrast to the situation in chickens, turkeys do respond to androgens with marked increases in growth rate, particularly of muscle, and with reductions in adipose tissue. However, androgens alone or with estrogens are not employed in turkey production.

β-AGONISTS

β-adrenergic agonists are compounds such as epinephrine (adrenaline) and norepinephrine (noradrenaline). The structures of some β-adrenergic agonists, such as ractopamine (Paylean), are shown in Figure 17.2. The effect of β-adrenergic agonists, such as ractopamine, on performance is direct action on muscle and adipose tissue (Table 17.6). Cimaterol (1 ppm) resulted in the following improved carcass composition in pigs (Moser et al. 1986):

- Increased muscle/lean, longissimus area, up 8.7%
- Decreased carcass fat:
  - Average backfat, down 9.3%
  - 10th rib fat depth, down 14.2%
  - Ham fat, down 7.9%
  - Loin fat, down 11.6%

L-644,969 (1 ppm) resulted in the following improved carcass composition in finishing steers (Moloney et al. 1990):

- Increased growth rate, up 16.7%
- Improved feed:gain, up 24.5%
- Increased carcass weight, up 9.3%
- Improved dressing percentage, up 4.0% (absolute)
- Increased muscle/lean:
  - M. Longissimus area, up 33.9%
  - M. Longissimus lean, up 13.1%
  - M. Longissimus protein, up? 4.3%
- Decreased carcass fat:
  - M. Longissimus fat, down 29.0% (by dissection)
  - M. Longissimus fat, down 50.0% (by analyis)

There is little involvement of changes in the release of growth related hormones (GH, IGF-I, and/or IGFBPs).

β-Adrenergic Receptors and Signal Transduction

β-adrenergic agonists act by binding to β-adrenergic receptors (also see Table 17.7). Three β-adrenergic receptors have been identified, namely β_1-, β_2-, and β_3-adrenergic receptors (β_1, β_2, and β_3AR), and a fourth might exist (β_4AR). The structure of these is established. They have seven transmembrane domains and are coupled to stimulatory G-proteins (reviewed e.g. Strosberg 1997). The sequence of amino-acid residues in livstock β_1, β_2, and β_3AR has been deduced from cDNA (porcine β_1AR: Cao et al. 1998; β_2AR: Liang et al. 1997; β_3AR: Smith et al. 2001) (bovine, ovine, and caprine β_3AR: Forrest and Hickford 2000). Both β_1AR and β_2AR bind ractopamine and other β-adrenergic agonists (Liang and Mills 2001; also see Table 17.7). The proportion of β_1, β_2, and β_3 adrenergic receptors in pig adipose tissue—based on β_1,

Table 17.6. Effect of feeding Paylean 9 (the β-agonist, ractopamine) (at 10 ppm) on performance of finishing swine

Feed:gain efficiency	↑ 7.8–15.2%
Average daily gain	↑ 6.3–20.6%
Carcass weight	↑ Increase of 10.6 lb. (4.8 kg)
Dressing percentage	↑ 1.3%
Fat-free lean estimate	↑ 1.3%

Source: Elanco Web site 2001 (http://www.elanco.com/us/products/paylean/paylean.html).

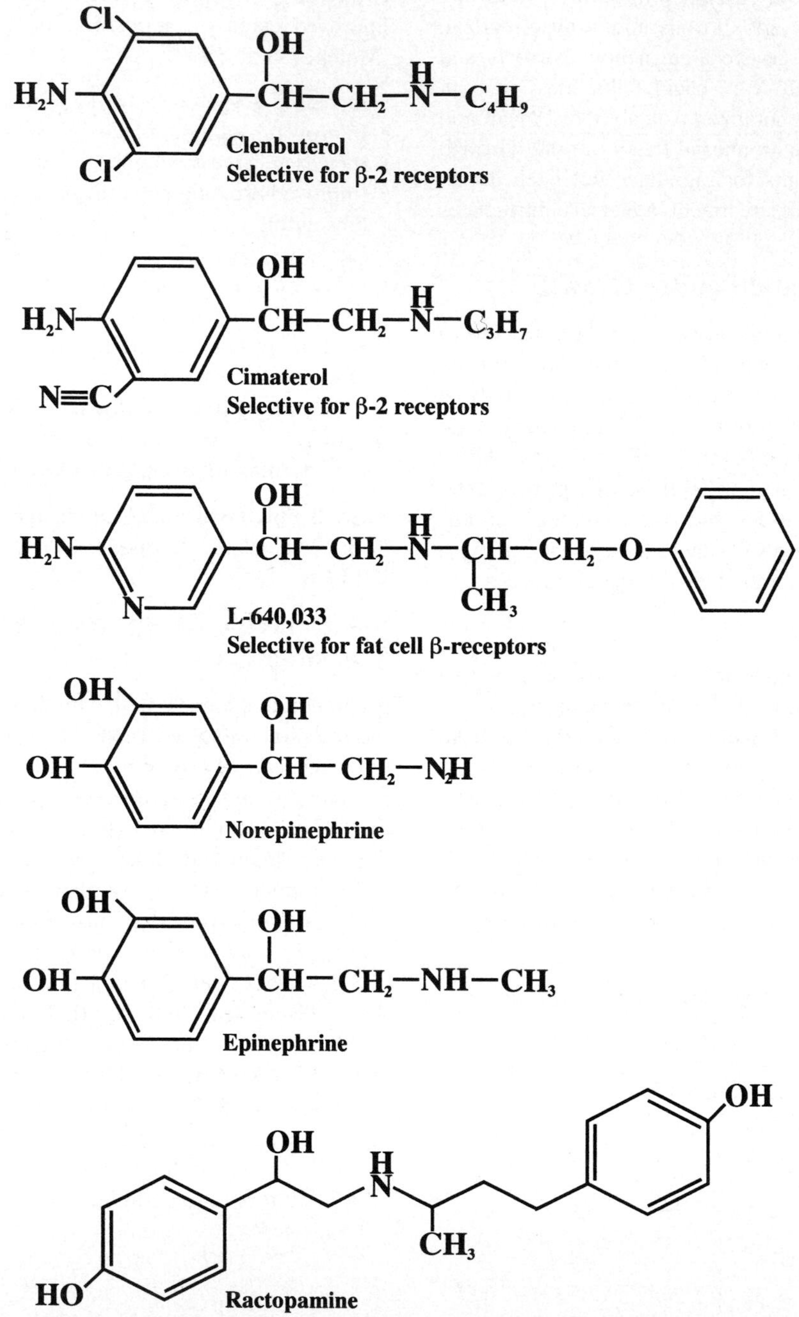

Figure 17.2. Structure of β-adrenergic agonists.

β$_2$ and β$_3$AR mRNA as determined by ribonuclease protection assay (McNeel and Mersmann 1999)—is the following: β$_1$AR 73%, β$_2$AR 20%, and β$_3$AR 7%.

The mechanism of action of β-adrenergic agonists is summarized in Figure 17.3. The β-adrenergic ago-

nist binds to β-adrenergic receptors on the surface of the adipose or muscle cells. This results (via G-proteins) in activation on another cell membrane associated with protein, adenylate cyclase. This, in turn, catalyzes the formation of cyclic AMP (cAMP) from

Table 17.7. Comparison of various ligands (binding affinities) for β-adrenergic receptors: porcine β₂-receptor expressed in Chinese hamster ovary cells or β receptors in pig adipose tissue (adapted from Liang and Mills, 2001).

	Ligand	Subtype Selectivity	Porcine β_2AR	Pig Adipose β Receptor(s)
Agonist				
	(−)Isoproterenol	1,2	340	66–280
	(+)Isoproterenol	1,2	9,820	750–2,000
	Epinephrine	1,2	1,060	9,993
	Norepinephrine	1,2	10,538	17,347
	Dobutamine	1	695	2,500
	Salbutamol	2	203	2,19
	Terbutaline	2	2,030	5,475
	Zinterol	2	13	
	BRL 37344	3	122	20 and 5,000
	Clenbuterol	2	11	5–154
	L-644,969	2	12	320
	Ractopamine	1	131	517
Antagonist				
	Propranolol	1,2	1.2	3.5
	Alprenolol	1,2	1.7	2.9
	Oxprenolol	1,2	0.9	
	ICI 118,551	2	48	80
	CGP 20712A	1	404	30
	Betaxolol	1	658	
	Bisoprolol	1	1,491	

ATP. The cAMP activates protein kinase A, which phosphorylates (activating or in some cases inactivating) key metabolic enzymes and changes gene expression of key proteins, including metabolic enzymes

β-Adrenergic Agonists and Growth/Performance in Livestock

There has been a very significant research effort on the effects of β-adrenergic agonists on growth and performance of livestock. A number of β-adrenergic agonists were used as different companies had proprietary interests in them. These include ractopamine (Elanco), clenbuterol, cimaterol (American Home Products), and L-644,969 (Merck Animal Health). At this time, the use of only one β-adrenergic agonist, ractomamine, has been approved in the U.S. by the FDA and only in finisher pigs. This is available commercially from Elanco

under the trade name, Paylean. It is likely that ractopamine acts via binding to β_1AR and β_2AR and perhaps β_3AR (Table 17.7).

Paylean 9 (Ractopamine)

In 2000, the FDA in the U.S. approved use of the β-agonist, ractopamine, for "finishing pigs" (150–240 lb). There are marked improvements in performance (see Table 17.8) by presence of ractopamine (10 ppm) in the feed. The addition of β-agonist to feed increases feed to gain efficiency, growth rate (average daily gain), carcass yield (dressing percentage), lean growth, and loin-eye area (10th rib), and decreases carcass fat and 10th rib backfat. The marked positive effect of ractopamine (Paylean 9) on pigs is exemplified in Tables 17.6 and 17.8. It is possible that ractopamine will be approved for turkeys and beef cattle, and for longer periods in pigs.

Figure 17.3. Mechanism of action of β-adrenergic agonists.

Cimaterol (1 ppm.) improved carcass composition in pigs:
- Increased muscle/lean:
- Longissimus area ↑ 8.7%
- Decreased carcass fat:
  - average backfat ↓ 9.3% ,
  - 10th rib fat depth ↓ 14.2%,
  - ham fat ↓ 7.9%,
  - loin fat ↓ 11.6%

(Moser *et al.*, 1986).

L-644,969 (1 ppm) improved carcass composition in finishing steers:
- Increased growth rate ↑ 16.7%;
- Improved feed to gain ↑ 24.5%;
- Increased carcass weight ↑ 9.3%;
- Improved dressing percentage ↑ 4.0% (absolute);
- Increased muscle/lean:
  - M. Longissimus area ↑ 33.9%;
  - M. Longissimus lean ↑ 13.1%;
  - M. Longissimus protein ↑? 4.3%.
  - Decreased carcass fat:
  - M. Longissimus fat ↓ 29.0% (by dissection);
  - M. Longissimus fat ↓ 50.0% (by analysis);

(Moloney *et al.*, 1990)

Table 17.8. Effect of feeding Paylean 9 (the β-agonist, ractopamine) (at 10 ppm) on performance of pigs slaughtered at 107 and 125 kilograms (235 or 275 lb.) (data from Crome et al., 1996)

	85 to 125 kg		68 to 107 kg	
	Control	Ractopamine 10ppm	Control	Ractopamine 10ppm
Average daily gain kg (% increase over control)	0.81	0.91(+12%)	0.84	0.95**(+13%)
Feed:gain ratio (% decrease from control)	3.52	3.07 (–13%)	3.87	3.22 (–17%)
Carcass dressing percentage	76.8	78.0	77.6	78.6**
10th rib fat—cm (% decrease from control)	2.62	2.44 (–7%)	3.18	2.89** (–8%)
Longissumus dorsi muscle area cm^2 (% increase over control)	34.7	40.3 (+16%)	35.2	42.5** (+21%)

**p<0.01 Significant ractopamine effect at both weights.

Adrenergic Agonists and Lipid Metabolism in Pigs

β-Adrenergic agonists profoundly influence fat metabolism, increasing lipolysis (breakdown of triglyceride) and reducing lipogenesis (fatty acid synthesis). Together, this reduces the amount of triglyceride stored in the adipose cell and hence the volume/weight of fat.

Lipolysis

Lipolysis or breakdown of triglycerides to fatty acids and glycerol is increased by the following β-adrenergic agonists: isoproterenol (Rule et al. 1987); epinephrine, isoproterenol, fenoterol, and dolbutamine (Hu et al. 1987); ractopamine but not clenbuterol (Liu et al. 1989); isoproterenol, cimaterol, ractopamine but not clenbuterol (Peterla et al. 1990).

Lipogenesis

Lipogenesis (synthesis of fatty acids) is inhibited by most β-adrenergic agonists: epinephrine, ractopamine but not clenbuterol(Mills and Liu 1990); isoproterenol, cimaterol, ractopamine but not consistently by clenbuterol (Peterla et al. 1990).

β-Adrenergic Agonists and Muscle/Protein Metabolism

β-adrenergic agonists consistently increase muscle weight in livestock species (see Figure 17.3, Tables 17.6, 17.8 through 17.10). For instance, clenbuterol (10 ppm) increased carcass protein in steers from 15.3% (control) to 17.3% (Ricks et al. 1984) with concomitant decreases in circulating concentrations of blood urea nitrogen. In pigs, there is clear evidence that the β-adrenergic agonist, ractopamine, increases muscle protein accretion by stimulating protein synthesis (see Table 17.9) (Bergen et al. 1989; Helferich et al. 1990). Although this is counter-intuitive, there may also be some increase in muscle protein degradation (see Table 17.9).

In ruminants, there is some evidence that β-adrenergic agonists increase muscle weight/protein content (Table 17.10, for example), at least partially by increasing protein synthesis. For instance, a marked tendency for increased protein synthesis was evident in lambs receiving clenbuterol (Claeys et al. 1989) (see Table 17.10). Similarly, clenbuterol decreased arterial concentrations of α-amino nitrogen in steers and increased tissue uptake of α-amino nitrogen (Eisemann et al. 1988).

β-*Adrenergic Agonists and Muscle Metabolism In Vitro*

Ractopamine, albeit at very high concentrations, increases protein synthesis by rat myotubes in vitro (Anderson et al. 1990), because of increases in ^{35}S-methionine incorporation into total proteins, 43-kDa proteins, and myosin heavy chain (Anderson et

Figure 17.4. Effect of β-adrenergic agonists on lipid metabolism in pigs.

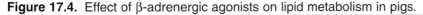

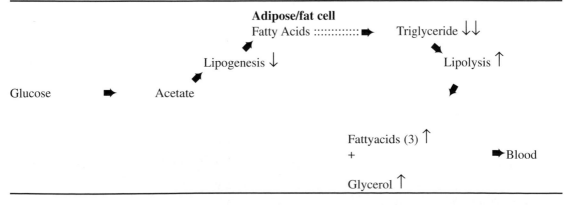

Table 17.9. Effect of the β-adrenergic agonist, ractopamine[1], on protein metabolism in the semi-tendinosus muscle in pigs

Parameter	Treatment			
	Control		β-adrenergic Agonist Ractopamine	Reference
Muscle weight	367	*	394	Bergen et al., 1989
Fractional synthesis (%/d)	4.4	+	6.1	Bergen et al., 1989
Fractional degradation rate (%/d)	3.4		4.9	Bergen et al., 1989
Fractional accretion rate (%/d)	1.0		1.2	Bergen et al., 1989
Synthesis rate (g/d)	2.8		4.3	Bergen et al., 1989
Degradation rate (g/d)	2.2		3.4	Bergen et al., 1989
Accretion rate (g/d)	0.64		0.86	Bergen et al., 1989
Synthesis				
Skeletal muscle a-actin				
Fractional synthesis rate (%/d)	2.9	*	4.5	Helferich et al., 1990
Skeletal muscle α-actin RNA				
Arbitrary units	1	*	2	Helferich et al., 1990
Degradation				
Calcium dependent protease	0.55		0.51	Bergen et al., 1989
Cathepsin B	24		24	Bergen et al., 1989
Cathepsin L	54	*	69	Bergen et al., 1989
Cathepsin H	142		160	Bergen et al., 1989

+$p<0.1$; *$p<0.05$.
[1] 20 ppm ractopamine was administered via the diet.

Table 17.10. Effect of the β-adrenergic agonist, clenbuterol, on in vivo muscle protein metabolism in lambs (data from Claeys et al., *1989*)

Parameters	Treatment		
	Control		β-Adrenergic Agonist
Semitendinosus muscle			
Weight (g)	52.4	*	65.2
Protein content (g/d)	11	+	15
Protein synthesis (g/d)	0.8	+	1.4
Protein degradation (g/d)	0.6		0.9
Longissimus			
Weight (g)	227		259
Protein content (g/d)	53	*	64
Protein synthesis (g/d)	5.8		6.6
Protein degradation (g/d)	3.3		4.6

+$p<0.1$; *$p<0.05$.

al. 1990). Other investigators have not observed this stimulatory effect (e.g., Reeds et al. 1986).

β-*Adrenergic Agonists and Blood Flow*

As might be anticipated, β-adrenergic agonists affect both heart rate and blood flow to organs. For instance, Eisemann and her colleagues (1988) observed chronic increases in both heart rate and blood flow to the hindquarters of steers receiving clebuterol for 9 days.

Illegal Use of β-Adrenergic Agonists

There have been documented problems of illegal use of β-adrenergic agonists in both the European Union and the United States. In the European Union (EU), β-adrenergic agonists have not been approved as growth promotants or repartitioning agents. In Spain in 1990 and 1991, there were two outbreaks of food poisoning from eating liver from cattle/calves that had received clenbuterol illegally (Martinez-Navarro 1990; Pulce et al. 1991). In the U.S., there have been cases of β-adrenergic agonists used in show cattle and of successful prosecutions for their use illegally as feed supplements (Mitchell and Dunnavan 1998). These events have led both the EU and U.S. regulatory agencies to have strict surveillance and monitoring. The incidence of illegal use of β-adrenergic agonists has fallen dramatically in the EU (Kuiper et al. 1998). While in the United States, the FDA has "policed" the industry with rigorous prosecutions to ensure that illegal use is not occurring (Mitchell and Dunnavan 1998).

ANTIBIOTICS (INCLUDING IONOPHORES, COPPER, ZINC)

Stokstad, Jukes, and colleagues (1949) first demonstrated that antibiotics (chlortetracycline) stimulated growth in chicks and young pigs. This effect is found in all domestic animals. Among the antimicrobial agents that are effective in increasing growth rate (and approved for use in the U.S.) are antibiotics including bacitracin, chlortetracycline, neomycin, oxytetracycline, penicillin, tylosin, and virginiamycin, and chemotherapeutics such as the arsenicals, arsanilic acid, roxarsone and carbadox, sulfametazine, and sulfathiazone.

Antimicrobial agents are widely employed by the livestock industry in the United States and many other countries. This is particularly the case with the prevalence of confinement facilities for animal production. Antimicrobial agents undergo regulatory approval by government agencies/departments to establish their safety. In the U.S., the FDA provides approval of individual and combinations of agents based on both the safety and efficacy of these antimicrobial agents. To reduce the problems of residues from antimicrobial agents, withdrawal periods may be required. There is considerable concern in both North America and Europe that the practice of using antibiotics in livestock production leads to the development of antibiotic resistance in bacteria that cause human disease.

Antibiotics consistently improve growth rate and feed:gain efficiency in livestock. Antibiotics exert a greater effect in studies on farms compared to research stations (e.g., universities, and agricultural experiment stations). This may reflect differences in management and sanitation. Cromwell (2001) reviewed many studies of the efficacy of antibiotics in young pigs (7–~26 kg). Combining data from 137 research station trials and 99 farm trials demonstrated improvements in average daily gain in the following manner: research station trials 16.7% and on-farm trials 26.4%; and for feed:gain efficiency: research station trials 6.8%; on-farm trials 11.5% (calculated from Cromwell 2001). Antibiotics are extensively employed for poultry and swine production. Marked improvements in performance (growth rate, feed to gain ratio) are consistently observed with subtherapeutic levels of antibiotics (see Table 17.11 for example study). Virginiamycin is used as a growth promoting antibiotic in pigs and poultry. In addition, it can improve feed efficiency and average daily gain in cattle (e.g., Rogers et al. 1995). It is probable that it exerts its effect in cattle by reducing lactic acid production in the rumen.

Ionophores

Ionophores influence growth in ruminants by shifting microbial fermentation in the rumen with reductions in the formation of methane together with acetate and butyrate but increases in propionate, the latter being the major gluconeogenic precursor. An example of an ionophore is monensin. This, marketed by Elanco as Rumensin, improves feed efficiency and prevents coccidiosis in cattle. Monensin also prevents coccidiosis in poultry (marketed under the name Coban). Tables 17.12 and 17.13 illustrate the effect of monensin on growth and feed efficiency in cattle.

Anthelmintics

In geographical areas where there are significant bovine nematodes present in pastures, anthelmintics

Table 17.11. Effect of antibiotics on the performance for five weeks of young pigs (34 days old) and circulating concentrations of the growth related hormone, IGF-I and IGFBP-3 (data from or calculated from Hathaway et al. 1996)

	Control		ASP-250
Gain—kg/d (as % change from control)	0.56	**	0.67 (+19%)
Feed:gain (as % change from control)	1.77	*	1.66 (−6.5%)
IGF-I—ng/ml (as % change from control)	105	***	133 (+27%)
IGFBP-3—units/ml (as % change from control)	10.5	*	5 (+59%)

*p<0.05; **p<0.01; ***p<0.001.

Diet supplemented with ASP-250 is chlortetracycline at 22.7ppm, sulfamethazine at 22.7 ppm, and penicillin at 11.4 ppm.

Table 17.12. Effect of monensin and tylosin on growth and feed efficiency in cattle (data from Stock et al., 1995)

	Treatment		
Parameter	Control		Monensin/Tylosin
Average daily gain kg	1.42	*	1.46
Feed:gain	6.21	**	5.96

*p<0.05; **p<0.01.

Table 17.13. Effects of feeding an ionophore (Monensin-Rumensin) and an anthelmintic (Ivermectin-Ivomec) on the performance of beef heifers (data from Purvis and Whittier, 1996)

	Control	Monensin	Ivermectin	Monensin + Ivermectin
Average daily gain (ADG) in kg/d	0.84	0.87	0.84	0.86
Feed:gain (as % change from control)	8.7[a]	7.5[c] (−13.5%)	8.1[b] (−7.3%)	7.2[c] (−16.7%)
Age at puberty, d	433[a]	425[b]	424[b]	425[b]

[a,b,c]Different superscripts indicate different p<0.05.

Dietary treatment for ~185 days, starting at 269 days old.

have marked stimulatory effects on growth rate. Discussion of the impact of parasitic infections is also discussed in Chapter 16.

Copper

The growth promoting effects of the addition of copper salts to the diets of young pigs is well established.

Table 17.14 provides an example of a study in which copper sulfate was added to the diet of young pigs and growth and feed-gain efficiency determined. Although it is well established that copper exerts a marked stimulatory effect on growth (17.14), the mechanism of action is not fully established. It is frequently assumed that the copper is affecting the intestinal microflora.

Table 17.14. Effect of copper sulfate on growth in weanling pigs (31 days) (data from Apgar et al., 1995)

	Treatment		
	Copper Sulfate (mg/kg diet)		
Parameter	0	100	200
Growth—average daily gain (as % of control)			
Weeks 1–2[a]	138 (100%)	181 (131%)	188 (136%)
Weeks 3–5[a]	403 (100%)	421 (105%)	452 (112%)
Feed efficiency (feed:gain)			
Weeks 1–2[a]	1.95	1.76	1.60
Weeks 3–5	1.71	1.80	1.70

[a]Linear copper effect $p < 0.05$.

Zinc

High concentrations of zinc in the diet enhance the performance of postweaning pigs (e.g., Poulsen 1989; Holm 1990; Hahn and Baker 1993; Carlson 1999; Hill et al. 2001). Table 17.15 shows the results of an extensive study (>50 replicate animals per treatment) on the effects of zinc oxide on postweaning growth. It would appear that zinc is acting both "as a growth promotant and as an aid in preventing postweaning diarrhea" (Hill et al. 2001). The mechanism of action of zinc is not fully understood. Probably several distinct aspects of growth promoting effects of zinc include ensuring the animal is zinc replete and changing in gut microorganisms.

PROBIOTICS

Probiotic bacteria are employed as feed supplements (reviewed Cromwell 2001). These probiotic microorganisms are either organisms that are widespread in the intestinal lumen or yogurt starter strains. These meet the requirements of the FDA as being "generally recognized as safe" (GRAS) and are referred to as *direct-fed microbials* (reviewed Cromwell 2001).

Table 17.15. Effect of zinc oxide on the performance of pigs (data from Hill et al., 2001)

Period	Age of Weaning	Control (0)		ZnO (2.0 g/kg)[+]
Gain				
0–28 days	<15 days	230	*	298
0–28 days	>21 days	466	*	513
Feed:Gain				
0–28 days	<15 days	1.61	**	1.50
0–28 days	<21 days	1.39	*	1.32

[+]Maximally effective dose.
*$p < 0.05$; **$p < 0.01$.

Lactobacilli and Poultry

It has been suggested that treatment of poultry with *Lactobacilli* (*Lactobacilli* including *Lactobacillus acidophilus*) as a probiotic would improve growth in a manner similar to antibiotics (Tortuero 1973) and promote the quality/safety of poultry products by reducing intestinal microorganisms e.g., coliforms, *Salmonella* (e.g., Adler and DaMassa 1980). The evidence for a growth promoting effect is somewhat equivocal with small but nonstatistically significant increases in growth observed in poultry. For instance, in turkey poults, a 3.1% improvement in growth was reported with *Lactobacilli* as a probiotic; this is identical to that observed with zinc bacitracin (Francis et al. 1978). Similarly in young chickens, a trend for a 2.5% increase in growth was observed with *Lactobacilli* (Adler and DaMassa 1980).

There is strong evidence that newly hatched chicks receiving cultures of cecal microorganisms from adult chickens show decreased colonization of *Salmonella* and pathogens (Nurmi and Rantala 1973; Snoeyenbos et al. 1978; Barnes et al., 1979). *Lactobacilli* and other probiotic microorganisms may reduce *Salmonella* and coliforms in young poultry by competitive exclusion, competing with the pathogen for binding sites on the intestine and by producing antibacterial substances (specific, e.g., Gusils et al. 1999a, 1999b; nonspecific such as volatile fatty acids, e.g., Barnes et al. 1979).

Growth Hormone Axis Hormones

The hormones of the hypothalamo-pituitary GH-IGF-I axis [namely, releasing hormone (GHRH), GH and IGF-I] play a critical role in the control of growth (see Chapter 5). Moreover, in cattle, GH is widely employed to increase milk yield and the efficiency of milk production (see Chapter 12).

There is substantial evidence for improvements in gain, feed efficiency, and carcass characteristics in pigs and cattle (see Chapter 5). At present, GH is, however, not approved to enhance growth/performance in the U.S. or most of the rest of the world. This is in part a commercial, not a regulatory, decision. It is unlikely that bGH will be marketed for beef cattle at a price that is below that for improvement of lactation efficiency in dairy cattle. Similarly, despite pGH improving growth/performance of pigs, it must compete with β-adrenergic agonists. These can be added to the feed rather than injected and may be less expensive to produce. The improvements in gain, feed efficiency, and carcass characteristics in pigs and cattle are due to increased muscle and reduced fat due, in turn, to decreased lipogenesis.

Growth Hormone

Porcine GH (Reporcin produced by Southern Cross Biotechnology in Australia) has been approved for use in pigs in Australia. Equine GH is approved and marketed by BresaGen in Australia as EquiGen. Its approved use is to aid nitrogen retention in aged horses. In addition, it is undergoing clinical trials to promote wound healing and recovery from injury. BresaGen is also conducting trials with canine GH as an agent to aid nitrogen retention in aged dogs.

Growth Hormone Releasing Hormone (GHRH)

The administration of a potent analogue of GHRH as twice daily injections has been found to improve growth, performance, and some but not all indices of carcass composition. For instance, Dubreil and colleagues (1990) reported that GHRH administration improves growth and performance of pigs:

- Increased growth rate, ↑ 6.8%
- Improved feed:gain, ↑ 25.9%
- Tendency for decreased carcass weight, ↓ 2.3%
- Reduced dressing percentage, ↑ 1.8% (absolute)
- Increased muscle/lean:
  - Loin area, ↑ 12.6%
  - Longissimus protein, ↑ 2.9%
  - Tendency for reduced fat, Longissimus, ↓ 28.9%

Similarly, GHRH administration was accompanied by marked improvement in carcass characteristics together with a reduction in fat in growing pigs (Pommier et al. 1990). As is the case with GH, GHRH has not been approved to enhance performance in livestock.

TRANSGENIC APPROACHES AND GROWTH

Biotechnology has been employed extensively since the 1930s to improve the genetics of animals. This in turn has the objective, in the case of livestock species, of improving the efficiency of production (particularly growth) and the quality of meat (muscle growth). For horses, the goal has been excellent athletic performance. A variety of techniques have been successfully introduced. These are illustrated in Table 17.16. Transgenic approaches offer tremendous scope for the future. It is now possible to develop a germline transgenic animal in which the transgene is incorporated into the genome in a stable manner and is capable of transfer to subsequent generations through reproduction. "Geneticists have long sought the ability to add or subtract individual genes from an organism's genome, or to be able to alter the level of expression of a targeted, developmentally and tissue-specific manner. The development of transgenic technology realized the possibilities." (Sokol and Murray 1996).

Potential uses of transgenic livestock have been reviewed by Pinkert and Murray (1999). These uses include increased efficiency of production, improved disease resistance, xenotransplantation, and livestock producing novel pharmaceuticals (*molecular "pharming"*)—e.g., production of human blood clotting factor IX (Schnieke et al. 1997) and human α_1-antitrypsin (reviewed Pinkert and Murray 1999). Transgenic livestock have been produced by microinjection of a gene to the egg pronucleus or of the nucleus from a cell that has been transformed in vitro and placed into an enucleated egg.

Microinjection of Genes into the Egg Pronucleus

Microinjection of the egg pronucleus with multiple copies of the putative transgene, the gene of interest together with appropriate promoters, was the initial technique employed in mice (Gordon et al. 1980) and livestock (cattle, sheep, and pigs) (reviewed Pursel and Rexroad 1993). Microinjection of eggs from livestock has inherent problems. Injection of fluid into the egg, along with the transgenes, can cause breaks in the chromosome. There is incorporation of the transgenes (during chromosome repair) at random integration sites (reviewed Wilmut et al. 1999).

Microinjection of Nuclei from Transformed Cells into Enucleated Eggs

Transgenic sheep have also been produced by targeted insertion of the transgene into somatic cells followed by nuclear transfer (McCreath et al. 2000). Similarly, pigs have been cloned using fetal fibroblast nuclei microinjected into enucleated oocytes and development induced by electroactivation (Onishi et al. 2000) or nuclear transfer from adult somatic cells (Polejaeva et al. 2000). Pig cloning has also been successful using the approach of microinjection of fetal fibroblast nuclei in denucleated ova (Onishi et al. 2000).

Cloning Livestock

There has been tremendous progress cloning cattle and sheep. Sheep have been cloned using nuclear transfer from cultured cells (Campbell et al. 1996), including cells derived from embryonic, fetal, and

Table 17.16. Biotechnology approaches and their application to domestic animals

Approach	Use
Artificial insemination (semen obtained and placed inseminated into cervix or uterus of recipient)	Very widely employed for cattle, pig, turkey, and some use for horses (e.g., in Standardbred but not Thoroughbred breeds) and broiler chickens.
Ova/embryo transfer (fertilized ova from a multiply ovulation female are placed in uterus/oviduct of recipient females)	Employed for cattle for improved production and maintaining genetic diversity (maintaining the germplasm of rare breeds).
Transgenic (foreign gene "inserted" in genome)	Successfully accomplished in sheep, cattle, pigs, and chickens as a research tool and for the production of pharmaceuticals.
Cloning (nucleus of adult cells inserted in denucleated ovum or embryonic ovum or embryonic stem cells to produce viable conceptus and offspring)	Successfully accomplished in sheep, pigs, and cattle. Potential for duplicating animals with unique or superior germplasm, particularly when coupled with trangenics.
Marker-assisted selection (identifying gene for specific trait and selecting for that gene)	Used for pigs and other livestock to improve production/quality traits.

adult mammary gland sources (Wilmut et al. 1997). Cloned transgenic calves have been produced using nuclear transfer from fetal fibroblast genetically modified with a marker gene (Cibelli et al. 1998). This approach appears to be considerably more efficient (see Table 17.17).

Transgenic Poultry

Producing transgenic poultry has proven to be more difficult than with livestock. This is due, in part, to the "laid" egg (prior to incubation) containing ~60,000 cells. Approaches that have been employed include retroviral insertion of transgenes (Bosselman et al. 1989) and transfer of genes into premordal germ cells (Wentworth et al. 1996; Petitte et al. 1997) or blastodermal cells in culture (Etches et al. 1997) or the entire embryo (reviewed Simkiss 1997). In the case of cells in culture, these are then replaced in developing embryos. In all cases, chimera may result. There then needs to be determination of which chimera and/or the next generation of individual chicks contain/express the transgene. Another approach involves injection of a gene of interest into a recently ovulated egg following by ex ova (in vitro) incubation (reviewed Bulfield 1997). The efficiency of producing transgenic gametes from chimeric chickens can be improved if the recipient's primoidal germ cells are destroyed by radiation or cytotoxic drugs (busulfan) (reviewed Simkiss 1997).

GH, GHRH, and IGF-I as Transgenes in Livestock

Transgenic livestock expressing GH have been successfully produced (reviewed Pursel et al. 1990; Pursel and Rexroad 1993). Some groups of transgenic pigs showed improved growth and feed efficiency (Pursel et al. 1989). There were, however, significant health problems, particularly in the adult (potential founder/breeder stock) with lameness, gastric ulcers, cardiomegaly, dermatitis, and reproductive problems (Pursel et al. 1989; reviewed Pursel et al. 1990). The abnormal animal appearance together with real and perceived welfare issues created a problem with the public, particularly in Europe. It is not clear the extent to whether the health problems result from the following: pharmacological levels of GH in inappropriate tissues expressing GH, wrong timing of expression/release (not in the normal episodic pattern), or promoter(s) that do not restrict expression of GH transgenes to the period during growth when GH could stimulate growth while not adversely affecting health (Pursel et al. 1990)

There have only been a few cases of sheep or pigs that express transgenes for either GHRH or IGF-I (reviewed Pursel and Rexroad 1993). This reflected the technical difficulties in producing transgenic livestock where there is expression of the transgene and translation to yield a biologically active protein/peptide. Moreover, there have been health problems and mortality (reviewed Pursel and Rexroad 1993).

An alternative approach has also been found to increase circulating concentrations of GH and hence growth by transfecting muscle cells with DNA for a protease-resistant GHRH as part of an injectable muscle-specific vector (Draghia-Akli et al. 1999).

Transgenic Fish

Transgenic fish have been produced that express GH and show enhanced growth (e.g., Martinez et al. 1996, 2000; Rahman et al. 1998).

REFERENCES

Adler, H.E., and DaMassa, A.J. 1980. Effect of ingested lactobacilli on *Salmonella infantis* and *Escherichia coli* and on intestinal flora, pasted vents, and chick growth. *Avian Diseases* 24:868–878.

Anderson, P.T., Helferich, W.G., Parkhill, L.C., Merkel, R.A., and Bergen, W.G. 1990. Ractopamine increases total and myofibrillar protein synthesis in cultured rat myotubes. *Journal of Nutrition* 120:1677–1683.

Table 17.17. Efficiency of production of transgenic livestock (based on Cibelli et al., 1998)

Technique	# of Embryos	Recipient Cows	# of Transgenic offspring
Micro-injection	500	500	1
Nuclear transfer from transformed cell line	9	4	1

Apgar, G.A., Kornegay, E.T., Lindemann, M.D., and Notter, D.R. 1995. Evaluation of copper sulfate and a copper lysine complex as growth promoters for weanling swine. *Journal of Animal Science* 73:2640–2646.

Baker, D.H., Jordan, C.E., Waitt, W.P., and Gouwens, D.W. 1967. Effect of a combination of diethylstilbesterol and methyltestosterone, sex and protein level on performance and carcass characteristics of finisher swine. *Journal of Animal Science* 26:1059–1066.

Barnes, E.M., Impey, C.S., and Stevens, B.J.H. 1979. Factors affecting the incidence and anti-salmonella activity of the anaerobic cecal flora of the young chick. *Journal of Hygiene* 82:263–283.

Bergen, W.G., Johnson, S.E., Skjaerlund, D.M., Babiker, A.S., Ames, N.K., Merkel, R.A., and Anderson, D.B. 1989. Muscle protein metabolism in finishing pigs fed ractopamine. *Journal of Animal Science* 67:2255–2262.

Bosselman, R.A., Hsu, R.-Y., Boggs, T., Hu, S., Bruszewski, J., Ou, S., Kozar, L., Martin, F., Green, C., Jacobsen, F., Nickolson, F., Schultz, J.A., Semon, K.M., Rishell,W., and Stewart, R.G. 1989. Germline transmission of exogenous genes in the chicken. *Science* 243:533–535.

Bulfield, G. 1997. Strategies for the future. *Poultry Science* 76:1071–1074.

Campbell, K.H.S., McWhir, J., Ritchie, W.A., and Wilmut, I. 1996. Sheep cloned by nuclear transfer from a cultured cell line. *Nature* 380:64–65.

Cao, H., Bidwell, C.A., Willilams, S.K., Liang, W., and Mills, S.E. 1998. Rapid communication: sequence of the coding region for the porcine β_1-adrenergic receptor gene. *Journal of Animal Science* 76:1720–1721.

Carlson, M.S., Hill, G.M., and Link, J.E. (1999) Early- and traditionally weaned nursery pigs benefit from phase-feeding pharmacological concentrations of zinc oxide: effect on metallothionein and mineral concentrations. *Journal of Animal Science* 77:1199–1207.

Cibelli, J.B., Stice, S.L., Golueke, P.J., Kane, J.J., Jerry, J., Blackwell, C., Ponce de Leon, F.A., and Robl, J.M. 1998. Cloned transgenic calves produced from nonquiescent fetal fibroblasts. *Science* 280:1256–1258.

Claeys, M.C., Mulvaney, D.R., McCarthy, F.D., Gore, M.T., Marple, D.N., and Sartin, J.L. 1989. Skeletal muscle protein synthesis and growth hormone secretion in young lambs treated with clenbuterol. *Journal of Animal Science* 67:2245–2254.

Crome, P.K., McKeith, F.K., Carr, T.R., Jones, D.J., Mowrey, D.H., and Cannon, J.E. 1996. Effect of ractopamine on growth performance, carcass composition, and cutting yields of pigs slaughtered at 107 and 125 kilograms. *Journal of Animal Science* 74:709–715.

Cromwell, G.L. 2001. Antimicrobial and promicrobial agents. In *Swine Nutrition*. A.J. Lewis and L.L. Southern, eds. Boca Raton, Florida: CRC Press.

Draghia-Akli, R., Fiorotto, M.L., Hill, L.A., Malone, P.B., Deaver, D.R., and Schwartz, R.J. 1999. Myogenic expression of an injectable protease-resistant growth hormone-releasing hormone augments long-term growth in pigs. *Nature Biotechnology* 17:1179–1183.

Dubreil, P., Petitclerc, G., Pelletier, G., Gaudreau, P. Farmer, C, Mowles, T.F., and Brazeau, P. 1990. Effect of dose and frequency of administration of a potent analog of human growth hormone-releasing factor on hormone secretion and growth in pigs. *Journal of Animal Science* 68:1254–1268.

Duckett, S.K., Wagner, D.G., Owens, F.N., Dolezal, H.G., and Gill, D.R. 1996. Effects of estrogenic and androgenic implants on performance, carcass traits, and meat tenderness in feedlot steers: A review. *Professional Animal Science* 12:205–214.

Duckett, S.K., Wagner, D.G., Owens, F.N., Dolezal, H.G., and Gill, D.R. 1999. Effect of anabolic implants on beef intramuscular lipid content. *Journal of Animal Science* 77:1100–1104.

Eisemann, J.H., Huntington, G.B., and Ferrell, C.L. 1988. Effects of dietary clenbuterol on metabolism of the hindquarters in steers. *Journal of Animal Science* 66:342–353.

Etches, R.J., Clark, M.E., Zajchowski, L., Speksnijder, G., Verrinder Gibbins, A.M., Kino, K., Pain, B., and Samarut, J. 1997. Manipulation of blastodermal cells. *Poultry Science* 76:1075–1083.

Forrest, RH., and Hickford, J.G.H. 2000. Rapid communication: Nucleotide sequences of the bovine, caprine, and ovine β_3-adrenergic receptor genes. *Journal of Animal Science* 78:1397–1398.

Francis, C., Janky, D.M., Arafa, A.S., and Harms, R.H. 1978. Interrelationship of lactobacillus and zinc bacitracin in the diets of turkey poults. *Poultry Science* 57:1687–1689.

Gordon, J.W., Scangos, G.A., Plotkin, D.J., Barbosa, J.A., and Ruddle, F.H. 1980. Genetic transformation of mouse embryos by microinjection of purified DNA. *Proceedings of the National Academy of Science, USA* 77:7380–7384.

Gusils, C., Gonzalez, S.N., and Oliver, G. 1999a. Some probiotic properties of chicken lactobacilli. *Canadian Journal of Microbiology* 45:981–987.

Gusils, C., Perez, A., Gonzalez, S.N., and Oliver, G. 1999b. Lactobacilli isolated from chicken intestines: potential use as probiotics. *Journal of Food Protection* 62:252–256.

Hahn, J.D., and Baker, D.H. 1993. Growth and plasma zinc responses of young pigs fed pharmacologic levels of zinc. *Journal of Animal Science* 71:3020–3024.

Hathaway, M.R., Dayton, W.R., White, M.E., Henderson, T.L., and Henningson, T.B. 1996. Serum insulin-like growth factor I (IGF-I) concentrations are increased in pigs fed microbials. *Journal of Animal Science* 74:1541–1547.

Hayden, J.M., Bergen, W.G., and Merkel, R.A. 1992. Skeletal muscle protein metabolism and serum growth hormone, insulin, and cortisol concentrations in growing steers implanted with estradiol-17β, trenbolone acetate, or estradiol-17β plus trenbolone acetate. *Journal of Animal Science* 70:2109–2119.

Helferich, W.G., Jump, D.B., Anderson, D.B., Skjaerlund, D.M., Merkel, R.A., and Bergen, W.G. 1990. Skeletal muscle a-actin synthesis is increased pretranslationally in pigs fed the phenethanolamine ractopamine. *Endocrinology* 126:3096–3100.

Hill, G.M., Mahan, D.C., Carter, S.D., Cromwell, G.L., Ewan, R.C., Harrold, R.L., Lewis, A.J., Miller, P.S.,

Shurson, G.C., and Veum, T.L. 2001. Effect of pharmacological concentrations of zinc oxide with or without the inclusion of an antibacterial agent on nursery pig performance. *Journal of Animal Science* 79:934–941.

Holgerholt, D.D., Crooker, B.A., Wheaton, J.E., Carlson, K.M., and Jorgenson, D.M. 1992. Effects of a growth hormone-releasing factor analogue and an estradiol-trenbolone acetate implant on somatotropin, insulin-like growth factor I, and metabolite profiles in growing hereford steers. *Journal of Animal Science* 70:1439–1448.

Holm, A. 1990. *E. coli* associated diarrhoea in weaned pigs: Zinc oxide added to the feed as a preventive measure? In *Proceedings 11ᵗʰ Congress International Pig Veterinary Society*, Lausanne, Switzerland.

Hu, C.Y., Novakofski, J., and Mersmann, H.J. 1987. Hormonal control of porcine adipose fatty acid release and cyclic AMP concentration. *Journal of Animal Science* 64:1031–1037.

Johnson, B.J., Anderson, P.T., Meiske, J.C., and Dayton, W.R. 1996a. Effect of a combined trenbolone acetate and estradiol implant on feedlot performance, carcass characteristics, and carcass composition of feedlot steers. *Journal of Animal Science* 74:363–371.

Johnson, B.J., Hathaway, M.R., Anderson, P.T., Meiske, J.C., and Dayton, W.R. 1996b. Stimulation of circulating insulin-like growth factor I (IGF-I) and insulin-like growth factor binding proteins (IGFBP) due to administration of a combined trenbolone acetate and estradiol implant in feedlot cattle. *Journal of Animal Science* 74:372–379.

Kuiper G.J.M., Lemmen J.G., Carlsson B., Corton J.C., Safe S.H., van der Saag P.T., van der Burg B., and Gustafsson J-A. 1998. Interaction of estrogenic chemicals and phytoestrogens with estrogen receptor beta. *Endocrinology* 139:4252–4263

Kuiper, H.A., Noordam, M.Y., van Dooren-Flipsen, M.M.H., Schilt, R., and Roos, A.H. (1998) Illegal use of β-adrenergic agonists: European community. *Journal of Animal Science* 76:195–207.

Liang, W., Bidwell, C.A., Williams, S.K., and Mills, S.E. 1997. Rapid communication: molecular closing of the porcine β_2-adrenergic receptor gene. *Journal of Animal Science* 75:2824.

Liang, W., and Mills, S. 2001. Profile of ligand binding to the porcine β_2-adrenergic receptor. *Journal of Animal Science* 79:877–883.

Liu, C.Y., Boyer, J.L., and Mills, S.E. 1989. Acute effects of beta-adrenergic agonists on porcine adipocyte metabolism in vitro. *Journal of Animal Science* 67:2930–2936.

Lucas, E.W., Wallace, H.D., Palmer, A.Z., and Combs, G.E. 1971. Influence of hormone supplementation, dietary protein level and sex on the performance and carcass characteristics of swine. *Journal of Animal Science* 33:780–786.

Marcus, A.I. 1994. *Cancer from Beef: DES, Federal Food Regulation, and Consumer Confidence*. Baltimore: Johns Hopkins University Press.

Martinez, R., Estrada, M.P., Berlanga, J., Guillen, I., Hernandez, O., Cabrera, E., Pimentel, R., Morales, R., Herrera, F., and Morales, A. 1996. Growth enhancement in transgenic tilapia by ectopic expression of tilapia growth hormone. *Molecular Marine Biology and Biotechnology* 5:62–70.

Martinez, R., Juncal, J., Zaldivar, C., Arenal, A., Guillen, I., Morera, V., Carrillo, O., Estrada, M., Morales, A., and Estrada, M.P. 2000. Growth efficiency in transgenic tilapia (*Oreochromis* sp.) carrying a single copy of an homologous cDNA growth hormone. *Biochemical Biophysical Research Communication* 267:466–472.

Martinez-Navarro, J.F. 1990. Food poisoning related to the consumption of illicit β-agonist in liver. *Lancet* 336:1311.

McCreath, K.J., Howcroft, J., Campbell, K.H.S., Colman, A., Schnieke, A.E., and Kind, A.J. 2000. Production of gene-targeted sheep by nuclear transfer from cultured somatic cells. *Nature* 405:1066–1069.

McNeel, R.L., and Mersmann, H.J. 1999. Distribution and quantification of beta₁-, beta₂-, and beta₃-adrenergic receptor subtype transcripts in porcine tissues. *Journal of Animal Science* 77:611–621.

Mills, S.E., and Liu, C.Y. 1990. Sensitivity of lipolysis and lipogenesis to dibutryl-cAMP and of ß adrenergic agonists in swine adipocytes in vitro. *Journal of Animal Science* 68:1017–1023.

Mitchell, G.A., and Dunnavan, G. 1998. Illegal use of β-adrenergic agonists in the United States. *Journal of Animal Science* 76:208–211.

Moloney, A.P., Allen, P., Ross, D.B., Olson, G., and Convey, E.M. 1990. Growth, feed efficiency and carcass composition of finishing Friesen steers fed the ß adrenergic agonist L-644,969. *Journal of Animal Science* 68:1269–1277.

Moser, R.L., Dalrymple, R.H., Cornelius, S.G., Pettigrew, J.E., and Allen, C.E. 1986. Effect of cimaterol (CL 263,780) as a repartitioning agent in the diet of pigs. *Journal of Animal Science* 62:21–26.

Nurmi, E., and Rantala, M. 1973. New aspects of salmonella infection in broiler production. *Nature* 241:210–211.

Onishi, A., Iwamoto, M., Akita, T., Mikawa, S., Takeda, K., Awata, T., Hanada, H., and Perry, A.C.F. 2000. Pig cloning by microinjection of fetal fibroblast nuclei. *Science* 289:1188–1190.

Peterla, T.A., Ricks, C.A., and Scanes, C.G. 1990. Effects of ß adrenergic agonists on lipolysis and lipogenesis by porcine adipose tissue in vitro. *Journal of Animal Science* 68:1024–1029.

Petitte, J.N., Karagenc, L., and Ginsburg, M. 1997. The origin of the avian germ line and transgenesis in birds. *Poultry Science* 76:1084–1092.

Pinkert, C.A., and Murray, J.D. 1999. *Transgenic Farm Animals*. J.D. Murray, G.B. Anderson, A.M. Oberbauer, and M.M. McGloughlin, eds. New York: CAB International.

Polejaeva, I.A., Chen, S.-H., Vaught, T.D., Page, R.L., Mullins, J., Ball, S., Dal, Y., Boone, J., Walker, S., Ayares, D.L., Colman, A., and Campbell, K.H. 2000. Cloned pigs produced by nuclear transfer from adult somatic cells. *Nature* 407:86–90.

Pommier, S.A., Dubreuil, P., Pelletier, G., Gaudreau, P., Mowles, T.F., and Brazeau, P. 1990. Effect of a potent analog of human growth hormone-releasing factor on carcass composition and quality of crossbred market pigs. *Journal of Animal Science* 68:1291–1298.

Poulsen, H.D. 1989. Zinc oxide for weaned pigs. In *Proceedings 40ʰ Annual Meeting European Association Animal Production*, Dublin, Ireland.

Pulce, C., Lamaison, D., Keck, G., Bostvironnois, C., Nicolas, and Descotes, J. 1991. Collective human food poisonings by clenbuterol residues in veal liver. *Veterinary and Human Toxicolicology* 33:480.

Pursel, V.G., Hammer, R.E., Bolt, D.J., Palmiter, R.D., and Brinster, R.L. 1990. Integration, expression and germ-line transmission of growth-related genes in pigs. *Journal of Reproductive Fertility, Supplement* 41:77–87.

Pursel, V.G., Pinkert, C.A., Miller, K.F., Bolt, D.J., Campbell, R.G., Palmiter, R.D., Brinster, R.L., and Hammer, R.E. 1989. Genetic engineering of livestock. *Science* 244:1281–1288.

Pursel, V.G., and Rexroad, C.E. 1993. Status of research with transgenic farm animals. *Journal of Animal Science* 71 (Suppl. 3):10–19.

Purvis, H.T., II, and Whittier, J.C. 1996. Effects of ionophore feeding and anthelmintic administration on age and weight at puberty in spring-born beef heifers. *Journal of Animal Science* 74:736–744.

Rahman, M.A., Mak, R., Ayad, H., Smith, A., and Maclean, N. 1998. Expression of a novel piscine growth hormone gene results in growth enhancement in transgenic tilapia (*Oreochromis niloticus*). *Transgenic Research* 7:357–369.

Reeds, P.J., Hay, S.M., Dorwood, P.M., and Palmer, R.M. 1986. Stimulation of muscle growth by clenbuterol: lack of effect on muscle protein synthesis. *British Journal of Nutrition* 56:249–258.

Ricks, C.A., Dalrymple, R.H., Baker, P.K., and Ingle, D.L. 1984. Use of a β-agonist to alter fat and muscle deposition in steers. *Journal of Animal Science* 59:1247–1255.

Rogers, J.A., Branine, M.E., Miller, C.R., Wray, M.I., Bartle, S.J., Preston, R.L., Gill, D.R., Pritchard, R.H., Stilborn, R.P., and Bechtol, D.T. 1995. Effects of dietary virginiamycin on performance and liver abscess incidence in feedlot cattle. *Journal of Animal Science* 73:9–20.

Rule, D.C., Smith, S.B., and Mersman, H.J. 1987. Effects of adrenergic agonists and insulin on porcine adipose tissue in vitro. *Journal of Animal Science* 65:136–149.

Schnieke, A.E., Kind, A.J., Ritchie, W.A., Mycock, K., Scott, A.R., Ritchie, M., Wilmut, I., Colman, A., and Campbell, K.H.S. 1997. Human factor IX transgenic sheep produced by transfer of nuclei from transfected fetal fibroblasts. *Science* 278:2130–2133.

Simkiss, K. 1997. Embryo manipulation of the germplasm. *Poultry Science* 76:1093–1100.

Smith, T.R., Bidwell, C.A., and Mills, S.E. 2001. Rapid Communication: Nucleotide sequence of the porcine β_3-adrenergic receptor gene. *Journal of Animal Science* 79:781–782.

Snoeyenbos, G.H., Weinack, O.M., and Smyser, C.F. 1978. Protecting chicks and poults from salmonellae by oral administration of "normal" gut microflora. *Avian Diseases* 22:273–287.

Sokol, D.L., and Murray, J.D. 1996. Antisense and ribozyme constructs in transgenic animals. *Transgenic Research* 5:363–371.

Stock, R.A., Laudert, S.B., Stroup, W.W., Larson, E.M., Parrott, J.C., and Britton, R.A. 1995. Effect of monensin and monensin and tylosin combination on feed intake variation of feedlot steers. *Journal of Animal Science* 73:39–44.

Stokstad, E.L.R., Jukes, T.H., Pierce, J., Page, A.C., and Franklin, A.L. 1949. The multiple nature of the animal protein factor. *Journal of Biological Chemistry* 180:647.

Strosberg, A.D. 1997. Structure and function of the β_3-adrenergic receptor. *Annual Review of Pharmacology and Toxicology* 37:424–450.

Tortuero, F. 1973. Influence of the implantation of lacto-bacillus acidophilus in chicks on the growth, feed conversion, malabsorption of fats syndrome and intestinal flora. *Poultry Science* 52:197–203.

Wentworth, B., Tsai, H., Wentworth, A., Wong, E., Proudman, J., and El Halawani, M. 1996. Primordial germ cells for genetic modification of poultry. In *Beltsville Symposia in Agricultural Research XX, Biotechnology's Role in the Genetic Improvement of Farm Animals*. R.H. Miller, V.G. Pursel, and H.D. Norman, eds. Champaign, Illinois: American Society of Animal Science.

Wilmut, I., Schnieke, A.E., McWhir, J., Kind, A.J., and Campbell, K.H.S. 1997. Viable offspring derived from fetal and adult mammalian cells. *Nature* 385:810–813.

Wilmut, I., Schnieke, A.E., McWhir, J., Kind, A.J., Colman, A., and Campbell, K.H.S. 1999. Nuclear Transfer in the Production of Transgenic Farm Animals. In *Transgenic Animals in Agriculture*. J.D. Murray, G.B. Anderson, A.M. Oberbauer, and M.M. McGloughlin, eds. New York: CAB International.

18
Immunological Manipulation of Growth

Rod A. Hill, Jennifer M. Pell, and David J. Flint

This chapter addresses ways our understanding of the immune system may be applied to target actions of critical molecules, including peptide hormones and receptors, which modulate growth, and specific cell types. This approach seeks to direct immune function to recognize specific "self-antigens" and influence growth processes by immunomodulation. The development of immunohistochemistry, radioimmunoassays, and enzyme-linked immunosorbent assays (ELISA) for detection and quantification of hormones, receptors, etc., required specific antibodies. It was quickly found that this was relatively straightforward. Antibodies against specific proteins from many species are available commercially and in laboratories. The ability to produce antibodies provoked study of their effects on hormone systems, etc., and immunomodulation of growth became an arena of scientific endeavor.

Animal scientists recognize that this approach has potential to enhance production. Harnessing the immune response against a molecule with endocrine activity provides a range of potential advantages:

• The amount of a substance needed to evoke a humoral immune response is very small; antibody production is induced by immunization of ruminants with as little as 10–50 µg. This represents >100-fold less than required for pharmacologically active compounds commonly used in animal production. Thus, the cost may be much lower. This issue has implications for market acceptance. Public awareness and resistance to the use of xenobiotic compounds in animal production is increasing. Immune stimulation using very small doses would result in little, if any, residue remaining in the meat.

• Because immunization results in a relatively long-lasting response, animals need to be treated only occasionally to receive an effective dose. Thus, management convenience and cost are optimized.

• Immunomodulation may be more specific than pharmacological agents. For example, pharmacological agents developed for one receptor sub-type may interact with additional receptor sub-types and have undesirable side effects. Antibodies can be highly specific and recognize discrete molecular domains.

The obvious question is the following: What growth/production vaccines are in commercial use today? The answer is very few. This chapter describes vaccine development and the challenges to be overcome to extend this to commercial development. We address the elements required to stimulate an appropriate immune response and consider the ways in which antibodies have been used to both inhibit and stimulate specific endocrine axes. The concepts underlying immune recognition and responses to homologous antigens are considered.

STIMULATING THE IMMUNE SYSTEM TO RECOGNIZE SELF-PROTEINS

How do we overcome the ability of the immune system to recognize self and remain recalcitrant to autoimmune responses? Are the pertinent antigens self-proteins or domains of self-proteins? Fortunately, the cellular and molecular mechanisms regulating humoral immune responses are relatively well understood—and are considered in the following sections.

Target Proteins

Immunomodulation requires antibody recognition (and thus binding) of a target molecule. These are almost exclusively proteins or peptides and may be hormones/growth factors, specific hormone binding proteins, hormone receptors, or other cell-associated molecules. In the cases of hormones/growth factors and binding proteins, these are soluble and the structures are usually well described. There are few problems in identifying suitable domains to be targeted for antibody recognition. Conversely, receptors are located in the cell membrane of the target tissue, and issues of antibody access to the interstitial space and obtaining a pure source of receptors must be considered.

Directing the Immune Response

Antigen Design: B-Cell Epitopes

As a first step in considering antigen design, interactions of antigen with the immune system are addressed. The B-cells are the lymphocytes, which, following stimulation by antigen binding and interactions with T-helper lymphocytes and associated cytokines, are stimulated to proliferate and differentiate into plasma cells—antibody producing "factories." The primary event is the binding of antigen to cell-associated immunoglobulin (Ig) class D (IgD) and class M (IgM) on the B-lymphocyte cell membrane. [IgD is absent from swine and ruminants (Butler 1998)]. Each B-lymphocyte expresses IgD/IgM, which has a single class of binding specificity in the antigen binding, hypervariable region of the molecule.

The aim is to evoke an immune response in an (production) animal, so that the antibodies produced will recognize a target protein in its native conformation. Targeting a hydrophobic domain (which is folded to an internal part of the molecule) is futile. Similarly, for a receptor, targeting an intracellular domain is inappropriate. Figure 18.1 shows the structure of the β_2-adrenoceptor (β_2-AR) and highlights the features of a domain suitable as an antigen (Hill et al. 1998b). In this example, the antigens were synthetic peptide analogues of an extracellular domain of the protein. For large molecules, such as receptors, the use of synthetic peptide analogues has several advantages. First, a suitable domain may be selected. Using the whole molecule as antigen would produce antibodies recognizing different domains of the receptor, many of which would be unsuitable. Second, a synthetic peptide representing a suitable domain is easily prepared, whereas purification of the receptor to homogeneity is both technically difficult and expensive. This approach has been widely used (Bahouth et al. 1991).

When using a synthetic peptide analogue, it is important to ensure that the antigen is large enough to fold into a tertiary structure so that it emulates the native molecule. This allows antibody recognition of "conformational epitopes," also known as configurational specificity (Roitt et al. 1993). Thus with β_2-AR, the 13-amino acid peptide antigen could not evoke antibodies recognizing a conformational epitope of β_2-AR but the 24-amino acid peptide was effective. There is not a defined number of amino acid residues that describe configurational specificity. The antigen epitope nestles in a cleft formed by the heavy and light chains of the antibody molecule (the paratope), where the antigen makes contact with 10–12 amino acid residues in the hypervariable regions of both chains (Roitt et al. 1993).

Generation of an Immune Response

It is not possible to evoke an immune response simply by injecting a protein or peptide containing epitopes recognized by B-cells. This is true for any protein, be it a vaccine or a "foreign" or homologous protein. It is necessary to emulate the features of an invading pathogen to stimulate the immune system. All vaccines rely on optimizing antigen presentation to evoke a sustained immune response. The following sections discuss inclusion of accessory molecules with the target protein to stimulate class II T-lymphocytes (T-helper lymphocytes), the roles of antigen presenting cells, activation of cytokines, and the use of adjuvants.

Adjuvants

Adjuvants are nonspecific stimulators of the immune system and are essential for stimulation of an immune response against a soluble antigen. There are two main types of adjuvants: water-in-oil emulsions and aluminium hydroxide precipitates. Both form a depot slowly releasing antigen from the injection site. Adjuvants traditionally contain substances to stimulate the lymphokines (cytokines, specific immune cell activators). Freund's Complete Adjuvant consisting of a mineral oil and heat-killed *Mycobacterium tuberculosis* is one of the most efficacious adjuvants. It is not used in humans and its use in animals is now restricted because it can induce severe granulomatous site reac-

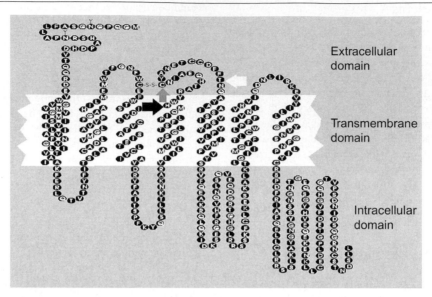

Figure 18.1. Model of the bovine β_2-adrenoceptor (β_2-AR). This membrane-bound receptor has been the target for a number of studies of immunomodulation (see References). In the study of Hill et al. (1998b), two synthetic peptide analogues representing part and all of an outer loop of the β_2-AR were used as antigens to raise antibodies. The larger peptide contained 24 amino acid residues—shown here commencing with Histidine 172 (black arrow) through to Threonine 195 (white arrow)—and the smaller peptide contained 13 amino acid residues commencing with Histidine 172 through to Cysteine 184 (gray arrow). Although antibodies were raised against both antigens, only antibodies against the longer peptide recognized (and activated) the β_2-AR. This illustrates the importance of conformation in antigen design (see text for details).

tions causing considerable irritation and pain. There are alternatives. Some contain the purified active component from *M. tuberculosis,* muramyl dipeptide or purified components from another nonspecific immune stimulator—e.g., heat-killed *Bordetalla pertussis.* Adjuvant design is becoming much more sophisticated. An active area of research is the inclusion of recombinant lymphokines in adjuvant formulations (Nash et al. 1993; Wood et al. 1994; Lofthouse et al. 1996). The adjuvant stimulates antigen recognition by immune cells—e.g., antigen presenting cells, T-lymphocytes, B-lymphocytes, and activation of these by lymphokines. This is directed to raising a specific immune response to a target protein.

Antigen Processing

Antigen is required in more than one form to stimulate antibody production. The antigen needs to contain conformational epitopes conferring configu-

rational specificity. It also needs to provide T-cell epitopes to activate T-helper cells and then to induce T-helper cell interaction with antigen-activated B-cells. To enhance this process, when attempting to stimulate B-cell recognition and response against a small peptide antigen (e.g., a hormone or receptor analogue), additional protein is chemically reacted or conjugated with the peptide. This is designed to increase the number of T-helper epitopes available. There is genetic restriction in the range of T-helper epitopes recognized by an individual of any species, and this is related to the major histocompatability complex (MHC) (Beh and Blattman 1994). A range of proteins has been characterized for MHC recognition, most thoroughly in the mouse and human. Relatively few are known for livestock. Only class II MHC molecules in the so-called "exogenous pathway" are involved in the humoral response leading to antibody production. Thus, we will focus on this mechanism.

The initial step in antigen processing (Figure 18.2) is internalization of antigen by antigen presenting cells and subsequent degradation by proteolytic enzymes within phagolysosomes. Thus much of the antigen is degraded. Linear sequences of 13–25 amino acid residues (Chicz and Urban 1994) constitute the class II peptide, which is then expressed at the cell surface in association with MHC molecules. The classes of cells processing antigens in this way (Figure 18.3) include mononuclear phagocytes, B-cells, and dendritic cells. The antigen presented in association with MHC is recognized by T-helper lymphocytes. These are then activated. This occurs at the site of immunization or in the lymph nodes draining the region. The T-epitopes and B-epitopes need not be mutually exclusive (Harris et al. 1996; Zhang et al. 1996). Thus simple antigens may be used to direct an immune response; however, the only responding animals will be those in which the antigen is compatible with the specific MHC haplotype. T-cell activation requires not only MHC-associated antigen, which binds the T-cell receptor, but also a complex interaction of other cell membrane-associated proteins and specific lymphokines (Figure 18.4). Antigen presenting cells also produce intercellular adhesion molecule-1 and lymphocyte functional antigen-3, which interact with T-cell proteins, lymphocyte functional antigen-1, and T-helper–specific antigen, CD2. Additionally, a complex array of lymphokines is involved in T-cell activation.

Antibody Production

Processes, including lymphokine actions, induce repeated B-cell division and differentiation to form the antibody producing plasma cells. This entire sequence requires "priming", because following an initial immunization, the primary response to a specific antigen is of relatively low magnitude and of limited duration. Initially, the antibodies produced are of the IgM isotype and have relatively low affinity. However, following a second immunization, optimally three to six weeks later, a response is evoked of a greatly increased magnitude and longevity. The antibodies generated are of the IgG isotype and have higher affinity for the antigen.

The Importance of a Sustained Response

To generate a useful production response, the active agent is the specific antibody generated by an appropriate immunization protocol. The goal is to generate and maintain antibody levels above some unknown, but critical, blood concentration for a minimum period (Pell and Aston 1995). (Usually longer is better.) This is a major challenge. Antibody concentration in blood is traditionally determined using serial dilution assays and thus is quantified by titer.

DETERMINATION OF ANTIBODY ACTION

Antibodies conventionally sequester antigen and inhibit antigen function. However in specific circumstances,

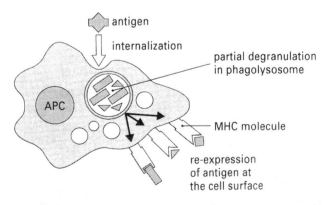

Antigen processing

antigen

internalization

partial degranulation in phagolysosome

APC

MHC molecule

re-expression of antigen at the cell surface

Figure 18.2. T-cell antigen processing. Antigens are internalized by antigen-presenting cells and are then degraded by proteolytic enzymes in specialized intracellular compartments. Antigenic peptides are linear fragments, which associate with class II MHC molecules as they are moved to the cell surface. (Reprinted from Roitt et al., 1993, by permission of the publisher, Mosby.)

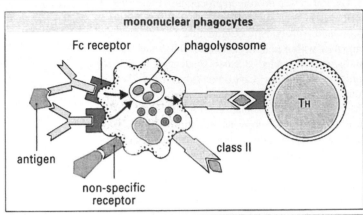

mononuclear phagocytes

Fc receptor   phagolysosome

antigen

non-specific
receptor

class II

T_H

Figure 18.3. Antigen presentation. Mononuclear phagocytes or macrophages (top), B cells (center), and dendritic cells (bottom) can all process and present antigen to MHC class II-restricted T cells. Macrophages take up antigen via nonspecific receptors or as immune complexes and probably process it internally before returning fragments to the cell surface in association with MHC class II molecules. Activated B cells can take up antigen via their surface immunoglobulin and present it to T cells alongside the class II molecules. Dendritic cells constituitively express class II molecules but are not phagocytic. Presumably they either take up antigen by pinocytosis or process it at the cell surface. (Reprinted from Roitt et al., 1993, by permission of the publisher, Mosby.)

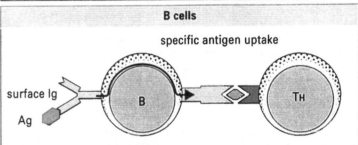

B cells

specific antigen uptake

surface Ig

Ag

B

T_H

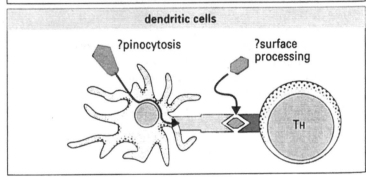

dendritic cells

?pinocytosis

?surface
processing

T_H

Figure 18.4. Molecular signaling in antigen presentation. The molecules are involved in the interaction between T cells and antigen-presenting cells. The various cytokines and their direction of action are shown. Not all factors are required in all circumstances. There are also additional signals involved in this interaction that have not been identified. (Reprinted from Roitt et al., 1993, by permission of the publisher, Mosby.)

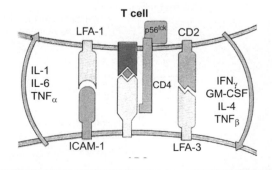

T cell

LFA-1   p56^{lck}   CD2

IL-1
IL-6
TNF_α

CD4

IFN_γ
GM-CSF
IL-4
TNF_β

ICAM-1   LFA-3

antibodies can surprisingly potentiate or enhance the activity of peptide hormones. Thus the strategy for antibody design depends on the hormone and how it might be manipulated to optimize animal production. Clearly, inhibitory agents in growth regulation—e.g., somatostatin (SRIF), would be the focus of design of inhibitory antibodies, whereas stimulatory factors—e.g., insulin-like growth factor-I (IGF-I), will be targeted for potentiation.

Temporal Effects

It is important to consider the time scale when designing immunization strategies. This is considered in the section "Passive and Active Immunization," later in this chapter.

Proportion of Responding Animals

There may be great variation between individuals in response to immunization, particularly when attempting to target the immune response to a specific epitope. Figure 18.5 illustrates an active immunization experiment and the importance of the proportion of animals immunized that are responders. The reasons for this variation are complex and only partially understood. One basis is the genetic restriction of the individual MHC haplotype, allowing only a limited range of class II peptide expression by antigen presenting cells. Thus in the example, only six of the seven immunized steers developed titers. Interpretation of physiological data is difficult; Gazzola and colleagues (1998) avoided

the problem of nonresponders by adopting a design in which animals were paired on feed intake. Out of eight steers immunized with leptin, only four responded. Data was analyzed for the responding steers and their paired controls. It is desirable to maximize the proportion of responders. However, should the production response be sufficient in most of the animals, a small proportion of nonresponders may have little effect on the economic benefit.

Control of Titer

Maintenance of the antibody at an effective titer is essential to achieving a growth response. For ruminants with a longer life cycle than other meat species, the intervention may be required to persist from several months to more than a year. Our understanding of what constitutes an effective dose is not clear and is determined empirically. In the example in Figure 18.5, steers developed only moderate titers following immunization with IGF-I. Antibody titers were detectable by ELISA two weeks after the second immunization. This is a typical pattern of antibody response, the primary response being too weak to be detected. The steers were feed restricted initially and their weight remained constant. During the compensatory growth phase, antibodies enhanced the effects of IGF-I.

In passive immunization, the amount of Ig administered to the target animal is regulated and therefore titer can be controlled. However, because the Ig must be injected, the volume that can be physically

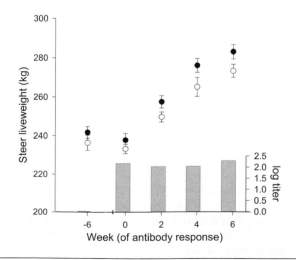

Figure 18.5. Weight gain and antibody titers in steers immunized against IGF-I. Steers (n = 7 per group) were immunized with an IGF-1 vaccine or sham, immunized on three occasions at 4-weekly intervals (weeks –6, –2, and 2). Antibody titers were developed in only six test steers (solid bars) and were persistent through to the end of the experiment. Liveweight gain was greater in the test group, commensurate with the development of antibody titers against IGF-I. Test steers were 11 kg heavier by the final week of the experiment (data obtained from Hill et al., 1998c).

administered is restricted and therefore will affect the antibody titer. The only restriction in active immunization is appropriate stimulation of the immune system. This, in theory, should generate higher titers than by passive immunization. Because the target protein is usually endogenous, it is necessary to develop strategies for the generation of high titers of antibodies against "self" molecules (reviewed Meloen 1995). There have been few systematic studies to optimize antibody production by varying the dose of antigen, the nature of the carrier molecule (e.g., ovalbumin, keyhole lympet hemocyanin, tetanus toxoid), and the immunostimulant (e.g., Freund's complete adjuvant, aluminium hydroxide). Responsiveness even to a single-dose combination of these three components may be very variable. For example, anti-placental lactogen (PL) antibody titer varied tenfold between two studies with similar immunization protocols (Leibovich et al. 2000). In contrast, even when the dose of antigen was varied, antibody responsiveness was not. Clearly, much work is needed to define immunization strategies. For full optimization, these may need to be specific for each antigen.

Importance of Antibody Affinity

In this section, we again use the example of antibodies raised against IGF-I. When the affinity of the antibody for IGF-I was similar to/less than that of the IGF-receptor for IGF-I, there appeared to be an IGF-enhancing effect. When the affinity of the antibody for IGF-I was considerably higher than IGF-receptor affinity for IGF-1, it appeared to be inhibitory. The dynamics of these interactions are complex. If we assume perhaps the simplest model of IGF-I binding to antibody, IGF-binding protein (IGFBP) and IGF-receptor, the distribution of bound IGF-I will be proportional to both the affinities of each of these interactions and the concentrations of each component (Figure 18.6). These interactions will be in dynamic equilibrium.

Peptide hormone receptors have affinities for their ligands of 10^9–10^{10} liters/mole whereas antibody affinities vary from 10^6 to 10^{10} liters/mole. It is generally assumed that antibodies with a higher affinity for the hormone than its cognate receptor inhibit the activity of the hormone (by competition for and sequestration of the peptide). Alternatively,

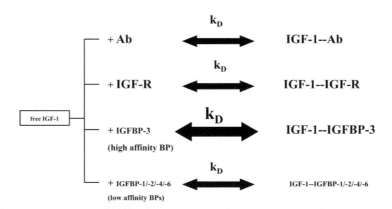

Figure 18.6. Interaction of IGF-I with antibody (Ab), specific IGF-binding proteins (IGFBPs), and the IGF-receptor (IGF-R). The distribution of bound and free IGF-I depends upon the concentration of each of the components and the affinities of each of the interactions. In IGF-I-immunized animals, this system will be in dynamic equilibrium in vivo. As physiological and metabolic changes influence each of the components, shifts in the distribution of each of the components will occur. The size of the font used for each component illustrates the notional distribution of each component. Thus there will be little free IGF-I. Although the affinity of the high affinity binding protein is much greater than those of the IGF-R and Ab, when the concentrations of the IGF-R and Ab exceed the concentration of IGFBP-3, the distribution of bound IGF-I among these forms will be similar. (In reality, other complex factors modify this simplistic model, which serves to illustrate the relative importance of concentration and affinity.)

if the antibody has an affinity for the peptide hormone that is less than that of the receptor, the receptor may be able to compete effectively for the pool of antibody-associated peptide. Further, the pool of available hormone could also be expanded by the presence of a large pool of low affinity antibody. In this situation, the antibody may be enhancing. Surprisingly, these hypotheses have not been formally tested. However, analogous examples are found in the relationship between IGF-I activity and modified IGFBPs. High affinity IGFBPs are inhibitory whereas low affinity IGFBPs potentiate IGF-I activity (reviewed Jones and Clemmons 1995). Similarly, antibodies potentiating IGF-I in vivo have a modest affinity for IGF-I (Stewart et al. 1993).

Circulating Immune Complexes

Even though antibody titers are measured in serum, this may not be their only site of action. If the aim of the administered Ig is to inhibit the activity of hormone, these measurements are appropriate. Similarly, if hormone-enhancing antibodies exert their effects simply by prolonging the half-life of the hormone, serum titers are most relevant. The degree to which hormones are complexed to antibodies depends on their relative concentrations and the affinity of the antibody. Immunoglobulins, particularly IgG, gain access to interstitial and pericellular spaces within tissues (Roitt et al. 1993; Zeitlin et al. 2000). Peripherally administered therapeutic antibodies against amyloid ß-peptide are found in the central nervous system (Bard et al. 2000). Enhancing antibodies to porcine GH (pGH) change the tissue distribution (Wang & Chard 1992; Tans et al. 1994). Only a proportion of exogenous hormone needs to be complexed to antibody for potentiation (Holder et al. 1985; Pell et al. 1989).

The way in which the immune system deals with circulating immune complexes is important to the efficacy of immunomodulation. Following binding to an antigen, an IgG molecule changes conformation, and recognition sites along the molecule, which were previously hidden, become exposed. These sites bind cell-associated proteins expressed by cells of the reticulo-endothelial system. When IgG is bound to a circulating hormone, the reticulo-endothelial system provides an alternative clearance mechanism. Figure 18.7 shows that in the presence of specific antibody, clearance of IGF-I was radically shifted from renal to hepatic; reticulo-endothelial clearance is highly active in the liver. This is not completely understood and is affected by IgG affinity for the hormone.

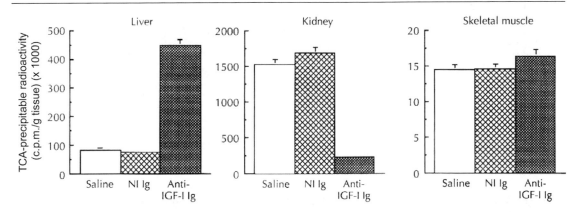

Figure 18.7. Clearance of IGF-I from dwarf rats that were pretreated with sheep anti-IGF-I Ig, nonspecific (nonimmune, NI-Ig), or saline. ^{125}I-IGF-I was used in this experiment as a tracer and shows the behavior of endogenous IGF-I. The huge effect of anti-IGF Ig on the clearance mechanism is clear. In the two control groups, the great majority of IGF-I is taken up by the kidneys, degraded and excreted. In the anti-IGF-I Ig-treated rats, much of the IGF-I is complexed with antibody. These "immune complexes" are cleared through the reticulo-endothelial system active in the liver. Interestingly, skeletal muscle tended to contain more IGF-I in the IGF-I Ig-treated rats, suggesting that this could provide a mechanism for improved muscle growth. (Reprinted from Hill et al., 1997, by permission of the Society for Endocrinology.)

Kinetics of Ig-Associated Peptide Hormones

The conventional role of antibodies in infection is to facilitate clearance of antigens. However, antibody-associated self-peptide hormone is cleared less rapidly and with different kinetic properties than non–antibody-associated hormone (Wang et al. 1992; Massart et al. 1993; Hill et al. 1997; Bealoye et al. 1999). Subcutaneous injection of pGH (pre-complexed to an enhancing monoclonal antibody) showed delayed absorption into the circulation prolonging exposure of tissues to GH (Wang et al. 1992). Unusual IGF kinetics were observed in animals receiving ^{125}I-labelled IGF-I precomplexed to enhancing anti-IGF-I polyclonal Ig (Hill et al. 1997). In a two-phase model, the clearance of IGF-I was decreased by ~50% but the half-life of IGF-I was decreased in the slower-decaying phase (Figure 18.8). The degradation rate was decreased suggesting that the Ig was protecting IGF-I from proteolysis. Enhancing antibodies can also change the interaction of hormone with its receptor. Prolonged receptor occupancy/activation by GH occurs when it is precomplexed to an enhancing MAb (Massart et al. 1993; Bealoye et al. 1999). Therefore, a key mechanism of antibody potentiation of hormone activity is prolonging the presence of bioavailable peptide hormone. Enhancing antibodies stimulate biological responses of a similar magnitude to that observed for GH where clearance is reduced by cotreatment with GH binding protein or by use of a long-acting form of GH conjugated with polyethylene glycol (Clark et al. 1996a, 1996b). Studies with antibody enhancement of IGF-I activity in vitro (Figure 18.9) suggest that other mechanisms are also important (Pell et al. 2000).

Site of Antibody Binding to Target

One reason for the (normally observed) inhibitory actions of polyclonal antisera is the binding of antibodies to multiple sites on the antigen. For hormone action, it is likely that the active site—i.e., the receptor binding site—will be obscured, preventing receptor interaction and activation. Enhancing antisera bind to peptide hormones at sites distant from the receptor-binding domain (Beattie and Holder 1994; Pell and James 1995; Hill and Pell 1998; Pell et al. 2000) (Figure 18.10). Thus it is advantageous to know the receptor binding site so that appropriate antigenic peptides can be designed.

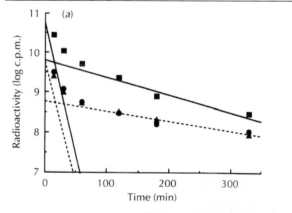
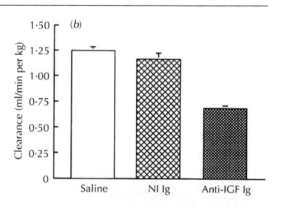

Figure 18.8. In A, the decay curves of IGF-I from the plasma of dwarf rats is shown. ^{125}I-IGF-I was used in this experiment as a tracer and shows the behavior of endogenous IGF-I. Dwarf rats were pretreated with anti-IGF-I Ig (■), nonimmune Ig (●), or saline (▲). In B, the clearance of IGF-I in dwarf rats pretreated with anti-IGF-I Ig, non-immune Ig, or saline is compared. The anti-IGF-I treatment has reduced the clearance rate of IGF-I, and more IGF-I remains in the circulation over time. Thus anti-IGF-I Ig treatment has increased the total pool of IGF-I. (Reprinted from Hill et al., 1997, by permission of the Society for Endocrinology.)

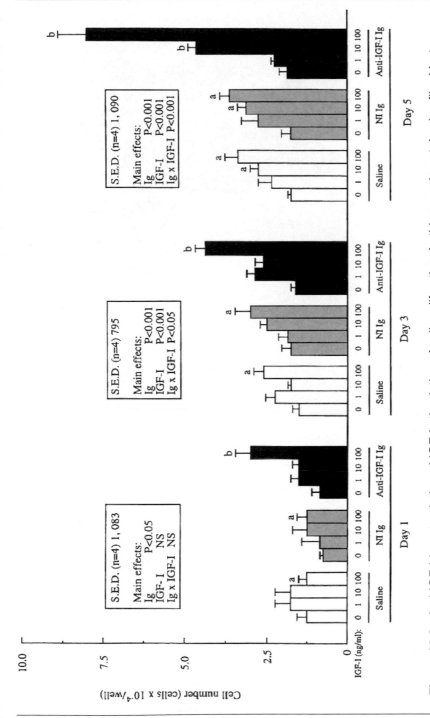

Figure 18.9. Anti-IGF-I Ig potentiation of IGF-I stimulation of cell proliferation. In this experiment, bovine fibroblasts were grown in cell culture. Fibroblasts were treated with a range of concentrations of IGF-I, from 0 to 100 ng/ml, and pretreated with either saline (open bars), nonimmune (NI) Ig (gray bars), or anti-IGF-I Ig (black bars), and the effects of these treatments on cell proliferation (increase in cell number) were determined after one, three, and five days. After one day of treatment, anti-IGF-I Ig treatment increased cell numbers at the highest concentration of IGF-I. The same effect was seen after three days of treatment. After five days of treatment, anti-IGF-I Ig increased proliferation at both 10 and 100 ng/ml IGF-I concentrations. Note also that after three and five days of treatment, IGF-I alone also increased cell proliferation and there was a combined effect of both anti-IGF-I Ig and IGF-I over the control treatments. (Reprinted from Hill et al., 2000, with permission of The Endocrine Society.)

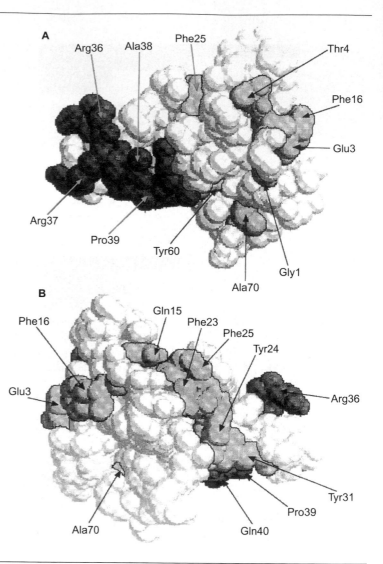

Figure 18.10. The structure of IGF-1 showing the regions that interact with IGF-binding proteins, anti-IGF-1 Ig, and the IGF receptor from two different perspectives. Residues important for IGF-binding protein interaction (Glu3, Thr4, Gln15, and Phe16), and IGF receptor binding ((Tyr24, Tyr31, and Tyr60) and the terminal residues, (Gly1 and Ala70) are shown in pale grey. Residues that have been epitope-mapped and interact with growth-enhancing anti-IGF-1 Ig (Arg36 to Ile43) are shown in dark grey. This evidence indicates that it may be possible for antibody to simultaneously bind IGF-1 while it is also bound to receptor or to binding proteins. (Reprinted from Hill et al., 1998, with permission of The Endocrine Society.)

PASSIVE AND ACTIVE IMMUNIZATION

There are two choices available for antibody administration: passive or active immunization. In passive immunization, antibodies are generated in an animal and are harvested. They may be purified and assessed. The target animal is "treated" with defined Ig and its immune system is not stimulated. In active immunization, the target animal is immunized directly with antigen and generates its own antibodies. The following are key differences between passive and active immunization:

- Passive immunization may be very controlled, whereas the response to active immunization is less predictable.
- Passive immunization is immediate but active immunization takes longer, because antibodies must be generated (>6 weeks).
- Passive immunization is readily reversible, but active immunization may not be.

Monoclonal Antibodies

An array of exciting new technologies is paving the way for the use of Monoclonal Antibodies (MAbs) as tools for passive immunization. MAbs are derived from a single clone and therefore generate just one Ig that defines a single epitope on the antigen, usually conformational rather than to a linear peptide sequence. Thus a part of the structure of the antigen is accurately mirrored, but this can be very difficult to define by techniques such as epitope scanning (Beattie and Holder 1994). A further benefit of MAbs is that their affinity will be precisely known. An obvious disadvantage of MAbs is their derivation from mouse cells. They are themselves antigenic, stimulating the production of anti-idiotypic antibodies that may interfere with the action of the original MAb.

A major advance in MAb technology is the development of genetically engineered antibodies (reviewed Hayden et al. 1997; Hudson 1999). This means that mouse antibodies can be "engineered" to be identical to the form of those from the "target" species, avoiding counterimmune responses. In theory, antibodies could be engineered for administration to any species. Antibody engineering has huge scope to modify and adapt antibody action, for example to change the half-life of defined antibody fragments (Chapman et al. 1999), to define peptides for subsequent active immunization (Vaiseman et al. 2000) or to change antibody affinity (Chowdhury and Pastan 1999). The major impact of this technology has been for therapeutic purposes in man—e.g., cancer therapy. To date most of these "humanized" MAbs have been inhibitory—for example. to block autoimmune diseases. However this could be applied to develop designer antibodies for immunological enhancement of hormones.

Active Immunization

Immunization using a self-protein requires multiple doses. A biological effect is observed when the antibody concentration is similar to the circulating concentration of the hormone or when immunizing against hormone receptors, antibody concentration and affinity must be sufficiently high so that the antibody can interact with the receptor in the presence of the cognate hormone. Another issue is variation in immune response.

EXPERIMENTAL APPROACHES TO IMMUNOMODULATION

Immunomodulation can influence hormone activity, either enhancing or inhibiting action.

Inhibition of Endocrine Axes

Antibodies can be used to inhibit hormone action.

Antibodies Against Somatostatin (SRIF)

SRIF inhibits GH release and is secreted by a range of tissues, including hypothalamic, gastric, and pancreatic sources. As such, SRIF might be expected to be a target for immunoneutralization and was one of the first hormones to be studied in this way, with anti-SRIF blocking the stress-induced decrease in blood GH in rats (Arimura et al. 1976). Many studies use SRIF antibodies to examine the physiology of SRIF or production responses. Early studies in unimproved breeds of sheep showed large improvements in feed efficiency and growth following immunization against SRIF (Spencer and Williamson 1981; Spencer et al. 1983a, 1983b). The mechanism may relate to SRIF action on gut peptides, improving digestion. In many cases, serum GH and IGF-I concentrations were increased, indicating that the mechanism may be more complex. Subsequent studies in improved breeds either failed to show these effects (Hoskinson et al. 1988) or the effects were smaller (Laarveld et al. 1986; Bass et al. 1987; Sun et al. 1990a, 1990b). Wynn and colleagues (1994a) proposed that the large improvement in growth and feed efficiency in unimproved breeds was due to enhancement of digestion in inefficient animals. In improved breeds with inherently better digestion, there was much less scope for improvement. Vaccination of pregnant ewes against SRIF improved growth in their lambs, probably due to increased lamb appetite for milk (Westbrook et al. 1993; Westbrook and McDowell 1994; Westbrook et al. 1994). The efficiency of feed utilization for milk production was also improved in the SRIF-vaccinated pregnant ewes (Westbrook et al. 1993; Sun et al. 1990b). Growth can be improved in SRIF-immunized lambs with muramyl dipeptide as an adjuvant (Westbrook and McDowell 1994; Figure 18.11).

Effects on feed efficiency and/or growth following SRIF immunization have also been reported for chickens (Spencer et al. 1986) and piglets for which the sow had been SRIF-immunized (Farmer et al. 1992). SRIF immunization also improved pregnancy rates in both sheep and pigs (Kirkwood et al. 1990). Thus, SRIF immunization appears to act through an immunoneutralization mechanism and may have potential to improve production.

Other Inhibitory Antibodies

Attempts have been made to invoke antibodies against adrenocorticotropic hormone (ACTH) or

Figure 18.11. The effects of immunization against somatostatin on liveweight in lambs. Lambs were immunized with somatostatin on three occasions (arrows), with different adjuvant formulations. Lambs were immunized with SRIF plus muramyl dipeptide (●) or plus Freund's incomplete adjuvant and muramyl dipeptide (■) or plus DEAE-dextran (○), or plus Quill A (□) or plus Freund's complete adjuvant (▲). In comparison to unimmunized control lambs (△), immunized lambs gained more liveweight over the 84 days of the experiment. (Reproduced from Westbrook and McDowell, 1994, by permission of CSIRO PUBLISHING.)

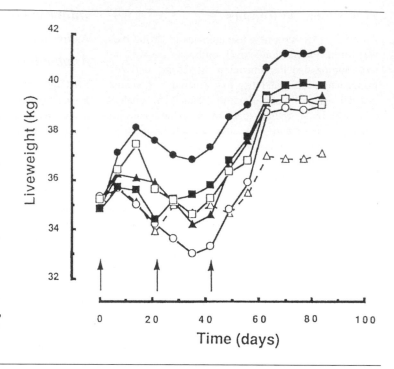

cortisol and, thereby, reduce growth inhibitory effects of stress. Although it is possible to raise antibodies against these hormones and the ACTH receptor, no production effects have been reported (reviewed Wynn et al. 1994b). Another potential target for immunomodulation is leptin (controlling appetite and energy expenditure). If leptin could be immunoneutralized, animal feed intake might be maximized, energy expenditure reduced, and efficiency improved. One study has reported a production response in beef cattle. Immunized animals on a poor quality diet gained more carcass fat but there was no effect on feed intake (Gazzola et al. 1998).

No treatment of immunomodulation of livestock production would be complete without mention of reproductive control vaccines. These were first developed as an alternative to spaying cull female cattle, which involves surgery and potentially high morbidity or even mortalities, especially in extensively grazed cattle. An immunization protocol was developed against gonadotropin releasing hormone (GnRH) and commercialized (Hoskinson et al. 1990). It has not been widely adopted by the cattle industry. The strategy is also effective for reversible castration of colts and spaying of fillies (Dowsett et al. 1993) and for boars, eliminating boar taint and

improving growth performance (Dunshea et al. 2001). Studies in feedlot bulls suggest it may be useful for some markets. The average daily gain and carcass weights were higher for untreated bulls, but GnRH-immunized bulls had numerically better feed efficiency and more tender rib-eye steaks (Cook et al. 2000).

Enhancement of Endocrine Axes

Antibodies can be used to enhance the apparent activity of hormones.

Antibodies Against Growth Hormone Releasing Factor (GHRH)

GHRH stimulates GH release. Potentiation of GHRH could increase GH secretion and hence growth. The receptor-binding region of GHRH resides in the N-terminal 29 residues (Coy et al. 1985). Specific site-directed anti-peptide antibodies have been generated against either the N- or C-terminal domains of GHRH (Pell and James 1995). Antibodies directed against the N-terminal region of GHRH inhibited GHRH activity, whereas antibodies directed against the C-terminal region enhanced GHRH activity in vivo and in vitro (Figure 18.12). Thus, the site of binding of the

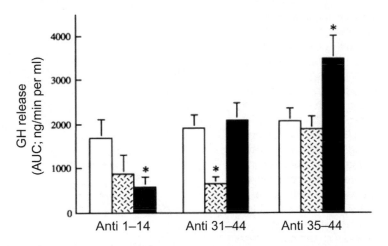

Figure 18.12. Growth hormone (GH) release into blood in sheep after treatment with growth hormone release factor (GHRH) and site-directed anti-peptide antibodies against GHRH. GH release was calculated as the area under the curve (AUC) of GH concentration versus time for each individual animal: GHRH alone (open bars), anti-peptide Ig alone (shaded bars), and GHRH preincubated with anti-peptide Ig (solid bars). Peptide sequences are given beneath each set of bars. Data are means ± S.E.M. (n = 5 per group). *P<0.05 is compared with the response for GHRH alone. GHRH-stimulated GH release is enhanced when GHRH is bound to antibodies directed against the nonreceptor binding C-terminal domain, but inhibited when bound to antibodies directed against the receptor-interacting N-terminal domain. (Reprinted from Pell and James, 1995, by permission of the Society for Endocrinology.)

antibody is important for subsequent hormone activity, and it appears that antibody-mediated enhancement may be demonstrated both in vivo and in vitro.

Antibodies Against Insulin-like Growth Factor-I (IGF-I)

Most studies have examined the effects of antibodies against IGF-I by passive immunization (Kerr et al. 1990; Spencer et al. 1991; Koea et al. 1992; Stewart et al. 1993; Bass et al. 1994; Hill et al. 1995; Pell et al. 1995, 1996; Hill et al. 1997; Manes et al. 1997a, 1997b; Hill et al. 1998a, 1998b; Hill and Pell 1998; Pell et al. 2000; Smith et al. 2000). Some of these reports have found an inhibitory effect of specific antibodies on IGF-I actions (Kerr et al. 1990; Spencer et al. 1991; Koea et al. 1992), although many of those cited above have described IGF-I-enhancing activity. One of the factors that has an important influence upon inhibition or enhancement of IGF-I actions is the affinity of the antibody for IGF-I (Smith & Hill 1999), although the range of epitopes recognized is also important.

The affinity of an enhancing anti-IGF-I antibody (Stewart et al. 1993) was similar to a potentiating IGFBP (~2 x 10^8 liters/mole). Therefore, it was proposed that the antibody provided an additional pool of bioavailable IGF-I, resulting in increased growth (Figure 18.13). The IGF-I epitopes recognized by the enhancing antibody have been determined, using epitope scanning techniques. In this approach, multiple short and overlapping peptides (typically hexamers or octamers) are synthesized that span the entire sequence of the peptide under investigation. These are then incubated with antibody and sites of interaction detected by ELISA techniques. The enhancing anti-IGF-I antiserum recognized a very specific region of IGF-I: residues Ser33 to Cys47 (Hill and Pell 1998). Antibodies that did not potentiate IGF-I activity do not recognize this region (Pell et al. 2000; Figure 18.14). This domain is situated on the opposite face of IGF-I to the receptor-binding site. This is consistent also with the location of antibodies that potentiate both GH and GHRH.

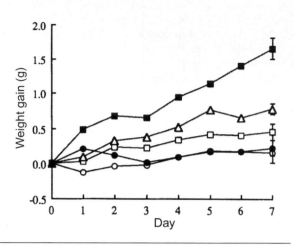

Figure 18.13. Weight gain in dwarf mice treated with IGF-I, anti-IGF-I Ig, or combined IGF-I and anti-IGF-I Ig. In this experiment, dwarf mice were treated with saline (open circles) passively immunized using sheep anti-IGF-I Ig alone (closed circles) or in combination with 20 µg IGF-I per day, which was precomplexed with the antibody, or with either saline (closed squares), 20 µg IGF-I per day alone (open squares), or 50 µg IGF-I per day alone (open triangles). Note that dwarf mice have very little endogenous IGF-I and there was no effect of anti-IGF-I Ig alone. However, mice dosed with combined IGF-I and anti-IGF-I Ig achieved a 3.5-fold increase in weight gain compared to mice treated with the same dose of IGF-I alone. (Reprinted from Stewart et al., 1993, with permission of The Endocrine Society.)

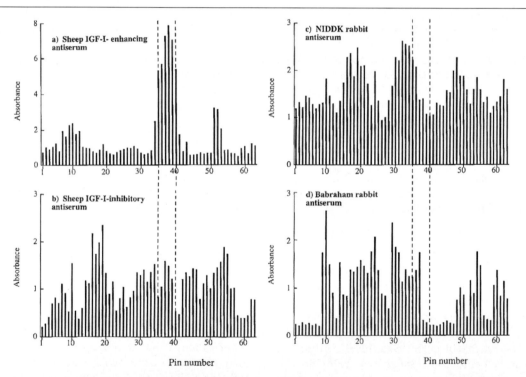

Figure 18.14. Scanning epitope analysis of the binding of different anti-IGF-I antibodies to sequential, 8-amino acid, linear peptides. In this experiment, anti-IGF-I antibodies from the various sources indicated were tested for binding to synthetic peptides (of eight amino acids), which in sum correspond to the whole IGF-I sequence. Peptide 1 corresponds to amino acids 1-8 of IGF-I, peptide 2 corresponds to amino acids 2-9 of IGF-I, and so on. The IGF-I-enhancing antibody binds a dominant epitope corresponding to the amino acid region between Arg36 and Ile43. (See also Figure 18.10.) In contrast, other antibodies appear to bind multiple regions of IGF-I. (Reprinted from Pell et al., 2000, with permission of The Endocrine Society.)

Antibodies as Enhancers of GH Activity

Antibodies usually neutralize antigenic molecules. For example, administration of polyclonal antibodies against GH reduce hormone activity (Flint et al. 1992; Palmer et al. 1994). However, certain MAb were surprisingly shown to increase GH action (Holder et al. 1985). There are potential benefits in devising methods whereby activity of GH is augmented because it leads to increased lean body mass and decreases fat deposition (Figure 18.15). The effect of GH was enhanced by precomplexing with MAb prior to administration to an animal model (Aston et al. 1986, 1987, 1989, 1991) (Figure 18.16). This finding had obvious agricultural implications to improve livestock growth. Potentiation of GH activity by MAb has been demonstrated for its lactogenic and diabetogenic properties in sheep (Pell et al. 1989). The use of anti-bGH MAbs for livestock is not currently feasible on grounds of cost and practicality. These antibodies, generally raised in mice, would be recognized as foreign protein and an anti-antibody response would be raised in the recipient species. This led to an alternative strategy using peptides derived from the sequence of the bovine GH molecule as vaccines to induce animals to generate self-antibodies, which would bind to, and enhance, endogenous GH activity. The feasibility of this approach was given further credence because antisera raised against fragments of both bovine and porcine GH enhanced hormone activity (Bomford and Aston 1990; Wang et al. 1990, 1994). Some studies employed GH-deficient animal models, and enhanced activity was demonstrated by complexing GH with anti-peptide antisera prior to administration. (This would have to happen in vivo in actual practice.)

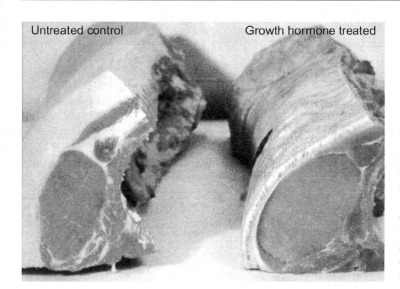

Untreated control

Growth hormone treated

Figure 18.15. Decreased fat accumulation in pigs given porcine GH treatment. This effect of growth hormone is observed in all livestock species studied to date. For maximum effect, a high plane of nutrition is required. The most dramatic effects may be seen in the pig. For more detailed information, see Chapter 5.

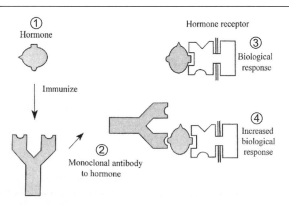

Figure 18.16. Monoclonal antibody (MAb) enhancement of hormone activity. The figure shows the mechanism that is believed to operate when site-specific MAbs directed against growth hormone (GH) interact in vivo. The MAb binds a site on GH discrete from the receptor binding site. The MAb then has a role in presenting GH to the receptor.

In an attempt to improve the development of a peptide vaccination, epitope mapping studies of the GH molecule were undertaken to identify regions of the GH molecule associated with enhancement. Previous GH peptides had been selected on the basis of computer algorithms predicting immunogenic regions. This resulted in the selection of many peptides contained in loop structures within/on the surface of the GH molecule. Antibodies generated from such peptides may bind better to native protein than those raised against elements within a protein. Initial mapping studies, with linear epitopes, showed that polyclonal antibodies raised against bGH contained major epitopes in all the loops joining the 4 α-helices as well as in the nonordered C-terminus of the protein (Beattie et al. 1992). Although many monoclonal antibodies could not be epitope-mapped using this technique, presumably because they recognized discontinuous epitopes, one anti-ovine GH enhancing antibody, MAb OA15, did bind to a continuous epitope lying between residues 91-102 of bGH in a loop between helices 2 and 3 of GH (Beattie and Holder 1994). The peptide epitope to which this enhancing MAb bound was used to produce a polyclonal antiserum, and this enhanced GH activity in a dwarf mouse model (Mockridge et al. 1998). Active immunization of lambs with a modified fragment, 134-154 of GH also increased carcass weight in lambs (Pell and Aston 1991).

The mechanisms of enhancement include increased half-life of the hormone-antibody complex, increased GH receptor occupancy time by hormone-antibody complexes, and the targeting of hormone to specific target tissues (e.g., liver) (Wang et al. 1992; Massart et al. 1993; Tans et al. 1994). A better understanding of the mechanism of enhancement would assist in the design of more effective agents.

Anti-Idiotypic Antibodies Against GH as Hormone Mimics

The anti-idiotypic network theory proposed by Jerne (1974) has led to attempts to use this to enhance hormone action. According to Jerne's theory, each antibody itself evokes an antibody response (i.e., anti-antibodies). A proportion of such antibodies may be mimics of the original immunogen (Figure 18.17). Polyclonal anti-idiotype antibodies raised in sheep against polyclonal anti-GH antiserum mimicked GH, stimulating growth in hypophysectomized rats (Gardner et al. 1990). In a similar fashion, an anti-idiotypic MAb raised against anti-pGH MAb promoted growth in hypophysectomized rats (Wang et al. 1994). Administration of a purified polyclonal rabbit antiserum against bGH to lactating cows increased "bGH-like" immunoreactivity in the sera but had no effect on either milk yield or serum IGF-I concentrations (Schalla et al. 1994).

Antibodies Against the GH Receptor (GHR) as Agonists

The concept is to produce antibodies to the site on the GH receptor (GHR) to which the hormone binds (Figure 18.18). GH activates its receptor by a homodimerization mechanism, two sites on GH interacting with two receptor molecules resulting in a 1:2 (hormone:receptor) complex (De Vos et al. 1992). This mechanism suggested that GHR activation might be achieved by binding a bivalent anti-GHR to two receptors. Such receptor-activating antibodies have been described for the prolactin receptor. These stimulate mammary gland casein synthesis in vitro and in vivo (Dusanter-Fourt et al. 1983, 1984). There are no reports of stimulatory

Figure 18.17. Using anti-idiotypic antibodies as hormones. The underlying principle here is that anti-antibodies are produced against the specific antigen binding region of a hormone-binding antibody. Thus these anti-antibodies have a specific binding site, which mimics the hormone. These are then capable of interacting with the receptor, mimicking hormone actions.

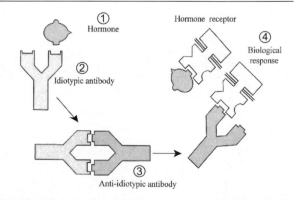

anti-GHR antibodies. Epitope mapping studies of the bovine GHR extracellular domain (Beattie et al. 1996) may assist in the selection of candidate GHR peptides for the generation of anti-GHR antibodies. These would need to facilitate receptor dimerization and signal transduction. Peptide antisera raised against linear sequences of the GHR recognize the GHR under denaturing conditions but not in its native state. An alternative strategy involves presenting putative peptide epitopes (e.g., from rat GHR) within the framework of the GHR derived from another species (e.g., sheep). When sheep are immunized with such peptides, the response to the chimeric protein should be targeted towards the rat sequences because the sheep are immunotolerant to their own GHR sequences. The use of such recombinant proteins as vaccines may overcome problems associated with the appropriate presentation of peptides. Studies with chimeric rat/ovine GH binding protein indicate that this approach is feasible (Allan et al. 1999).

Antibodies as Enhancers of β-Adrenoceptor Actions

β-agonists are anabolic in cattle, sheep, and pigs. β-agonists have a short half-life in vivo and, to be effective, regular dosing is necessary. Also β-agonists are thermally stable and there may be concern about residue even in cooked meat. These factors prompted the investigation of immunomodulation of the β_2-AR. Immunomodulation offers treatment over extended periods. Moreover, antibodies are not thermally stable and are destroyed by cooking.

There is an extensive literature on antibodies raised against the β-adrenoceptor including mechanistic, fundamental and clinical studies. There are a few studies of β-AR antibodies addressing livestock production. Antibody actions are clearly demonstrated in vitro and in model species with a consistent mechanism across species and β-AR sub-types. Despite this, there are no reports of production responses in livestock.

Antibodies Against Synthetic Peptide Analogues of β-AR

Synthetic peptide antigens are useful only if the structures of the protein are known. Fortunately the structure of the β-AR has been elucidated. Rabbit antibodies to extracellular domains of the hamster β_2-AR have been raised recognizing β_2-AR in immunoblots and precipitating radiolabelled β_2-AR (Theveniau et al. 1989). Anti-peptide antibodies have been raised in rabbits using 26 amino acid sequences corresponding to outer loop 2 of the β_1- and β_2-AR (Magnusson et al. 1989, 1990, 1991, 1994). The main focus was the β_1-AR, because this is the predominant sub-type in the heart. Anti-β_1-AR antibodies incubated with C6 glioma cell membranes (rich in β_1-AR) were able to enhance isoprotenerol binding. However, anti-β_2-AR antibodies did not show any effects on ligand binding when incubated with A431 cell membranes rich in

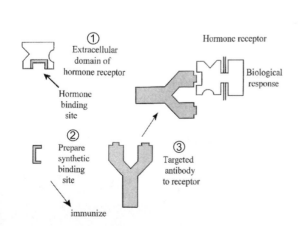

Figure 18.18. Using anti-receptor antibodies as pseudo-hormones. The mechanism of action of anti-receptor antibodies is thought to involve antibody binding to extracellular domains of the receptor, not necessarily the hormone binding site. This principle has been demonstrated for both the growth hormone receptor and for β-adrenoceptors (see the next section). Synthetic peptide mimics of an outer domain of the receptor are used to immunize animals and evoke antibodies, which bind to this receptor domain. On antibody binding, a change in receptor conformation is induced. This leads to an intracellular response, utilizing the usual second messenger pathway.

β$_2$-AR (Magnusson et al. 1989). Interestingly, anti-β$_1$-AR also produced an agonist-like chronotropic effect in an in vitro bioassay, isolated, neonatal rat cardiomyocytes (Magnusson et al. 1991). This was blocked by preincubation with the β$_1$-peptide and was antagonized by a β$_1$-selective antagonist but not by a β$_2$- selective antagonist.

These findings of antibody having a biological effect (at the β$_1$-AR) led to study of the β$_2$-AR. These earlier findings were very encouraging for the ultimate development of a peptide-based "growth vaccine." Hill and colleagues (1998b) produced anti-β$_2$-AR antibodies by immunizing rabbits with a peptide preparation. These antibodies were biologically active, increasing the affinity of a β-antagonist and causing a leftward shift in the concentration-response curve for isoproterenol-induced bovine smooth muscle relaxation (Figure 18.19). Possible mechanisms by which the antibodies exert their effects at the β$_2$-AR include the following: Antibodies might behave similarly to the conventional agonists in causing a conformational change in the receptor protein upon binding. β-agonists bind to side-chains of amino acid residues within the cleft formed by the seven transmembrane domains of the receptor (see Figure 18.1). The mechanism of antibody binding and activation of the β$_2$-AR is likely to be different. Sterically, anti-

bodies would be precluded from binding to the conventional ligand binding site deep within the receptor; the molecular mass of conventional agonists is ~0.001 that of IgG. Assuming that antibodies bind to the sequence corresponding to the synthetic peptide used as antigen, their effects must be mediated via the second outer loop, which joins transmembrane domains 4 and 5 (Figure 18.1). Both these domains play a role in conventional ligand binding. This evidence suggests that the binding of antibodies to outer loop 2 may induce a conformational change in the receptor, analogous to that following binding of a conventional agonist. This proposed conformational change then may lead to receptor activation. This is consistent with that for activation of human β$_1$-AR. Despite demonstration of biological activity, there are no reports of production effects in livestock.

Antibodies Against Placental Lactogen (PL)

Placental lactogen (PL) has been implicated in prenatal growth regulation, possibly by stimulating repartitioning of nutrients to the fetus and also by stimulating the fetus to utilize these substrates (Byatt et al. 1992; Anthony et al. 1995). Leibovich and colleagues (2000) actively immunized ewes with PL at 5 months of age, generating anti-PL

Figure 18.19. The effects of anti-β$_2$-adrenoceptor (β$_2$-AR) antibodies on the relaxation of bovine smooth muscle in vitro. In this experiment, bovine tracheal smooth muscle was incubated in an organ bath and suspended such that its contraction could be measured. Isoproterenol is a β$_2$-agonist drug, which causes relaxation of muscle (closed circles). The figure shows that in the presence of specific anti-β$_2$-AR antibody (open circles) the dose response curve for isoproterenol is left-shifted. This shows that when the antibody is present, less of the drug is needed for similar effect. Thus the antibody has increased the action of the drug. Note also that antibody alone also caused relaxation of the tissue. This may be due to antibody action on the receptor in the presence of endogenous epinephrine, the hormone that activates the β$_2$-AR in vivo. (Reprinted from Hill et al., 1998, with permission.)

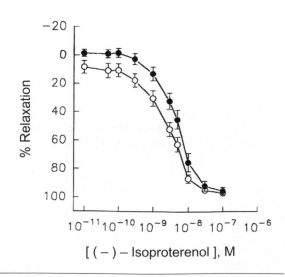

antibodies that were active in an in vitro assay and which maintained a pool of antibody-bound hormone in vivo. In a subsequent pregnancy, lamb birth weight and maternal milk yield were increased.

Other Immunization Strategies

Antibodies to Adipocyte Plasma Membranes

The problem of excess fat deposition has been targeted for immunomodulation. Antibodies are used in their more classical role of targeting molecules and cells for destruction by the immune system—for example, via complement-mediated cell lysis. Antibodies directed against the plasma membranes of adipocytes induce their destruction and thereby limit the storage capacity for fat. Successful depletion of fat has been achieved in rats, sheep, and pigs in both passive and active immunization.

Passive Immunization

Early studies demonstrated lysis of isolated adipocytes in vitro (Flint et al. 1986). and these antibodies were also effective in vivo. Within the first week of treatment, adipocyte destruction and invasion by macrophages were evident (Figure 18.20) and following this, a 75% decrease in adipocyte mass 2 months later (Futter and Flint 1987). There were also unexpected effects, appetite, protein deposition, and food conversion efficiency all increased after treatment (Panton et al. 1990). There were, however, also side effects, including reduced food intake on the day of treatment and transient sedative effects lasting several hours. Activation of the immune system, along with depletion of serum complement, occurs rapidly after treatment and could explain these side effects. If so, a slow release formulation might reduce or eliminate these unwanted effects. Subsequent studies were undertaken in sheep, pigs, chickens, and rabbits. In sheep, passive immunization against adipocyte plasma membranes produced modest effects, reducing both fat content and liveweight gain (Moloney and Allen 1989; Nassar and Hu 1991). In rabbits, more dramatic effects were achieved 1 week after treatment but there was an ability to replete fat stores 2 months later (Dulor et al. 1990). The most promising studies in an agricultural species have been achieved in pigs. Subcutaneous injections produced total fat depletion at injection sites lasting over 3 months (Kestin et al. 1993) (Figure 18.21). Intraperitoneal injection produced a 30% decrease in back fat thickness, a 25% decrease in fat content of the forelimb, and an increase in muscle mass.

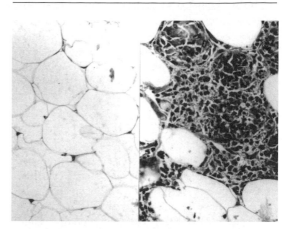

Figure 18.20. Normal adipose tissue (left) and adipose tissue undergoing macrophage infiltration one week after immunization with antibodies to adipocytes. The destruction of adipocytes is mediated by antibody binding and activation of the complement pathway, which leads to adipocyte cell lysis. The released fat is then utilized in the body for metabolic processes.

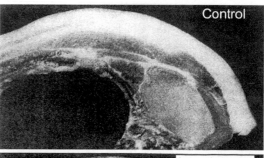

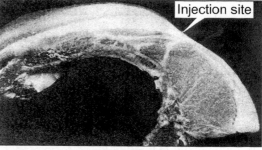

Figure 18.21. Localized destruction of adipose tissue three months after injection of antibodies to adipocytes (lower panel). Upper panel shows a control injection site in the same pig.

Ideally treatment should be given early in life, because, if dosing is on a body weight basis, it will be more economical. Given that treatment requires an active complement system, this must be sufficiently mature in the young animal. Thus these two factors would need to be considered in a treatment regime.

Active Immunization

Active immunization, using adipocyte plasma membranes as an immunogen, to provoke an autoimmune response against adipose tissues has been assessed in rats, sheep, and pigs. Although reductions in adipocyte cell numbers were achieved in rats, the effects were offset by compensatory increases in adipocyte volume (Futter et al. 1992), reducing the effect on adipose tissue mass. Studies in sheep either failed to have any effects or to decrease liveweight gain, as well as that of fat and lean tissues (Nassar and Hu 1991). By contrast, in pigs, immunization produced significant decreases in body fat content (Kestin et al. 1993).

Mechanism of Action of Antibodies

Early studies demonstrated that antibodies induce lysis of adipocytes in vitro solely in the presence of complement (Flint et al. 1986). In vivo studies involved cellular infiltration of adipose tissue. These suggest a role for cell-mediated responses (Futter and Flint 1987). Studies in complement-deficient rats clearly demonstrated that antibodies were completely ineffective in the absence of complement (Futter et al. 1992).

Antibody Specificity

Antisera to adipocyte plasma membranes cross-react with other tissues and this could provoke unwanted side effects. The relative specificity for adipose tissue is better than may be imagined. Identifying "adipocyte-specific" cell surface antigens nevertheless remains a priority to avoid adverse side effects due to cross-reactions with other tissues.

Development of an Anti-Obesity Therapy

Although originally developed for use in livestock species, this approach could be considered for clinical use to treat obesity. The antibody however would need to be a monoclonal antibody, probably with absolute specificity for the adipocyte. Obesity is not simply a cosmetic problem but a considerable and increasing health risk based upon the strong association between obesity, diabetes, and cardiovascular disease. Studies were conducted in the "cafeteria-fed" rat as a model of obesity. After consuming a high fat diet and increasing their body weight by almost 50%, animals were treated with antisera to adipocytes. The response to treatment was a 10% decrease in body weight and a 30–40% reduction in body fat, which lasted for at least 3 months after treatment (Flint 1998; Figure 18.22). There was also improvement in a factor associated with obesity, serum leptin; concentrations were decreased from the very high levels in untreated obese rats.

The search for suitable antibodies has begun (Vaughan et al. 1996). A panel of over 100 different

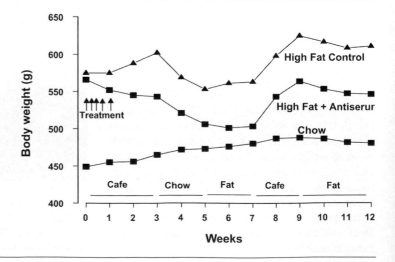

Figure 18.22. Changes in body weight after treatment (arrows) with antibodies to adipocytes in rats fed a cafeteria diet. Diets were switched to low fat (chow) and intermediate fat (fat) and back to a high fat diet (cafe) showing that the loss of weight was maintained independently of the diet.

human single-chain Fv (scFv) antibodies binding human adipocyte plasma membranes have been isolated (Edwards et al. 2000). Three of these were selected based upon their additional cross-reaction with rat adipocytes. Each scFv was reformatted as a rat chimaeric IgG2b, and the ability to induce lysis of rat adipocytes in vitro and reduction of serum complement levels in vivo was determined. Each of these antibodies, both singly and in combination, was able to induce adipocyte lysis in vitro, and they were also effective in vivo where they reduced serum complement levels indicating adipocyte lysis (Dickinson et al. 2002). Taken together these results suggest that single monoclonal antibodies could be used therapeutically and that the massive adipocyte lysis occurring over several weeks is well tolerated at least in obese rodents.

CONCLUSIONS

Our understanding of the processes and interactions in immunomodulation of growth is incomplete. However in some cases it has been possible to obtain useful production responses. In order to develop this technology to its full potential, advances in understanding of the immune systems of livestock species are required. Mapping of T-cell epitopes for each species will especially aid design of accessory molecules to help direct the immune response to the target protein. Novel approaches to vaccine formulation, such as the inclusion of lymphokines may also enhance the desired response. At present, the major challenges for the technology are to provide the following:

- A maximum proportion of responding animals
- Control of titer, so that animals respond with antibody production at a sufficiently high level to allow biological interaction of antibody with the target protein
- Persistence of the response so that antibodies remain at a useful titer for a period of time that allows the interaction to result in a meaningful biological change in metabolism, resulting in a production advantage

Public resistance to the use of drugs in agriculture is increasing, although these arguments are sometimes emotive and not based in fact. Immunomodulation provides animal scientists with an alternative tool for improving the productive efficiency of livestock, with large potential benefits for the future.

REFERENCES

Allan, G.J., Shand, J.H., Beattie, J., and Flint, D.J. 1999. Identification of novel sites in the ovine growth hormone receptor involved in binding hormone and conferring species specificity. *European Journal of Biochemistry* 261:555–562.

Anthony, R. V., Liang, R., Kayl, E. P., and Pratt, S. L. 1995. The growth hormone prolactin family in ruminant placenta. *Journal of Reproduction and Fertility* 49Suppl.1:83–95.

Arimura, A., Smith, W.D., and Schally, A.V. 1976. Blockade of the stress-induced decrease in blood GH by anti-somatostatin serum in rats. *Endocrinology* 98:540–543.

Aston, R., Cowden, W.B., and Ada, G.L. 1989. Antibody-mediated enhancement of hormone activity. *Molecular Immunology* 26:435–46.

Aston, R., Holder, A.T., Ivanyi, J., and Bomford, R. 1987. Enhancement of bovine growth hormone activity in vivo by monoclonal antibodies. *Molecular Immunology* 24:143–150.

Aston, R., Holder, A.T., Preece, M.A., and Ivanyi, J. 1986. Potentiation of the somatogenic and lactogenic activity of human growth hormone with monoclonal antibodies. *Journal of Endocrinology* 110:381–388.

Aston, R., Rathjen, D.A., Holder, A.T., Bender, V., Trigg, T.E., Cowan, K., Edwards, J.A., and Cowden, W.B. 1991. Antigenic structure of bovine growth hormone: location of a growth enhancing region. *Molecular Immunology* 28:41–50.

Bahouth, S.W., Wang, H., and Malbon, C.C. 1991. Immunological approaches for probing receptor structure and function. *Trends in Pharmacological Sciences* 12:338–343.

Bard, F., Cannon, C., Barbour, R., Burke, R.-L., Games, D., Grajeda, H., Guido, T., Hu, K., Huang, J., Johnson-Wood, K., Khan, K., Kholodenko, D., Lee, M., Lieberburg, I., Motter, R., Nguyen, M., Soriano, F., Vasquez, N., Weiss, K., Welch, B., Seubert, P., Schenk, D., and Yednock, T. 2000. Peripherally administered antibodies against amyloid ß-peptide enter the central nervous system and reduce pathology in a mouse model of Alzeimer disease. *Nature Medicine* 6:916–919.

Bass, J.J., Gluckman, P.D., Fairclough, R.J., Peterson, A.J., Davis, S.R., and Carter, W.D. 1987. Effect of nutrition and immunization against somatostatin on growth and insulin-like growth factors in sheep. *Journal of Endocrinology* 112:27–31.

Bass, J.J., Hodgkinson, S.C., and Spencer, G.S.G. 1994. Effects of immunisation against insulin-like growth factors. In *Vaccines in Agriculture. Immunological Applications to Animal Health and Production.* P.R. Wood, P. Willadsen, J.E. Vercoe, R.M. Hoskinson, and D. Demeyer, eds. Melbourne: CSIRO.

Bealoye, V., Muaku, S.M., Lause, P., Portetell, D., Renaville, R., Robert, A.R., Ketelslegers, J.M., and Maiter, D. 1999. Monoclonal antibodies to growth hormone (GH) prolong liver GH binding and GH-induced IGF/IGFBP-3 synthesis. *American Journal of Physiology* 277:E308–E315.

Beattie, J., Fawcett, H.A., and Flint, D.J. 1992. The use of multiple-pin peptide synthesis in an analysis of the continuous epitopes recognised by various anti-(recombinant bovine growth hormone) sera. Comparison with predicted regions of immunogenicity and location within the three-dimensional structure of the molecule. *European Journal of Biochemistry* 210:59–66.

Beattie, J., and Holder, A.T. 1994. Location of an epitope defined by an enhancing monoclonal antibody to growth hormone: some structural details and biological implications. *Molecular Endocrinology* 8:1103–1110.

Beattie, J., Shand, J.H., and Flint, D.J. 1996. An immobilised peptide array identifies antibodies to a discontinuous epitope in the extracellular domain of the bovine growth hormone receptor. *European Journal of Biochemistry* 239:479–486.

Beh, K.J., and Blattman, A.N. 1994. The major histocompatibility complex system of vertebrates. In *Vaccines in Agriculture. Immunological Applications to Animal Health and Production.* P. R. Wood, P. Willadsen, J.E. Vercoe, R.M. Hoskinson, and D. Demeyer, eds. Melbourne: CSIRO.

Bomford, R., and Aston, R. 1990. Enhancement of bovine growth hormone activity by antibodies against growth hormone peptides. *Journal of Endocrinology* 125:31–38.

Butler, J.E. 1998. Immunoglobulin diversity, B-cell and antibody repertoire development in large farm animals. *Revue Scientifique et Technique* 17:43–70.

Byatt, J.C., Warren, W.C., Eppard, P.J., Staten, N.R., Krivi, J.J., and Collier, R.J. 1992. Ruminant placental lactogens: structure and biology. *Journal of Animal Science*, 70:2911–2923.

Chapman, A.P., Antoniw, P., Spitali, M., West, S., Stephens, S., and King, D.J. 1999. Therapeutic antibody fragments with prolonged in vivo half-lives. *Nature Biotechnology*, 17:780–3.

Chicz, R.M., and Urban, R.G. 1994. Analysis of MHC-presented peptides: applications in autoimmunity and vaccine development. *Immunology Today*, 15:155–160.

Chowdhury, P.S., and Pastan, I. 1999. Improving antibody affinity by mimicking somatic hypermutation in vitro. *Nature Biotechnology*, 17:568–572.

Clark, R., Olson, K., Fuh, G., Marian, M., Mortensen, D., Teshima, G., Chang, S., Chu, H., Mukku, V., Canova-Davis, E., Somers, T., Cronin, M., Winkler, M., and Wells, J. A. 1996a. Long-acting growth hormones produced by conjugation with polyethylene glycol. *Journal of Biological Chemistry*, 271:21969–21977.

Clark, R.G., Mortensen, D.L., Carlsson, L.M., Spencer, S.A., McKay, P., Mulkerrin, M., Moore, J., and Cunningham, B.C. 1996b. Recombinant human growth hormone (GH)-binding protein enhances the growth-promoting activity of human GH in the rat. *Endocrinology*, 137:4308–4315.

Cook, R.B., Popp, J.D., Kastelic, J.P., Robbins, S., and Harland, R. 2000. The effects of active immunization against GnRH on testicular development, feedlot performance, and carcass characteristics of beef bulls. *Journal of Animal Science*, 78:2778–2783.

Coy, D.H., Murphy, W.A., Sueiras-Diaz, J., Coy, E.J., and Lance, V.A. 1985. Structure activity studies on the N-terminal region of growth hormone releasing factor. *Journal of Medicinal Chemistry*, 28:181–185.

De Vos, A.M., Ultsch, M., and Kossiakoff, A.A. 1992. Human growth hormone and extracellular domain of its receptor: crystal structure of the complex. *Science*, 255:306–312.

Dickinson, K., North, T.J., Telford, G., Smith, S.E., Edwards, B.M., Main, S.H., Field, R., Hatton, D., Vaughan, T.J., Flint, D.J., and Jones, R.B. 2002. Antibody-induced lysis of isolated rat epididymal adipocytes and complement activation in vivo. *Obesity Research*, 10:122–127.

Dowsett, K.F., Tshweng, U., Knott, L.M., Jackson, A.E., and Trigg, T.E. 1993. Immunocastration of colts and immunospeying of fillies. *Immunology and Cell Biology*, 71:501–508.

Dulor, J.P., Reyne, Y., and Nougues, J. 1990. In vivo effects of treatment with antibodies to adipocyte plasma membranes in the rabbit. *Reproduction Nutrition et Developpement*, 30:49–58.

Dunshea, F.R., Colantoni, C., Howard, K., McCauley, I., Jackson, P., Long, K.A., Lopaticki, S., Nugent, E.A., Simons, J.A., Walker, J., and Hennessy, D.P. 2001. Vaccination of boars with a GnRH vaccine (Improvac) eliminates boar taint in increases growth performance. *Journal of Animal Science*, 79:2524–2535.

Dusanter-Fourt, I., Djiane, J., Houdebine, L.M., and Kelly, P.A. 1983. In vivo lactogenic effects of anti prolactin receptor antibodies in pseudopregnant rabbits. *Life Sciences*, 32:407–412.

Dusanter-Fourt, I., Djiane, J., Kelly, P.A., Houdebine, L.M., and Teyssot, B. 1984. Differential biological activities between mono- and bivalent fragments of anti-prolactin receptor antibodies. *Endocrinology* 114:1021–1027.

Edwards, B.M., Main, S.H., Cantone, K.L., Smith, S.D., Warford, A., and Vaughan, T.J. 2000. Isolation and tissue profiles of a large panel of phage antibodies binding to the human adipocyte cell surface. *Journal of Immunological Methods* 245:67–78.

Farmer, C., Petitclerc, D., Pelletier, G., Gaudreau, P., and Brazeau, P. 1992. Carcass composition and resistance to fasting in neonatal piglets born of sows immunized against somatostatin and/or receiving growth hormone-releasing factor injections during gestation. *Biology of the Neonate* 61:110–117.

Flint, D.J. 1998. Effects of antibodies to adipocytes on body weight, food intake, and adipose tissue cellularity in obese rats. *Biochemical and Biophysical Research Communications* 252:263–268.

Flint, D.J., Coggrave, H., Futter, C.E., Gardner, M.J., and Clarke, T.J. 1986. Stimulatory and cytotoxic effects of an antiserum to adipocyte plasma membranes on adipose tissue metabolism in vitro and in vivo. *International Journal of Obesity*, 10:69–77.

Flint, D.J., Tonner, E., Beattie, J., and Panton, D. 1992. Investigation of the mechanism of action of growth hormone in stimulating lactation in the rat. *Journal of Endocrinology*, 134:377–383.

Futter, C.E., and Flint, D.J. 1987. Long-term reduction of adiposity in rats after passive immunization with antibodies to rat fat cell plasma membranes. In *Recent Advances in Obesity Research V.* E.M. Berry, ed. London: John Libbey.

Futter, C.E., Panton, D., Kestin, S., and Flint, D.J. 1992. Mechanism of action of cytotoxic antibodies to adipocytes on adipose tissue, liver and food intake in the rat. *International Journal of Obesity and Related Metabolic Disorders* 16:615–622.

Gardner, M.J., Morrison, C.A., Stevenson, L.Q., and Flint, D.J. 1990. Production of anti-idiotypic antisera to rat GH antibodies capable of binding to GH receptors and increasing body weight gain in hypophysectomized rats. *Journal of Endocrinology* 125:53–59.

Gazzola, C., Hill, R.A., Herd, R.M., and Oddy, V.H. 1998. Effect of immunization against leptin on growth rate and fat deposition in cattle. In *Proceedings of the Nutrition Society of Australia*, Adelaide, Australia.

Harris, D.P., Vordemeier, H.-M., Arya, A., Bogdan, C., Moreno, C., and Ivanyi, J. 1996. Immunogenicity of peptides for B cells is not impaired by overlapping T-cell epitope topology. *Immunology* 88:348–354.

Hayden, M.S., Gilliland, L.K., and Ledbetter, J.A. 1997. Antibody engineering. *Current Opinion in Immunology* 9:201–212.

Hill, R.A., Dye, S., Sheldrick, E.L., Flick-Smith, H.C., and Pell, J.M. 1995. Regulation of plasma clearance and tissue distribution of insulin-like growth factor-1 (IGF-I) by an IGF-I enhancing antibody. *Journal of Endocrinology* 144Supp.l:P63.

Hill, R.A., Flick-Smith, F.C., Dye, S., and Pell, J.M. 1997. Actions of an IGF-I-enhancing antibody on IGF-I pharmacokinetics and tissue distribution: increased IGF-I bioavailability. *Journal of Endocrinology* 152:123–130.

Hill, R.A., Gazzola, C., Herd, R.M., and Oddy, V.H. 1998a. An insulin-like growth factor-1 based vaccine changes body composition in Angus steers. *Proceedings of the Nutrition Society of Australia* 22:176.

Hill, R.A., Hoey, A.J., and Sillence, M.N. 1998b. Functional activity of antibodies at the bovine β_2-adrenoceptor. *Journal of Animal Science* 76:1651–1661.

Hill, R.A., and Pell, J.M. 1998. Regulation of insulin-like growth factor 1 (IGF-I) bioactivity in vivo: further characterisation of an IGF-I-enhancing antibody. *Endocrinology* 139:1278–1287.

Hill, R.A., Smith, N.N., and Holmes, M.A. 1998c. An insulin-like growth factor-1 (IGF-I) based vaccine improves growth rate in steers. *Animal Production in Australia* 22:321.

Holder, A.T., Aston, R., Preece, M.A., and Ivanyi, J. 1985. Monoclonal antibody-mediated enhancement of growth hormone activity in vivo. *Journal of Endocrinology* 107:R9–R12.

Hoskinson, R.M., Djura, P., Welch, R.J., Harrison, B.E., Brown, G.H., Donnelly, J.B., and Jones, M.R. 1988. Failure of antisomatostatin antibodies to stimulate the growth of crossbred lambs. *Australian Journal of Experimental Agriculture* 28:161–165.

Hoskinson, R.M., Rigby, R.D.G., Mattner, P.E., Huynh, V.L., D'Occhio, M.J., Neish, A., Trigg, T.E., Moss, B.A., Lindsay, M.J., and Coleman, G.D. 1990. Vaxtreate: an anti-reproductive vaccine for cattle. *Australian Journal of Biotechnology* 4:166–170.

Hudson, P.J. 1999. Recombinant antibody constructs in cancer therapy. *Current Opinions in Immunology* 11:548–557.

Jerne, N.K. 1974. Toward a network theory of the immune system. *Annales d' Immunologie (Paris)* 125C:373–389.

Jones, J.I., and Clemmons, D.R. 1995. Insulin-like growth factors and their binding proteins: biological actions. *Endocrine Reviews* 16:3–34.

Kerr, D.E., Laarveld, B., and Manns, J.G. 1990. Effects of passive immunization of growing guinea-pigs with an insulin-like growth factor-I monoclonal antibody. *Journal of Endocrinology* 124:403–415.

Kestin, S., Kennedy, R., Tonner, E., Kiernan, M., Cryer, A., Griffin, H., Butterwith, S., Rhind, S., and Flint, D. 1993. Decreased fat content and increased lean in pigs treated with antibodies to adipocyte plasma membranes. *Journal of Animal Science* 71:1486–1494.

Kirkwood, R.N., Korchinski, R.S., Thacker, P.A., and Laarveld, B. 1990. Observations on the influence of active immunization against somatostatin on the reproductive performance of sheep and pigs. *Journal of Reproductive Immunology* 17:229–238.

Koea, J.B., Gallaher, B.W., Breier, B.H., Douglas, R.G., Hodgkinson, S., Shaw, J.H.F., and Gluckman, P.D. 1992. Passive immunisation against circulating insulin-like growth factor-I (IGF-I) increases protein catabolism in lambs: Evidence for a physiological role for circulating IGF-I. *Journal of Endocrinology* 135:279–284.

Laarveld, B., Chaplin, R.K., and Kerr, D.E. 1986. Somatostatin immunization and growth of lambs. *Canadian Journal of Animal Science* 66:77–83.

Leibovich, H., Gertler, A., Bazer, F.W., and Gootwine, E. 2000. Active immunization of ewes against ovine placental lactogen increases birth weight of lambs and milk production with no adverse effect on conception rate. *Animal Reproduction Science* 64:33–47.

Lofthouse, S.A., Andrews, A.E., Elhay, M.J., Bowles, V.M., Meeusen, E.N.T., and Nash, A.D. 1996. Cytokines as adjuvants for ruminant vaccines. *International Journal for Parasitology* 26:835–842.

Magnusson, Y., Hoyer, S., Lengagne, R., Chapot, M.P., Guillet, J.-G., Hjalmarson, A., Strosberg, A.D., and Hoebeke, J. 1989. Antigenic analysis of the second extracellular loop of the human β-adrenergic receptors. *Clinical and Experimental Immunology*, 78:42–48.

Magnusson, Y., Marullo, S., Hoyer, S., Waagstein, F., Anderrson, B., Vahine, A., Guillet, J., Strosberg, A.D., Hjalmarson, A., and Hoebeke, J. 1990. Mapping of a functional autoimmune epitope on the β_1-adrenergic receptor in patients with idiopathic dilated cardiomyopathy. *Journal of Clinical Investigation* 86:1658–1663.

Magnusson, Y., Wallukat, G., Guillet, J., Hjalmarson, A., and Hoebeke, J. 1991. Functional analysis of rabbit anti-peptide antibodies which mimic autoantibodies against the β_1-adrenergic receptor in patients with idioipathic dilated cardiomyopathy. *Journal of Autoimmunity* 4:893–905.

Magnusson, Y., Wallukat, G., Waagstein, F., Hjalmarson, A., and Hoebeke, J. 1994. Autoimmunity in idiopathic dilated cardiomyopathy. Characterization of antibodies against the β_1-adrenoceptor with positive chronotropic effect. *Circulation* 89:2760–2767.

Manes, S., Kremer, L., Albar, J.P., Mark, C., Llopis, R., and Martinez-A, C. 1997a. Functional Epitope Mapping of Insulin-Like Growth Factor I (IGF-I) by Anti-IGF-I Monoclonal Antibodies. *Endocrinology* 138:905–915.

Manes, S., Kremer, L., Vangbo, B., Lopez, A., Gomez-Mouton, C., Peiro, E., Albar, J.P., Mendel-Hartvig, I.B., Llopis, R., and Martincz, C. 1997b. Physical mapping of human insulin-like growth factor-I using specific monoclonal antibodies. *Journal of Endocrinology* 154:293–302.

Massart, S., Maiter, D., Portetelle, D., Adam, E., Renaville, R., and Ketelslegers, J.-M. 1993. Monoclonal antibodies to bovine growth hormone potentiate hormonal activity in vivo by enhancing growth hormone binding to hepatic somatogenic receptors. *Journal of Endocrinology* 139:383–393.

Meloen, R.H. 1995. Basic aspects of immunomodulation through active immunisation. *Livestock Production Science* 42:135–145.

Mockridge, J.W., Aston, R., Morrell, D.J., and Holder, A.T. 1998. Cross-linked growth hormone dimers have enhanced biological activity. *European Journal of Endocrinology / European Federation of Endocrine Societies* 138:449–459.

Moloney, A.P., and Allen, P. 1989. Growth and weights of abdominal and carcass fat in sheep immunized against adipose cell membranes. In *Proceedings of the Nutrition Society.*

Nash, A.D., Lofthouse, S.A., Barcham, G.J., Jacobs, H.J., Ashman, K., Meeusen, E.N.T., Brandon, M.R., and Andrews, A.E. 1993. Recombinant cytokines as immunological adjuvants. *Immunology and Cell Biology* 71:367–379.

Nassar, A.H., and Hu, C.Y. 1991. Growth and carcass characteristics of lambs passively immunised with antibodies developed against ovine adipocyte plasma membranes. *Journal of Animal Science* 69:578–586.

Palmer, R.M., Loveridge, N., Thomson, B.M., Mackie, S.C., Tonner, E., and Flint, D.J. 1994. Effects of a polyclonal antiserum to rat growth hormone on circulating insulin-like growth factor (IGF)-I and IGF-binding protein concentrations and the growth of muscle and bone. *Journal of Endocrinology* 142:85–91.

Panton, D., Futter, C.E., Kestin, S., and Flint, D.J. 1990. Increased growth and protein deposition in rats treated with antibodies to adipocytes. *American Journal of Physiology* 258:E985–E989.

Pell, J.M., and Aston, R. 1991. Active immunisation with a synthetic peptide region of growth hormone increased lean tissue growth. *Journal of Endocrinology* 131:R1–R4.

Pell, J.M., and Aston, R. 1995. Principles of immunomodulation. *Livestock Production Science* 42:123–133.

Pell, J.M., Flick-Smith, H.C., Dye, S., and Hill, R.A. 1995. Further characterisation of an IGF-I enhancing antibody: actions on IGF-induced hypoglycaemia and interaction with the analogue LR3IGF-I. *Progress in Growth Factor Research* 6:367–375.

Pell, J.M., Flick-Smith, H.C., Stewart, C.E.H., and Hill, R.A. 1996. Peptide mimics for a major binding site on IGF-I for an IGF-I-enhancing antibody. *Journal of Endocrinology* 151Supp.l:P32.

Pell, J.M., Hill, R.A., Stewart, C.E.H., Weston, C.R., and Flick-Smith, H.C. 2000. Enhancement of IGF-I activity by novel antisera: potential structure/function interactions. *Journal of Endocrinology* 141:741–751.

Pell, J.M., and James, S. 1995. Immuno-enhancement and -inhibition of GH-releasing factor by site-directed and anti peptide antibodies in vivo and in vitro. *Journal of Endocrinology* 146:535–541.

Pell, J.M., Johnson, I.D., Puller, R.A., Morrell, D.J., Hart, I.C., Holder, A.T., and Aston, R. 1989. Potentiation of growth hormone activity in sheep using monoclonal antibodies. *Journal of Endocrinology* 120:R15–R18.

Roitt, I.M., Brostoff, J., and Male, D.K. 1993. *Immunology*. London: Mosby.

Schalla, C.L., Roberge, S., Wilkie, B.N., McBride, B.W., and Walton, J. S. 1994. Production of anti-idiotypic antibodies resembling bovine somatotropin by active immunisation of lactating cows. *Journal of Endocrinology* 141:203–208.

Smith, N.N., and Hill, R.A. 1999. Binding characterisation of anti-insulin-like growth factor-1 (IGF-I) antibodies raised in cattle and sheep. *Proceedings of the Endocrine Society of Australia* 42:73.

Smith, N.N., Hill, R.A., Pegg, G.G., and Pell, J.M. 2000. Passive immunisation with anti-IGF-I antibodies increases feed intake during nutritional restriction. *Asian-Australasian Journal of Animal Sciences* 13Supp.lC:154.

Spencer, G.S., Harvey, S., Audsley, A.R., Hallett, K.G., and Kestin, S. 1986. The effect of immunization against somatostatin on growth rates and growth hormone secretion in the chicken. *Comparative Biochemistry and Physiology. Part A, Physiology* 85:553–556.

Spencer, G.S. G., Garssen, G.J., and Bergström, P.L. 1983a. A novel approach to growth promotion using auto-immunisation against somatostatin II. Effects on appetite, carcass composition and food utilisation in lambs. *Livestock Production Science* 10:469–477.

Spencer, G.S.G., Garssen, G.J., and Hart, I.C. 1983b. A novel approach to growth promotion using auto-immunisation against somatostatin. I. Effects on growth and hormone levels in lambs. *Livestock Production Science* 10:25–37.

Spencer, G.S.G., Hodgkinson, S.C., and Bass, J.J. 1991. Passive immunisation against insulin-like growth factor-I does not inhibit growth hormone-stimulated growth in dwarf rats. *Endocrinology* 128:2103–2109.

Spencer, G.S.G., and Williamson, E.D. 1981. Increased growth in lambs following auto-immunization against somatostatin. *Animal Production*, 32:376.

Stewart, C.E., Bates, P.C., Calder, T.A., Woodall, S.M., and Pell, J.M. 1993. Potentiation of insulin-like growth factor-I (IGF-I) activity by an antibody: supportive evidence for enhancement of IGF-I bioavailability in vivo by IGF binding proteins. *Endocrinology*, 133:1462–1465.

Sun, Y.X., Drane, G.L., Currey, S.D., Lehner, N.D., Gooden, J.M., Hoskinson, R.M., Wynn, P.C., and McDowell, G.H.

1990a. Immunization against somatotropin release inhibiting factor improves digestibility of food, growth and wool production of crossbred lambs. *Australian Journal of Agricultural Research*, 41:401–411.

Sun, Y.X., Sinclair, S.E., Wynn, P.C., and McDowell, G.H. 1990b. Immunization against somatotropin release inhibiting factor increases milk yield in ewes. *Australian Journal of Agricultural Research*, 41:393–400.

Tans, C., Dubois, F., Zhong, Z.D., Jadot, M., Wattiaux, R., and Wattiaux-De Coninck, S. 1994. Uptake by rat liver of bovine growth hormone free or bound to a monoclonal antibody. *Biologie Cellulaire*, 82:45–49.

Theveniau, M.A., Raymond, J.R., and Rougon, G. 1989. Antipeptide antibodies to the β_2-adrenergic receptor confirm the extracellular orientation of the amino-terminus and the putative first extracellular loop. *Journal of Membrane Biology*, 111:141–153.

Vaiseman, N., Nissim, A., Klapper, L.N., Tirosh, B., Yarden, Y., and Sela, M. 2000. Specific inhibition of the reaction between a tumor-inhibitory antibody and the ErbB-2 receptor by a mimotope derived from a phage display library. *Immunology Letters*, 75:61–67.

Vaughan, T.J., Williams, A.J., Pritchard, K., Osbourn, J.K., Pope, A.R., Earnshaw, J.C., McCafferty, J., Hodits, R.A., Wilton, J., and Johnson, K.S. 1996. Human antibodies with sub-nanomolar affinities isolated from a large non-immunized phage display library. *Nature Biotechnology*, 14:309–314.

Wang, B.S., Lumanglas, A.L., Szewczyk, E., McWilliams, W., Loullis, C.C., and Hart, I.C. 1992. A proposed mechanism of action of a growth hormone-specific monoclonal antibody in the enhancement of hormonal activity. *Molecular Immunology*, 29:313–317.

Wang, B.S., Szewczyk, E., Shieh, H.M., and Hart, I.C. 1990. Potentiation of the growth-promoting activity of porcine growth hormone (pGH) with an antibody generated in rabbits to the peptide sequence pGH110-118. *Journal of Endocrinology*, 127:481–485.

Wang, B.S., Zhang, R.J., Bona, C.A., and Moran, T.M. 1994. Promotion of animal growth with a monoclonal anti-idiotype specific to anti-porcine growth hormone antibody. *Molecular Immunology*, 31:651–656.

Wang, H.S., and Chard, T. 1992. The role of insulin-like growth factor-I and insulin-like growth factor-binding protein-1 in the control of human fetal growth. *Journal of Endocrinology*, 132:11–19.

Westbrook, S.L., Chandler, K.D., and McDowell, G.H. 1993. Immunization of pregnant ewes against somatotropin release inhibiting factor increases growth of twin lambs. *Australian Journal of Agricultural Research*, 44:229–238.

Westbrook, S.L., and McDowell, G.H. 1994. Immunization of lambs against somatotropin release inhibiting factor to improve productivity: comparison of adjuvants. *Australian Journal of Agricultural Research*, 45:1693–1700.

Westbrook, S.L., Mohammed Ali, A., and McDowell, G.H. 1994. Passively acquired antibodies to somatotropin release inhibiting factor (SRIF) increase appetite and growth of milk-fed lambs. *Australian Journal of Agricultural Research*, 45:293–302.

Wood, P.R., Seow, H.-F., and Rothel, J.S. 1994. Cytokines and regulation of the immune response. In *Vaccines in Agriculture. Immunological Applications to Animal Health and Production.* P.R. Wood, P. Willadsen, J.E. Vercoe, R.M. Hoskinson, and D. Demeyer, eds. Melbourne: CSIRO.

Wynn, P.C., Behrendt, R., Jones, M.R., Rigby, R.D.G., Bassett, J. R., and Hoskinson, R.M. 1994a. Immuno-modulation of hormones controlling growth. *Australian Journal of Agricultural Research*, 45:1091–1109.

Wynn, P.C., Behrendt, R., Pattison, S.T., Jones, M.R., Shahneh, A., Yacoub, C., Sheehy, P.A., Rigby, R.D.G., Bassett, J.R., and Hoskinson, R.M. 1994b. Immunomodulation of hormones of the hypothalamic-pituitary-adrenal axis and animal productivity. In *Vaccines in Agriculture. Immunological Applications to Animal Health and Production.* P.R. Wood, P. Willadsen, J.E. Vercoe, R.M. Hoskinson, and D. Demeyer, eds. Melbourne:CSIRO.

Zeitlin, L., Cone, R.A., Moench, T.R., and Whaley, K.J. 2000. Preventing infectious disease with passive immunization. *Microbes and Infection* 2:701–8.

Zhang, L., Yang, M., Chong, P., and Mohapatra, S.S. 1996. Multiple B- and T-cell epitopes on a major allergen of Kentucky Bluegrass pollen. *Immunology* 87:283–290.

19
Growth of Livestock

Rod A. Hill, Frank R. Dunshea, and Michael V. Dodson

Chapters 1 through 18 of this text describe many aspects of animal growth and development, and have set the stage for applying these principles to livestock species.

This chapter presents an overview of the growth and development of cattle, sheep, and pigs, and the technology aimed at improving their growth. We also highlight the important issues that challenge this technology: to improve growth efficiency, to reduce the cost of production, to minimize the impact of production on the environment, and to produce a healthy product.

WORLD MEAT CONSUMPTION

Meat is a good source for vitamins, minerals, and high-quality protein. It is becoming more affordable to all peoples, and world consumption of meat is increasing, with the main continent of growth being Asia. As the world population increases, so also does the demand for meat products. Production of pork and poultry in Asia represents a large response to this demand. International trade in meat has been increasing during the past decade and is forecast to further increase in the early part of this century (Figure 19.1). Production in countries that have low labor and land costs provides them with a potential advantage in terms of meat products. Developed countries, such as the United States of America, which is a net exporter of meats, need to develop and implement more efficient production strategies to offset disadvantages in world terms, such as high labor costs.

DOMESTIC MEAT CONSUMPTION

Consumers' preferences for meat products have changed over the course of the past 10–15

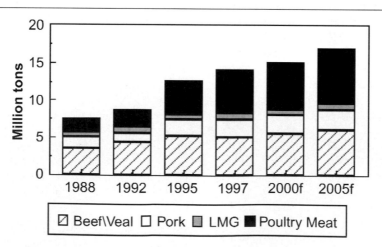

Figure 19.1. Growth in world meat trade for beef/veal, pork, lamb/mutton/goat meat (LMG), and poultry meat for the years 1988 to forecast 2005 (USDA).

years. Traditional red meat cuts are slowly being replaced by white meats (chicken, fish, and pork), and fish products are becoming popular. Many consumers desire meat products that they can prepare quickly, are low in fat, and are perceived as being healthy. Commercial food processing companies are now producing specialty meat products in which variables of consumer preference—such as quality, palatability, preparation time, and nutrient composition—are being optimized. Clearly, producers must align their production to consumer preference. In the past, efficiency and rate of growth have been important. A further challenge is to produce high-quality meat that is healthy and produced in an environmentally friendly manner.

Regardless of the extent of manipulation of growth or development, the one factor that must be considered to be a primary goal, either as an animal scientist, growth biologist, or producer, is to make more money than was spent on purchase price, maintenance, and production of livestock. Economies of scale related to the high cost of capital equipment and land needed for grazing have led to the demise of the small, family-operated businesses. Many of those remaining in the business have persevered on lower incomes and primarily for other quality of life reasons.

MANAGEMENT SYSTEMS FOR RUMINANTS AND PIGS

Technology has had a large impact on livestock production efficiency. As might be expected, the species in which the greatest gains have been made are those with a short generation interval, which also happen to be the intensively managed species.

Traditionally, the costs of production of intensively managed livestock animals were high, due to housing, feed, and labor costs that were much greater than for other animals. As our understanding of the basic physiology of animal growth and development has improved, refinements in management (breeding, housing, nutrition, and behavior) have allowed us to manipulate animal management with much greater precision. Intensive livestock management also affords tight control of environmental variables. The rate of technological advances might be summarized as poultry>pigs>beef/sheep. Because there are fundamental differences in the physiology, and production management systems, of these animals, each of these groups is considered separately in this chapter. Where possible, some comparisons and contrasts are used to illustrate particular points.

GROWTH OF RUMINANTS

Ruminants are highly adapted for the utilization of a diet high in fiber and low in protein, and they are able to thrive under conditions where simple-stomached animals may barely survive. This is due in part to the ability of rumen microflora to utilize cellulose, and the ability of the ruminant host to utilize the nutrients provided by the digestion of the rumen microflora and their byproducts.

Fundamentals of Ruminant Energy Metabolism

There are major differences in energy utilization pathways between ruminants and nonruminants. No evidence is available to suggest an evolution of biochemical pathways that might be unique to ruminants. However, ruminants have evolved a metabolism that can utilize nutrients from low-quality feedstuffs and that is directly related to the output from the rumen. For example, ruminants are able to tolerate high circulating concentrations of VFA. As such, acetate is a major precursor of fatty acid synthesis, which occurs mainly in adipose tissue. Unlike ruminants, nonruminants utilize glucose as the main precursor of fatty acid synthesis.

Ruminants are less reliant than nonruminants in using glucose as an energy source. In all animal species, however, glucose is the major nutrient utilized by the brain and central nervous system. In order to maintain adequate plasma glucose concentrations, gluconeogenesis is a major metabolic activity in beef cattle in both the fasted and fed states (Annison 1976). In addition, ruminant tissues are much less sensitive to insulin than the tissues of the monogastric animals, such as pigs (Pethick and Dunshea 1996).

The classes of metabolites, which may be utilized by the hind limb muscle of sheep at rest and during exercise, are shown in Figure 19.2. Glucose and acetate provide the greatest proportion of substrates at rest, but during exercise, FFA become the major substrates (Hocquette et al. 1998; Pethick 1993; Pethick and Dunshea 1993). Perhaps it is no surprise that compared to other livestock species, ruminants have much lower growth rates. This is a reflection of their adaptation to tolerance of poor nutrition.

Growth Efficiency

Growth efficiency may be defined in general terms as the gross nutrition units required to increase the liveweight of an animal by a defined unit amount. A

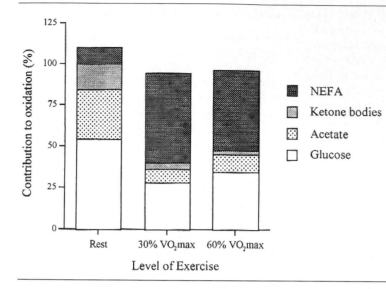

Figure 19.2. Metabolite utilization by sheep hind-limb muscle at rest and during exercise. Note that during moderate exercise, similar to that during grazing behavior, the role of free fatty acids (non-esterified fatty acids, NEFA) increases in importance compared to glucose, when the animal is at rest. Not shown here is the increase in total energy requirement during exercise. (Reprinted from Hocquette et al., 1998, with permission from Elsevier Science.)

common term used is the feed conversion ratio, which may be expressed as the units of kg dry feed consumed over a prescribed time period divided by the change in liveweight of the animal (in kg) over the same time period:

$$FCR = FI \ (kg) \ / \ \Delta \ LW \ (kg)$$

where FCR = feed conversion ratio, FI = feed intake of a specified diet, and Δ LW = change in liveweight.

For sheep and cattle growing under "normal" conditions (and depending on the energetic and protein quality of the feed and the stage of maturity of the animal), this ratio may be between 7:1 and 12:1 and is very different from those for poultry and pigs, which may be 1.5:1, but is more usually around 3:1. An important aspect of this difference is that poultry and pigs are offered a high-quality diet throughout their life cycle. Where all other factors are held constant, improving the quality of the feed offered improves the FCR.

Feed conversion ratio is just one way to describe growth efficiency. Additional terms may be added to the formula to take into account the production system. Primary producers are interested in the cost of raising their product. They may assign a value to the cost of the feed and add further real costs. These include the following:

• The cost of breeding and maintaining the animal's parent generation

• The cost of maintaining the infrastructure needed to keep the animal, including a component for the use of the "real estate"
• Any supplements
• Husbandry costs

Use of these values allows the cost of production per kg of animal raised to be determined. The difference between this cost and the realized sale price per kg of the animal is the producer's profit. Thus, keeping costs to a minimum and efficiency to a maximum is of great interest to the primary producer.

Another applied estimate of growth efficiency in beef cattle, is net feed efficiency (NFE), which is often quantified in terms of net feed intake (NFI) or residual feed intake (Archer et al. 1999). This is a term describing individual animal efficiency within a population. It is most useful when the gene pool is well defined and applied to animals of the same age, cohort, sex, and management history. As with feed conversion ratio, the two central variables are the amount of feed consumed and the change in liveweight of the animal. The NFI of an individual animal is the difference between its actual feed intake and that predicted over a defined time period (usually 10 weeks) using a modeling routine. The components of the model include the liveweights of the animals recorded weekly and the metabolic weights of the animals at the midpoint of the test (metabolic weight is the liveweight raised to the power of 0.73). Individual daily feed intake is modeled by multiple linear regres-

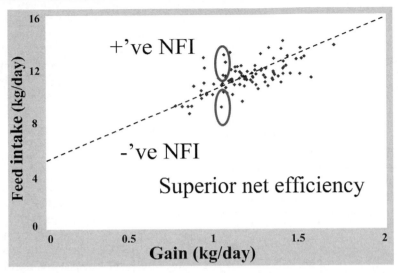

Figure 19.3. Net feed intake (NFI) is determined from a plot of feed intake against gain in live weight. In this example, 100 Angus bulls were tested for NFI in a 140-day standard test at the Trangie Research Station, New South Wales, Australia. The circles show bulls that gained at the same rate, but which varied in feed intake. The dotted line shows the regression of intake against gain. Negative NFI indicates that these animals required less feed for similar gain, compared to animals with positive NFI, which required more feed for similar gain. (Figure provided by pers. comm. Dr Robert Herd, New South Wales Agriculture Department, Australia.)

sion, including terms for weight gain and metabolic weight (Figure 19.3). NFI for each animal is calculated as the residual error after fitting the multiple regression model to actual feed intake (Parnell et al. 1995). Thus NFI is either positive, when an animal consumes more feed than expected for a given weight gain; or negative, when an animal consumes less feed than expected for a given weight gain. In theory, the most desirable animals are those with a negative NFI, meaning that the animals are consuming less feed for an equivalent liveweight gain. This test is theoretically independent of animal liveweight and growth rate, and thus selection using this method should not alter frame size (Herd et al. 1998). In contrast, selection for improved feed conversion ratio has had the effect of selecting for animals with a higher frame size and growth rate. This is undesirable, because larger framed animals often fall outside of market specifications, having less fat cover at market weight.

Maintenance and Growth

When evaluating the energetic cost of growth, it is important to consider that in order for an animal to survive, it must first maintain its primary functions. The ability to move to obtain feed and water, to find shelter during harsh environmental conditions, to avoid predators or other stressors, and to digest food are basal metabolic functions. Basal metabolism is the energy/nutrition required for the animal to survive, without the incorporation of a growth component.

Total energy/nutrition requirements are defined as the sum of that required for growth plus that required for maintenance:

$$E_T = E_m + E_g$$

where E_T = total energy requirement, E_m = energy requirement for maintenance, and E_g = energy requirement for growth.

Because ruminants develop more slowly than other animals, more of the resources consumed are required for maintenance than for growth. Due to the increased cost of maintenance, spread over a greater time period, ruminants characteristically show lower feed conversion ratios than do other animals.

Growth Rate, Frame Size, and Composition

An animal growing at a fast rate is more efficient than an animal growing at a slow rate. Thus it follows that providing optimum nutrition will improve production efficiency. However, this must be balanced against the cost of providing the feed. In the case of ruminant production, a management system has evolved with two main phases. For the phase in which lean growth is predominant (early growth), lower-quality nutrition is provided by grazing pasture, and for the finishing period, in which fat deposition is relatively greater and lean growth is relatively less, a higher-quality (feedlot) diet is provided. As muscle is energetically less expensive to deposit than fat (Lindsay et al. 1993), this system appears logical. However, it must be remembered that the metabolic rate of muscle is generally much greater than for fat. In addition each unit of muscle protein deposited requires the addition of about 3.5 units of water; whereas each unit of fat deposited requires only about 0.1 units of water. Thus although muscle is less expensive to deposit, it is more expensive to maintain over time in terms of both its inherent metabolic demands and in the energetic cost of "carrying" the additional water which is integral in its composition. A further factor, which affects growth rate, is the potential mature size of the animal. For beef cattle, the larger breeds, such as Simmental and Charolais, have a large mature size and a high potential growth rate. It must be remembered, however, that at a given liveweight, larger-framed breeds will be less mature than smaller-framed breeds and thus have relatively less fat. Although more efficient growth is important, it is equally important that the animal meets market specifications.

Low Quality Nutrition

The ability of a production animal to regulate its basal metabolic rate must be considered in a production regimen. For ruminants, especially those adapted to low quality nutrition, this is an important survival mechanism. All mammals, including man, can adapt to a persistent change in the level of nutrition over the medium term. When nutrition is plentiful, basal metabolic rate is increased, and the body's ability to process nutrients more rapidly is enhanced. Conversely, when nutrition is limiting, basal metabolic rate is reduced, the body processes the available nutrients more slowly, and less of the resource is required to maintain basal functions. However, under nutritionally limiting conditions, proportionately more of the resources will be needed for maintenance. As the plane of nutrition is further reduced, growth rate is also reduced and (ultimately), if nutrition is further reduced, the body begins to utilize stored energy and tissue components for maintenance. This is known as a catabolic state, and if protracted, leads to chronic atrophy and may lead finally to the death of the animal.

Cattle have evolved over a wide range of environmental conditions. The breeds that are best adapted to the harshest nutritional restrictions are the tropical breeds and are represented by both *Bos taurus* and *B. indicus* breeds (Frisch et al. 1997). Brahman cattle adapt very well to limiting nutrition. They may down-regulate their basal requirements to a lower level than European or British breeds. This advantage becomes a disadvantage at the opposite end of the nutrition "spectrum." Under feedlot conditions, where nutrition is maximized, the Brahman is unable to up-regulate its metabolism to the same level as European or British breeds. Brahmans are unable to develop the same level of appetite, and grow more slowly under feedlot conditions (Frisch and Vercoe ; 1969; Vercoe 1970; Vercoe and Frisch 1970; Frisch 1981).

For the purposes of the following discussion, *B. indicus* serves as an example of a tropically adapted animal, and *B. taurus* represents temperate breeds, such as Hereford, Angus, Charolais. As depicted in Figure 19.4, during severe undernutrition, although animals may down-regulate their maintenance requirement, nutrition is insufficient to maintain basal processes. Thus the body begins to metabolize tissues (first, gut protein and fat and then, muscle protein). This is a catabolic state. As *B. taurus* breeds generally have a higher basal metabolic rate, they catabolize tissue reserves more quickly than the *B. indicus* breeds, a situation that continues until nutrition reaches a critical level, above which each type may recommence growth. When very high-quality feed is available, the *B. indicus* is unable to up-regulate its metabolism to the same degree as the *B. taurus*, and thus is unable to utilize the available nutrition. In this case, the *B. taurus* will outperform the *B. indicus* in growth rate. Thus the *B. taurus* has the higher growth potential, but the environment must be favorable for it to realize that potential. In the tropics, where nutrition is often limiting, *B. indicus* cattle will outperform *B. taurus*.

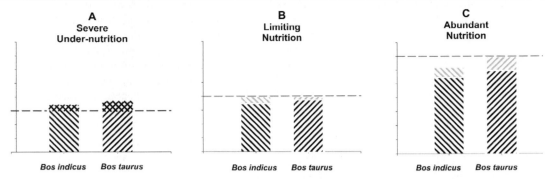

Figure 19.4. Effect of level of nutrition on the realized growth of *Bos indicus* and *Bos taurus* cattle. In each figure, the dashed horizontal line indicates the relative level of nutrition available; the dark hatch represents the maintenance requirement, and the light hatch represents the growth requirement. In A, severe under-nutrition, maintenance requirements are not met. Although each breed has down-regulated BMR, maintenance requirements (represented by the entire bar in each case) exceed available nutrition. Thus the body begins to catabolize reserves to meet this requirement (crosshatch). Because *B. taurus* animals have a greater maintenance requirement, they will lose proportionately more of their liveweight under these conditions. In B, when nutrition is limiting, animals with a lower maintenance requirement will grow at a slightly better rate than animals with a higher maintenance requirement. In C, when the level of nutrition is abundant, both groups up-regulate their metabolism, increasing the maintenance requirement and growth rate. Most *B. taurus* breeds can up-regulate to a higher level than most *B. indicus*, and thus have a greater growth potential.

Growth Promotants/Growth Factors

Specific effects of hormonal growth promotants and growth factors are addressed in detail elsewhere. A brief discussion is offered here of three categories of hormone treatments/strategies that improve growth efficiency. The first category includes those that may reduce basal metabolic rate, providing additional energy for growth. Anabolic steroids are an example of this category. Under nutritional restriction, treatment with the synthetic steroid, trenbolone acetate further reduced maintenance energy requirements by 10–15%, providing additional energy for preservation of body mass (Hunter and Vercoe 1987). This effect was also augmented by a concomitant improvement in nitrogen retention. Treatment with combined estradiol and trenbolone acetate improved feed efficiency in feedlot cattle. The effects were large, with improvements in steers being of the order of 13–23%, and in heifers, 26% (Popp et al. 1997). The mechanism of action of these agents, however, is not clear. Even though blood insulin-like growth factor-I (IGF-I) concentrations were increased (Johnson et al. 1996a,

1996b), at least one study has shown no effect on muscle protein degradation (Hayden et al. 1992).

A second category of growth promotants demonstrates more efficient utilization of available nutrients, via repartitioning of fat to protein or preservation of protein mass through reduced protein turnover. Although reducing protein turnover is not mutually exclusive from reducing basal metabolic rate, it is a more closely specified subset of the latter. Repartitioning of fat to protein is invoked by treatment with both growth hormone and β-agonists. However, responses to growth hormone are reliably invoked in animals only on a high plane of nutrition. Responses in both heifers (Schwartz et al. 1993) and steers (Moseley et al. 1992) to moderate doses of bovine somatotropin (bST) result in repartitioning of fat to lean and an improvement in nitrogen retention, with little improvement in weight gain. The major benefit is an improvement in feed efficiency of the order of 12%. The β-agonists selectively partition protein to skeletal muscle, at the expense of fat and/or gut protein. Thus, they are potentially useful in meat production but may have production drawbacks in terms of other physiological processes, such as fiber or milk production. β-agonists also reduce protein turnover (Bohorov et al. 1987, Sillence et al. 1993). There are other mechanisms within this category that may be important in understanding variation in efficiency. Some treatments reduce protein degradation rate, such as IGF-I (Walton et al. 1995; Hill et al. 1999) and stimulation of the GH axis via dosing with GHRH (Etherton et al. 1986). During normal growth, protein turnover is an essential process for cell function, growth, and repair. When the rate of protein synthesis exceeds the rate of protein degradation, the animal is in an anabolic phase (Figure 19.5). Small reductions in protein turnover can have significant effects on the protein "economy" of an animal. As noted by MacRae and Lobley (1991), protein accretion and degradation reactions considerably exceed those of absorption through the intestine and protein deposition and amino acid oxidation. As Figure 19.6 shows, for steers fed at 1.6× maintenance, the rates of synthesis and degradation exceeded absorption by 1.8-fold, and protein deposition exceeded by a factor of 17. In steers fed at maintenance, the rates of synthesis and degradation exceeded absorption by 2.4-fold, and protein deposition by a factor of 64 (Lobley et al. 1987). It must be remembered that in this scenario, feeding at maintenance will result in very little protein deposition. However, as can be seen from the example of growing steers (Figure 19.6), small changes in the rate of synthesis or degradation may have a large effect on net protein gain. The potential advantage appears to be exag-

gerated as the level of nutrition is reduced. This suggests that improved feed efficiency through reduced protein degradation may have considerable benefits where cattle are exposed to conditions of restricted nutrient intake. In the context of improving growth efficiency, a reduction in protein degradation rate is a more beneficial process, because it requires relatively little or no additional energy input, whereas an increase in protein anabolism requires additional nutritional and energetic inputs.

A third category of growth promotants improves the efficiency of digestion of feed. This mechanism has been invoked in treatments that affect the somatostatin (SRIF) axis. As well as its effects on GH release, SST is known to affect other hormones, including a possible action at the gut. For example, passive vaccination with SST antibodies reduced digesta flow (Fadlalla et al. 1985). Studies of ruminant utilization of nutrients suggest that there is great potential for improvement of feed digestibility with this agent. Westbrook and colleagues (1993) suggested that SST vaccination of pregnant ewes resulted in improved growth in their lambs, and from this and another study using active immunization of lambs (Spencer et al. 1983), there appears to be an increase in appetite of lambs for milk, which improves their growth. Later in their lives, this is replaced by an increased efficiency of feed utilization. Furthermore, the efficiency of feed utilization for milk production was also demonstrated in actively vaccinated pregnant ewes (Westbrook et al. 1993, Sun et al. 1990). The poten-

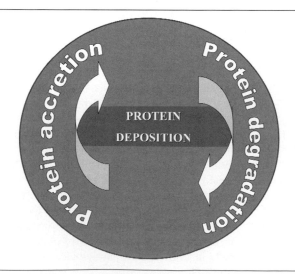

Figure 19.5. Protein deposition. When the rate of protein accretion exceeds the rate of protein degradation, the animal is in an anabolic phase. The rate of protein turnover plays an important role in determining the cost in terms of energy and amino acids required for the process.

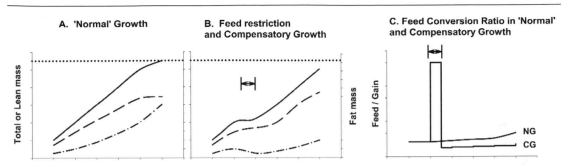

Figure 19.7. Composition of growth during "normal" feeding (A) or the effects of a short period of feed restriction (arrows) on composition of growth (B) and feed conversion ratio (feed:gain, C). Total mass (solid curve) and lean mass (long dash) are shown on the same scale, and fat mass (dash, dot) is shown on an expanded scale to more clearly show relative changes in fat and lean growth. In A, during "normal" growth, lean mass increases at a relatively constant rate in the younger animal. As the animal approaches mature size, relative rates of growth change, lean growth reducing and fat growth increasing. In B, during feed restriction, gut and fat mass are lost and if feed restriction is not severe or prolonged, muscle mass may be conserved. When animals are returned to a normal diet, lean growth increases, but fat mass does not usually recover. A and B also show that animals do not recover live weight at the same age, even after an extended period of compensatory growth (dotted line). *Note:* during the refeeding phase, the slope of the lean growth curve (long dash) during compensatory growth is steeper than that during normal growth. In C, during "normal" growth (NG), feed:gain slowly increases as maintenance requirements increase. During feed restriction, feed:gain increases rapidly as the denominator approaches 0. Following refeeding, maintenance requirement is reduced and lean mass increases rapidly with a reduced feed requirement (CG). Animals that have been subjected to a short period of feed restriction are often attractive to feedlot operators.

are now aimed at maximizing protein deposition. As a consequence, an excellent understanding is unfolding regarding the nutritional constraints to protein deposition. Numerous factors are being determined—such as genotype, sex, age, and environment—which impact lean tissue growth and development. As discussed for ruminants, the relationships between absorbed nutrient supply and protein deposition also hold true for pigs.

Interrelationships Between Dietary Protein and Energy on Protein Deposition

Theoretical responses to dietary protein intake are shown in Figure 19.8. This depicts the two phases of protein deposition: an initial protein-dependent phase where protein deposition increases linearly with protein intake regardless of energy intake, and an energy-dependent phase in which protein deposition increases only if additional energy is provided. When pigs of a given weight (sex, genotype, etc.) are fed increasing amounts of a protein of constant composition at a set level of energy intake (E_1), protein deposition increases linearly until a maximum (M_1) is reached at a protein intake of P_1. Beyond this protein intake, the rate of protein deposition will increase only if additional energy is provided (i.e., energy-dependent phase). If extra energy is provided (E_2), protein deposition increases linearly up to a new plateau at a higher protein intake (P_2). If the intrinsic ceiling for protein deposition is M_2, neither extra energy nor protein will further increase protein deposition. However, the ratio of protein:energy required to maximize protein deposition will decrease. Although these theoretical relationships have been confirmed for a very homogeneous group of pigs (see SCA 1987), a normal population of pigs contains individual pigs that exhibit individual linear/plateau responses. When these individual response curves are combined, the population response may be curvilinear. Fitting a quadratic or asymptotic rather than linear/plateau model to these data generally results in increasing the estimate of

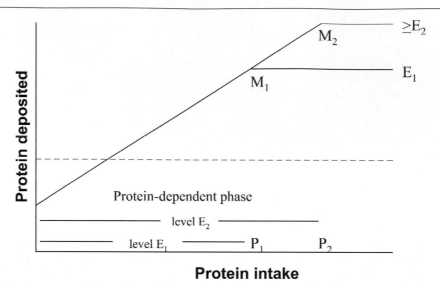

Figure 19.8. Relationship between protein deposition and intake of protein (levels P_1 and P_2) and energy (levels E_1 and E_2) (SCA 1987).

protein requirement. One approach when using the quadratic or asymptotic models is to take the protein requirement at the point where 95% of the asymptote was achieved (King et al. 2000). Although this often raises concerns in the interpretation of experimental data because both model types may describe the data equally well, the interpretation of the biology of the system is generally the same.

The slope of the ascending portion of the curves depicted in Figure 19.8 is the efficiency with which dietary protein is deposited. This slope is determined by the digestibility of dietary protein and by how well the pattern of absorbed amino acids matches the pattern of requirements for tissue deposition and maintenance. When considering protein requirements of the pig, it should be borne in mind that the pig does not have a requirement for protein per se but rather for an appropriate level and balance of individual amino acids, particularly the essential amino acids. Any imbalance in the amino acids profile will result in the catabolism of the excess amino acids. The carbon skeletons from relatively minor amino acid excesses will be incorporated into additional fat deposition. However, substantial amino acid excesses result in a decrease in performance because there is an energetic cost in excreting nitrogen. In an effort to ease the complexity of diet formulation, the ARC (1981) adopted the concept of

the "ideal" protein. Because amino acids are used predominantly for protein deposition, the composition of the ideal protein closely resembles that of muscle (Wang and Fuller 1989). The concept of ideal protein has to some extent successfully shifted the focus of feed manufacturers and producers away from individual amino acid requirements (e.g., lysine, threonine) toward thinking in terms of an adequate balance of amino acids in the diet. As an animal grows, the composition of the ideal protein also changes as the usage (maintenance versus growth) and source of amino acids change. Metabolic modifiers likely change the ratio of amino acids deposited to amino acids used for maintenance, and this will affect the pattern of amino acids required. Nevertheless, these will, for the large part, be subtle changes.

Effect of Energy Intake on Protein Deposition Under Conditions of Protein Adequacy

Knowledge of the relationship between protein deposition and energy intake is crucial to determining optimum feeding strategies for different classes of pigs. These relationships are outlined in Figures 19.9 and 19.10. In this model, total energy deposition increases linearly with increasing energy intake

(Figure 19.9). Energy retained as protein also increases linearly up to a maximum at an energy intake of Q, beyond which further energy has no effect on the rate of protein deposition. Fat deposition also increases linearly until an energy intake of Q, after which a sharp increase in the rate of fat deposition occurs. At zero energy balance (R), protein gain is still marginally positive and fat deposition is negative. The potential impact of energy intake upon body composition is very much related to what intake, if any, corresponds to Q for a particular pig. This is perhaps more clearly demonstrated in Figure 19.10, which depicts the ratio of fat to protein in tissue gain. Protein deposition increases linearly with energy intake, but the ratio of fat to protein deposited increases curvilinearly, rising steeply initially before approaching an asymptote. However, after a plateau in protein deposition is reached, there is a sharp linear increase in the ratio of fat to protein deposited (beyond energy intakes of Q). Therefore, whether protein deposition continues to respond linearly up to the limit of appetite or reaches a plateau at an intermediate energy intake can have profound effects upon the composition of weight gain, body composition and FCE.

Effect of Live Weight on Protein Deposition

The relationships between protein intake and protein deposition were elegantly illustrated in the study of Campbell et al. (1985a), where young growing pigs were fed 8 levels of ideal protein at 3 levels of energy intake between 20 and 45 kg liveweight (Figure 19.11). For example, for pigs fed 3.5 Mcal DE/d, protein deposition increased linearly until it reached a maximum of 68 g/d at a protein intake of 208 g/d. Beyond this protein intake, the rate of protein deposition is increased only if extra energy is provided. Hence, for pigs fed 4.4 and 5.4 Mcal DE/d, protein deposition increases linearly up to maximal rates of 83 and 101 g/d at protein intakes of 245 and 294 g/d, respectively (Figure 19.12). When these rates of protein deposition are graphed against protein content of the diets, maximum protein deposition at the 3 levels of energy intake occurs at similar protein:energy ratios, and therefore the point of inflection for each level of energy intake is the same (52 g CP/Mcal DE; Figure 19.13). For young boars, voluntary intake is not sufficient to maximize protein deposition, so the inflection point remains constant. Campbell and colleagues (1984) also conducted a similar study in older boars that were fed 8 levels of dietary protein at 2 levels of energy intake. Again, protein deposition increased in a linear manner, with increasing level of protein intake before reaching a plateau that was dependent upon energy intake (i.e., at protein deposition rates of 125 and 135 g/d for 6.4 and 8.1 Mcal DE/d, respectively). Therefore, when the data are expressed in terms of dietary protein:energy, the

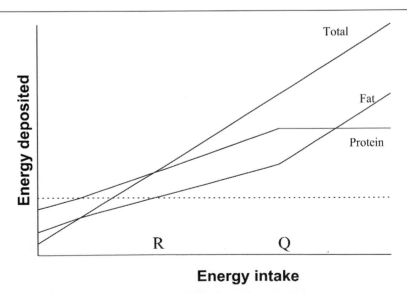

Figure 19.9. Effect of energy intake on total energy and energy deposited as protein (SCA 1987). (Q is maximum energy retained as protein; R is zero energy balance.)

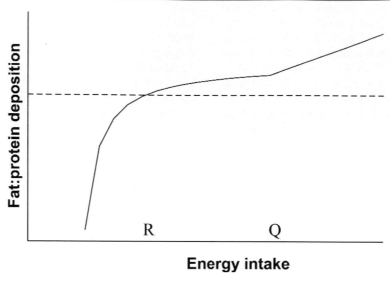

Figure 19.10. Effect of energy intake on the ratio of fat to protein deposition (SCA 1987). (Q is maximum energy retained as protein; R is zero energy balance.)

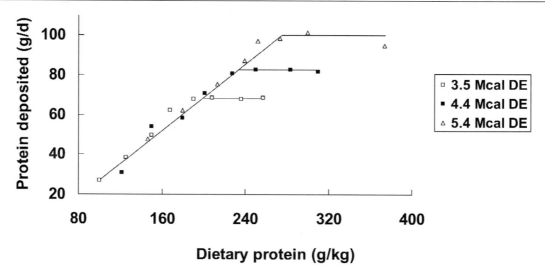

Figure 19.11. Relationship between protein deposition and protein intake in boars fed three levels of feed intake between 20 and 45 kg (Campbell et al. 1985a).

minimum requirement decreases at the higher energy intake. With these energy intakes, it is more appropriate to talk in terms of daily requirements for protein.

If the data from a series of studies conducted with a similar unimproved genotype are collated, the effects of liveweight on energy intake and protein deposition may be seen (Figure 19.13). For pigs up to about 50 kg liveweight, protein deposition is limited by energy intake, because the relationship between energy intake and protein deposition is linear with no sign of a plateau. Management practices that maximize feed intake should be utilized for these animals if protein deposition is to be maximized. However, for this genotype, ad libitum energy intake can exceed that required to maximize protein deposition when the

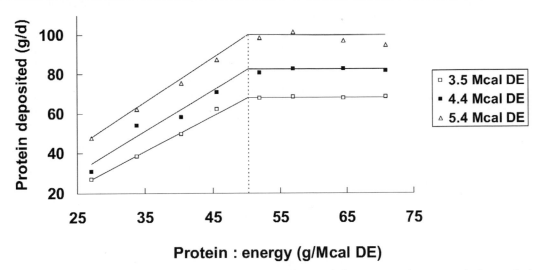

Figure 19.12. Relationship between protein deposition and dietary protein:energy in boars fed three levels of feed intake between 20 and 45 kg (Campbell et al. 1985a).

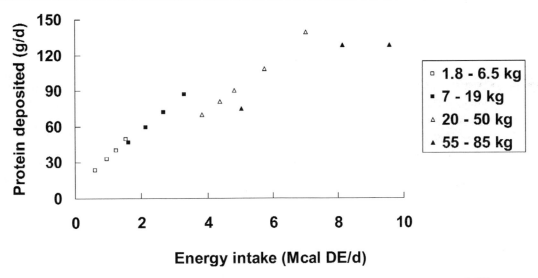

Figure 19.13. Relationship between protein deposition and energy intake in pigs of different weights (same genotype) (Campbell et al. 1984, 1985a, 1985b).

pigs get beyond 55 kg liveweight, as indicated by the plateau in protein deposition. In these animals, it may be necessary to restrict feed intake to below about 8 Mcal DE/d in order to ensure that pigs do not become over-fat. Also note that as animals get bigger the linear ascending portion of the relationship between energy intake and protein deposition moves to the

right, and the slope decreases as more energy is diverted to maintenance of the larger body.

Effect of Sex on Protein Deposition

There are well-established differences in growth performance between boars, gilts, and barrows (Campbell et al. 1989, 1990; Dunshea et al. 1993b,

1998a; King et al. 2000). Similarly to ruminants, males (boars) deposit more protein and generally less fat than either castrates (barrows) or females (gilts). Also, the maximal rates of protein deposition and the liveweight at which it occurs differs between the sexes (Whittemore et al. 1988; Suster et al. 2001). Another important observation is that the slope of the relationship between energy intake and protein deposition is steeper for boars than for gilts or castrates (King et al. 1997; Dunshea et al. 1998a). Older data suggest that, for finisher pigs (>55 kg liveweight), a plateau in protein deposition is achieved in all sex classes of pigs at an intake of around 8 Mcal DE/d. Recent studies have been conducted with genetically improved pigs. These suggest that the plateau occurs at higher feed intakes, or in the case of elite boars, not at all (Rao and McKracken et al. 1992; Dunshea et al. 1998a; King et al. 1997). The practical message from these studies is that improved boars and some gilts can be fed ad libitum to maximize protein deposition without the pigs getting over-fat. This is particularly so when it is realized that feed intake is generally lower under commercial conditions than it is in the individually housed pigs that have been used for many of these studies (Black et al. 2001). One implication from these findings is that the growth performance and rate of lean tissue deposition of the improved pig is vulnerable to any factors that reduce feed intake. The situation is not so clear with finisher barrows, because they have a similar maximal rate of protein deposition as gilts but a higher voluntary feed intake (Dunshea et al. 1993a). However, at liveweights below about 50 kg, improved boars and barrows have a similar potential to deposit lean tissue (Suster et al. 2001) and can be fed ad libitum. The greater rate of protein deposition of boars as compared to gilts and barrows would suggest that boars have a greater protein requirement than the latter sex classes.

Effect of Genotype on Protein Deposition

There have been enormous improvements in the pig industry over the last two decades, and much of this can be attributed to heavy selection pressure for lean tissue growth. The selection pressure has most likely been on mature body weight, although pigs are rarely grown out to mature body size to confirm this. Generally, genotypes that are heavier at maturity grow faster and contain less fat than do animals of smaller mature size. The discussion to date has already alluded to the impact of improved genetics

on the effects of liveweight and sex on the relationships between protein deposition and protein and energy intake. To summarize, improved pigs deposit more protein and less fat at any particular energy intake than unimproved pigs. Also, the slope of the ascending portion of the curve relating protein deposition to energy intake is greater in the improved genotypes. Some improved genotypes cannot consume sufficient energy to maximize protein deposition even during the finishing phase. As a consequence, growth performance and rate of lean tissue deposition of the improved pig is vulnerable to any factors that reduce feed intake, particularly since genetic pressure on reduced carcass fatness has indirectly meant selection pressure against feed intake.

Effect of Metabolic Modifiers

Somatotropin/Growth Hormone

In the grower pig (30–60 kg) it appears that pST has very little, if any, effect on dietary protein requirements. However, there is an increase in the efficiency of utilization of dietary protein (Campbell et al. 1990; Caperna et al. 1990; Krick et al. 1993) of the order of 25%. Therefore, it appears that conventional starter/grower diets (180 g/kg crude protein) may be sufficient to allow the expression of the benefits on pST in grower pigs (25–60 kg). In this class of pigs, energy intake is more likely to be limiting than protein intake.

The effects of pST on the protein requirements of finisher pigs (60–90kg), in which increases in protein deposition are greater, are more equivocal. In order to assess how the protein requirements of finisher pigs are affected by pST, King et al. (2000) conducted a study with heavy improved pigs typical of those used in better production systems. It appeared that there was little effect of pST on the efficiency of use of dietary lysine and that the increase in lysine requirement appeared to be commensurate with the increase in protein deposition.

The relationship between energy intake and protein deposition is linear in the grower pig fed protein-adequate diets. This was confirmed in the study of Campbell et al. (1988), which demonstrated that protein deposition increased with energy intake in young pigs treated with excipient or pST. At all levels of energy intake, protein deposition was higher and fat and total energy deposition lower in the pigs treated with pST. Extrapolation of the relationship between total energy deposition and energy intake to zero energy retention suggests that maintenance energy requirement (MER) is increased during pST treatment. The increases in energy requirements are at least in part due to increased protein synthesis in muscle and in visceral tissues, such as gut and liver, which are increased in mass during pST treatment. Also, ad libitum energy intake was 10% lower in pigs treated with pST. In older pigs, where ad libitum feed intake is greater, the relationship between energy intake and protein deposition is more typically a linear-plateau one. Although for pST-treated boars, the relationship was linear (see Campbell et al. 1991). Therefore, if the full benefits of exogenous pST are to be achieved commercially, feed intake needs to be maximized, particularly for improved boars.

β-Agonists

As for pST-treated pigs, the β-agonist ractopamine (RAC, recently commercialized as Paylean) has no effect on nutrient digestibility. Consequently, its effects must be post-absorptive. The limited information, obtained only in finishing pigs, suggests that the increased protein deposition rates (observed in response to β-agonists) increase the dietary requirement for protein. The increased dietary protein requirement during dietary RAC treatment has been confirmed in an experiment in which 6 levels of dietary protein were fed in restricted amounts (7.2 Mcal DE/d) to finisher gilts (Dunshea et al. 1993b). This study found that the efficiency of use of dietary protein was not altered by RAC, because protein deposition increased with protein content at a similar rate for both the control and RAC-treated pigs over at least the two lowest levels of dietary protein (<110 g/kg crude protein). However, at higher dietary protein contents, the plateau or maximal protein deposition rate was 23% higher in the gilts receiving RAC (96 vs. 118 g/d for control and RAC-treated pigs, respectively). The levels of dietary protein required for maximum protein deposition were 127 g/kg for the control and 158 g/kg for the RAC-treated pigs. At dietary protein contents, which maximize protein deposition in the control gilts, there is no difference in performance between the control and the RAC-treated gilts. As dietary protein level is increased, there is no further improvement in protein deposition in the control gilts. However, protein deposition is increased in gilts treated with dietary RAC. Unlike pST, RAC and other β-agonists stimulate protein deposition only in skeletal muscle. Metabolically active visceral tissue—such as gut, heart, and liver—are often reduced in mass, often resulting in an improvement in dressing percentage.

Restrictively fed gilts did not respond as well to dietary RAC as ad libitum–fed gilts, suggesting that the responses to dietary RAC may also be limited by dietary energy intake. To test this, Dunshea and colleagues (1998a) investigated the interactions between dietary energy intake and protein and fat deposition in RAC-treated finisher gilts and boars. The relationship between protein deposition and DE intake for the control gilts was of the linear-plateau form, with carcass protein deposition reaching a plateau at 140 g/d at an energy intake of 8.6 Mcal DE/d. However, in RAC-treated gilts, protein deposition increased linearly with increasing energy intake, up to a maximum of 191 g/d, at an ad libitum DE intake of 11.3 Mcal DE/d. Supplementation of the diet with RAC increased protein deposition at every level of energy intake. The slope of the linear ascending portions of the curve were not different, and the improvement in protein deposition due to dietary RAC was 21 g/d up until a DE intake of 8.6 Mcal/d. For boars receiving either 0 or 20 ppm of RAC, the relationship between protein deposition and energy intake was linear up until ad libitum DE intakes of approximately 11.0 Mcal/d. Although the slopes of these lines were the same, the benefit to protein deposition in boars (19 g/d) was similar to that observed in gilts. Therefore, dietary RAC increases protein deposition in both gilts and boars at every level of energy intake, but ad libitum intakes are necessary to maximize protein deposition in improved genotypes treated with RAC. Also, the differences in protein deposition between boars and gilts are still evident during RAC treatment. Despite an increase in protein deposition, dietary RAC had no effect on MER. This may be due to the energy requirements of an increased skeletal muscle mass being offset by a reduced visceral mass.

The lean tissue responses to β-agonists reduce with time, being most pronounced over the first 2 weeks and diminishing over subsequent weeks (Dunshea 1991; Dunshea et al. 1993a). This process, called down-regulation, is due to extended exposure to the ß–agonist and occurs in response to many compounds. However, it is quite possible that a controlled incremental approach with RAC may be one way of ensuring a more consistent and sustained response.

Conjugated Linoleic Acid

Over the past decade there has been escalating interest in this group of fatty acids because of their apparent potent antioxidative and anticarcinogenic properties. Another biological effect of CLA relates to fat accretion and nutrient partitioning. In general, these studies have suggested that backfat depth is reduced (Dugan et al. 1997; Dunshea et al. 1998b). The carcass protein accretion response to dietary CLA appears to be quadratic in nature (Ostrowska et al. 1999), with protein accretion maximized at a dietary CLA supplement of 5.0 g/kg. Carcass fat accretion decreased linearly with increasing CLA supplement rates. At the highest level of CLA, there was a 30% reduction (–86 g/d) in carcass fat accretion. Dietary CLA had no significant effect on average daily gain or feed intake throughout the study. However, feed:gain was improved by 0.2 kg/kg (–6.5%) in pigs fed diets containing CLA. The improvements in feed:gain were a combination of the small but nonsignificant changes in both growth rate and feed intake. More recently, a study was conducted with a leaner genotype of pig, housed under commercial conditions, to assess the effects of feeding 4.0 g/kg CLA. CLA had no significant effect upon feed intake and daily gain, but the small changes in both resulted in a reduction in (–0.10 g/g, P = 0.10) feed:gain (Dunshea et al. 2002). Although there was no significant effect of CLA on ultrasonic backfat depths, there was a significant decrease in carcass P2 (–1.0 mm, P = 0.014) and estimated carcass fat (–7 g/kg, P = 0.049), with responses being greater in gilts than in boars.

Betaine

Betaine is a naturally occurring substance, found in a wide variety of plant and invertebrate species. Vertebrates have a limited ability to produce betaine. Consequently, uptake of betaine is mainly from ingested plant material (Burg 1994). One of its major roles is to act as an osmoregulator to aid in maintenance of cellular water balance, as well as a methyl group donor. It was in this latter role that betaine was first investigated as a partial replacement for choline in pig and poultry diets, because it is less expensive and less corrosive than choline. As an additional benefit, it was found that carcass fat was reduced in chickens receiving supplemental betaine, but not when receiving supplemental choline or methionine (Saunderson and Mackinlay 1990). More recently, the effects in pigs have been investigated. Cadogan and colleagues (1993) found that betaine had no effect on growth performance of finisher gilts. However, backfat at the P2 region was decreased from 17.6 to 15.0 mm. Given that there was no change in ADG or feed intake, this suggested that there was a repartitioning of adipose tissue fat. Recently, Wang and Xu (1999) found that

betaine increased ADG by up to 15% and decreased backfat by up to 18% in grower gilts and barrows. In another study, Smith et al. (1994) found that betaine did not alter growth performance, LEA, or backfat. Likewise, Overland and colleagues (1999) also found that betaine had no effect upon growth performance or carcass characteristics in limit-fed pigs. These types of findings and variable responses on livestock animals have somewhat confused researchers and producers alike.

Results from a slaughter balance study suggested that betaine may have an energy sparing effect, through reducing the pigs' maintenance requirement (Campbell et al. 1997). These researchers fed various levels of energy (from 3.70 to 6.5 Mcal DE/d) to finisher gilts and observed that supplemental betaine tended to increase ADG and fat deposition and decreased FCR, but had no effect on protein deposition. Improvements in performance were most pronounced in pigs fed energy levels below ad libitum. However, a study by Matthews et al. (1998) examining interactions between dietary protein, betaine, and energy suggested that the interactions may be very complex. These workers found that betaine increased ADG in pigs fed low protein–low energy diets and high protein–high energy diets but decreased ADG in pigs fed low protein–high energy diets and high protein–low energy diets.

One class of pig in which energy intake may be limiting lean tissue accretion is the pST-treated boar, particularly if feed intake is restricted by high stocking density or temperature. In order to study these interactions, Suster and colleagues (2002) investigated the effect of betaine and pST in boars fed approximately 80% of ad libitum feed intake (ca. 2.7 kg) from 64 kg liveweight. Both pST and betaine increased daily gain and lean tissue deposition and reduced back fat, and the effects were to a large extent additive. Although these feed intakes were 80% of ad libitum for individually housed pigs, they are probably at the high end of feed intakes observed in group-housed pigs under commercial conditions. Therefore, it is likely that when energy intake is limiting the potential for lean tissue deposition, betaine alone—or in combination with pST—can increase growth performance and lean tissue deposition.

Androgens

Unlike ruminant animals, androgen implants appear to have little effect upon growth performance and carcass quality in pigs.

CONCLUSION

The growth of livestock is complex, and optimizing growth is a primary goal of industry, animal scientists, and government. Technology has had an enormous impact on the efficiency of production of livestock, at all levels. Management practices based upon sound scientific investigation have been adopted in all animal industries. Two of the primary determinants of the performance of an animal are its genetic potential and the environmental factors that mold this potential. The role of animal science will be to continue to improve quality and efficiency of production of a diverse array of livestock food sources. In order to do this, we need to gain greater understanding of the underlying mechanisms of growth biology. In the pig and in ruminants, there is potential to modify or tailor growth at all stages of the life cycle. There is a lack of understanding of the factors affecting growth potential, particularly in early stages of development. Technology has improved efficiency of production and quality of the meat produced from cattle, sheep, and pigs. One universal lesson that animal scientists have learned is that although science has taught us much of what we know, we understand relatively little of the complex process of growth and development. There is much yet to be discovered.

REFERENCES

Annison, E.F. 1976. Energy utilization in the body. In *Principles of Cattle Production*. H. Swan., and W.H. Broster, eds. London: Butterworth & Co. Ltd.

ARC (Agricultural Research Council). 1981. The Nutrient Requirements of Pigs. Slough, U.K.: Commonwealth Research Bureaux.

Archer, J.A., Richardson, E.C., Herd, R.M., and Arthur, P.F. 1999. Potential for selection to improve efficiency of feed use in beef cattle: a review. *Australian Journal of Agricultural Research* 50:147–161.

Bell, A.W. 1993. Pregnancy and fetal metabolism. In *Quantitative Aspects of Ruminant Digestion and Metabolism*. J.M. Forbes and J. France, eds. Cambridge: CAB International.

Black, J.L., Giles, L.R., Wynn, P.C., Knowles, A.G., Kerr, C.A., Jones, M.R., Strom, A.D., Gallagher, N.L., and Eamens, G.J. 2001. A review—factors limiting the performance of growing pigs in commercial environments. In *Manipulating Pig Production VIII*. P.D. Cranwell, ed. Werribee, Australia: Australasian Pig Science Association.

Bohorov, O., Buttery, P.J., Correia, J.H.R.D., and Soar, J.B. 1987. The effect of the β_2-adrenergic agonist clenbuterol or implantation with oestradiol plus trenbolone acetate on protein metabolism in wether lambs. *British Journal of Nutrition* 57:99–107.

Bryson, J.M., Phuyal, J.L., Swan, V., and Caterson, I.D. 1999. Leptin has acute effects on glucose and lipid metabolism in both lean and gold thioglucose-obese mice. *American Journal of Physiology Endocrinology and Metabolism* 277:E417–422.

Burg, M.B. 1994. Molecular basis for osmoregulation of organic osmolytes in renal medullary cells. *Journal of Experimental Zoology* 268:171–175.

Buskirk, D.D., Faulkner, D.B., Hurley, W.L., Kelser, D.J., Ireland, F.A., Nash, T.G., Castree, J.C., and Vicini, J.L. 1996. Growth, reproductive performance, mammary development, and milk production of beef heifers as influenced by prepubertal dietary energy and administration of bovine somatotropin. *Journal of Animal Science* 74:2649–2662.

Buskirk, D.D., Faulkner, D.B., and Ireland, F.A. 1995. Increased postweaning gain of beef heifers enhances fertility and milk production. *Journal of Animal Science* 73:937–946.

Cadogan, D.J., Campbell, R.G., Harrison, D., and Edwards, A.C. (1993). The effects of betaine on the growth performance and carcass characteristics of female pigs. In *Manipulating Pig Production IV*. E.S. Batterham, ed. Attwood, Australia: Australasian Pig Science Association:).

Campbell, R.G., Johnson, R.J., King, R.H., Taverner, M.R., and Meisinger, D.J. 1990. Interaction of dietary protein content and exogenous porcine growth hormone administration on protein and lipid accretion rates in growing pigs. *Journal of Animal Science* 68:3217–3225.

Campbell, R.G., Johnson, R.J., Taverner, M.R., and King, R.H. 1991. Interrelationships between exogenous porcine somatotropin (pST) administration and dietary protein and energy intake on protein deposition capacity and energy metabolism of pigs. *Journal of Animal Science* 69:1522–1531.

Campbell, R.G., Morley, W.C., and Zabaras-Krick, B. 1997. The effects of betaine on protein and energy metabolism of growing pigs. In *Manipulating Pig Production VI*. P.D. Cranwell, ed. Werribee, Australia: Australasian Pig Science Association, .

Campbell, R.G., Steele, N.C., Caperna, T.J., McMurtry, J.P., Solomon, M.B., and Mitchell, A.D. 1988. Interrelationships between energy intake and exogenous growth hormone administration on the performance, body composition and protein and energy metabolism of growing pigs weighing 25 to 55 kilograms body weight. *Journal of Animal Science* 66:1643–1655.

Campbell, R.G., Steele, N.C., Caperna, T.J., McMurtry, J.P., Solomon, M.B., and Mitchell, A.D 1989. Interrelationships between sex and exogenous porcine growth hormone administration and performance, body composition and protein and fat accretion of growing pigs. *Journal of Animal Science* 67:177–186.

Campbell, R.G., Taverner, M.R., and Curic, D.M. 1984. Effect of feeding level and dietary protein content on the growth, body composition and rate of protein deposition in pigs growing from 45 to 90 kg. *Animal Production* 38:233–240.

Campbell, R.G., Taverner, M.R., and Curic, D.M. 1985a. The influence of feeding level on the protein requirements of pigs between 20 and 45 kg liveweight. *Animal Production* 40:489–496.

Campbell, R.G., Taverner, M.R., and Curic, D.M. 1985b. Effects of sex and energy intake between 48 and 90 kg on protein deposition in growing pigs. *Animal Production* 40:497–504.

Caperna, T.J., Steele, N.C., Komarek, D.R., McMurtry, J.P., Rosebrough, R.W., Solomon, M.B., and Mitchell, A.D. 1990. Influence of dietary protein and recombinant porcine somatotropin administration in young pigs: growth, body consumption and hormone status. *Journal of Animal Science* 68:4243–4252.

Ceddia, R.B., William, W.N.J., and Curi, R. 1999. Comparing effects of leptin and insulin on glucose metabolism in skeletal muscle; evidence for an effect of leptin on glucose uptake and decarboxylation. *International Journal of Obesity* 23:75–82.

Dagogo-Jack, S., Fanelli, C., Paramore, D., Brothers, J., and Landt, M. 1996. Plasma leptin and insulin relationships in obese and nonobese humans. *Diabetes* 45:695–698.

Dugan, M.E.R., Aalhus, J.L., Schaefer, A.L., and Kramer, J.K.G. 1997. The effects of linoleic acid on fat to lean repartitioning and feed conversion in pigs. *Canadian Journal of Animal Science* 77:723–725.

Dunshea, F.R. 1991. Factors affecting efficacy of ß-agonists for pigs. *Pig News and Information* 12:227–231.

Dunshea, F.R., Eason, P.J., King R.H., and Campbell, R.G. 1998a. Interrelationships between dietary ractopamine, dietary energy and sex on protein and fat deposition in growing pigs. *Australian Journal of Agricultural Research* 49:565–574.

Dunshea, F.R., King, R.H, and Campbell, R.G. 1993a. Interrelationships between dietary protein and ractopamine on protein and lipid deposition in finishing gilts. *Journal of Animal Science* 71:2931–2941.

Dunshea, F.R., King, R.H., Campbell, R.G., Sainz, R.D., and Kim, Y.S. 1993b. Interrelationships between sex and ractopamine on protein and lipid deposition in rapidly growing pigs. *Journal of Animal Science* 71:2919–2930.

Dunshea, F.R., Ostrowska, E., Luxford, B., Smits, R.J. Campbell, R.G., D'Souza, D.N., and Mullan, B.P. 2002. Dietary conjugated linoleic acid can decrease backfat in pigs housed under commercial conditions. *Asian Australasian Journal of Animal Science* (in press).

Dunshea, F.R., Ostrowska, E., Muralitharan, M., Cross, R., Bauman, D.E., Pariza, M.W., and Skarie, C. 1998b. Dietary conjugated linoleic acid decreases backfat in growing gilts. *Journal of Animal Science* 76Suppl.1:131.

Dwyer, C.M., Fletcher, J.M., and Stickland, N.C. 1993. Muscle cellularity and postnatal growth in the pig. *Journal of Animal Science* 71:3339–3343.

Ehrhardt, R.A., Slepetis, R.M., Bell, A.W., and Boisclair, Y.R. 2001. Maternal leptin is elevated during pregnancy in sheep. *Domestic Animal Endocrinology* 21:85–96.

Etherton, T.D., Wiggins, J.P., Chung, C.S., Evock, C.M., Rebhun, J.F., and Walton, P.E. 1986. Stimulation of pig growth performance by porcine growth hormone and growth hormone-releasing factor. *Journal of Animal Science* 63:1389–1399.

Fadlalla, A.M., Spencer, G.S.G., and Lister, D. 1985. The effect of passive immunization against somatostatin on marker retention time in lambs. *Journal of Animal Science* 61:234–239.

Freetly, H.C., and Cundiff, L.V. 1998. Reproductive performance, calf growth, and milk production of first-calf heifers sired by seven breeds and raised on different levels of nutrition. *Journal of Animal Science* 76:1513–1522.

Freetly, H.C., Ferrell, C.L., and Jenkins, T.G. 2000. Timing of realimentation of mature cows that were feed-restricted during pregnancy influences calf birth weights and growth rates. *Journal of Animal Science* 78:2790–2796.

Freetly, H.C., Ferrell, C.L., and Jenkins, T.G. 2001. Production performance of beef cows raised on three different nutritionally controlled heifer development programs. *Journal of Animal Science* 79:819–826.

Frisch, J.E. 1981. Changes occurring in cattle as a consequence of selection for growth rate in a stressful environment. *Journal of Agricultural Science, Cambridge* 96:23–38.

Frisch, J.E., Drinkwater, R., Harrison, B., and Johnson, S. 1997. Classification of the southern African sanga and East African shorthorned zebu. *Animal Genetics* 28: 77–83.

Frisch, J.E., Munro, R.K., and O'Neill, C.J. 1987. Some factors related to calf crops of Brahman, Brahman Crossbred and Hereford x Shorthorn cows in a stressful tropical environment. *Animal Reproduction Science* 15:1–26.

Frisch, J.E., and Vercoe, J.E. 1969. Liveweight gain, food intake, and eating rate in Brahman, Africander, and Shorthorn x Hereford cattle. *Australian Journal of Agricultural Research* 20:1189–1195.

Frisch, J.E., and Vercoe, J.E. 1977. Food intake, eating rate, weight gains, metabolic rate and efficiency of feed utilization in *Bos taurus* and *Bos indicus* crossbred cattle. *Animal Production* 25:343–358.

Gatford, K.L., Owens, J.A., Campbell, R.G., Boyce, J.M., Grant, P.A., De Blasio, M.J., and Owens, P.C. 2000. Treatment of underfed pigs with GH throughout the second quarter of pregnancy increases fetal growth. *Journal of Endocrinology* 166:227–234.

Greenwood, P.L., Hunt, A.S., Hermanson, J.W., and Bell, A.W. 1998. Effects of birth weight and postnatal nutrition on neonatal sheep: I. Body growth and composition, and some aspects of energetic efficiency. *Journal of Animal Science* 76:2354–2367.

Hayden, J.M., Bergen, W.G., and Merkel, R.A. 1992. Skeletal muscle protein metabolism and serum growth hormone, insulin, and cortisol concentrations in growing steers implanted with estradiol-17ß, trenbolone acetate, or estradiol-17ß plus trenbolone acetate. *Journal of Animal Science* 70:2109–2119.

Herd, R.M., Archer, J.A., Arthur, P.F., and Richardson, E.C. 1998. Reducing the cost of beef production through the genetic improvement of net feed efficiency. In *Proceedings of the British Society of Animal Science*.

Hetzel, D.J.S., Mackinnon, M.J., Dixon, R., and Entwistle, K.W. 1989. Fertility in a tropical beef herd divergently selected for pregnancy rate. *Animal Production* 49:73–81.

Hill, R.A., Hunter, R.A., Lindsay, D.B., and Owens, P.C. 1999. Action of long(R^3)-insulin-like growth factor-1 on protein metabolism in beef heifers. *Domestic Animal Endocrinology* 16:219–229.

Hocquette, J.F., Ortigues-Marty, I., Pethick, D., Herpin, P., and Fernandez, X. 1998. Nutritional and hormonal regulation of energy metabolism in skeletal muscles of meat-producing animals. *Livestock Production Science* 56:115–143.

Hornick, J.L., Van Eenaeme, C., Gerard, O., Dufrasne, I., and Istasse, L. 2000. Mechanisms of reduced and compensatory growth. *Domestic Animal Endocrinology* 19:121–132.

Hunter, R.A., and Vercoe, J.E. 1987. Reduction of energy requirements of steers fed on low-quality-roughage diets using trenbolone acetate. *British Journal of Nutrition* 58:477–483.

Johnson, B.J., Anderson, P.T., Meiske, J.C., and Dayton, W.R. 1996a. Effect of a combined trenbolone acetate and estradiol implant on feedlot perfomance, carcass characteristics, and carcass composition of feedlot steers. *Journal of Animal Science* 74:363–371.

Johnson, B.J., Hathaway, M.R., Anderson, P.T., Meiske, J.C., and Dayton, W.R. 1996b. Stimulation of circulating insulin-like growth factor I (IGF-I) and insulin-like growth factor finding proteins (IGFBP) due to administration of a combined trenbolone acetate and estradiol implant in feedlot cattle. *Journal of Animal Science* 74:372–379.

King, R.H., Campbell, R.G., Morley, W.C., Ronnfeldt, K., and Dunshea, F.R. 1997. The response of pigs between 80–120 kg live weight to energy intake. In *Manipulating Pig Production VI*. P.D. Cranwell, ed. Werribee, Australia: Australasian Pig Science Association.

King, R.H., Campbell, R.G., Smits, R.J., Morley, W.C. Ronnfeldt, K., Butler, K., and Dunshea, F.R. 2000. Interrelationships between dietary lysine, sex and porcine somatotropin administration on growth performance and protein deposition in pigs between 80 and 120kg live weight. *Journal of Animal Science* 78:2639–2851.

Krick, B.J., Boyd, R.D., Roneker, K.R., Beermann, D.H., Bauman, D.E., Ross, D.A., and Meisinger, D.J. 1993. Porcine somatropin affects the dietary lysine requirement and net lysine utilization for growing pigs. *Journal of Nutrition* 123:1913–1922.

Lindsay, D.B., Hunter, R.A., Gazzola, C., Spiers, W.G., and Sillence, M.N. 1993. Energy and Growth. *Australian Journal of Agricultural Research* 44:875–899.

Lobley, G.E., Connell, A., and Buchan, V. 1987. Effect of food intake on protein and energy metabolism in finishing beef steers. *British Journal of Nutrition* 57:457–465.

MacRae, J.C., and Lobley, G.E. 1991. Physiological and metabolic implications of conventional and novel methods for the manipulation of growth and production. *Livestock Production Science* 27:43–59.

Mantzoros, C.S., Liolias, A.D., Tritos, N.A., Kaklamani, V.G., Doulgerakis, D.E., Griveas, I., Moses, A., and Flier, J.S. 1998. Circulating insulin concentrations, smoking, and alcohol intake are important independent predictors of leptin in young healthy men. *Obesity Research* 6:179–186.

Masuzaki, H., Ogava, Y., Sagawa, N., Hosoda, K., Matsumoto, T., Mise, H., Nishimura, H., Yoshimasa, Y., Tanaka, I., Mori, T., and Nakao, K. 1997. Nonadipose tissue production of leptin; Leptin as a novel placenta-derived hormone in humans. *Nature Medicine* 3:1029–1033.

Matthews, J.O., Southern, L.L., Pontif, J.E., Higbie, A.D., and Bidner, T.D. 1998. Interactive effects of betaine, crude protein, and net energy in finishing pigs. *Journal of Animal Science* 76:2444–2455.

Moseley, W.M., Paulissen, J.B., Goodwin, M.C., Alaniz, G.R., and Clafin, W.H. 1992. Recombinant bovine somatotropin improves growth performance in finishing beef steers. *Journal of Animal Science* 70:412–425.

Muoio, D.M., Dohm, G.L., Fiedorek, F.T., Tapscott, E.B., and Coleman, R.A. 1997. Leptin directly alters lipid partitioning in skeletal muscle. *Diabetes* 46:1360–1363.

Muoio, D.M., Dohm, G.L., Tapscott, E.B., and Coleman, R.A. 1999. Leptin opposes insulin's effects on fatty acid partitioning in muscle isolated from obese ob/ob mice. *American Journal of Physiology* 276:E913–E921.

Myers, S.E., Faulkner, D.B., Ireland, F.A., and Parrett, D.F. 1999. Comparison of three weaning ages on cow-calf performance and steer carcass traits. *Journal of Animal Science* 77:323–329.

Neville, W.J., Richardson, K.L., Williams, D.J.R., Mullinix, B.G.J., and Utley, P.R. 1990. Subsequent reproduction and calf performance of nonpregnant cows compared with pregnant cows and replacement females. *Journal of Animal Science* 68:2188–2197.

Neville, W.J., Richardson, K.L., Williams, D.J.R., and Utley, P.R. 1987. Cow breeding and calf growth performance as affected by pregnancy status the previous year. *Journal of Animal Science* 65:345–350.

Oddy, V.H., Harper, G.S., Greenwood, P.L., and McDonagh, M.B. 2001. Nutritional and developmental effects on the intrinsic properties of muscles as they relate to the eating quality of beef. *Australian Journal of Experimental Agriculture* 41:921–942.

Ostrowska, E., Muralitharan, M., Cross, R.F., Bauman, D.E., and Dunshea, F.R. 1999. Dietary conjugated linoleic acid increases lean tissue and decreases fat deposition in the growing pig. *Journal of Nutrition* 129:2037–2042.

Overland, M., Rorvik, K.A., and Skrede, A. 1999. Effect of trimethylamine oxide and betaine in swine diets on growth performance, carcass characteristics, nutrient digestibility, and sensory quality of pork. *Journal of Animal Science* 77:2143–2153.

Parnell, P.F., Herd, R.M., Arthur, P.F., and Wright, J. 1995. Breeding for improved net feed conversion efficiency in beef cattle. *Proceedings of the Australian Association of Animal Breeding and Genetics* 11:384–388.

Pethick, D.W. 1993. Carbohydrate and lipid oxidation during exercise. *Australian Journal of Agricultural Research* 44:431–441.

Pethick, D.W., and Dunshea, F.R. 1993. Fat metabolism and turnover. In *Quantitative Aspects of Ruminant Digestion and Metabolism*. J.M. Forbes and J. France, eds. Cambridge: CAB International.

Pethick, D.W., and Dunshea, F.R. 1996. The partitioning of fat in farm animals. *Proceedings of the Nutrition Society of Australia* 20:3–13.

Popp, J.D., McAllister, T.A., Burgevitz, W.J., Kastelic, J.P., and Cheng, K.-J. 1997. Effect of trenbolene acetate/estradiol implants and estrus suppression on growth performance and carcass characteristics of beef heifers. *Canadian Journal of Animal Science* 77:325–328.

Ramsey, W.S., Hatfield, P.G., and Wallace, J.D. 1998. Relationships among ewe milk production and ewe and lamb forage intake in Suffolk and Targhee ewes nursing single or twin lambs. *Journal of Animal Science* 76:1247–1253.

Ramsey, W.S., Hatfield, P.G., Wallace, J.D., and Southward, G.M. 1994. Relationships among ewe milk production and ewe and lamb forage intake in Targhee ewes nursing single or twin lambs. *Journal of Animal Science* 72:811–816.

Rao, D.S., and McKracken, K.J. 1992. Energy:protein interactions in growing boars of high genetic potential for lean growth. 2. Effects on chemical composition of gain and whole-body protein turn-over. *Animal Production* 54:83–93.

Rehfeldt, C., Kuhn, G., Nurnberg, G., Kanitz, E., Schneider, F., Beyer, M., Nurnberg, K., and Ender, K. 2001a. Effects of exogenous somatotropin during early gestation on maternal performance, fetal growth, and compositional traits in pigs. *Journal of Animal Science* 79:1789–1799.

Rehfeldt, C., Kuhn, G., Vanselow, J., Furbass, R., Fiedler, I., Nurnberg, G., Clelland, A.K., Stickland, N.C., and Ender K. 2001b. Maternal treatment with somatotropin during early gestation affects basic events of myogenesis in pigs. *Cell Tissue Research* 306:429–440.

Robinson, J.J., Sinclair, K.D., and McEvoy, T.G. 1999. Nutritional effects on foetal growth. *Animal Science* 68:315–331.

Saunderson, C.L., and Mackinlay, J.H. 1990. Changes in body-weight, composition and hepatic enzyme activities in response to dietary methionine, betaine and choline levels in growing chicks. *British Journal of Nutrition* 63:339–349.

SCA (Standing Committee on Agriculture). 1987. Feeding standards for Australian Livestock. *Pigs*. CSIRO.

Schwartz, F.J., Schams, D., Röpke, R., Kirchgessner, M., Kögel, J., and Matzke, P. 1993. Effects of somatotropin treatment on growth performance, carcass traits, and the endocrine system in finishing beef heifers. *Journal of Animal Science* 71:2721–2731.

Sillence, M.N., Hunter, R.A., Pegg, G.G., Brown, L., Matthews, M.L., Magner, T., Sleeman, M., and Lindsay, D.B. 1993. Growth, nitrogen metabolism, and cardiac responses to clenbuterol and ketoclenbuterol in rats and underfed cattle. *Journal of Animal Science* 71:2942–2951.

Smith, J.W., Owen, K.Q., Nelssen, J.L., Goodband, M.D., Tokach, M.D., Lohrmann, T.L., and Blum, S.A. 1994. The effects of dietary carnitine, betaine and chromium nicotinate supplementation on growth and carcass characteristics in growing-finishing pigs. *Journal of Animal Science* 72 (Suppl. 1):274.

Snowder, G.D., and Glimp, H.A. 1991. Influence of breed, number of suckling lambs, and stage of lactation on ewe milk production and lamb growth under range conditions. *Journal of Animal Science* 69:923–930.

Snowder, G.D., Knight, A.D., Van Vleck, L.D., Bromley, C.M., and Kellom, T.R. 2001. Usefulness of subjective ovine milk scores: I. Associations with range ewe characteristics and lamb production. *Journal of Animal Science* 79:811–818.

Spencer, G.S.G., Garssen, G.J., and Bergström, P.L. 1983. A novel approach to growth promotion using auto-immunisation against somatostatin II. Effects on appetite, carcass composition and food utilisation in lambs. *Livestock Production Science* 10:469–477.

Sun, Y.X., Sinclair, S.E., Wynn, P.C., and McDowell, G.H. 1990. Immunization against somatotropin release inhibiting factor increases milk yield in ewes. *Australian Journal of Agricultural Research* 41:393–400.

Suster, D., King, R.H., Mottram, M., Leury B.J., and Dunshea, F.R. 2002. Dietary betaine (Betafin) and porcine somatotropin (Reporcin) have additive effects upon growth performance in restrictively-fed boars. *Journal of Animal Science* 80(Suppl. 1): (in press).

Suster, D., Leury, B.J., Kerton, D.J., Borg, M.L., and Dunshea, F.R. 2001. Boars deposit more lean and less fat than barrows under two housing conditions. In *Manipulating Pig Production VIII*. P.D. Cranwell, ed. Werribee, Australia: Australasian Pig Science Association.

Vercoe, J.E. 1970. The fasting metabolism of Brahman, Africander and Hereford x Shorthorn cattle. *British Journal of Nutrition*, 24:599–606.

Vercoe, J.E., and Frisch, J.E. 1970. Digestibility and nitrogen metabolism in Brahman, Africander and Shorthorn x Hereford cattle fed lucerne hay. *Proceedings of the Australian Society of Animal Production*, 8:131–135.

Walton, P.E., Dunshea, F.R., and Ballard, F.J. 1995. In vivo actions of IGF analogues with poor affinities for IGFBPs: metabolic and growth effects in pigs of different ages and GH responsiveness. *Progress in Growth Factor Research* 6: 385–395.

Wang, T.C., and Fuller, M.F. 1989. The optimum dietary amino acid pattern for growing pigs. 1. Experiments by amino acid deletion. *British Journal of Nutrition* 62:77–89.

Wang, Y.Z., and Xu, Z.R. (1999). Effect of feeding betaine on weight-gain and carcass trait of barrows and gilts and approach to mechanism. *Journal of Zhejiang Agricultural University* 25:281–285.

Westbrook, S.L., Chandler, K.D., and McDowell, G.H. 1993. Immunization of pregnant ewes against somatotropin release inhibiting factor increases growth of twin lambs. *Australian Journal of Agricultural Research* 44:229–238.

Whittemore, C.T., Tulis, J.B., and Emmans, G.C. 1988. Protein growth in pigs. *Animal Production* 46:437–445.

Wolter B.F. and Ellis M. 2001. The effects of weaning weight and rate of growth immediately after weaning on subsequent pig growth performance and carcass characteristics. *Canadian Journal of Animal Science* 81:363–369.

Yambayamba, E.S.K., Price, M.A., and Jones, S.D.M. 1996. Compensatory growth of carcass tissues and visceral organs in beef heifers. *Livestock Production Science*, 46: 19–32.

20
Growth of Poultry

Colin G. Scanes

Broiler consumption as a percentage of chicken consumed in the United States of America is increasing dramatically, as can be seen from the following: 4% in 1934 to >99% in 2000. Prior to the advent of the broiler industry, chicken meat was "spent" or old laying hens or young males. The number of broiler chickens produced in the U.S. increased from 34 million in 1934 (Ensminger 1992) to >6 billion produced in 2001 (National Agricultural Statistics Service USDA). Correcting for the increased size of broiler chickens today, *production has increased by ~299 fold in 67 years.* Analogous increases in turkey production have occurred, particularly in North America and the United Kingdom. Since the 1960s, turkey consumption per capita in the U.S. has risen approximately four-fold.

Recently, major increases in broiler production and chicken consumption have also been seen in many countries/areas of the world, including China, Southeast Asia, European Union, Australia, and Latin America. Increases in poultry meat consumption may surprisingly reduce utilization of cereal feed-stuffs if the rise is at the expense of pork and beef, poultry having a superior feed:gain ratio.

Ratites, ostriches, and emus have been grown commercially for many years, particularly in their countries of origins, respectively South Africa and Australia. There is substantial interest in them in Europe and North America as producers of "exotic" meat, together with use of the hide and feathers (reviewed e.g., Gillespie and Schupp 1998).

This chapter briefly discusses the changes in the poultry industry and in production during the twentieth century. The tremendous progress was facilitated by focused research. Examples of the changes in the biology of the chickens is included. In addition, the use of growth curves in chickens and

turkeys is considered; other aspects on the biology of growth of poultry are covered throughout this volume. Finally, growth in ratites (ostriches and emus) is considered.

CHANGES IN POULTRY PRODUCTION IN THE LAST SEVENTY YEARS

There have been tremendous improvements in poultry produced, and hence in the industry. Table 20.1 summarizes the improvements in growth rate and feed efficiency since 1935. Improvements of broiler chicken performance involved can be ascribed to the following. Poultry breeders and geneticists have employed the high heritability (~0.4) for body weight and conformation and heterosis (hybrid vigor) gained by crossing different parent stocks (viewed Cahaner and Siegel 1986; Siegel and Dunnington 1987) to improve poultry growth. Nongenetic improvements include housing, nutrition for optimal growth, subtherapeutic antibiotics, vaccines for disease prevention (reduced mortality and alleviation of growth suppression), etc.

It might be questioned as to what relative contribution nutrition and genetics have made in the improved growth of poultry. This important question has been evaluated. Direct comparisons were made of growth in random-bred "1950s" chickens (Athens-Canadian) and "1990s" broiler chickens reared on either 1950s diets or 1990s diets (Havenstein et al. 1994a). Growth rate was much greater in the 1990s broiler chickens. This is summarized in Table 20.2. It is clear that there was a 3.4-fold greater body weight/growth rate in the genetically improved chickens on the superior diet. If we assume this is typical of the industry, it is clear from the data presented in Table 20.2 that about

Table 20.1. Changes in characteristics of broiler production with time (based on Horton, 1951; Cahaner and Siegel, 1986; and USDA)

Year	Age at Market (Weeks)	Live Weight at Market (kg)	Feed:Gain Ratio
1935	13.5	1.3	4.3
1951	12	1.6	3.5
2002	6–7	>2.2	~1.8

Table 20.2. The relative contribution of improvements in breeding/genetics and nutrition on the growth of broiler chickens; direct comparison of 1957 and 1990s genetics (respectively, Athens-Canadian Randombred Control and Arbor Acres chicks) fed either typical diets of the 1950s or 1990s (data from Havenstein et al., 1994a, 1994b)

Body weight (kg) at 42 days (mean male and female)

	1950s Diet	1990s Diet (as % increase over 1950s diet) [as % increase over 1950s genetics]
1950s chickens—Athens-Canadian random-bred control chicks	0.51	0.63
1990s chickens—Arbor Acres chicks	1.77	2.13 (20.2) [240]

Feed conversion at 42 days (mean male and female)

	1950s diet	1990s diet (as % decrease over 1950s diet) [as % decrease over 1950s genetics]
1950s chickens—Athens-Canadian random-bred control chicks	3.00	2.51
1990s chickens—Arbor Acres chicks	2.28	2.04 (10.5) [18.7]

Breast muscle weight as percentage of live body weight at 43 days (mean male and female)

	1950s diet	1990s diet (as % decrease over 1950s diet) [as % decrease over 1950s genetics]
1950s chickens—Athens-Canadian random-bred control chicks	11.2	11.6
1990s chickens—Arbor Acres chicks	12.7	14.9 (17.3) [28.4]

three-quarters of the improvement in broiler chicks is due to genetics and one-quarter to improvement in nutrition. It might also be noted that with selec-tion, there were marked performance improvements in feed conversion efficiency and breast muscle per-centage (Table 20.2), but reduced immune functioning (antibody production) (Qureshi and Havenstein 1994).

GROWTH AND GROWTH EQUATIONS

Growth in Chickens

Growth in chickens has been described using general growth models including the Gompertz equation, logistics, and saturation kinetics/Michaelis-Menton kinetics (Rogers et al. 1987; López et al. 2000). All models accurately described broiler chicken growth, but the Gompertz model appeared the most accurate (Rogers et al. 1987) and has been employed in numerous research reports (e.g., Anthony et al. 1991; Knizetova et al. 1991). The heritabilities of Gompertz growth curve parameters have been determined and range from 0.31–0.54 (Mignon-Grasteau et al. 1999). Use selection for shape of the Gompertz growth curve has been proposed as an approach to reduce sexual dimorphism of growth (Mignon-Grasteau et al. 2000).

Gous and colleagues (1999) recently reported analyses of chicken growth using the Gompertz equation. There were marked sex differences in growth. For instance, males have a 16.1% higher mature live weight (males—6.1 kg; females—5.2) in one cross. Changes in body components (protein, lipid, water, muscle, feathers, etc.) have also been subject to analysis using the Gompertz equation (Gous et al. 1999).

Muscle Growth

Breast muscle growth is not allometric, with the percentage of breast meat increasing with larger eviscerated carcass weights (Gous et al. 1999).

Growth in Turkeys

The Gompertz equation growth has been used to describe growth in turkeys (e.g., Anthony et al. 1991). The model has been employed in the evaluation of turkey genetics, management, and nutrition. For instance, Nicholas turkeys had more rapid growth rate and an earlier point of inflection on the Gompertz growth curve than British United Turkeys (Lilburn and Emmerson 1993). Supplementary lysine and methionine above NCR requirements improved growth rate but had little effect on functions from the Gompertz growth curve (Lilburn and Emmerson 1993). In contrast, although lighting regimen did not significantly affect growth as indicated by body weight at 16 weeks of age with "step-up" lighting (increasing the ambient photoperiod/

daylength) tending to be superior than "step-down," significant differences were reported for Gompertz functions (Lilburn et al. 1992).

GROWTH IN OSTRICHES AND EMUS (RATITES)

Growth of ratites appears to require optimal nutrition, vaccination, and care. Growth has been measured (in ostriches, e.g., Cilliers et al. 1995; Deeming et al. 1996; Mushi et al. 1998) (in emu, Blache et al. 2001). There is little, if any, sexual dimorphism of growth in the ostrich. No differences were observed between male and female ostriches in hatching weight (0.8–0.9 kg), rate of growth/maturing, age of maximal weight gain, or mature body weights (~120 kg) (Cilliers et al. 1995). Incubation can profoundly affect posthatching growth. Ostrich chicks, where hatching has been assisted, have markedly poorer survival and growth rate even after 35 days (Deeming and Ayres 1994).

Growth Equations

Growth of one ratite, the ostrich, has been mathematically described using the Gompertz model (Cilliers et al. 1995). The age of maximal growth rate is ~180–200 days of age [approximately one-third of the time to maturity/plateaued body weight (602 and 664 days in male and female ostriches, respectively)].

Hormones and Growth

Limited information is available on the relationship between hormones and growth in ratites There are reports on the developmental changes in circulating concentrations of growth hormone, thyroxine, and tri-iodothyronine in both the ostrich and emu (Dawson et al. 1996; Blache et al. 2001). There is some evidence to link the abnormally low thyroid function with the neotenous appearance (juvenile-like) of adult ratites.

REFERENCES

Anthony, N.B., Emmerson, D.A., Nestor, K.E., Bacon, W.L., Siegel, P.B., and Dunnington, E.A. 1991. Comparison of growth curves of weight selected populations of turkeys, quail, and chickens. *Poultry Science* 70:13–19.

Blache, D., Blackberry, M.A., Van Cleeff ,J., and Martin, G.B. 2001. Plasma thyroid hormones and growth hormone in embryonic and growing emus (*Dromaius novaehollandiae*). *Reproduction Fertility and Development* 13:125–32.

Cahaner, A., and Siegel, P.B. 1986. Evaluation of industry breeding programs for meat-type chickens and turkeys. In *3rd World Congress on Genetics Applied to Livestock*. 337–346.

Cilliers, S.C., du Preez, J.J., Maritz, J.S., and Hayes, J.P. 1995. Growth curves of ostriches (*Struthio camelus*) from Oudtshoorn in South Africa. *Animal Science* 61:161–164.

Dawson, A., Deeming, D.C., Dick, A.C., and Sharp, P.J. 1996. Plasma thyroxine concentrations in farmed ostriches in relation to age, body weight, and growth hormone. *General and Comparative Endocrinology* 103:308–315.

Deeming, D.C., and Ayres, L. 1994. Factors affecting the rate of growth of ostrich (*Struthio camelus*) chicks in captivity. *Veterinary Record* 135:617–622.

Deeming, D.C., Sibly, R.M., and Magole, H. 1996. Estimation of the weight and body condition of ostriches (*Struthio camelus*) from body measurements. *Vet Rec* 139:210–213.

Gillespie, J.M., and Schupp, A.R. 1998. Ratite production as an agricultural enterprise. *Veterinary Clinics of North America: Food Animal Practice* 14:373–386.

Gous, R.M., Moran, E.T., Jr., Stilborn, H.R., Bradford, G.D., and Emmans, G.C. 1999. Evaluation of the parameters needed to describe the overall growth, the chemical growth, and the growth of feathers and breast muscles of broilers. *Poultry Science* 78:812–821.

Havenstein, G.B., Ferket, P.R., Scheideler, S.E., and Larson, B.T. 1994a. Growth, livability, and feed conversion of 1957 vs 1991 broilers when fed "typical" 1957 and 1991 broiler diets. *Poultry Science* 73:1785–1794.

Havenstein, G.B., Ferket, P.R., Scheideler, S.E., and Rives, D.V. 1994b. Carcass composition and yield of 1991 vs 1957 broilers when fed "typical" 1957 and 1991 broiler diets. *Poultry Science* 73:1795–1804.

Horton, D.H. 1951. *Broiler Growing*. Long Island Agricultural and Technical Institute.

Knizetova, H., Hyanek, J., Knize, B., and Roubicek, J. 1991. Analysis of growth curves of fowl. I. Chickens. *British Poultry Science* 32:1027–1038.

Lilburn, M.S., and Emmerson, D. 1993. The influence of differences in dietary amino acids during the early growing period on growth and development of Nicholas and British United Turkey Toms. *Poultry Science* 72:1722–1730.

Lilburn, M.S., Renner, P.A., and Anthony, N.B. 1992. Interaction between step-up versus step-down lighting from four to sixteen weeks on growth and development in turkey hens from two commercial strains. *Poultry Science* 71:419–426.

López, S., France, J., Gerrits, W.J.J., Dhanoa, M.S., Humphries, D.J., and Dijkstra, J. 2000. A generalized Michaelis-Menten equation for the analysis of growth. *Journal of Animal Science* 78:1816–1828.

Maruyama, K., Potts, W.J., Bacon, W.L., and Nestor, K.E. 1998. Modeling turkey growth with the relative growth rate. *Growth Development and Aging* 62:123–139.

Mignon-Grasteau, S., Beaumont, C., Le Bihan-Duval, E., Poivey, J.P., de Rochambeau, H., and Ricard, F.H. 1999. Genetic parameters of growth curve parameters in male and female chickens. *British Poultry Science* 40:44–51.

Mignon-Grasteau, S., Piles, M., Varona, L., de Rochambeau, H., Poivey, J.P., Blasco, A., and Beaumont, C. 2000. Genetic analysis of growth curve parameters for male and female chickens resulting from selection on shape of growth curve. *Journal of Animal Science* 78:2515–2524.

Mushi, E.Z., Isa, J.F., Chabo, R.G., and Segaise, T.T. 1998. Growth rate of ostrich (*Struthio camelus*) chicks under intensive management in Botswana. *Tropical Animal Health and Production* 30:197–203.

Qureshi, M.A., and Havenstein, G.B. 1994. A comparison of the immune performance of a 1991 commercial broiler with a 1957 randombred strain when fed "typical" 1957 and 1991 broiler diets. *Poultry Science* 73:1805–1812.

Rogers, S.R., Pesti, G.M., and Marks, H.L. 1987. Comparison of three nonlinear regression models for describing broiler growth curves. *Growth* 51:229–239.

Siegel, P.B., and Dunnington, E.A. 1987. Selection for growth in chickens. *CRC Critical Reviews in Poultry Biology* 1:1–24.

21
Growth of Companion Animals

Karyn Malinowski and Colin G. Scanes

This chapter addresses growth of companion animals. Unlike the situation with many livestock that are marketed for meat at a specific age/weight, there is interest in growth in companion animals throughout growth and maturation. Interest in growth of companion animals comes from a desire to ensure a healthy adult animal that has had optimal nutrition during the growth period. This is critical to performance, for instance, with the equine athlete.

Studies of growth are expensive and there is considerably less funding available for companion animals than for livestock or for biomedical models. There is, however, a good body of information on the growth of companion animals.

GROWTH OF HORSES

Growth of horses is of considerable interest due to the economic importance of the equine athlete. Performance is most probably linked to optimal growth of both the skeletal system and musculature. Table 21.1 summarizes growth in two breeds of horses.

The strength of the skeleton is essential for the success of the equine athlete. Bone fractures and other musculo-skeletal injuries are frequently associated with the end of the career of the equine athlete. There are growth-related changes in skeletal strength. These have been characterized, e.g., in Glade et al. (1986).

Gender and Growth

There are effects of gender on growth in horses. In the period following birth (2–22 days of age), the male foal is slightly larger/heavier (1.3–2.0%) than the female (Hintz et al. 1979; McKeever et al. 1981; Thompson and Smith 1994). This difference is even smaller at 66 days of age (Hintz et al. 1979) (Table 21.2). Thereafter the difference becomes more marked with colts being >4.5% heavier than fillies and ~1.4% taller (Hintz et al. 1979) (Table 21.2). Differences in growth rate between fillies and geldings (castrated males) are also evident (McCann et al. 1992). This would be indicative of female hormones inhibiting growth rather that testicular hormones enhancing growth in the colt. These differences, albeit of a small magnitude, may be critically important to the performance of the equine athlete at racing venues.

Effect of Dam on Growth

In addition to the genetic effect of the dam, there are effects of dam age on growth of the foal (Hintz et al. 1979). Foals from young and old mares are somewhat smaller and grow at a lower rate (Hintz et al. 1979) (see Table 21.3). These differences may reflect fetal growth and/or quality/quantity of milk produced. There is evidence that nutrition can influence milk quality of the lactating broodmare and thereby affect growth of the foal (Glade and Luba 1990). Feeding mares a diet with soybean meal resulted in increases in milk protein, elevated circulating concentrations of free amino acids in the foals, and increased skeletal growth in foals (Glade and Luba 1990).

Breed and Growth

There are profound differences in the size/weight of horses in different breeds. Table 21.4 lists a number of examples. The magnitude of the differences is less though than that in the dog. Moreover, there do not appear to be obvious hormonal differences with size of breed (Malinowski et al. 1996), unlike the situation in the dog (see below).

Table 21.1. Growth of Percheron horses and Thoroughbred horses[1] (data from Brody, 1945; Hintz et al., 1979)

| Age(Days/Month) | Percheron | | Thoroughbreds[1] | |
	Body Weight(kg)	Height (cm)	Cannon Bone Length (cm)	Body Weight (kg)
2 d	75	100.3	12.4	54
21/22 d	100	107.6	13.2	85
2.3 m	175	120.4	14.8	143
4 m	250	128.4	15.7	188
6 m	300	133.4	16.6	236
8 m	336	138.8	18.1	288
299 d	357	142.9	18.6	318
352 d	370	145.0	19.1	337
404 d	394	147.8	19.8	364
464 d	414	150.8	20.4	403
524 d	438	152.7	20.7	428
644 d	480	155.5	21.1	459

[1]n = ~2000.

Table 21.2. Differences in growth between female and male Thoroughbred horses (data from or calculated from Hintz et al., 1979)

Age (Days)	Δ Body Weight— Difference Between Fillies and Colts Δ kg (Δ%)	Δ Skeletal Growth— Difference Between Height Between Fillies and Colts cm (Δ%)
22	+1.1[*] (+1.3%)	0.4[*] (+0.4%)
66	+1.3[*] (+0.9%)	0.3 (+0.2%)
118	+3.3[**] (+1.8%)	0.8[**] (+0.6%)
178	+8.3[**] (+3.6%)	1.3[**] (+1.0%)
239	+10.9[**] (+3.9%)	1.4[**] (+1.0%)
299	+14.1[*] (+4.6%)	1.4[**] (+1.0%)
358	+15.9[**] (+4.8%)	1.7[**] (+1.2%)
419	+17.3[**] (+4.7%)	2.0[**] (+1.4%)
510	+22.6[**] (+5.5%)	2.1[**] (+1.4%)

[*]$p<0.05$; [**]$p<0.01$.
n = ~1000 colts and ~1000 fillies.

Growth Curves

Equine growth is most frequently characterized by average daily gain, by indices of skeletal growth, etc.

Nutrition (Including Environmental Toxicants) and Growth

Growth in horses requires optimal nutrition. The recommendations for equine nutrition are published (NRC 1978). There is some additional information

that suggests diets can be further improved. For instance, weanling Quarter horses grew more (gained more weight) when receiving a diet containing 125% of the NRC recommendation for both protein and energy than on diets containing either 100% of protein and 100% of energy or 100% of protein and 125% of energy (Topliff et al. 1988). There was some tendency for increased growth diet of weanling foals receiving diets containing added fat (Davison et al. 1991). Although young growing

Table 21.3. Effect of mare's age in foal growth (calculated from Hintz et al., 1979)

Age of Dam (Years)	Body Weight of Foal[1,2] (kg)		
	22 Days	66 Days	178 Days
3–4	78[a] (–8.7%)	133[a] (–7.5%)	223 (–3.7%)
7	85[b] (0%)	143[b] (0%)	232 (0%)
12–15	88[c] (+3.2%)	148[c] (+4.7%)	236 (+1.7%)
19–20	84[b] (–0.2%)	141[b] (–1.6%)	227 (–2.2%)

[1]n = >200 foals per age except 19–20 years; male n = 43.
[2]Percentage increase/decrease compared to 7-year-old dams.
[a,b,c]Different superscripts indicate different $p<0.05$.

Table 21.4. Differences in body weight, height, and circulating concentrations of IGF-I in different breeds of horses (data from Malinowski et al., 1996)

Breed	Weight kg[1]	Height cm[1]	IGF-I ng/ml[1]
Miniature	90	85	184[c]
Shetland	115	115	309[a,b]
Welsh pony A	270	120	196[b,c]
Welsh pony B	320	135	263[a,b,c]
Standardbred	455	155	231[a,b,c]
Thoroughbred	455	160	244[a,b,c]
Friesen	590	170	324[a]
Draft (Belgian and Percheron)	640	170	198[b,c]

[a,b,c]Different superscript letters indicate different $p<0.05$.
[1]Data from National Breed Registries.

horses retain considerably more nitrogen when receiving a diet containing soybean meal compared to alfalfa, this difference was not reflected in average daily gain or skeletal growth (Wall et al. 1997). There is, however, no discernable difference between growth rate in yearling horses fed an oats/alfalfa diet compared to concentrates and alfalfa (Gibbs et al. 1989). Forage type/quality influences growth of horses—for instance, growth of yearling horses is superior on Bermuda than Klein grass pastures (Webb et al. 1990).

Nutrition not only influences overall growth but also development of skeletal strength. For instance, Glade and colleagues (1986) determined that young horses receiving a diet meeting only 70% of NRC-recommended levels was associated with reduced medio-lateral diameter and medial-lateral cortical thickness of the metacarpal bones compared to horses on a 100% NRC diet.

Growth of horses can be influenced by environmental toxicants. For instance, growth of yearling horses was lower when fed tall fescue infected with high levels of endophyte compared with fescue with low infestation (Aiken et al. 1993), ADG being 0.56 kg/d on low level and 0.24 kg/d on high levels of endophyte investation (Aiken et al. 1993). In another study, there was no difference in growth rate in yearlings fed endophyte-infected fescue, albeit at somewhat lower levels (McCann et al. 1992).

The Equine Hypothalamo-Pituitary (GH)-IGF-I Axis

The hypothalamo-pituitary (GH)-IGF-I axis in the horse appears to function in a manner very similar to that in other domestic animals. The major form of equine GH has been characterized (Conde et al. 1973). In addition, there is variant that lacks the sequence of amino-acid residues between 76 and 92

(Cascone et al. 1992). The physiological significance of this form is not known. In the equine pituitary gland, GH is synthesized by somatotropes and
by a subset of cells producing GH and prolactin
(Rahmanian et al. 1997).

Secretion of GH is under the control of the hypothalamus; the releasing factor, GHRH, increases circulating concentrations of GH (e.g., Christensen et
al. 1997). In the growing horse, GH is released in a
pulsatile/episodic manner (Christensen et al. 1997)
but with no difference with stage of growth
(Thomas et al. 1998).

The effects of GH administration have been examined in adult horses. As would be expected with a
functional hypothalamo-pituitary (GH)-IGF-I axis,
circulating concentrations of IGF-I are elevated following GH administration (Buonomo et al. 1996)
(Table 21.5). A concomitant increase in musculature
is also observed (Malinowski et al. 1997) (Table
21.5). In addition, some diabetogenic effect of GH is
observed with elevated circulating concentrations of
glucose and insulin (Buonomo et al. 1996) (Table
21.5). There are marked changes in the circulating

concentration of IGF-I during growth (Malinowski et
al. 1996) (Table 21.6).

Other Hormones and Equine Growth—Glucocorticoids

It is likely that environmental stresses impair equine
growth. This is supported by the almost complete
suppression of growth of foals receiving administration of the synthetic glucocorticoid, dexamethasone
(Glade et al. 1981). Stresses elevate release of cortisol, the endogenous glucocorticoid. For instance,
transportation stress increases circulating concentrations of cortisol (Stull and Rodiek 2000), as does
fasting (Glade et al. 1984). There is also an interaction between the stress-induced cortisol secretion
and inadequate nutrition. Fasting induces a greater
elevation in the circulating concentrations of cortisol in horses that had been previously compared on
a low plane to those on a high plane of nutrition
(respectively 80% and 160% of the National
Research Council recommendation) (Glade et al.
1984).

Table 21.5. Effect of GH administration on horses

Parameters	Age of Horses	Control		GH
Study A (Buonomo et al. 1996)				
Circulating IGF-I ng/ml	adult	185±20	*	818±20
Blood urea nitrogen mg/dl	adult	12.9±0.9	*	7.6±0.9
Serum glucose mg/dl	adult	93±7	*	122±6
Serum insulin uIU/ml	adult	52±9	*	105±9
Study B (Malinowski et al. 1997)				
Increase body weight (kg)	Aged (20–26 years)	+10		+19
Musculature score	Aged (20–26 years)	0.7±0.4	*	2.5±0.6
Study C (Julen Day et al. 2000)				
Calcium				
Intake (g/d)	2-year-old	38.2±1.7		37.4±1.4
Fecal (g/d)	2-year-old	11.2±1.0		11.0±1.0
Urinary (g/d)	2-year-old	6.1±1.1	*	4.2±0.3
Retention (g/d)	2-year-old	20.9±1.6		21.7±1.1
Phosphate				
Intake (g/d)	2-year-old	19.4±1.2		19.0±1.1
Fecal (g/d)	2-year-old	16.5±1.5	*	12.0±0.9
Urinary (g/d)	2-year-old	0.08±0.01		0.09±0.01
Retention (g/d)	2-year-old	2.8±0.8	*	6.8±0.8

*Significant difference—$p<0.05$

Table 21.6. Changes in circulating concentrations of IGF-I during growth of female Standardbred horses (data from Malinowski et al., 1996)

Age	IGF-I[1] ng/ml
0	285[c]
1 d	320[c]
7 d	506[a,b]
14 d	572[a,b]
1 m	597[a]
2 m	604[a]
4 m	535[a,b]
6 m	453[a,b,c]
9 m	530[a,b]
Adult (5–8 y)	369[b,c]
Adult (16–22 y)	295[c]

[1]Pooled S.E.M = 50.
[a,b,c]Different superscripts indicate different $p<0.05$.

Table 21.7. Effect of the glucocorticoid, dexamethasone, on growth in foals (data from Glade et al., 1981)

Parameters	Control		Dexamethasone (5 mg/100 kg)
A. *Horse foals*[1]			
Body weight (kg±S.E.M.)	229±21	*	304±6
Height at withers cm	135±3	*	143±2
Heart girth (cm)	140±4	*	152±2
B. *Pony foals*[2]			
Nitrogen absorption (% of intake)	82		82
Nitrogen excretion (% of intake)	41	*	81
Nitrogen retention	41	*	2

*Significant difference $p<0.05$.
[1]Dexamethasone was administered daily to groups of 6-month-old Standardbred and Thoroughbred foals for 20 weeks.
[2]Dexamethasone was administered from 6 months for 10 months.

Growth almost completely abated in foals receiving dexamethasone irrespective of whether growth was measured as body weight or indices of skeletal growth (Glade et al. 1981) (see Table 21.7). Moreover, dexamethasone administration is associated with an almost doubling in nitrogen excretion (Table 21.7). It can be estimated that nitrogen retention is reduced by >95% by glucocorticoid (Table 21.7).

Effect of Season on Growth

There are marked effects of the month of a foal's birth and its subsequent growth (Hintz et al. 1979). Foals born in late Spring/early Summer are larger at 22 days of age than those born in January through April (Hintz et al. 1979). This difference in body weight is maintained throughout growth (Hintz et al. 1979) (see Table 21.8 for body weights at representative ages). The basis for these differences may be fetal growth, quality/quantity of the dam's milk (possibly due to improved nutrition), and/or the absence of cold stress with the higher ambient temperatures.

GROWTH OF DOGS

Man's association with dogs is extremely ancient; dogs were the first domestic animals and companion animals. They can be working animals. Their working

Table 21.8. Effect of season on foal growth (data from Hintz et al., 1979)

Month/Season	Body Weight of Foal[1]—kg		
	22d	66d	178d
January–March	82[a]	140[a]	230[a]
April	85[b]	144[b]	232[b]
May, June, July	88[c]	145[b]	234[b]

[1]n ≥ 500 per month/season.
[a,b,c]Different superscripts indicate different $p<0.05$.

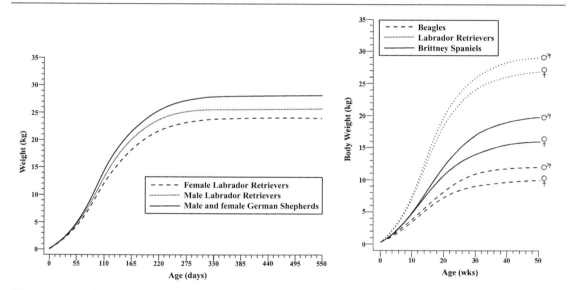

Figure 21.1. Growth of dogs. (Data adapted from Allard et al. 1988; Helmink et al. 2000.)

uses include in hunting, in agriculture (e.g., herding and estrus determination), in racing (e.g., greyhounds), in law enforcement, in aiding the handicapped (e.g., seeing-eye dogs for the visually impaired, etc.) and as laboratory animals. They may also be acquired for companionship and emotional support.

There has been significant interest in growth—its control and pathological abnormalities—in dogs. There are tremendous differences in growth between breeds of dogs of different sizes, which range from the "toy" to the "giant," with a 100-fold difference in adult body weight being observed from ~1 kg to >100 kg (Burger and Johnson 1991). Based on the rate of growth/scaling of specific organs and particularly the brain, Kirkwood (1985)

suggested that "the toy breeds are like pups whose development and growth has been curtailed." An analogous argument can be made for the giant breeds with growth/development being extended.

Quantitative aspects of growth have been reported in the scientific literature only for a relatively small numbers of breeds: beagles, Brittany spaniels, German shepherd dogs, and Labrador retrievers (Allard et al. 1988; Helmink et al. 2000; see Figure 21.1). It should be noted that these determinations of growth have been made under standardized conditions. The quantitative data is almost completely limited to body weight. with little attention focused on skeletal growth. An exception to this is the comprehensive study by Kirkwood (1985).

Fetal Growth

There is only a modest amount of information on fetal growth in dogs. Some relationship between fetal growth and maternal size exists (Kirkwood 1985). Breed differences exist between birth weight but these are of a smaller magnitude than in the adult (Kirkwood 1985). There is little difference in gestational length among breeds (Kirkwood 1985), and thus fetal growth will show tremendous breed differences. Sex differences in body weight are not apparent in newborn puppies (Allard et al. 1988).

Gender and Growth

There is significant sexual dimorphism in growth rates in dog with the male achieving a plateau in body weight that is 17–19% higher than in the female. Moreover, males grow for a somewhat longer period; for instance, adult body weight is achieved at 24 weeks in female beagles and 30 weeks in males (Allard et al. 1988). Male dogs have a slightly later point of inflection of the Gompertz growth curve (Helmink et al. 2000).

Weaning and Growth

In a comprehensive study of canine growth where puppies had free access to solid food during weaning, Allard and colleagues (1988) observed no reduction in growth.

Breed and Growth

Smaller breeds reach plateau body weight earlier than larger breeds. For instance, male Labrador retrievers reached their adult weight at 44 weeks of age, and male beagles require only 30 weeks (Allard et al. 1988).

There have been a few studies on the hormonal basis of growth differences in various breeds. These are summarized in Table 21.9. There appears to be a relationship between the circulating concentration of IGF-I and growth rate. For instance, it is clear that although toy and miniature poodles have aberrantly low circulating concentrations of IGF-I (Table 21.9). Circulating concentrations of GH are somewhat elevated (Table 21.9). The low circulating concentrations of IGF-I may reflect a breed difference at the level of the GH receptor and hence IGF-I production. Moreover, there is a marked tendency that the larger the breed, the higher the circulating concentration of IGF-I (Table 21.9).

Hip and elbow dysplasia are fairly common heritable diseases in dogs. These are particularly prevalent in large breeds where there is very rapid growth and considerable body weight to be supported (reviewed Mäki et al. 2000).

Growth Curves

Much but not all growth can be described as a linear function, but overall the Gompertz growth curve provides a superior fit. Linear growth is reported between 4 and 24 weeks of age in Labrador bitches (Chakraborty et al. 1983). Gompertz growth curves have been constructed for beagles, Brittany spaniels, German shepherd dogs, and Labrador retrievers (Allard et al. 1988; Helmink et al. 2000) (see Figure 21.1). Male dogs have a slightly later point of inflection of the curve (Table 21.10) (Helmink et al. 2000). This has been applied to growth of both dogs and cats. It is interesting to note that the average mature weight (Table 21.10) for male Labrador retrievers is close to the maximal optimum weight (32 kg) for guide dogs (e.g., seeing-eye dogs). Hence, many male Labrador retrievers are likely to be rejected from the program due to excess weight/size (Helmink et al. 2000).

Nutrition and Growth

Adequate nutrition is obviously required for normal growth, but there is a problem with canine obesity. The quality of commercial dog food allows puppies to grow at a rapid rate (Hirakawa and Baker 1988). Table 21.11 summarizes the growth rate and retention of nutrients in young puppies receiving a commercial dog chow or three experimental diets: casein-based, corn-soybean-based, or a semi-synthetic diet with nitrogen provided as crystalline amino acids. The chow provided sufficient nutrients for as strong growth as the semi-synthetic diet and superior growth to the corn-soy diet. Puppies fed the casein-based diet show maximal growth due to nutrient composition, high palatability, and digestibility (Table 21.11).

The pattern of feeding or time of food availability influences growth. For instance, growth in puppies was compared feeding a calorie-dense diet either free-choice/self-feeding (ad libitum feed availability) or time-restricted manner ("time restricted meal fed") (Alexander and Wood 1987). Body weight gain was depressed in the puppies who had food available only during two meal times per day, but skeletal growth (forelimb length and body length) was not affected by feeding regimen (Alexander and Wood 1987). This may represent an approach to reduce excessive weight gain.

Breed and, in particular, size/weight affect nutritional requirements. In the adult dog, the digestible energy requirement has been estimated (Burger and Johnson 1991) as 678 $W^{0.64}$ kJ/d for resting energy

Table 21.9. Circulating concentrations of hormones related to growth in dogs with different growth characteristics (±S.E.M.)

Breed	Body Weight (kg)	Plasma Hormone Concentration (ng/ml)		
		GH	(Peak GH[2])	IGF-I
Study A (Eigenmann et al. 1984a)				
Standard Poodle	20.9±1.6[a]	1.6±0.3[a]	17.3±3.0[a]	96±15[a]
Miniature Poodle[1]	6.2±0.4[b]	5.7±2.1[a]	33.3±9.5[a]	24±5[b]
Toy Poodle[1]	3.0±0.2[c]	2.2±1.0[a]	29.1±6.7[a]	16±4[b]
Study B (Eigenmann and Eigenmann 1981; Eigenmann et al. 1984b)				
German Shepherd	32.1±1.5[a]	1.5±1.2[a]	44.4±0.09[a]	280±23[a]
Dwarf German Shepherd	8.4±0.6[b]	0.5±0.1[a]	0.6±0.1[b]	11±2[b]
Study C (Eigenmann et al. 1984c)				
Cocker spaniels	12.4±1.1[a]	-	-	36±9.5[a]
Beagles	14.7±1.8[a,b]	-	-	87±10.4[b]
Keeshonden	17.2±1.8[b]	-	-	117±10.8[b]
German Shepherds	35.8±2.4[c]	-	-	280±6.4[c]
Dogs with GH elevated	-			700±90[d]
Dogs with acromegaly				679±116[d]

[1]n = 10 per group of adult dogs.
[2]Peak circulating GH concentrations in response to clonidine.
[a,b,c,d]Different superscript letters indicate different $p<0.05$.

Table 21.10. Gompertz function for growth of dogs (based on Helmink et al. 2000)

Breed-Sex	Mature Weight, kg	Point of Inflection, Day
German Shepherd dog		
Female	24.4	84.0
Male	29.1	86.6
Labrador retriever		
Female	26.8	82.7
Male	31.4	87.4

Gompertz function $W_t = W_{max} \exp\{-e^{[-(t-c)/b]}\}$
Where
W_t = weight at time, t
W_{max} = mature body weight
b = proportional to duration of growth
c = age at point of inflection
t = age in days

An alternative expression of the Gompertz function is the following:

$W_t = W_o{}^* e^{k(1-e-\alpha t)}$

Where W_t = weight at time, t
W_o = birth weight
k = the growth parameter
α = the expotential rate of decline in growth

expenditure, 655 $W^{0.69}$ kJ/d for moderate activity, and 643 $W^{0.73}$ kJ/d for higher activity (W is the body weight in kg).

There is some consensus that the commonly accepted value of 0.75 for the mass exponential is not applicable to dogs (Heusner 1991). The influ-

Table 21.11. Effect of diet on growth in puppies[1] (data from Hirakawa and Baker, 1988)

Parameter	Chow[2]	Casein-Based Diet	Corn-Soybean Diet	Synthetic/Crystalized Amino-Acid–Based Diet
Growth (average daily gain g)	93[b]	111[a]	53[c]	87[b]
Food intake (g/day)	199[a]	182[a,b']	155[b]	158[b]
Digestibility (%)				
Nitrogen	71.7[b]	93.8[a]	64.8[b]	93.2[a]
Energy	75.4[b]	91.3[a]	75.8[b]	93.6[a]

[1]7-week-old fed diets for 21 days.
[2]Purina Puppy Chow.
[a,b,c]Different superscript letters indicate different $p < 0.05$.

Table 21.12. Effect of GH or the GH-RP analogue MK-0677 in growth and circulating concentrations of IGF-I in dogs (adapted from Prahalada et al., 1999)

Treatment	Body Weight (kg±S.E.M.)	Δ (Increase in) Body Weight (kg)	IGF-I (ng/ml)
O	10.3±1.5	0.2	196[a]
MK-0677	10.8±0.4[*]	0.8	310[b]
GH	11.5±0.6[*]	0.9	507[c]

[*]Different from prior to treatment.
[a,b,c]Different letters indicate different $p < 0.05$.

ence of breed on growth of puppies is exemplified by the improved growth rate of Great Danes on a diet containing higher levels of protein than National Research Council recommendations (Nap et al. 1991)

The Canine Hypothalamo-Pituitary (GH)-IGF-I Axis

The dog has a fully functioning hypothalamo-pituitary (GH)-IGF-I axis. Based on the sequence of cDNA, canine GH is identical to porcine GH (Ascacio-Martinez et al. 1994). Secretion of GH in the dog is controlled by hypothalamic releasing factors being increased by GHRH and decreased by SRIF (Cella et al. 1993; Cowan et al. 1984). Secretion of GH from the dog pituitary is stimulated analogues of GH-releasing peptide (GH-RP) (acutely: Jacks et al. 1996; chronically: Prahalada et al., 1999), by clonidine (acting at the level of the hypothalamus) (Eigenmann et al. 1983), and by nutritional deprivation. Fasting increases circulating concentrations of GH (Eigenmann and de Bruijne 1985). Except under pathological situations (see below), there does not appear to be a strong or consistent relationship between circulating concentrations of GH and growth rate (Chakraborty et al. 1983). However, a temporal relationship between serum GH concentrations and both longitudinal bone growth and circulating concentrations of IGF-I has been reported in growing dogs but with a one-day time lag (Conzemius et al. 1998). In addition, plasma concentrations of GH but not IGF-I were recently reported to be higher in young dogs of a large breed (Great Dane) than of a smaller breed (beagles) (Favier et al. 2001) (also see above for breed differences).

Both growth and circulating concentrations of IGF-I are elevated with either the chronic administration of porcine GH or the analogue of GH-RP (Prahalada et al. 1999) (Table 21.12). The GH or GHRP analogue was administered daily (for 2 weeks) to male beagle dogs (42–46 weeks old)—an age when growth/body weight had effectively plateaued (Allard et al. 1988). Similar increases in body weight with GH administration have been observed previously by the same group, with the

Table 21.13. Effects (including pathological) of GH administration[1] in adult dogs (data calculated from Prahalada et al., 1998; Laroque et al., 1998; Molon-Noblot et al., 1998)

Parameters	Vehicle		GH
Body weight gain (kg)	0.4	*	4.7
Muscle fibers			
type 1 (% increase)	100±4	*	134±4
type 2 (% increase)	100±2	*	119±4
Red Blood Cells (10^6/mm^3)	7.1±0.2[2]	*	4.8±0.14
Insulin (area under curve) for 8 hours			
including postprandial	0.10±0.01	*	1.92±0.09
Liver (kg)	0.31±0.01	*	0.65±0.05
Pituitary wt (mg)	75±3	*	100±5
Histopathologies			
Stomach	0/8	*	8/8
Liver	0/8	*	8/8
Spleen	1/8	*	8/8
Skin	0/8	*	8/8

*$p<0.05$.
[1]0.56 GH/kg was administered daily for 14 weeks to beagle dogs (54–69 weeks) (per treatment: 4 male, 4 female).
[2]± S.E.M.

increase in body weight being due to greater muscling (Laroque et al. 1998) (also see Table 21.13) and to changes in internal organs, such as the liver (hepatomegaly) (Prahalada et al. 1998).

Pathologies with GH Administration

There are marked pathological changes in dogs with excessive GH. Dogs are sensitive to the diabetogenic effects of GH with excess GH, due to hypersecretion, for instance, following administration of the progestagen, medroxyprogesterone (Eigennmann et al. 1983) or exogenous GH administration. For instance, circulating concentrations of insulin are greatly elevated in dogs receiving chronic GH administration (Prahalada et al. 1998) (see Table 21.13). The circulating concentration of red blood cells declined in dogs receiving GH (Prahalada et al. 1998) (Table 21.13). Moreover, histopathologies are observed in all dogs receiving a high dose of GH (Prahalada et al. 1998) (Table 21.13).

Extra-Pituitary Synthesis of GH

There is evidence canine mammary tissue expresses GH, and this can affect mammary and/or tumor development via an autocrine/paracrine loop (van Garderen et al. 1997, 2001).

Dwarfism

Dogs can have marked GH deficiency. This dwarfism is most frequently reported in German shepherds. The symptoms include reduced growth and abnormal hair growth (retension of lanugo or secondary hairs, lack of primary hairs, and alopecia) (Kooistra et al. 2000). Dogs exhibit hypopituitary dwarfism due to the congenital GH deficiency, together with hyposecretion of other adenohypophyseal hormones (e.g., Andresen and Willeberg 1976). Cases of this have been demonstrated to be due to a simple autosomal recessive abnormality, which results in the anterior pituitary lobe not being fully formed (Nicholas 1978). Another form of congenital hyposomatotropinemia has been reported in which there is hyposecretion of GH, prolactin, thyrotropin, and gonadotropins, but normal ACTH secretion (Kooistra et al. 2000). This is due presumably to a mutation that impedes pituitary stem cell expansion after the appearance of the corticotropes (Kooistra et al. 2000). Dogs with hypopituitary dwarfism have very low circulating concentrations of the hormone mediating GH's effect, namely IGF-I (see Table 21.9 and Figure 21.2) (Eigenmann et al. 1984b; Eigenmann and Eigenmann 1981).

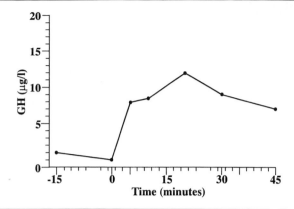

Figure 21.2. Response of dogs to GHRH. (Data adapted from Kooistra et al., 2000.)

Adrenergic Agonists and Lipid Metabolism

Canine adipose tissue appears to respond to adrenergic agonists (epinephrine, norepinehrine, together with synthetic adrenergic-agonists) in a manner similar to the situation in other species (see Chapter 15). β-adrenergic agonists induce increased lipolysis and decreased lipogenesis. Both α_2-agonists and adenosine depress lipolysis (Rudman et al. 1963; Fredholm and Sollevi, 1981; Berlan et al., 1982). The canine β_2-adrenergic receptor has been characterized based on sequencing of the cDNA (Emala et al. 1996).

GROWTH OF CATS

Cats are among the most popular companion animals. Not only are they held in high esteem for companionship and emotional support, but they also have been extensively employed in vermin control. They are also used as laboratory animals.

There are a number of reports describing and/or quantifying the growth of cats (Latimer and Ibsen 1932; Rosenstein and Berman 1973; Douglass et al. 1988;). In cats, there is not a post-birth reduction in body weight and growth continues unabated (Latimer and Ibsen 1932).

Fetal Growth

There is relatively little information on fetal growth. There is a consistency in gestational length irrespective of birth weight (Hall and Pierce 1934). Early studies would also suggest that maternal size (and presumably nutritional status) have little effect on fetal growth (Hall and Pierce 1934). Some rela-

tionship between number of fetuses and fetal growth is possible; the highest birth weights are observed with a litter size of 5 compared to small litters (2) or very large litters (6) (Hall and Pierce 1934). There is no evidence of sexual dimorphism in fetal growth in cats based on birth weights (Table 21.14).

Gender and Growth

There is a marked difference in the growth rate and mature body weight between male and female cats (Table 21.14). Males grow to >25% greater mature body weights (Table 21.14), which is somewhat greater than the situation in dogs (males having ~20% greater body weights).

Growth Curves

There are two studies that have quantitatively described the growth of cats employing Gompertz function (Douglass et al. 1988; Rosenstein and Berman 1973). These studies are summarized in Figure 21.3 and Table 21.15. The growth parameter (k) is consistently 14% greater in male than female cats (Table 21.15) (Douglass et al. 1988; Rosenstein and Berman 1973). The divergence between growth in males and female cats begins at 7–8 weeks of age (Latimer et al. 1932).

The Feline Hypothalamo-Pituitary (GH)-IGF-I Axis

There is little information in the literature about the feline hypothalamo-pituitary (GH)-IGF-I axis. There is no reason, however, to doubt that the cat does not have a fully functioning hypothalamo-pituitary (GH)-IGF-I axis.

Table 21.14. Sexual dimorphism in growth in cats

	Male		Female
Study A (Rosenstein and Berman 1972)			
Birth weight g±S.D.	103±19		97±15
Adult weight kg±S.D.	3.3±1.0	*	2.6±0.4
(% increase in males compared to females)	(+29%)		
Study B(Douglass et al. 1988)			
Birth weight g±S.D.	106±18		99±14.0
Adult weight kg±S.D.	4.5±0.6	*	2.8±0.5
(% increase in males compared to females)	(+61%)		

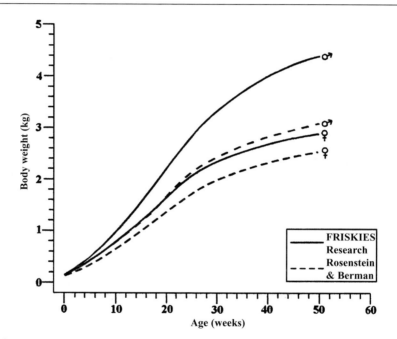

Figure 21.3. Growth of cats. (Data adapted from Rosenstein and Berman, 1973.)

Dwarfism/Stunting of Growth—Feline GM1 Gangliosidosis

Cats with feline GM1 gangliosidosis show stunting of growth, premature thymic involution, and progressive neural dysfunction. This disease is an autosomal recessive defect of lysosomal β-galactosidase and hence reduced catabolism of GM1 gangliosides together with glycoproteins and glycolipids (reviewed Cox et al. 1999). Cats with feline GM1 gangliosidosis show disturbance to the hypothal-amo-pituitary-GH axis with progressively lower circulating concentrations of IGF-I than not-mutant cats (Cox et al. 1999) (see Table 21.16).

Adrenergic Agonists and Lipid Metabolism

Cat adipose tissue responds to adrenergic agonists (epinephrine, norepinehrine, together with synthetic adrenergic-agonists) in a manner similar to the situation in other species (see Chapter 17). β-

Table 21.15. Characteristics of growth in dogs and cats

	k	α	Predicted		
	(Growth Parameter)	(Decline in Growth Rate)	Wo (g)	W_{max} (kg)	Reference
Dogs					
Beagle					
female	3.52	0.116	0.308	10.4	Allard et al., 1988
male	3.64	0.112	0.327	12.7	Allard et al., 1988
Brittany spaniel					
female	3.89	0.110	0.333	16.3	Allard et al., 1988
male	4.12	0.108	0.327	20.2	Allard et al., 1988
Labrador retriever					
female	3.94	0.117	0.525	26.7	Allard et al., 1988
male	3.98	0.115	0.555	29.8	Allard et al., 1988
Cats					
female	2.93	0.080	97	251	Rosenstein and Berman, 1973
	3.21	0.092	99	2.87	Douglass et al., 1988
male	3.32	0.074	103	3.20	Rosenstein and Berman, 1973
	3.66	0.073	106	4.62	Douglass et al., 1988

Table 21.16. Effect of feline GM1 gangliosidosis on the hypothalamo-pituitary GH-IGF-I axis in cats (data from Cox et al., 1999)

	Normal		Mutant
Pituitary			
GH mRNA (200 d)	143	*	58
Circulating IGF-I			
~60 days	132		114
~160 days	253	***	129
~270 days	451	***	96
Liver IGF-I mRNA (> 200 d)	136	**	64
Circulating IGFBPs			
IGFBP-2	0.3	***	2.3
IGFBP-3	14.7	**	6.7

$p<0.05$; **$p<0.01$; ***$p<0.001$.

adrenergic agonists (epinephrine and isoproterenol) increase lipolysis, and these effects are suppressed in the presence of the β-antagonist, propranolol (Table 21.17) (Ng 1985). There is also evidence that both epinephrine acting via the α_2-adrenergic G_i-linked receptor and adenosine acting via the adenosine G_i-linked receptor depress lipolysis (Ng 1985).

Table 21.17. Effect of β-adrenergic agonists on lipolysis by cat adipocytes in vitro (adapted from Ng, 1985)

Treatment	Lipolysis (Glycerol Release as a Percentage of Control)
Control	100±34[a]
Epinephrine	212±28[b]
Isoproterenol (β agonist)	328±7[c]
Epinephrine + Propranolol (β antagonist)	89±13[a]
Isoproterenol + Propranolol	97±37[a]

[a,b,c]Different superscript letters indicate different p<0.05.

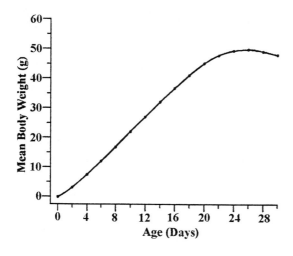

Figure 21.4. Growth of parakeets. (Data adapted from Earle and Clarke, 1991.)

GROWTH OF FERRETS

The ferret—or more specifically the European ferret (*Mustela putorius*)—is a companion animal with distinct popularity. In addition, they are employed in hunting and trapping, as fur-bearing animals, and as laboratory animals. There is a definitive study of growth in ferrets (Shump and Shump 1978). Ferrets reach a mature weight/size at about 20 weeks of age.

Weaning and Growth

There does not appear to be a reduction in growth at the time of weaning (Shump and Shump 1978).

Gender and Growth

There are considerable differences in the growth rate and mature body weight between male and female ferrets. Males grow to >75% greater mature

body weights. This is much greater than the situation in dogs (males having ~20% greater body weights) and cats (males having ~25% greater body weights).

Growth Curves

There are no studies reporting ferret growth described by the Gompertz function.

The Hypothalamo-Pituitary (GH)-IGF-I Axis

There is no specific information about the ferret hypothalamo-pituitary (GH)-IGF-I axis, but it is reasonable to assume a fully functioning axis.

GROWTH OF RABBITS

Rabbits are used as both livestock animals for meat and fur and as companion animals. Diet is, as expected, important to optimal growth/performance of growing rabbits. For instance, inclusion of alfalfa in rabbit diet is accompanied by an improved growth rate and reduced mortality (Cheeke and Patton 1978).

CAGED BIRDS

There are a number of species of caged birds, including parakeets or budgerigars, canaries, and parrots. Parakeets or budgerigars (*Melopisittacus undulatus*) originate from Australia. They are a very popular companion animal and are certainly the most numerous species of caged bird.

Parakeets or budgerigars are rapidly growing birds. The growth of parakeets or budgerigars has been described (Figure 21.4) (Earle and Clarke 1991). Moreover, their nutritional requirements are becoming established (Earle and Clarke 1991).

REFERENCES

Aiken, G.E., Bransby, D.I., and McCall, C.A. 1993. Growth of yearling horses compared to steers on high- and low-endophyte infected tall fescue. Journal of Equine Veterinary Science 13:26–28.

Alexander, J.E., and Wood, L.H. 1987. Growth studies in Labrador Retrievers fed a caloric-dense diet: Time-restricted versus free-choice feeding. Canine Practice 14:41–47.

Allard, R.L., Douglass, G.M., and Kerr, W.W. 1988. The effects of breed and sex on dog growth. Companion Animal Practice 2:25–19.

Andresen, E., and Willeberg, P. 1976. Pituitary dwarfism in German shepherd dogs: additional evidence of simple, autosomal recessive inheritance. Nordic Veterinary Medicine 28:481–486.

Ascacio-Martinez, J.A., and Barrera-Saldana, H.A. 1994. A dog growth hormone cDNA codes for a mature protein identical to pig growth hormone. Gene 143:277–280.

Berlan, M., Carpene, C., Lafontan, M., and Dang Tran, L. 1982. Alpha$_2$-adrenergic antilipolytic effect in dog fat cells: incidence of obesity and adipose tissue localization. Hormones and Metabolic Research 14:257–260.

Brody, S. 1945. Bioenergetics and growth. Baltimore: Waverly Press.

Buonomo, F.C., Ruffin, D.S., Brendemeuhl, J.P., Veenhuizen, J.J., and Sartin, J.L. 1996. The effects of bovine somatotropin (bST) and porcine somatotropin (pST) on growth factor and metabolic variables in horses. Journal of Animal Science 74:886–894.

Burger, I.H., and Johnson, J.V. 1991. Dogs large and small: The allometry of energy requirements within a single species. Journal of Nutrition 121:S18–S21.

Cascone, O., Fukushima, J.G., Mihajlovich, V., Santome, J.A., and De Jimenez Bonino, M.B. 1992. An equine growth hormone molecular species lacking the 76–92 peptidic fragment. International Journal of Peptide Protein Research 39:397–400.

Cella, S.G., Arce, V.M., Pieretti, F., Locatelli, V., Settembrini, B.P., and Müller, E.E. 1993. Combined administration of growth-hormone-releasing hormone and clonidine restores defective growth hormone secretion in old dogs. Neuroendocrinology 57:432–438.

Chakraborty, P.K., Stewart, A.P., and Seager, S.W.J. 1983. Relationship of growth and serum growth hormone concentration in the prepubertal Labrador bitch. Laboratory Animal Science 33:51–55.

Cheeke, P.R., and Patton, N.M. 1978. Effect of alfalfa and dietary fiber on the growth performance of weanling rabbits. Laboratory Animal Science 28:167–172.

Christensen, R.A., Malinowski, K., Hafs, H.D., and Scanes, C.G. 1997. Pulsatile release of somatotropin related to meal feeding and somatotropin response to secretagogues in horses. Journal of Animal Science 75:2770–2777.

Conde, R.D., Paladini, A.C., Santome, J.A., and Dellacha, J.M. 1973. Isolation, purification and characterization of equine growth hormone. European Journal of Biochemistry 32:563–8.

Conzemius, M.G., Cimino Brown, D., Brabec, M., Smith, G.K., Washabau, R., LaFond, E., and Chakraborty, P.K. 1998. Correlation between longitudinal bone growth, growth hormone, and insulin-like growth factor-I in prepubertal dogs. American Journal of Veterinary Research 59:1608–1612.

Cowan, J.S., Gaul, P., Moor, B.C., and Kraicer, J. 1984. Secretory bursts of growth hormone secretion in the dog may be initiated by somatostatin withdrawal. Canadian Journal of Physiology and Pharmacology 62:199–207.

Cox, N.R., Morrison, N.E., Sartin, J.L., Buonomo, F.C., Steele, B., and Baker, H.J. 1999. Alterations in the growth hormone/insulin-like growth factor I pathways in feline GM1 gangliosidosis. Endocrinology 140:5698–5704.

Davison, K.E., Potter, G.D., Evans, J.W., Greene, L.W., Hargis, P.S., Corn, C.D., and Webb, S.P. 1991. Growth, nutrient utilization, radiographic bone characteristics and postprandial thyroid hormone concentrations in weanling horses fed added dietary fat. Journal of Equine Veterinary Science 11:119–125.

Douglass, G.M., Kane, E., and Holmes, E.J. 1988. A profile of male and female cat growth. Companion Animal Practice 2:9–12.

Earle, K.E., and Clarke, N.R. 1991. The nutrition of the Budgerigar (Melopsittacus undulatus). Journal of Nutrition 121:S186–S192.

Eigenmann, J.E., and de Bruijne, J.J. 1985. Insulin-like growth factor I and growth hormone in canine starvation. Acta Endocrinologica 108:161–166.

Eigenmann, J.E., and Eigenmann, R.Y. 1981. Radioimmunoassay of canine growth hormone. Acta Endocrinologica 98:514–520.

Eigenmann, J.E., Eigenmann, R.Y., Rijnberk, A., van der Gaag, I., Zapf, J., and Froesch, E.R. 1983. Progesterone-controlled growth hormone overproduction and naturally occurring canine diabetes and acromegaly. Acta Endocrinologica 104:167–176.

Eigenmann, J.E., Patterson, D.F., and Froesch, E.R. 1984a. Body size parallels insulin-like growth factor I levels but not growth hormone secretory capacity. Acta Endocrinologica 106:448–453.

Eigenmann, J.E., Patterson, D.F., Zapf, J., and Froesch, E.R. 1984c. Insulin-like growth factor I in the dog: a study in different dog breeds and in dogs with growth hormone elevation. Acta Endocrinologica 105:294–301.

Eigenmann, J.E., Zanesco, S., Arnold, U., and Froesch, E.R. 1984b. Growth hormone and insulin-like growth factor I in German Shepherd dwarf dogs. Acta Endocrinologica 105:289–293.

Emala, C.W., Kuhl, J., Hirshman, C.A., and Levine, M.A. 1996. Cloning and sequencing of a canine β2-adrenergic receptor cDNA. Journal of Animal Science 74:2285.

Favier, R.P., Mol, J.A., Kooistra, H.S., and Rijnberk, A. 2001. Large body size in the dog is associated with transient GH excess at a young age. Journal of Endocrinology 170:479–484.

Fredholm, B.B., and Sollevi, A. 1981. The release of adenosine and inosine from canine subcutaneous adipose tissue by nerve stimulation and noradrenaline. Journal of Physiology 313:351–367.

Gibbs, P.G., Sigler, S.H., and Foehring, T.B. 1989. Influence of diet on growth and development of yearling horses. Journal of Equine Veterinary Science 9:215–218.

Glade, M.J., Gupta, S., and Reimers, T.J. 1984. Hormonal responses to high and low planes of nutrition in weanling thoroughbreds. Journal of Animal Science 59:658–665.

Glade, M.J., Krook, L., Schryver, H.F., and Hintz, H.F. 1981. Growth inhibition induced by chronic dexamethasone treatment of foals. Journal of Equine Veterinary Science 1:198–201.

Glade, M.J., and Luba, N.K. 1990. Benefits to foals of feeding soybean meal to lactating broodmares. Journal of Equine Veterinary Science 10:422–428.

Glade, M.J., Luba, N.K., and Schryver, H.F. 1986. Effects of age and diet on the development of mechanical strength by the third metacarpal and metatarsal bones of young horses. Journal of Animal Science 63:1432–1444.

Hall, V.E., and Pierce, G.N., 1934. Litter size, birth weight and growth to weaning in the cat. Anatomical Record 60:111–124.

Helmink, S.K., Shanks, R.D., and Leighton, E.A. 2000. Breed and sex differences in growth curves for two breeds of dog guides. Journal of Animal Science 78:27–32.

Heusner, A.A. 1991. Body mass, maintenance and basal metabolism in dogs. Journal of Nutrition 121:S8–S17.

Hintz, H.F., Hintz, R.L., and Van Vleck, L.D. 1979. Growth rate of thoroughbreds, effect of age of dam, year and month of birth, and sex of foal. Journal of Animal Science 48:480–487.

Hirakawa, D.A., and Baker, D.H. 1988. Comparative performance as well as nitrogen and energy metabolism of young puppies fed three distinctly different experiment dog foods and one commercial product. Companion Animal Practice 2:25–32.

Jacks, T., Smith, R., Judith, F., Schleim, K., Frazier, E., Chen, H., Krupa, D., Hora, D., Nargund, R., Patchett, A., and Hickey, G. 1996. MK-0677, a potent, novel, orally active growth hormone (GH) secretagogue: GH, insulin-like growth factor I, and other hormonal responses in beagles. Endocrinology 137:5284–5289.

Julen Day, T.R., Potter, G.D., Morris, E.L., Greene, L.W., and Simmons, J.B. 2000. Effects of exogenous equine somatotropin on mineral balance in two-year-old horses in race training. Journal of Equine Veterinary Science 20:201–206.

Kirkwood, J.K. 1985. The influence of size on the biology of the dog. Journal of Small Animal Practice 26:97–110.

Kooistra, H.S., Voorhout, G., Mol, J.A., and Rijnberk, A. 2000. Combined pituitary hormone deficiency in German Shepherd dogs with dwarfism. Domestic Animal Endocrinology 19:177–190.

Laroque, P., Molon-Noblot, S., Prahalada, S., Stabinski, L.G., Hoe, C.-M., Peter, C.P., Duprat, P., and Van Zwieten, M.J. 1998. Morphological changes in the pituitary gland of dogs chronically exposed to exogenous growth hormone. Toxicologic Pathology 26:201–206.

Latimer, H.B., and Ibsen, H.L. 1932. The postnatal growth in body weight of the cat. Anatomical Record 52:1–5.

Mäki, K., Liinamo, A.-E., and Ojala, M. 2000 Estimates of genetic parameters for hip and elbow dysplasia in Finnish Rottweilers. Journal of Animal Science 78:1141–1148.

Malinowski, K., Christensen, R.A., Hafs, H.D., and Scanes, C.G. 1996. Age and breed differences in thyroid hormones, insulin-like growth factor (IGF)-I and IGF binding proteins in female horses. Journal of Animal Science 74:1936–1942.

Malinowski, K., Christensen, R.A., Konopka, A., Scanes, C.G., and Hafs, H.D. 1997. Feed intake, body weight, body condition score, musculation, and immunocompetence in aged mares given equine somatotropin. Journal of Animal Science 75:755–760.

McCann, J.S., Heusner, G.L., Amos, H.E., and Thompson, D.L. 1992. Growth rate, diet digestibility, and serum prolactin of yearling horses fed non-infected and infected tall fescue hay. Equine Veterinary Science 12:240–243.

McKeever, K., Heusner, G., and Sperling, D. 1981. Quarter horse foal growth—Effect of month of birth, age of dam, and sex of foal. Sixth Equine Nutrition and Physiology Proceedings.

Molon-Noblot, S., Laroque, P., Prahalada, S., Stabinski, L.G., Hoe, C.-M., Peter, C.P., Duprat, P., and Van Zwieten, J. 1998. Effect of chronic growth hormone administration on skeletal muscle in dogs. Toxicologic Pathology 26:207–212.

Nap, R.C., Hazewinkel, A.W., Voorhout, G., Van Den Brom, W.E., Goedegebuure, S.A., and Van'T Klooster, A.T. 1991. Growth and skeletal development in great Dane pups fed different levels of protein intake. Journal of Nutrition 121:S107–S113.

Ng, T.B. 1985. Adrenergic control of lipolysis in adipocytes of several mammalian species. Comparative Biochemistry and Physiology 82C:463–466.

Nicholas, F. 1978. Pituitary dwarfism in German Shepherd dogs: a genetic analysis of some Australian data. Journal of Small Animal Practice 19:167–174.

NRC. 1978. Nutrient Requirements of Domestic Animals No. 6. Nutrient requirements of horses (4th revised ed), National Academy of Sciences National Research Council, Washington, D.C.

Prahalada, S., Block, G., Handt, L., DeBurlet, G., Cahill, M., Hoe, C.M., and van Zwieten, M.J. 1999. Insulin-like growth factor-1 and growth hormone (GH) levels in canine cerebrospinal fluid are unaffected by GH or GH secretagogue (MK-0677) administration. Hormones and Metabolic Research 31:133–137.

Prahalada, S., Stabinski, L.G., Chen, C.Y., Morrissey, R.E., De Burlet, G., Holder, D., Patrick, D.H., Peter, C.P., and Van Zwieten, M.J. 1998. Pharmacological and toxicological effects of chronic porcine growth hormone administration in dogs. Toxicologic Pathology 26:185–200.

Rahmanian, M.S., Thompson, D.L., and Melrose, P.A. 1997. Immunocytochemical localization of prolactin and growth hormone in the equine pituitary. Journal of Animal Science 75:3010–3018.

Rosenstein, L., and Berman, E. 1973. Postnatal body weight changes of domestic cats maintained in an outdoor colony. American Journal of Veterinary Research 34:575–577.

Rudman, D., Brown, S.J., and Malkin, F. 1963. Adipokinetic action of adrenocorticotropin, thyroid stimulating hormone vasopressin, α- and β-melanocyte stimulating hormones, Fraction H, epinephrine and norepinephrine in the rabbit, guinea-pig, hamster, rat, pig and dog. Endocrinology 72:527–543.

Shump, A.U., and Shump, K.A. 1978. Growth and development of the European ferret (mustela putorius). Laboratory Animal Science 28:89–91.

Stull, C.L., and Rodiek, A.V. 2000. Physiological responses of hormones to 24 hours of transportation using a commercial van during summer conditions. Journal of Animal Science 78:1458–1466.

Thomas, M.G., Bennett-Wimbush, K., Keisler, D.H., and Loch, W.E. 1998. Plasma concentrations of growth hormone and insulin-like growth factor-I in prepuberal quarter horses and ponies. Journal of Equine Veterinary Science 18:52–55.

Thompson, K.N., and Smith, B.P. 1994. Skeletal growth patterns of thoroughbred horses. Journal of Equine Veterinary Science 14:148–151.

Topliff, D.R., Boren, S.R., Freeman, D.W., Bahr, R.J., and Wagner, D.G. 1988. Growth of weanling quarter horses fed varying energy and protein levels. Journal of Equine Veterinary Science 8:371–375.

van Garderen, E., de Wit, M., Voorhout, W.F., Rutteman, G.R., Mol, J.A., Nederbragt, H., and Misdorp, W. 1997. Expression of growth hormone in canine mammary tissue and mammary tumors. Evidence for a potential autocrine/paracrine stimulatory loop. American Journal of Pathology 150:1037–1047.

van Garderen, E., Swennehuis, J.F., Hellmén, and Schalken, J.A. 2001. Growth hormone induces tyrosyl phosphorylation of the transcription factors Stat5a and Stat5b in CMT-U335 canine mammary tumor cells. Domestic Animal Endocrinology 20:123–135.

Wall, L.H., Potter, G.D., Gibbs, P.G., and Brumbaugh, G.W. 1997. Growth of yearling fillies fed alfalfa or soybean meal. Journal of Equine Veterinary Science 18:266–269.

Webb, G.W., Hussey, M.A., Conrad, B.E., and Potter, G.D. 1990. Growth of yearling horses grazing Klein grass or Bermuda grass pastures. Journal of Equine Veterinary Science 10:195–198.

Index